Symptoms, Diagnosis and Treatment of Ovarian Cancer

Symptoms, Diagnosis and Treatment of Ovarian Cancer

Editor: Lester Price

FOSTER
ACADEMICS

www.fosteracademics.com

www.fosteracademics.com

FOSTER ACADEMICS

Cataloging-in-Publication Data

Symptoms, diagnosis and treatment of ovarian cancer / edited by Lester Price.
p. cm.
Includes bibliographical references and index.
ISBN 978-1-63242-497-6
1. Ovaries--Cancer. 2. Ovaries--Cancer--Diagnosis. 3. Ovaries--Cancer--Treatment. 4. Symptoms.
I. Price, Lester.
RC280.O8 S86 2017
616.994 65--dc23

Foster Academics,
118-35 Queens Blvd., Suite 400,
Forest Hills, NY 11375, USA

ISBN 978-1-63242-497-6 (Hardback)

Printed and bound in China.

Contents

Preface

In my initial years as a student, I used to run to the library at every possible instance to grab a book and learn something new. Books were my primary source of knowledge and I would not have come such a long way without all that I learnt from them. Thus, when I was approached to edit this book; I became understandably nostalgic. It was an absolute honor to be considered worthy of guiding the current generation as well as those to come. I put all my knowledge and hard work into making this book most beneficial for its readers.

This book talks in detail about ovarian cancer. It gives knowledgeable insights about this area of study. Ovarian cancer is the cancer which affects the ovaries. It is hard to detect at the initial stage, like most other cancers but the symptoms become clear as it progresses. The treatment includes chemotherapy, radiotherapy and surgery. This book consists of contributions made by international experts. It strives to provide a fair idea about this discipline and to help develop a better understanding of the latest advances within this field. For all those who are interested in the study of ovarian cancer, this text can prove to be an essential guide. Researchers and students engaged in this field will be assisted by this book.

I wish to thank my publisher for supporting me at every step. I would also like to thank all the authors who have contributed their researches in this book. I hope this book will be a valuable contribution to the progress of the field.

Editor

Upregulation of miR-21 in Cisplatin Resistant Ovarian Cancer via JNK-1/c-Jun Pathway

Ileabett M. Echevarría-Vargas[1,2], Fatma Valiyeva[1], Pablo E. Vivas-Mejía[1,2]*

1 Comprehensive Cancer Center, University of Puerto Rico, San Juan, Puerto Rico, **2** Department of Biochemistry, University of Puerto Rico, San Juan, Puerto Rico

Abstract

Cisplatin has been the most accepted drug for the treatment of ovarian cancer for almost 40 years. Although the majority of patients with ovarian cancer respond to front-line platinum combination chemotherapy, many patients will develop cisplatin-resistance disease, which is extremely rapid and fatal. Although various mechanisms of cisplatin resistance have been postulated, the key molecules involved in such resistance have not been identified. MiRNAs are endogenously expressed small non-coding RNAs, which are evolutionarily conserved and function as post-transcriptional regulators of gene expression. Dysregulation of miRNAs have been associated with cancer initiation, progression and drug resistance. The oncogenic miRNA-21, one of the best-studied miRNAs, is upregulated in almost all human cancers. However, the regulation of miR-21 in cisplatin resistant ovarian cancer cells has not been assessed. In this study, we measured the miR-21 expression by real-time PCR and found upregulation of miR-21 in cisplatin resistant compared with cisplatin sensitive ovarian cancer cells. Chromatin immunoprecipitation studies demonstrated the association of the c-Jun transcription factor to the pri-mir-21 DNA promoter regions. Blocking the JNK-1, the major activator of c-Jun phosphorylation, reduced the expression of pre-mir-21 and increased the expression of its well-known target gene, PDCD4. Overexpression of miR-21 in cisplatin sensitive cells decreased PDCD4 levels and increased cell proliferation. Finally, targeting miR-21 reduced cell growth, proliferation and invasion of cisplatin resistant ovarian cancer cells. These results suggest that the JNK-1/c-Jun/miR-21 pathway contributes to the cisplatin resistance of ovarian cancer cells and demonstrated that miR-21 is a plausible target to overcome cisplatin resistance.

Editor: Alfons Navarro, University of Barcelona, Spain

Funding: This project was supported partially by the NIH/NCI (1K22CA166226-01A1) to PEVM, institutional seed funds from the University of Puerto Rico Comprehensive Cancer Center (PEVM), National Institute of Health, and Minority Biomedical Research Support (MBRS) RISE Grant Number R25-GM061838 (IEV). The funders had no role in study design, data collection and analysis, decision to publish, or preparation of the manuscript.

Competing Interests: The authors have declared that no competing interest exist.

* E-mail: pablo.vivas@upr.edu

Introduction

Ovarian cancer (OvCa) accounts for near 3% of all cancers in the Western world [1]. Typical treatment for women with OvCa is cytoreduction followed by chemotherapy [2]. Despite the high initial response rate to cisplatin-based compounds as the first-line chemotherapy, most ovarian carcinomas relapse [2],[3]. Postulated mechanisms of cisplatin resistance include decreased intracellular accumulation of cisplatin, increased intracellular levels of certain sulfur-containing macromolecules, and increased DNA repair [4]. Evidence suggests that inactivation of intrinsic cell death pathways, activation of cell survival pathways, and dysregulation of oncogenes, tumor suppressor genes, and microRNAs, contribute to the cisplatin resistance of ovarian cancer cells [3],[5],[6]. However, the exact mechanism by which ovarian cancer cells become resistant to cisplatin treatment is presently unknown.

MicroRNAs (miRNAs) are naturally occurring small (21–22 base pairs) non-coding RNAs, which recognizes mainly the 3′-UTR region of messenger RNA (mRNA) and inhibit protein synthesis [7]. Recent reports indicate that dysregulation of miRNAs, and their target genes, promote cancer initiation, progression and drug resistance [6],[8],[9]. For these reasons, miRNAs have been proposed as a diagnostic, prognostic and targets for cancer therapy [10]. One of the best studies miRNAs is miR-21 which is overexpressed in most cancers and displays oncogenic activity [11]. In HER2(+) breast cancers overexpression of miR-21 conferred resistance to trastuzumab therapy [12]. Nam et al., found miR-21, miR-203, and miR-205 as overexpressed in serous ovarian carcinoma versus normal ovarian tissue; miR-21 being present in 85% samples [13]. Xie et al. observed that in the A2780 human ovarian cancer cells, miR-21 modulates the hypoxia-inducible factor-1α (HIF-1α), and the resistance of paclitaxel [14]. MiR-21 exerts its biological role by targeting key genes controlling cell growth and proliferation. However, in solid tumors including ovarian cancer, the tumor suppressor gene programmed cell death 4 (PDCD4) appears to be one of the most important functional miR-21 targets [15],[16],[17]. The central role of PDCD4 in ovarian cancer is further supported by observations that lower levels of this tumor suppressor correlate directly with poor prognosis of ovarian cancer patients [15]. More recently, Chan et al. showed that miR-21 is overexpressed in cisplatin sensitive compared with cisplatin resistant cells, and that miR-21 inhibition induced apoptosis and increases PDCD4 levels [18].

The upstream molecular events that accounts for the miR-21 overexpression in ovarian cancer cells need further study. Reports indicate that the pri-mir-21 DNA promoter regions contain recognition elements for c-Jun and STAT3 transcription factors [19]. In colon cancer cells, curcumin reduced miR-21 via AP-1 (transcription factor complex composed of c-Jun and c-Fos, mainly) regulation, and in the human promyelocytic cell line, HL-60, phorbol 12-myristate 13-acetate (PMA) induced miR-21 expression by AP-1 activation [17],[20]. MiR-21 upregulation by AP-1 was also observed in certain chemoresistant side populations of cancer stem cells [21].

Because the recognized role of miR-21 in cancer initiation, progression and drug resistance, we investigated the regulation of miR-21 in cisplatin resistant ovarian cancer cells. We used real-time polymerase chain reaction (PCR) and found that cisplatin resistant ovarian cancer cells express higher miR-21 levels compared with cisplatin sensitive cells. We then analyzed the possible mechanism of miR-21 upregulation. Treatment of cells with SP600125, an inhibitor of the c-Jun phosphorylation, reduced pre-mir-21 expression in cisplatin resistant ovarian cancer cells. Chromatin immunoprecipitation (ChIP) studies showed higher c-Jun phosphorylation (p-c-Jun) protein levels bound to the pri-mir-21 DNA promoter region in cisplatin resistant compared with cisplatin sensitive ovarian cancer cells. Overexpression of miR-21 in cisplatin sensitive cells, increased cell proliferation, and decreased the PDCD4 protein levels. Opposite, miR-21 oligonucleotide inhibitor (antagomir), significant inhibited cell growth, proliferation and the invasion ability of A2780CP20 cells. This data demonstrate that upregulation of the JNK-1/c-Jun pathway leads to the aberrant increasing of miR-21, and propose to miR-21 as a potential target to overcome cisplatin resistance of ovarian cancer cells.

Materials and Methods

Chemicals and reagents

Cisplatin was purchased from Sigma-Aldrich (St. Louis, MO) and reconstituted in 0.9% NaCl. SP600125 (Sigma-Aldrich, St. Louis, MO) was reconstituted in 100% DMSO up to final concentration of 10 mM. When added to the cells, the final concentration of DMSO on the culture medium was less than 0.1%.

Cells and culture conditions

The human ovarian epithelial cancer cells SKOV3ip1, HEYA8, and A2780CP20 cells have been described elsewhere [22],[23],[24],[25],[26]. A2780 and A2780CIS cells were purchased from the European Collection of Cell Cultures (ECACC). The cells were propagated *in vitro* in RPMI-1640 medium (Thermo Scientific, Logan, UT, USA) supplemented with 10% fetal bovine serum (FBS) (Thermo Scientific) and 0.1% antibiotic/antimycotic solution (Thermo Scientific) and maintained at 37°C in 5%CO_2/95% air. All tumor cell lines were screened using Mycoplasm removal agent as described by the manufacturer (AbD Sertotec, NC, USA). *In vitro* assays were performed at 70–85% cell density. A2780CP20 cells (5×10^5 cells/dish) were treated with 10 µmol/L of SP600125 for eight hours. Cisplatin concentrations inhibiting 50% of cell growth (IC_{50}) were calculated after 72-hr drug incubation (cisplatin doses: 100, 10, 1, 0.1, and 0.01 µM, final concentrations). Cell growth was measured with the Alamar blue dye as previously described [27].

Microarray analysis of gene expression

Total RNA was isolated from A2780 and A2780CP20 ovarian cancer cell lines with the GenElute Mammalian Total RNA Purification Kit (Sigma-Aldrich). The RNA concentration was read in a nanodrop. RNA quality was verified in a Bioanalyzer (Agilent Technologies, Inc., Santa Clara, CA). One hundred nanograms of total RNA were used to cDNA synthesis. Complementary cDNA was synthesized, labeled, fragmented and hybridized to the Affymetrix GeneChip Gene 1.0 ST Human Array. After 16 hours of incubation at 45°C, the arrays were washed, stained and scanned (Affymetrix Model 3000 scanner), and data was analyzed using the Partek Genomics Suited (Partek, St. Louis, MO). Experiments were performed in duplicate. Two-way ANOVA was used to determine differences in gene expression ($p<0.05$ fold change 2). 1359 probes (4%) sets showed ±2-fold change between A2780CP20 and A2780 cells. Additional filtering (±3-fold change, and $p<0.003$) showed 321 probes (0.96%) changed between A2780CP20 and A2780 cells.

RNA isolation and cDNA synthesis

Total RNA (including miRNAs) was isolated using the *mir*Vana miRNA isolation kit from Ambion (Life Technology, Grand Island, NY). RNA was converted into cDNA with the Enhanced Avian RT first strand synthesis kit from Sigma-Aldrich. In brief, total RNA (1 µg), 500 µM dNTP and 3.5 µM oligo$(dT)_{23}$ were mixed and water was added up to 10 µL total volume. Samples were mixed, centrifuged and heated at 70°C for 10 min. This mixture was combined with 1 µL enhanced avian RT, 2 µL 10X buffer, 1 µL RNase inhibitor, and water up to 20 µL final volume. Samples were incubated at 25°C for 15 min following by 45°C for 50 minutes. cDNA synthesis to detect mature miRNAs was performed with the All-in-One miRNA qRT-PCR detection kit (GeneCopoeia, Rockville, MD). In brief, cDNA synthesis mixture contained 1 µg of total RNA, 1 µL Poly(A) Polymerase, 1 µL RTase Mix, 5 µL 5X PAP/RT Buffer and water up to 25 µL final volume. The revere transcription reaction was incubated at 37°C for 60 min, and 85°C for 5 min in a Veriti thermal cycler (Applied Biosystems, Carlsbad, CA).

Polymerase Chain Reaction (PCR) and SYBR-I-based real-time PCR

PCR was performed in a Verity 96 wells thermal cycler (Applied Biosystems). In brief, 12.5 µL JumpStart REDTaq ReadyMix 1X (Sigma), 0.5 µL forward, and 0.5 µL reverse primers (0.4 µM final concentration of each), 2 µL of the cDNA product, and water up to 50 µL final volume. The cycling conditions were one cycle at 94°C for 5 min, followed by 30 cycles at 95°C for 15 sec (denaturation), 60°C for 30 sec (annealing), and 72°C for 30 sec (extension). A final extension step was performed at 72°C for 10 min. PCR products were separated by electrophoresis in 1% agarose gel. Images were obtained (after gel staining with ethidium bromide) in a FluorChem 8900 (Alpha Innotech). SYBR-I-real time PCR to assess the mature miR-21 levels were performed with the All-in-One miRNA qRT-PCR detection kit (GeneCopoeia) in a StepOne plus real-time PCR thermal cycle system (Applied Biosystems). The PCR reactions mix contained 10 µl 2X All-in-One qPCR Mix, 2 µl All-in-One miRNA qPCR primer, 2 µL universal adaptor PCR primer, 2 µL first strand cDNA, and 4 µL of water. Specific primers for miR-21 and U6 (internal standard) were used (GeneCopoeia). Cycling conditions: one cycle of 15 min at 95°C, and 40 cycles of 15 sec at 94°C, 30 sec at 60°C and 30 sec at 72°C [28]. Melt curve analysis was always performed at the end of the PCR reaction. Relative miR-21 expression was calculated with the ΔΔCt-method [29],[30],[31].

Western blot analysis

Cells were collected and washed twice with Phosphate Buffer Saline (PBS), harvested and stored at −80°C until processed. For cytosolic and nuclear extraction, cells were resuspended in cytoplasmic buffer (0.5% Nonidet P-40, 10 mM KCl, 10 mM Hepes, pH 7.9, and 1X protease inhibitor) for 15 min on ice and centrifuged at 14,000 rpm at 4°C [32]. The supernatants (containing the cytoplasmic fraction) were collected. The remaining pellets were washed twice with the cytoplasmic buffer following by the addition of nuclear buffer (400 mM NaCl, 20 mM Hepes, pH 7.9 and 1X protease inhibitor). Samples were incubated for 15 min on ice, centrifuged for 10 min at 4°C and supernatant (containing the nuclear protein fractions) were collected. For total proteins extraction, cells were lysed with lysis buffer (150 mM NaCl, 1% Triton-X, 0.4 mM NaF, 0.4 mM $NaVO_4$, 25 mM Tris-HCl, pH 7.6 and 1X protease inhibitor) for 45 min on ice, centrifuged for 10 min at 4°C and the supernatants were collected. Protein concentration was determined using Bio-Rad Protein Reagents (Bio-Rad, Hercules, CA). Protein lysates (50 μg) were separated by SDS-PAGE, blotted onto membranes, and probed with the appropriate dilution of each primary antibody. Membranes were rinsed and incubated with the appropriate horseradish peroxidase-conjugated secondary antibody, rinsed again, and the bound antibodies were detected using enhanced chemiluminescence (GE Healthcare, Piscataway, NJ) following by autoradiography in a FluorChem 8900 (Alpha Innotech Corporation, San Leandro, CA). Primary anti-bodies: anti-phospho-SAPK/JNK (Thr183/Tyr185), anti-SAPK/JNK, anti-phospho-c-Jun (Ser73), anti-c-Jun, anti-phospho-ERK (Thr202/Tyr204), anti-ERK kinase, anti-STAT3, anti-histone H3 (Cell Signaling, Danvers, MA), anti-PDCD4 (Rockland, Gilbertsville, PA) and anti-β-actin (Sigma-Aldrich). Secondary antibodies used were anti mouse and anti rabbit IgG horseradish peroxidase (HRP)-linked, anti rabbit (Cell Signaling).

Chromatin immunoprecipitation (ChIP)

A2780CP20 and A2780 cells were collected and crosslinked with 1% formaldehyde for 10 min at 37°C. Cells were lysed in sodium dodecyl sulfate (SDS) lysis buffer (1% SDS, 10 mM EDTA, 50 mM Tris, pH 8.1 and protease and phosphatase inhibitors). Samples were sonicated (4°C) using a Branson 250 sonicator with 10 continued pulses of 10 seconds (sec) each. The sonicated lysates were pre-cleared with protein A or G magnet beads overnight at 4°C. Lysates were immunoprecipitated with 5 or 10 μg of antibody/magnet beads against p-c-Jun, Pol-II (Santa Cruz), c-Jun (BD Transduction laboratory, Franklin Lakes, New Jersey, USA) or IgG (Abcam, Cambridge, MA, USA) overnight at 4°C. Samples were washed five times for 5 min each at 4°C with wash buffer (RIPA) (50 mM Hepes-KOH pH 7.6, 500 mM LiCl, 1% NP-40, 0.7% deoxycholic acid, 1 mM EDTA, and 1X protease and 1X phosphatase inhibitors). Samples were washed once with 1X TE buffer and eluted with SDS elution buffer (1% SDS, 10 mM EDTA, 50 mM Tris pH 8.1, and 1X protease and 1X phosphatase inhibitors). Following elution, samples were reverse cross-linked at 65°C for 4 hours, treated with RNase A (0.2 μg/ml) at 37°C for 2 hours, mixed with $CaCl_2$ (300 mM $CaCl_2$ in 10 mM Tris pH 8.0) and Proteinase K (0.2 mg/ml) at 37°C overnight. The immunoprecipitated DNA was isolated using QiAquick PCR Purification Kit (Qiagen). DNA was quantified by SYBR-1-based real-time PCR using a StepOne Plus Thermocycler (Applied Biosystems). In brief, PCR reaction mix contained 10 μL SYBR-green, 0.5 μL forward primer, 0.5 μL reverse primer (0.25 nM final concentration), 2 μL of DNA sample and 7 μL of nuclease free water. Cycling conditions: one cycle of 10 min at 95°C, and 40 cycles of 30 sec at 95°C, 30 sec at 60°C and 30 sec at 72°C.

Transient and stable transfections

Ectopic miR-21 expression was performed in A2780 cells. Briefly, A2780 (2×10^4 cell/ml) cells were seeded in six well plates. For each well, 1 μg of pCMV-MIR21 or 1 μg of empty vector (pCMV-EV) (both from OriGene Technologies, Inc. Rockville, MD) and 1 μL of MegaTran 1.0 transfection reagent (OriGen) were diluted in 98 μL of Opti-MEM I (Life Technologies). pCMV vector contains a green fluorescein protein (GFP) cassette. The mixture was incubated for 10 min at room temperature and added to the cells. Twenty-four hours later, the medium was replaced with fresh RPMI-1640 (10% FBS, 0.1% antibiotic/antimycotic solution and 500 μg/mL G418 disulfate salt solution). After 2–3 weeks, independent colonies were picked and cultured separately as independent clones. The transfection efficiency was monitored by immunofluorescence as follows: A2780 clones were seeded in microscope slides overnight. Then, cells were fixed with 4% paraformaldehyde, blocked with 0.3% H_2O_2 in methanol for 10 min and 10% FBS for 20 min. Cells were incubated with anti-GFP antibody (dilution 1:250) or DAPI (dilution 1:5000 from Santa Cruz Biotechnology Inc., Dallas, Texas, USA) overnight. The next day, slides were washed, and the secondary antibody anti-rabbit (dilution 1:5000) was added. Cover slips were placed on the microscope slides and fixed with Aqueous-mounting medium (Abcam). Cells were visualized and photographed in an Olympus IX71 inverted microscope (Center Valley, PA). To inhibit miR-21, we transiently transfect A2780CP20 cells with a miR-21 oligonucleotide (Life Technology, Grand Island, NY, USA) and a negative oligonucleotide inhibitor as a control (Life Technology). MiRNA inhibitors were always mixed with HiPerfect transfection reagent (Qiagen, Valencia, CA, USA), and Opti-MEM I growth medium (Life Technologies).

Small interference RNA (siRNA) transfection

To silence human c-Jun (NM_002228) two siRNAs targeting the sequences: 5′-CCTTCTATGACGATGCCCT-3′, and 5′-GATGGAAACGACCTTCTAT-3′ were used (Sigma-Aldrich). A non-silencing siRNA (NC-siRNA) was used as the negative control (Sigma-Aldrich). In brief, A2780CP20 (2.25×10^5 cells) were seeded in petri dishes. Twenty-four hours later, 200 nM of siRNA (final concentration) were mixed with HiPerfect transfection reagent (Qiagen) at 1:2 ratio (siRNA:transfection reagent) in Opti-MEM I growth medium. The mix was incubated for 15 minutes at room temperature and added to the cells. Cells were collected after 24 hours and store at -80°C until use.

Cell growth and proliferation

A2780CP20 (2×10^4 cell/ml) were seeded in six well plates. Twenty-four hours later a transfection reaction mix containing miR-21 inhibitor (Life Technology) (50 nM final concentration) and HiPerfect transfection reagent (Qiagen) in a 1:4 ratio, was added to the cells. Six hours later, the cultured medium was removed and replaced by RPMI-1640 medium (10% FBS). To assess cell viability, seventy-two hours after transfection, live cells were collected and counted in the presence of 0.5% Trypan blue using a Countess automated cell counter (Invitrogen, Grand Island, NY). Cell proliferation was assessed with a colony formation assay. Briefly, eight hours after transfection, 1000 cells were seeded in 10 cm-Petri dishes. Ten days later, colonies were stained with 0.5% crystal violet in methanol, and counted using the microscope Nikon eclipse TS100.

In vitro invasion assay

Cells (2.5×10^4 cells/ml) were plated in a petri dish. Twenty-four hours later a transfection reaction mix containing miR-21 inhibitor (Life Technology) (50 nM final concentration) and HiPerfect transfection reagent (Qiagen) in a 1:2 ratio, was added to the cells. The next day, 600 μL of diluted matrigel (serum-free RPMI medium) was putted into upper chamber of 6-well Transwell plates (Corning Incorporated, Lowell, MA). The chamber was incubated at 37°C at least 4 to 5 hours for gelling. MiR-21 inhibitor-transfected cells were collected and resuspended in serum-free RPMI-1640 medium at a density of 1.5×10^5 cells/ml. The matrigel was gently washed with warmed serum free-RPMI-1640 medium, and 1.0 mL of the cell suspension was putted onto the matrigel. The lower chamber of the transwell was filled with 1.0 mL RPMI-1640 medium (10% FBS), and the plate was incubated at 37°C for 48- hr. The transwells were removed from the 6-well plates and stained with the PROTOCOL HEMA 3 Stain set (Fisher Scientific Company, Kalamazoo, MI). The non-invaded cells were scraped off on the top of the transwell with a cotton swab. The number of invaded cells was counted in four microscope fields (10X) per condition. Percentage of invasion was calculated relative to the number of invaded cells in the control miRNA inhibitor well, which was taken as 100%.

Statistical analysis

Student's t-test was performed using GraphPad Prism version 5.04 for Windows, GraphPad Software, San Diego California USA, www.graphpad.com. All experiments were performed in triplicate and p-value <0.05 for a two-sided test was considered statistically significant.

Results

Expression of miR-21 and miR-21-related molecules in ovarian cancer cells

In a preliminary microarray analysis performed in our laboratory, we identified 320 genes differentially expressed (fold change >3 and p-value < 3×10^{-4}) in A2780CP20 (cisplatin resistant) *vs.* A2780 (cisplatin sensitive) cells (Table S1). The microarray data was deposited in the Gene Expression Omnibus (GEO): accession: http://www.ncbi.nlm.nih.gov/geo/query/acc.cgi?acc = GSE51683. Whereas miR-21 and c-Jun were upregulated, PDCD4 was downregulated in A2780CP20 compared with A2780 cells (Table S1). RT-PCR experiments corroborated the microarray data (Figure 1A). MiR-21 gene is located in the intron 10 of the TMEM-49 gene [17]. The messenger RNA (mRNA) levels of TMEM-49 and β-actin were not different in A2780CP20 and A2780 cells (Figure 1A), which corroborate previous finding that pre-mir-21 and TMEM-49 are independently regulated [33]. Figure 1B shows that the miR-21 levels correlate with the sensitivity of ovarian cancer cells to cisplatin treatment (IC_{50}, Figure 1B). Western blot analysis (Figure 1C) showed that the total c-Jun and p-c-Jun protein levels were higher in A2780CP20 compared with A2780 cells. However, the PDCD4 protein levels showed opposite results (Figure 1C). In other cell lines, the Signal Transducer and Activator of Transcription 3 (STAT3) regulate miR-21 expression [17]. However, the STAT3 protein levels were similar in A2780CP20 and A2780 cells (Figure S1), which rule out the possibility that STAT3 account for the higher miR-21 levels in A2780CP20 compared with A2780 cells. These results suggest that c-Jun is responsible for miR-21 expression levels in cisplatin resistant ovarian cancer cells.

It is well known that the major activator of c-Jun is JNK-1 [34]. Thus, we assessed the protein levels of JNK in A2780 and A27870CP20 cells. The total JNK-1 and nuclear p-JNK-1protein levels were higher in A2780CP20 compared with A2780 cells. The protein levels of p-JNK-2/3 and total JNK-2/3, the two other JNK-1 isoforms, were similar in both cells lines (Figure 1D), which suggest that the JNK-1/c-Jun cascade regulate miR-21 in A2780CP20 cells. Evidence indicates that the extracellular signal regulated kinase, ERK can activate c-Jun [35],[36]. Although the total ERK protein levels were similar in both cells lines, the p-ERK protein levels were lower in A2780CP20 compared with A2780 cells ruled out the possibility that activated ERK account for the higher miR-21 levels in A2780CP20 compared with A2780 cells.

Effect of JNK-1/c-Jun inhibition in miR-21 and PDCD4 expression

To further determine whether JNK-1 regulates c-Jun and miR-21 expression in cisplatin resistant cells, we treated A2780CP20 cells with SP600125, a well-known chemical inhibitor of c-Jun phosphorylation by JNK-1 [34]. Incubation of A2780CP20 cells with SP600125 decreased the p-c-Jun levels, as expected (Figure 2A). No significant changes in the protein levels of c-Jun, total and p-JNK-1 or total and p-JNK-2/3 were observed following treatment of A2780CP20 cells with SP600125 inhibitor (Figure 2A). Real-time PCR showed a significant reduction (60% and *$p<0.05$) in the pre-mir-21 levels following treatment of A2780CP20 cells with SP600125 (Figure 2B). The same inhibitor caused an increase in the PDCD4 protein levels as observed in the western blot of Figure 2C. Furthermore, inhibition of miR-21 with a miR-21 specific oligonucleotide inhibitor (antagomiR) increased the PDCD4 protein levels (Figure 2D), which confirmed previous results that miR-21 regulates PDCD4 in ovarian cancer cells [37],[18]. Furthermore, transient transfection of A2780CP20 cells with a siRNA against c-Jun significantly (**$p<0.01$) inhibited pre-miR-21 expression (Figure 2E). Western blot analysis showed that treatment of the cisplatin sensitive A2780 cells with SP600125 did not affect the levels of p-JNK-1, JNK-1, p-JNK-2/3, JNK2/3, c-Jun, pre-miR-21 or PDCD4 (Figure S2). These results suggest that JNK-1/c-Jun pathway lead to miR-21 overexpression in cisplatin resistant ovarian cancer cells.

Analysis of the c-Jun binding to miR-21 DNA promoter regions

To definitely demonstrate that c-Jun is responsible of the higher miR-21 levels in A2780CP20 compared with A2780 cells, we assessed the pri-mir-21 promoter DNA regions associated with p-c-Jun by ChIP analysis. The amount of DNA immunoprecipitated with p-c-Jun antibody in both cell lines was amplified with a pair of primers encompassed the c-Jun recognition elements in the pri-mir-21 promoter region (Figure S3 and Table S2). Other pair of primers amplifying a DNA region far from the c-Jun recognition sites was used as a control (Table S2). More than five times of DNA levels were pulling out in A2780CP20 than in A2780 cells after immunoprecipitation with the p-c-Jun antibody (Figure 3A). No significant differences in DNA amounts were observed after immunoprecipitation with c-Jun, Pol- II or IgG antibodies (Figure 3A) which demonstrated that p-c-Jun binds specifically to pri-mir-21 promoter regions, and that more p-c-Jun protein levels are higher in A2780CP20 than in A2780 cells. No significant differences in the DNA levels were observed when the PCR was performed with the non-promoter DNA primers after immuno-precipitation with the p-c-Jun antibody (Figure 3B).

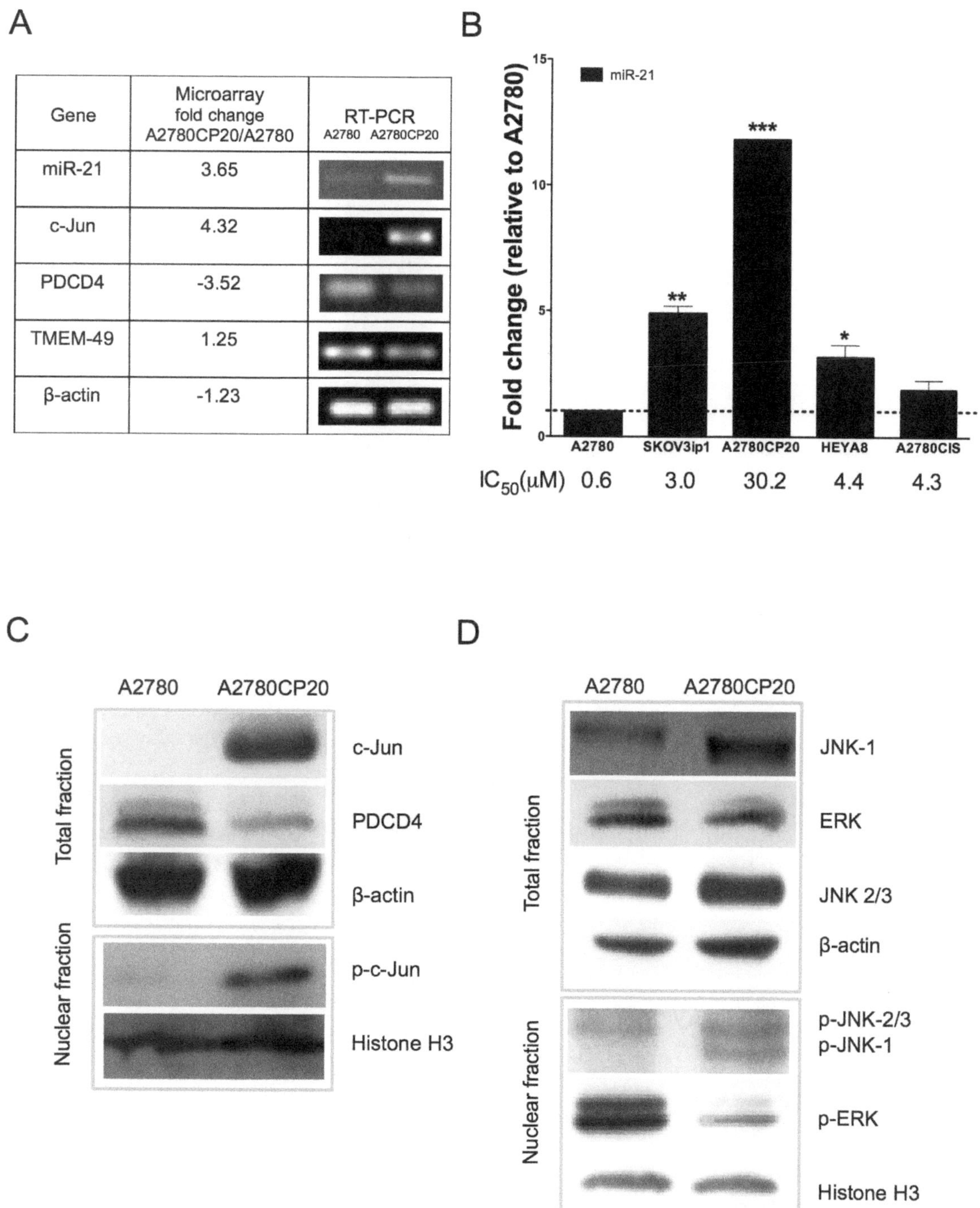

Figure 1. RT-PCR and western blot analysis of miRNA-21-related molecules. (**A**) Validation of microarrays by RT-PCR. (**B**) MiR-21 levels in a panel of ovarian cancer cells. MiR-21 levels were expressed relative to the A2780 cells miR-21 levels. IC50s were calculated after 72-hr treatment of cells with different concentrations of cisplatin as described in the "Material and Methods" section. (**C**) Evaluation of c-Jun and p-c-Jun protein expression in A2780 and A2780CP20 cells. (**D**) Protein expression analysis of MAPKs in total and nuclear fractions of A2780 and A2780CP20 cells. Expression level in Figures A, C and D are without cisplatin treatment. *$p<0.05$, **$p<0.01$, ***$p<0.001$ compared to control. Columns represent the means of triplicates ± S.E.M.

Effect of miR-21 overexpression in the sensitivity of ovarian cancer cells to cisplatin treatment

To test whether miR-21 contributes to the cisplatin resistance of ovarian cancer cells, we ectopically expressed pre-mir-21 in A2780 cells (Figure S4 and S5). Figure 4A, shows that compared with untransfected A2780 cells or with the empty vector (clone 1, Figure S4), stable transfection of pre-mir-21 (clone 1, Figure S4) increased the miR-21 mature levels. The PDCD4 protein levels were also significantly decreased (69%, ***$p<0.001$) in the pre-mir-21 A2780 clone (A2780-miR-21) compared with the empty vector clone (A2780-EV) (Figure 4B). Ectopic expression of pre-

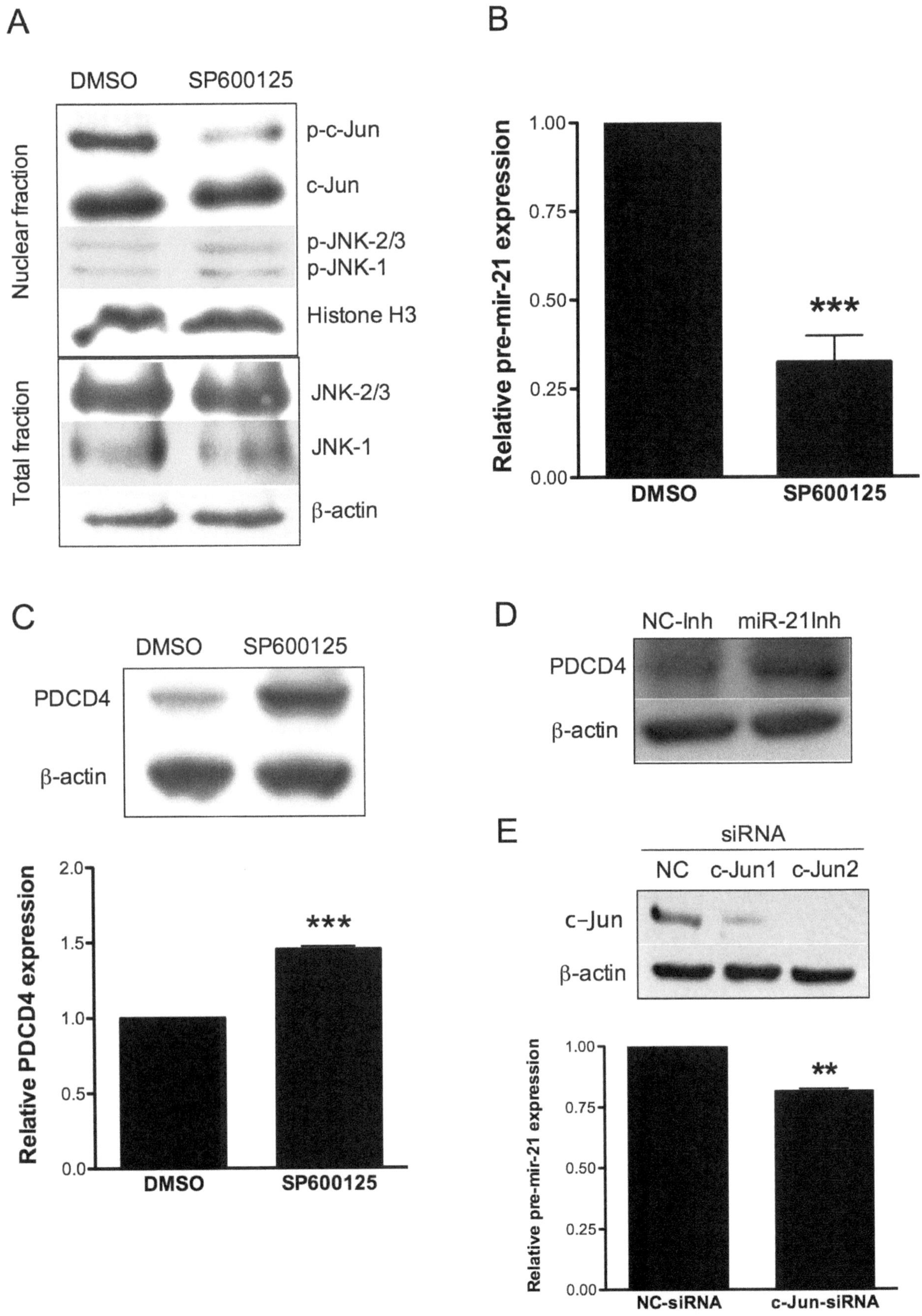
A
DMSO
SP600125
Nuclear fraction
p-c-Jun
c-Jun
p-JNK-2/3
p-JNK-1
Histone H3
Total fraction
JNK-2/3
JNK-1
β-actin
B
Relative pre-mir-21 expression
1.00
0.75
0.50
0.25
0.00
***
DMSO
SP600125
C
DMSO
SP600125
PDCD4
β-actin
Relative PDCD4 expression
2.0
1.5
1.0
0.5
0.0
***
DMSO
SP600125
D
NC-Inh
miR-21Inh
PDCD4
β-actin
E
siRNA
NC
c-Jun1
c-Jun2
c-Jun
β-actin
Relative pre-mir-21 expression
1.00
0.75
0.50
0.25
0.00
**
NC-siRNA
c-Jun-siRNA

Figure 2. Effect of JNK-1 inhibition in miR-21 and PDCD4 expression. A2780CP20 cells were treated with 10 μM SP600125. (**A**) Western blot shown the inhibition of p-c-Jun after treatment with SP600125 in A2780CP20 cells compared to control (DMSO). (**B**) SYBR-I-based real-time PCR was performed to calculate the relative pre-mir-21 expression in A2780CP20 cells after treatment with SP600125 inhibitor. (**C**) Western blot and densitometric analysis of PDCD4 protein expression levels after treatment of A2780CP20 cells with SP600125. (**D**) PDCD4 protein expression levels after transfection of A2780CP20 with miR-21 oligonucleotide inhibitor. (**E**) A2780 CP20 cells were transiently transfected with two c-Jun-targeted siRNAs as described in the "Materials and Methods" section. Western blot analysis shows that both c-Jun-siRNAs decreased the c-Jun levels. SYBR-I-based real-time PCR was performed (see "Materials and Methods" section) to calculate the relative pre-mir-21 expression levels in A2780CP20 cells after siRNA-mediated c-Jun silencing. $^{*}p<0.05$, $^{**}p<0.01$, $^{***}p<0.001$ compared to control. Columns represent the means of triplicates ± S.E.M.

mir-21 in A2780 cells resulted in a significant increase in cell proliferation (15.4%, $^{***}p<0.001$) compared with A2780-EV cells (Figure 4C). In addition, cisplatin treatment (1 μM) of A2780-miR-21 cells resulted in significant (approximately 15%, $^{**}p<0.01$) reduction of cell growth inhibition compared the cisplatin treatment of A2780-EV cells (Figure 4D).

A

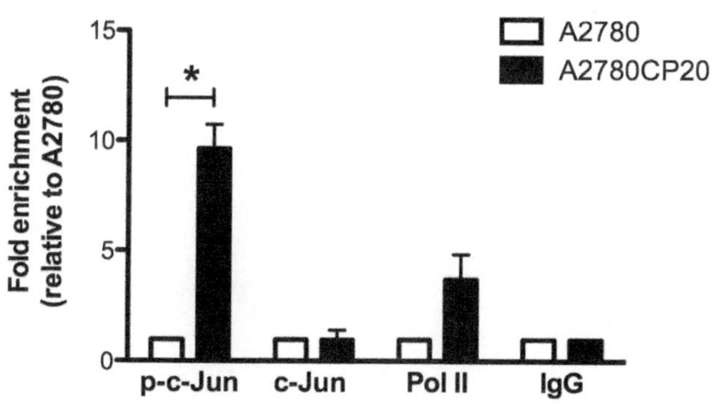

B

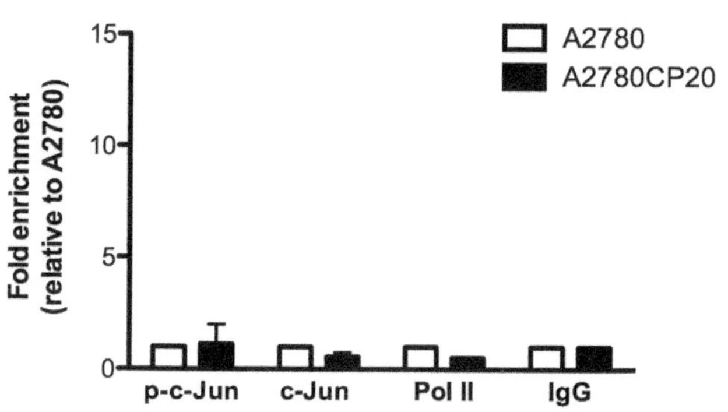

Figure 3. Chromatin immunoprecipitation assay (ChIP). ChIP assay was performed as described in the "Materials and Methods" section. (**A**) SYBR-I-based real-time PCR amplification of the region containing the c-Jun recognition sequence in the pri-miR-21 DNA. The phospho-c-Jun levels bound to the pri-miR-21 promoter was higher in A2780CP20 cells compared with A2780 cells. (**B**) SYBR-I-based real-time PCR amplification of a DNA region far of the pre-mir-21 promoter was performed as a control. $^{*}p<0.05$ compared to control. Columns represent the means of triplicates ± S.E.M.

Effect of miR-21 inhibition in cell growth, proliferation and invasion

We next assessed the effect of miR-21 inhibition in cell growth and proliferation of A2780CP20 cells. For this set of experiments, we first confirmed the downregulation of miR-21 expression ($^{**}p<0.001$) by the miR-21-Inh (Figure 5A). Comparing with a negative control miRNA inhibitor (NC-Inh), transient transfection of A2780CP20 with the miR-21 antagomir (miR-21-Inh) significantly reduced (35%, $^{**}p<0.01$) cell survival (Figure 5B). MiR-21 inhibition induced long-term effects in cell growth and proliferation. In a colony formation assay, transient transfection of miR-21 inhibitor in A2780CP20 cells reduced significantly (33%, $^{*}p<0.05$) the number of colonies formed compared with the NC-Inh transfected cells (Figure 5C).

Increased levels of miR-21 have been associated with accelerated metastatic rate of various tumors. Thus, we assessed whether miR-21 inhibition reduced the metastatic potential of A2780CP20 cells [16],[35],[36],[37]. Invasion assays confirmed that 50 nM of miR-21-Inh reduced significantly (50%, $^{*}p<0.05$) the invasion ability of A2780CP20 cells compared with 50 nM of NC-Inh (Figure 5D). This data suggest that increased miR-21 levels are associated with the metastatic potential of cisplatin resistant ovarian cancer cells, and that miR-21 is a potential target to overcome the cisplatin resistance of highly metastatic ovarian cancer cells.

Discussion

The major findings of this study were that the JNK-1/c-Jun pathway regulates the miR-21 expression in the cisplatin resistance of ovarian cancer cells, and that targeting miR-21 inhibited cell growth and proliferation of these cells. MiR-21, one of the most commonly upregulated miRNAs in tumor cells, is endowed with oncogenic properties, and promotes cell proliferation, invasion, and migration of cancer cell populations [11],[37],[38],[39]. MiR-21 overexpression has also been associated with drug resistance [40]. The regulation of miR-21 in cisplatin resistant ovarian cancer cells had not been well studied.

We found that the miR-21 levels correlated well with the sensitivity of ovarian cancer cells to cisplatin treatment. In addition, the total and phospho JNK-1 and c-Jun protein levels were higher in A2780CP20 compared with their parental sensitive A2780 cells. Inhibition of c-Jun phosphorylation with the JNK-1 specific inhibitor SP600125 in A2780CP20 cells decreased the pre-mir-21 mRNA and increased the PDCD4 protein levels. These effects were not observed in the cisplatin sensitive A2780 cells. Furthermore, the ChIP experiments confirmed that c-Jun binds physically to the pri-mir-21 DNA promoter regions and activates pri-mir-21 expression. In colon cancer, human promyelocytic, and in certain chemoresistant side populations of cancer stem cells, regulation of miR-21 (under different treatments) was AP-1-mediated, which is in agreement with our findings that the JNK-1/c-Jun/miR-21 pathway is activated in cisplatin resistant ovarian cancer cells.

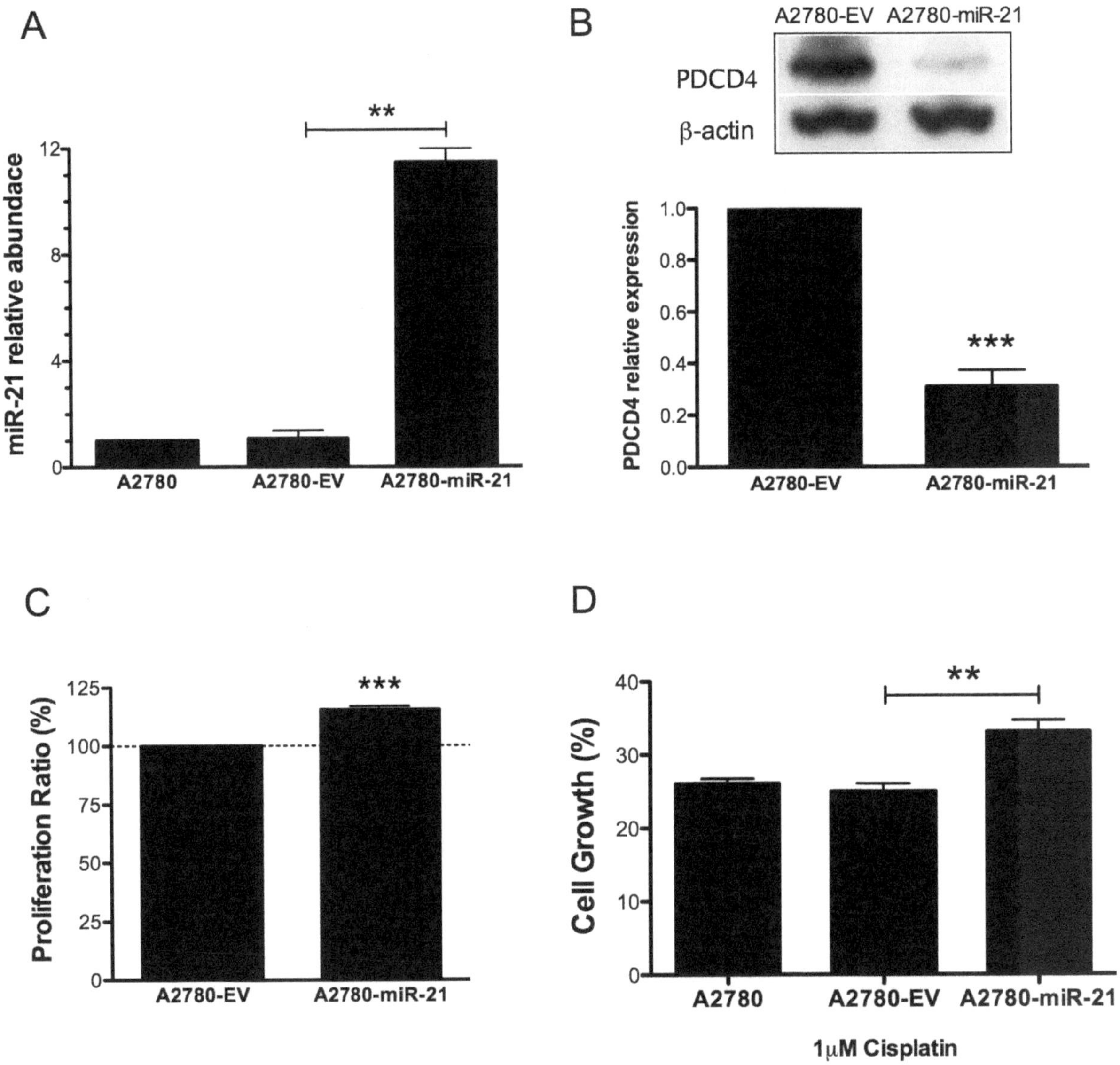

Figure 4. Effect of pre-mir-21 overexpression in A2780 cells. (**A**) A2780 cells were stably transfected with pCMV-miR21 or empty pCMV-EV vectors. The miR-21 expression was quantified by qRT-PCR. (**B**) Western blot analysis shows a decreased expression of PDCD4 levels in A2780-miR-21 compared with A2780-EV cells. (**C**) Overexpression of miR21 increased cell proliferation (13%, ***$p<0.001$) in A2780-miR-21 compared with A2780-EV cells. (**D**) A2780-miR-21 overexpressed clones were more resistant to cisplatin-induced cell death compared with untransfected A2780 cells or with the A2780-EV cells. **$p<0.01$. Columns represent the means of triplicates ± S.E.M.

Several miRNAs have been reported as differentially abundant in cisplatin sensitive and cisplatin resistant ovarian cancer cells [41],[42]. For example, miR-214 overexpression was associated with cisplatin resistance of ovarian cancer cells [43],[44]. Intriguing, our preliminary microarray studies (Table S1) showed lower miR-214 levels in A2780CP20 compared with A2780 cells. In other cell lines downregulation of miR-214 was associated with tumor aggressiveness [45],[46]. Thus, the miR-214 expression levels in the context of drug resistance need further analysis. Overexpression of miR-141 and downregulation of its target gene the Kelch-Like ECH-Associated Protein 1 (KEAP1) have also been associated with cisplatin resistance [47]. However, in human esophageal squamous cell carcinoma cells miR-141 appears to induce cisplatin resistance through the Yes-Associated Protein 1 (YAP1) [47],[48]. By using next generation sequencing approaches, several other differentially expressed miRNA have been identified in cisplatin sensitive and cisplatin and resistant ovarian cancer cells [41],[43],[49],[50]. However, the upstream molecular mechanism leading to dysregulation of such number of miRNAs in cisplatin resistant ovarian cancer cells remains unclear. Our study is the first showing that overexpression of miR-21 in cisplatin resistant ovarian cancer cells is a secondary event associated with the activation of the JNK-1/c-Jun pathway in these cells. This hypothesis is further supported by studies showing that the phosphorylation level of JNK-1 correlates well with progression free survival and overall survival of ovarian cancer patients [51]. Nevertheless, targeting miR-21 inhibited cell growth, proliferation and the invasion ability of cisplatin resistant cells, which demonstrates that miR-21, could be considered as a potential target to overcome the cisplatin resistance of highly metastatic ovarian cancer tumors. This idea is supported by recent reports of Chan et al whom using "The cancer Genome Atlas" (TCGA)

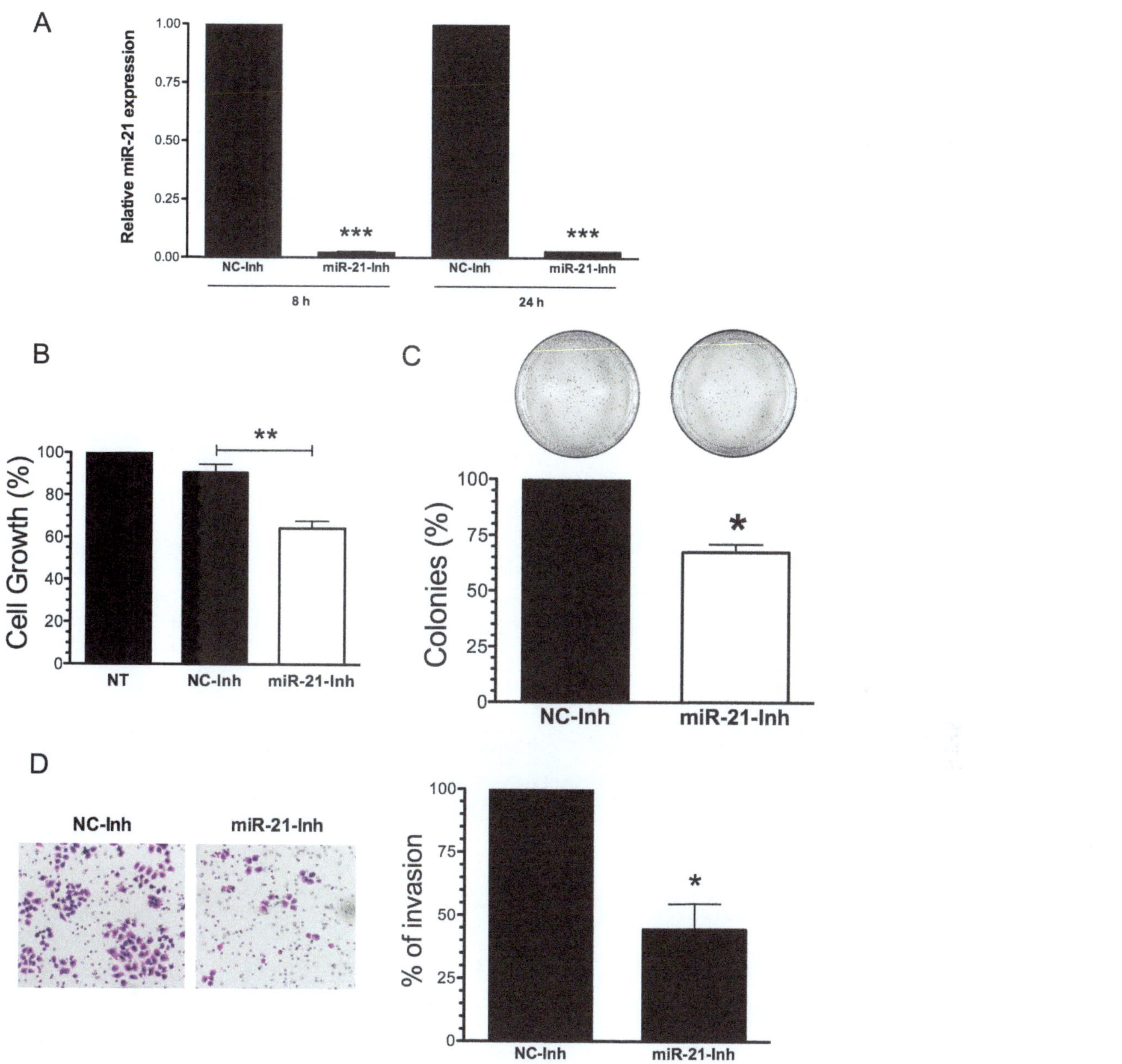

Figure 5. Effect of miR-21 inhibition in cell growth, proliferation and invasion. (**A**) A2780CP20 cells were transiently transfected with a miR-21 antagomir or with a negative antagomir (-) as described in the "Materials and Methods" section. Eight and 24 hours after transfection cells were collected and RNA (including miRNAs) was isolated as described in the "Materials and Methods" section. (**B**) MiR-21 inhibition reduced cell growth compared to untreated cells (NT) or with the negative control inhibitor (NC-Inh). (**C**) A2780CP20 cells were transfected as in 5A. A thousand cells were seeded in Petri dishes. Ten days later, the colonies were stained and counted. Inhibition of miR-21 decreased the ability of cells to undergo unlimited division compared with the NC-Inh. (**D**) Cell invasion was carried out as described in the "Materials and Methods" section. The number of invaded cells was expressed in percentages, taken the NC-Inh as 100%. *$p<0.05$, **$p<0.01$ compared to NC-Inh. Columns represent the means of triplicates ± S.E.M.

database found that women with tumors overexpressing miR-21 exhibited shorter progression-free survival [18].

Taken together, we showed that JNK-1/c-Jun pathway is activated in cisplatin resistant ovarian cancer cells and promote miR-21 upregulation in these cells. Overexpression of miR-21, in turn activates its cognate targets, including the tumor suppressor gene, PDCD4. All of these molecular events play a pivotal role in the cisplatin resistance of ovarian cancer cells. The upstream molecular events of many other miRNAs differentially abundant in drug resistant and drug sensitive ovarian cancer cells needs to be further investigated. This could provide an explanation of how several miRNAs are dysregulated not only in ovarian cancer but also in many other tumor types.

Supporting Information

Figure S1 STAT3 protein levels in A2780CP20 and A2780 cells. Protein extraction and Western blot analysis was performed as described in the "Methods" section. The STAT3 protein levels were similar in A2780CP20 and A2780 cells.

Figure S2 Effect of JNK-1 inhibition in pre-mir-21 and PDCD4 expression. A2780 cells were treated with 10 μM SP600125 as described in the "Materials and Methods" section. RNA, protein extraction, real-time PCR and western blots were performed as described in the "Material and Methods" section. **(A)** Western blot analysis showing that treatment of A2780 cells with SP600125 did not affect the total or the phosphorylation levels of JNK-1, JNK-2/3 or c-Jun. **(B)** SYBR-I-based real-time PCR was performed to assess the relative pre-mir-21 expression levels in A2780 cells following SP600125 treatment. A small, no significant increasing, rather than a decreasing in pre-mir-21 levels was observed in SP600125-treated cells compared with DMSO-treated cells. **(C)** Western blot and densitometric analysis showed not visible changes in the PDCD4 protein levels after treatment of A2780 cells with SP600125.

Figure S3 MiR-21 promoter region. Primers were designed to amplify a DNA region encompassing the AP-1 binding sites (grey shadows) in the miR-21 promoter region. The other pair of primers amplifies a DNA outside of the AP-1 promoter region.

Figure S4 PDCD4 expression in miR-21 and empty vector clones. Protein extraction and Western blot analysis was performed as described in the "Methods" section. A2780-EV: empty vector clones. A2780-miR-21: miR-21 overexpressed clones.

Figure S5 Visualization of the pre-miR-21 stable transfection in A2780 cells. Stable transected A2780 cells were was monitored by the tGFP signal. Red: GFP. Blue: DAPI.

Table S1 Microarray data analysis. Two way-ANOVA was used to calculate genes with fold changes of +/− 3 in A2780CP20 vs. A2780 cells.

Acknowledgments

We wish to thank Dr. Carmen Cadilla and Jessica Renta of the Molecular Genetics Core Facility for helping us with the processing and analysis of the microarray data; and to Krizia Rohena for helping us with the immunofluorescence protocol.

Author Contributions

Conceived and designed the experiments: IEV PEV. Performed the experiments: IEV FV PEV. Analyzed the data: IEV PEV. Contributed reagents/materials/analysis tools: PEV. Wrote the paper: IEV PEV.

References

1. Siegel R, Naishadham D, Jemal A (2013) Cancer Statistics, 2013. 63: 11–30.
2. Bast RC, Hennessy B, Mills GB (2009) The biology of ovarian cancer: new opportunities for translation. Nature reviews Cancer 9: 415–428.
3. Vasey PA (2003) Resistance to chemotherapy in advanced ovarian cancer: mechanisms and current strategies. British journal of cancer 89 Suppl 3: S23–8.
4. Galluzzi L, Senovilla L, Vitale I, Michels J, Martins I, et al. (2011) Molecular mechanisms of cisplatin resistance. Oncogene: 1869–1883.
5. Kikuchi Y (2001) [The mechanism of cisplatin-resistance in ovarian cancer]. Human cell 14: 115–133.
6. Sorrentino A, Liu C-G, Addario A, Peschle C, Scambia G, et al. (2008) Role of microRNAs in drug-resistant ovarian cancer cells. Gynecologic oncology 111: 478–486.
7. Slezak-Prochazka I, Durmus S, Kroesen B-J, Van den Berg A (2010) MicroRNAs, macrocontrol: regulation of miRNA processing. RNA (New York, NY) 16: 1087–1095.
8. Bartel DP (2004) MicroRNAs: genomics, biogenesis, mechanism, and function. Cell 116: 281–297.
9. Ma J, Dong C, Ji C (2010) MicroRNA and drug resistance. Cancer gene therapy 17: 523–531.
10. Nana-Sinkam SP, Croce CM (2013) Clinical applications for microRNAs in cancer. Clinical pharmacology and therapeutics 93: 98–104.
11. Pan X, Wang Z-X, Wang R (2010) MicroRNA-21: a novel therapeutic target in human cancer. Cancer biology & therapy 10: 1224–1232.
12. Gong C, Yao Y, Wang Y, Liu B, Wu W, et al. (2011) Up-regulation of miR-21 mediates resistance to trastuzumab therapy for breast cancer. The Journal of biological chemistry 286: 19127–19137.
13. Nam EJ, Yoon H, Kim SW, Kim H, Kim YT, et al. (2008) MicroRNA expression profiles in serous ovarian carcinoma. Clinical cancer research 14: 2690–2695.
14. Xie Z, Cao L, Zhang J (2013) miR-21 modulates paclitaxel sensitivity and hypoxia-inducible factor-1α expression in human ovarian cancer cells. Oncology letters 6: 795–800.
15. Wei NA, Liu SS, Leung THY, Tam KF, Liao XY, et al. (2009) Loss of Programmed cell death 4 (Pdcd4) associates with the progression of ovarian cancer. Molecular cancer 8: 70.
16. Talotta F, Cimmino a, Matarazzo MR, Casalino L, De Vita G, et al. (2009) An autoregulatory loop mediated by miR-21 and PDCD4 controls the AP-1 activity in RAS transformation. Oncogene 28: 73–84.
17. Mudduluru G, George-William JN, Muppala S, Asangani IA, Kumarswamy R, et al. (2011) Curcumin regulates miR-21 expression and inhibits invasion and metastasis in colorectal cancer. Bioscience reports 31: 185–197.
18. Chan JK, Blansit K, Kiet T, Sherman A, Wong G, et al. (2014) The inhibition of miR-21 promotes apoptosis and chemosensitivity in ovarian cancer. Gynecologic oncology 132: 739–744.
19. Krichevsky AM, Gabriely G (2009) miR-21: a small multi-faceted RNA. Journal of cellular and molecular medicine 13: 39–53.
20. Fujita S, Ito T, Mizutani T, Minoguchi S, Yamamichi N, et al. (2008) miR-21 Gene expression triggered by AP-1 is sustained through a double-negative feedback mechanism. Journal of molecular biology 378: 492–504.
21. Misawa A, Katayama R, Koike S, Tomida A, Watanabe T, et al. (2010) AP-1-Dependent miR-21 expression contributes to chemoresistance in cancer stem cell-like SP cells. Oncology research 19: 23–33.
22. Apte SM, Bucana CD, Killion JJ, Gershenson DM, Fidler IJ (2004) Expression of platelet-derived growth factor and activated receptor in clinical specimens of epithelial ovarian cancer and ovarian carcinoma cell lines. Gynecologic oncology 93: 78–86.
23. Schmandt RE, Bennett M, Clifford S, Thornton A, Jiang F, et al. (2006) The BRK tyrosine kinase is expressed in high-grade serous carcinoma of the ovary. Cancer biology & therapy 5: 1136–1141.
24. Skilling JS, Squatrito RC, Connor JP, Niemann T, Buller RE (1996) p53 gene mutation analysis and antisense-mediated growth inhibition of human ovarian carcinoma cell lines. Gynecologic oncology 60: 72–80.
25. Sood AK, Seftor EA, Fletcher MS, Gardner LM, Heidger PM, et al. (2001) Molecular determinants of ovarian cancer plasticity. The American journal of pathology 158: 1279–1288.
26. Behrens BC, Hamilton TC, Masuda H, Grotzinger KR, Whang-Peng J, et al. (1987) Characterization of a cis-diamminedichloroplatinum(II)-resistant human ovarian cancer cell line and its use in evaluation of platinum analogues. Cancer research 47: 414–418.
27. Al-Nasiry S, Geusens N, Hanssens M, Luyten C, Pijnenborg R (2007) The use of Alamar Blue assay for quantitative analysis of viability, migration and invasion of choriocarcinoma cells. Human reproduction 22: 1304–1309.
28. Peltier HJ, Latham GJ (2008) Normalization of microRNA expression levels in quantitative RT-PCR assays: identification of suitable reference RNA targets in normal and cancerous human solid tissues. RNA (New York, NY) 14: 844–852.
29. Schmittgen TD, Livak KJ (2008) Analyzing real-time PCR data by the comparative C(T) method. Nature protocols 3: 1101–1108.
30. Vivas-Mejia PE, Rodriguez-Aguayo C, Han H-D, Shahzad MMK, Valiyeva F, et al. (2011) Silencing survivin splice variant 2B leads to antitumor activity in taxane—resistant ovarian cancer. Clinical cancer research 17: 3716–3726.
31. Echevarria-Vargas I, Vivas-Mejia P (2013) Assessment of mRNA Splice Variants by qRT-PCR. Ovarian Cancer. Malek A, Tchernitsa O, editors Totowa, NJ: Humana Press. p . 171–186.
32. Vivas-Mejía PE, Ozpolat B, Chen X, Lopez-Berestein G (2009) Downregulation of the c-MYC target gene, peroxiredoxin III, contributes to arsenic trioxide-induced apoptosis in acute promyelocytic leukemia. International journal of cancer 125: 264–275.
33. Kumarswamy R, Volkmann I, Thum T (2011) Regulation and function of miRNA-21 in health and disease. RNA biology 8: 706–713.

34. Bennett BL, Sasaki DT, Murray BW, O'Leary EC, Sakata ST, et al. (2001) SP600125, an anthrapyrazolone inhibitor of Jun N-terminal kinase. Proceedings of the National Academy of Sciences of the United States of America 98: 13681–13686.
35. Leppä S, Saffrich R, Ansorge W, Bohmann D (1998) Differential regulation of c-Jun by ERK and JNK during PC12 cell differentiation. The EMBO journal 17: 4404–4413.
36. Karin M (1995) The regulation of AP-1 activity by mitogen-activated protein kinases. The Journal of biological chemistry 270: 16483–16486.
37. Lou Y, Cui Z, Wang F, Yang X, Qian J (2011) miR-21 down-regulation promotes apoptosis and inhibits invasion and migration abilities of OVCAR3 cells. Clinical and investigative medicine 34: E281.
38. Si M-L, Zhu S, Wu H, Lu Z, Wu F, et al. (2007) miR-21-mediated tumor growth. Oncogene 26: 2799–2803.
39. Lou Y, Yang X, Wang F, Cui Z, Huang Y (2010) MicroRNA-21 promotes the cell proliferation, invasion and migration abilities in ovarian epithelial carcinomas through inhibiting the expression of PTEN protein. International journal of molecular medicine 26: 819–827.
40. Chen Y, Tsai Y-H, Fang Y, Tseng S-H (2012) Micro-RNA-21 regulates the sensitivity to cisplatin in human neuroblastoma cells. Journal of pediatric surgery 47: 1797–1805.
41. Di Leva G, Croce CM (2013) The Role of microRNAs in the Tumorigenesis of Ovarian Cancer. Frontiers in oncology 3: 153.
42. Chen Y, Zhang L, Hao Q (2013) Candidate microRNA biomarkers in human epithelial ovarian cancer: systematic review profiling studies and experimental validation. Cancer cell international 13: 86.
43. Yang H, Kong W, He L, Zhao J-J, O'Donnell JD, et al. (2008) MicroRNA expression profiling in human ovarian cancer: miR-214 induces cell survival and cisplatin resistance by targeting PTEN. Cancer research 68: 425–433.
44. Braun R, Finney R, Yan C, Chen Q-R, Hu Y, et al. (2013) Discovery analysis of TCGA data reveals association between germline genotype and survival in ovarian cancer patients. PloS one 8: e55037.
45. Derfoul A, Juan AH, Difilippantonio MJ, Palanisamy N, Ried T, et al. (2011) Decreased microRNA-214 levels in breast cancer cells coincides with increased cell proliferation, invasion and accumulation of the Polycomb Ezh2 methyl-transferase. Carcinogenesis 32: 1607–1614.
46. Peng R-Q, Wan H-Y, Li H-F, Liu M, Li X, et al. (2012) MicroRNA-214 suppresses growth and invasiveness of cervical cancer cells by targeting UDP-N-acetyl-α-D-galactosamine:polypeptide N-acetylgalactosaminyltransferase 7. The Journal of biological chemistry 287: 14301–14309.
47. Imanaka Y, Tsuchiya S, Sato F, Shimada Y, Shimizu K, et al. (2011) MicroRNA-141 confers resistance to cisplatin-induced apoptosis by targeting YAP1 in human esophageal squamous cell carcinoma. Journal of human genetics 56: 270–276.
48. Van Jaarsveld MTM, Helleman J, Boersma AWM, Van Kuijk PF, Van Ijcken WF, et al. (2013) miR-141 regulates KEAP1 and modulates cisplatin sensitivity in ovarian cancer cells. Oncogene 32: 4284–4293.
49. Integrated genomic analyses of ovarian carcinoma. (2011). Nature 474: 609–615.
50. Wyman SK, Parkin RK, Mitchell PS, Fritz BR, O'Briant K, et al. (2009) Repertoire of microRNAs in epithelial ovarian cancer as determined by next generation sequencing of small RNA cDNA libraries. PloS one 4: e5311.
51. Vivas-Mejia P, Benito JM, Fernandez A, Han H-D, Mangala L, et al. (2010) c-Jun-NH2-kinase-1 inhibition leads to antitumor activity in ovarian cancer. Clinical cancer research: 16: 184–194.

2

The MyD88+ Phenotype Is an Adverse Prognostic Factor in Epithelial Ovarian Cancer

Charles J. d'Adhemar[1☯], Cathy D. Spillane[1☯], Michael F. Gallagher[1☯], Mark Bates[1], Katie M. Costello[2], Jacqui Barry-O'Crowley[2], Kathryn Haley[3], Niamh Kernan[2], Ciara Murphy[2], Paul C Smyth[1], Ken O'Byrne[4], Stephen Pennington[5], Aoife A. Cooke[1], Brendan Ffrench[1], Cara M. Martin[1], Dearbhaile O'Donnell[6], Bryan Hennessy[7], Britta Stordal[1], Stephen Finn[1], Amanda McCann[5], Noreen Gleeson[3], Tom D'Arcy[3], Brian Flood[1], Luke A. J. O'Neill[8], Orla Sheils[1], Sharon O'Toole[1,3¶]*, John J. O'Leary[1,2¶]

1 Department of Histopathology, Trinity College Dublin, Dublin, Ireland, **2** Department of Pathology, Coombe Women's & Infants University Hospital, Dublin, Ireland, **3** Department of Obstetrics and Gynaecology, Trinity College Dublin, Dublin, Ireland, **4** Translational Research Institute, Princess Alexandra Hospital, Brisbane, Australia, **5** College of Health Sciences, University College Dublin, Belfield, Dublin, Ireland, **6** Department of Medical Oncology, St. James's Hospital, Dublin, Ireland, **7** Department of Medical Oncology, Royal College of Surgeons, Dublin, Ireland, **8** Department of Biochemistry, Trinity College Dublin, Ireland

Abstract

The prognosis of epithelial ovarian cancer is poor in part due to the high frequency of chemoresistance. Recent evidence points to the Toll-like receptor-4 (TLR4), and particularly its adaptor protein MyD88, as one potential mediator of this resistance. This study aims to provide further evidence that MyD88 positive cancer cells are clinically significant, stem-like and reproducibly detectable for the purposes of prognostic stratification. Expression of TLR4 and MyD88 was assessed immunohistochemically in 198 paraffin-embedded ovarian tissues and in an embryonal carcinoma model of cancer stemness. In parallel, expression of TLR4 and MyD88 mRNA and regulatory microRNAs (miR-21 and miR-146a) was assessed, as well as in a series of chemosensitive and resistant cancer cells lines. Functional analysis of the pathway was assessed in chemoresistant SKOV-3 ovarian cancer cells. TLR4 and MyD88 expression can be reproducibly assessed via immunohistochemistry using a semi-quantitative scoring system. TLR4 expression was present in all ovarian epithelium (normal and neoplastic), whereas MyD88 was restricted to neoplastic cells, independent of tumour grade and associated with reduced progression-free and overall survival, in an immunohistological specific subset of serous carcinomas, $p<0.05$. MiR-21 and miR-146a expression was significantly increased in MyD88 negative cancers ($p<0.05$), indicating their participation in regulation. Significant alterations in MyD88 mRNA expression were observed between chemosensitive and chemoresistant cells and tissue. Knockdown of TLR4 in SKOV-3 ovarian cells recovered chemosensitivity. Knockdown of MyD88 alone did not. MyD88 expression was down-regulated in differentiated embryonal carcinoma (NTera2) cells, supporting the MyD88+ cancer stem cell hypothesis. Our findings demonstrate that expression of MyD88 is associated with significantly reduced patient survival and altered microRNA levels and suggest an intact/functioning TLR4/MyD88 pathway is required for acquisition of the chemoresistant phenotype. *Ex vivo* manipulation of ovarian cancer stem cell (CSC) differentiation can decrease MyD88 expression, providing a potentially valuable CSC model for ovarian cancer.

Editor: Chiara Romualdi, University of Padova, Italy

Funding: This work was supported by Cancer Research Ireland (grant reference number ICS CRP09OLE), the Meath foundation, The Royal City of Dublin Hospital Trust, BDI-2 (10/CE/B1821), the Emer Casey foundation, the Irish Cancer Society, and a Marie Curie European Union grant. The funders had no role in study design, data collection and analysis, decision to publish, or preparation of the manuscript.

Competing Interests: The authors have declared that no competing interests exist.

* Email: shotoole@tcd.ie

☯ These authors are joint first authors on this work.

¶ These authors are joint senior authors on this work.

Introduction

Ovarian cancer is one of the most common and lethal cancers in women [1,2], with incidences and mortality predicted to increase in western countries [3]. Epithelial ovarian cancers (EOCs) comprise the vast majority of adult ovarian malignancies, which are most commonly serous carcinomas [4,5]. As ovarian cancer is often asymptomatic in its early stages or presents with vague symptoms mimicking extra-ovarian disease; most patients (70–75%) present with widespread disease at diagnosis with a resulting high mortality rate [6]. Current treatment options include surgery and platinum and/or taxane-based chemotherapy [7]. Although EOC typically responds very well to standard chemotherapy, with initial 70–80% response rates, this is frequently followed by recurrence that is often chemoresistant [8,9]. Predicting and overcoming this chemoresistance remains a key challenge in treatment, however there are currently no available biomarkers (serum or tissue) that are truly predictive of behavior or chemoresponsiveness.

Toll-like receptors (TLRs) function as essential components of the innate immune system. They are membrane-bound receptors that recognize components of exogenous pathogens, such as bacterial lipopolysaccharide (LPS) and viral RNAs, leading to an inflammatory response. TLRs may also be activated by endogenous ligands including cellular debris derived from cancer progression [10–13]. Most TLRs signal via the myeloid differentiation primary response gene 88 (MyD88) and are expressed in both lymphoid and non-lymphoid tissues (predominantly in the former), with increasing evidence that they play important roles in cancer pathogenesis [14,15]. The net effect of TLR signalling (+/−MyD88) is transcription factor activation, including nuclear factor-κB (NF-κB). NF-κB is a universally expressed transcription factor that is particularly important both as part of the normal inflammatory response and in tumourigenesis, regulating the expression of various inflammatory, apoptotic and oncogenic genes [16]. Ultimately NF-κB activation leads to increased production of cytokines, chemokines and growth factors. The activity of this pathway is normally kept in check, during the normal immune response, in part through microRNA regulation of TLR4 signaling, examples of which include microRNA 21 (miR-21) and miR-146a [17,18,19].

The TLR4/MyD88 pathway has in recent years been proposed as a risk factor for carcinogenesis and chemoresistance in ovarian cancer [20,21]. While it has been observed that TLR4 expression is ubiquitous in EOC cells, a subgroup differentially expressing MyD88 has demonstrated increased cytokine/chemokine production and cellular proliferation upon activation of TLR4 [20]. Chen et al. [21] have used this differential expression to subdivide EOC into MyD88 positive and MyD88 negative. MyD88 positive EOCs have a functioning TLR4/MyD88 pathway and may represent an ovarian cancer stem cell (CSC) that is highly resistant to pro-apoptotic signaling and which can recruit leukocytes to actively promote a pro-inflammatory, pro-proliferative microenvironment [22]. MyD88 negative EOCs in contrast lack MyD88 and may represent more differentiated tumours that are less biologically aggressive [20,23]. Alvero et al. [12] demonstrated that CSCs derived from ovarian tumour samples have a unique CD44+/MyD88+ phenotype, which facilitated resistance to both tumour necrosis factor (TNF) induced apoptosis and cytotoxic therapy. More recently MyD88 protein expression was shown to be a significantly poor prognostic factor in EOC [24].

The differential classification of MyD88 positive and negative EOC has implications for current therapeutic strategies. Although cisplatin-resistance occurs in a minority of women during their initial treatment (30%), it subsequently develops in all women receiving treatment for recurrent disease [9], and is most likely due to resistance to apoptotic signalling in MyD88 positive cells [12,25,26]. In addition, paclitaxel (a taxane-based agent) is a TLR4 ligand and can activate the TLR4/MyD88 pathway in MyD88 positive cells, actually inducing their proliferation [20,27]. Such MyD88 competent cancer cells are theoretically able to exploit current chemotherapeutic strategies, by not only resisting their cytotoxic effects but also by using paclitaxel-ligation to facilitate their growth and that of the surrounding stroma via enhanced NF-κB production. Therefore current evidence suggests that paclitaxel may in fact be disadvantageous in patients whose tumours contain MyD88 positive EOC cells, despite retaining its cytotoxic effects in MyD88 negative cells [20,27]. It is also possible that recurrent disease may represent a pool of more aggressive cancer cells (CSCs), which have effectively been 'selected out' by paclitaxel treatment.

We hypothesise that MyD88+ cancer cells represent a subpopulation of cells in EOC that confer more aggressive biological behaviour and chemoresistance. To date relatively small numbers of ovarian cancer samples, or isolated cancer cell lines, have been examined with respect to TLR4/MyD88 expression [20,23,27,28]. The aim of this study was to comprehensively characterise the distribution and clinical significance of TLR4 and MyD88 expression in a cohort of ovarian neoplasms, which includes all common histologic subtypes and represents the largest such series studied to date [20,23,24,27,28]. The expression of two microRNAs known to regulate the TLR4/MyD88 pathway was also evaluated in a subset of malignant tumour samples to explore their role as epigenetic modulators of this pathway. Knockdown of TLR4/MyD88 was assessed to dissect the functional role of these genes. In parallel with the above experiments, TLR4/MyD88 expression was assessed in undifferentiated and differentiated embryonal carcinoma cells to provide further evidence of the cancer stem cell hypothesis in ovarian cancer.

Results

TLR4 and MyD88 Expression in the Test Series

The primary test series of malignant ovarian tumours comprised 20 patients with serous adenocarcinomas that were matched for grade (high-grade) and stage (FIGO III), and who had received platinum-based adjuvant chemotherapy. TLR4 expression was universally present and scored as positive (immunoscore >4) in all tumours (20/20). In contrast, positive immunostaining for MyD88 was observed in only 12/20 cases, and the remainder (8/20) were classified as MyD88 negative. Clinical follow-up data was available for all patients, 12 of whom had died at the time of this study, and retrospective analysis was performed to determine whether MyD88 expression was associated with patient survival. Progression free survival (PFS) and overall survival (OS) were assessed. Figure 1 demonstrates that MyD88 expression was associated with significantly shortened PFS and OS ($p<0.05$). The median time to recurrence (from the time of surgery) for patients with MyD88 positive tumours was 16 months, whereas MyD88 negative tumours recurred at a median time of 42 months ($p = 0.018$). MyD88 positive tumours were also associated with a markedly shorter OS. The median OS time for patients with MyD88 positive tumours was 43 months, compared to 108 months for MyD88 negative tumours ($p = 0.008$).

TLR4 and MyD88 in the Validation Series

Expression of TLR4 and MyD88 was then assessed in 178 patient samples in order to validate the test series findings and to examine expression in non-malignant ovarian tissue and different histologic subtypes of EOC. These samples included normal ovaries ($n = 50$), benign cysts ($n = 15$), borderline tumours ($n = 28$) and malignant tumours ($n = 85$). Average patient age at time of surgery was 51 years for borderline tumours (range, 20-81) and 59 years for all malignant tumours (range, 23–94). The majority of malignant tumours were high-grade, with 62% assigned a grade of 3 (predominantly serous carcinomas), and high stage (51.3% FIGO stage IIIC, 8.1% stage IV). All tumours that were staged IIB and higher were serous carcinomas. The immunophenotype of each tissue type is summarized in Table 1.

The expression of both TLR4 and MyD88 was most uniform and strongest in serous neoplasms, particularly borderline and malignant serous tumours. Examples of TLR4 and MyD88 IHC expression are shown in Figures 2 & 3. Normal ovarian surface epithelium (NOSE) showed variable expression of TLR4 (7/50) but was uniformly negative for MyD88 (0/50). Approximately half of the benign cysts were TLR4 positive (7/15, mixed subtypes) but only a minority were MyD88 positive (3/15, all serous). The majority of borderline serous tumours were both TLR4 and MyD88 positive (12/15), with strong staining observed in 7/12. In

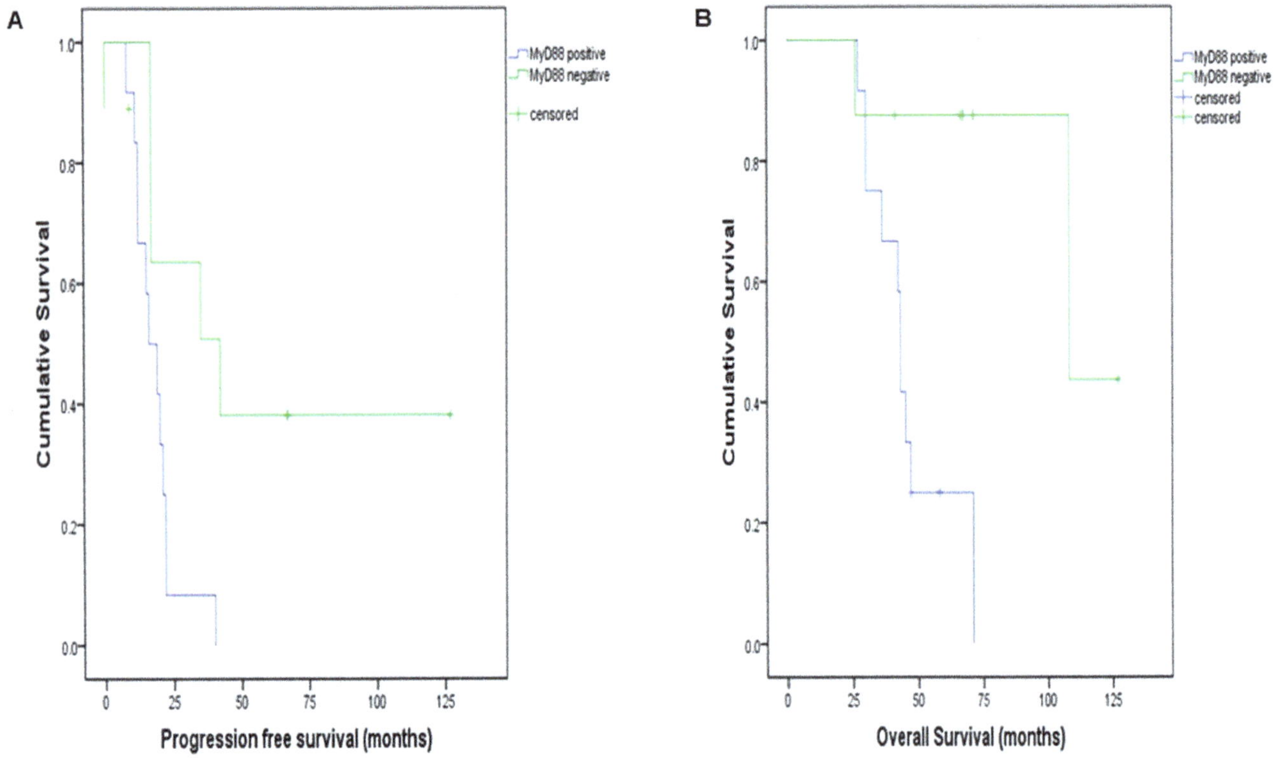

Figure 1. MyD88 expression and survival (Kaplan-Meier curves: median survival time shown in months). MyD88 positive tumours (n = 12) had significantly reduced progression-free survival (A) and overall survival (B) (p = 0.018 and p = 0.008, respectively).

contrast all borderline mucinous tumours were MyD88 negative. While 73% (62/85) of malignant tumours were TLR4 positive (mixed subtypes), co-expression of MyD88 was observed in only 47% cases, which were all serous carcinomas. All non-serous carcinomas (mucinous, clear cell and endometrioid) were MyD88 negative. This data generated 40 MyD88 positive and 45 MyD88 negative cancers. MyD88 expression was observed in both poorly- and well-differentiated tumour cells, and was strong near areas of necrosis. As shown in Table 2 there was no correlation between patient age or overall grade of differentiation and TLR4 or MyD88 expression. Collectively, the TLR4+/MyD88- phenotype was associated with all types of tissue, including non-dysplastic epithelium, while TLR4+/MyD88+ (co-expression) was associated only with ovarian neoplasms.

Table 1. Distribution of TLR4 & MyD88 protein expression in all patient samples.

Ovarian Tissue	TLR Positive[†]	MyD88 Positive[†]
NOSE (n = 50)	7 (14%)	0
Benign (n = 15)	7 (47%)	3 (20%)
Serous (n = 5)	3 (60%)	3 (60%)
Mucinous (n = 5)	2 (40%)	0
Brenner (n = 5)	2 (40%)	0
Borderline (n = 28)	17 (61%)	12 (43%)
Serous (n = 15)	12 (80%)	12 (80%)
Mucinous (n = 13)	5 (38%)	0
Malignant (n = 85)	62 (73%)	40 (47%)
Serous (n = 69)	55 (80%)	40 (58%)
Mucinous (n = 6)	2 (33%)	0
Clear Cell (n = 5)	3 (60%)	0
Endometrioid (n = 5)	2 (40%)	0

Abbreviations: SD, standard deviation; FIGO, Federation International of Gynecology & Obstetrics; NOSE, normal ovarian surface epithelium.
[†]TLR4, MyD88 expression by immunohistochemistry (score >4 = positive).

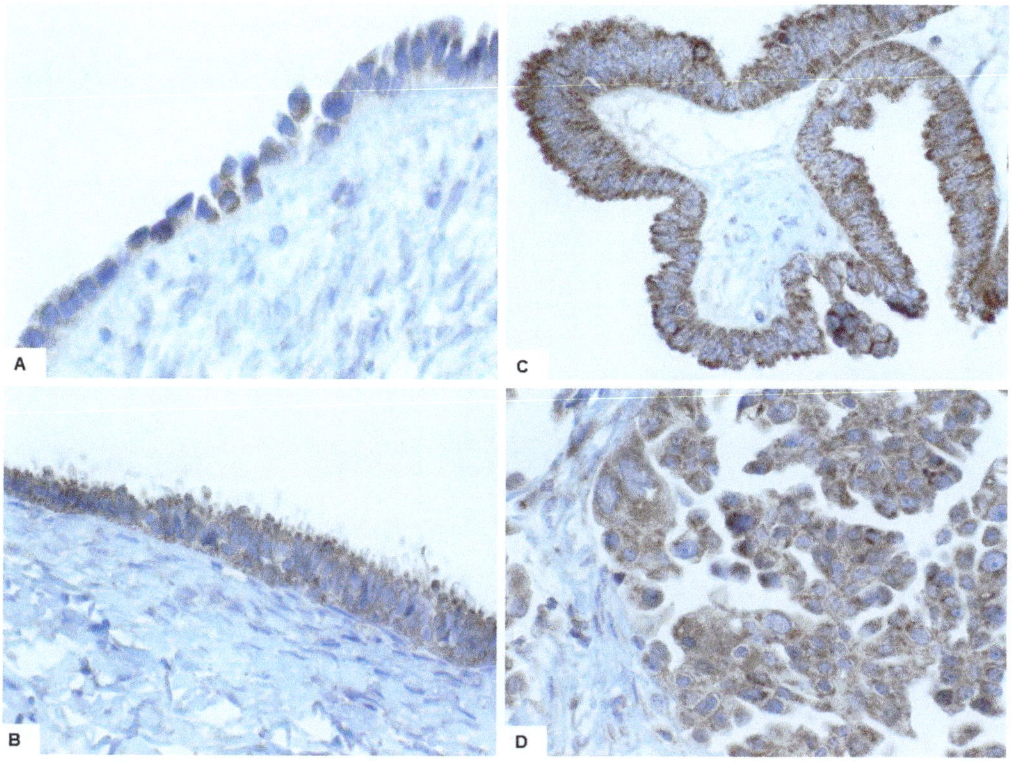

Figure 2. TLR4 expression pattern. A: focal weak staining in normal ovarian surface epithelium (40x); B: diffuse moderate staining in a benign serous cystadenoma (20x); C: diffuse strong staining in a borderline serous tumour (10x); D: diffuse strong staining in a (grade 2) serous carcinoma (40x).

Retrospective analysis was performed to determine whether TLR4/MyD88 expression influenced patient survival in this larger series. Clinical follow-up data was available for 39 patients with malignant tumours, 33 of whom had died at the time of this study. Cases excluded from follow-up included non-serous carcinomas (all MyD88 negative), those with recurrent disease (n = 2), patients who died of post-operative complications or unrelated causes (n = 2) and patients lost to follow-up (further treatment and follow-up at a different institution). Selected cases were classified into 2 groups based on MyD88 protein expression: Group 0 (MyD88 negative); Group 1 (MyD88 positive). All cases were grade and stage-matched (grade 3, FIGO III/IV), were optimally debulked and patients had received adjuvant platinum-based chemotherapy with (n = 28) or without (n = 11) paclitaxel. As illustrated in Figures 4 & 5, TLR4 and MyD88 expression were both associated with significantly shortened progression-free survival (PFS), and MyD88 expression was associated with reduced overall survival ($p<0.05$). The median time to recurrence for patients with tumours that expressed TLR4 was 12 months (n = 20), whereas TLR4 negative tumours recurred in a median time of 27 months (n = 19); $p = 0.016$. Similarly, median time to recurrence for MyD88 positive tumours was 13 months (n = 21), compared to 31 months if MyD88 negative (n = 18); $p = 0.02$. The difference in OS between TLR4 positive (n = 19) and TLR4 negative tumours (n = 14) was not statistically significant ($p = 0.312$). The median OS time for patients with MyD88 positive EOC was 28 months (n = 21), while patients with MyD88 negative tumours (n = 12) had significantly longer overall survival (47 months, $p = 0.029$). MyD88 positive malignancies therefore were associated with reduced patient survival and disease-free intervals.

MicroRNA Expression in the Test Series

EOC samples from the initial test series were divided into two groups based on previous immunohistochemical results (MyD88 positive, n = 11; MyD88 negative, n = 9). As shown in Figure 6, the average expression of miR-21 and miR-146a in MyD88 negative cancers was increased relative to the average of the MyD88 positive group ($p<0.001$).

Gene and microRNA Expression in the Validation Series

Selected malignant patient tumour samples were divided into two groups based on previous IHC results (MyD88 positive, n = 10; MyD88 negative, n = 12). Expression of miR-21 and miR-146a was analyzed in parallel with TLR4 and MyD88 gene expression analysis. Figure 7 shows that, similar to the test series, expression of both microRNAs was significantly increased in MyD88 negative cancers relative to the MyD88 positive group (miR-21, $p = 0.0046$; miR-146a, $p = 0.0191$), with more biological heterogeneity observed with miR-146a levels. The associated levels of TLR4 & MyD88 mRNA were statistically unaltered between the MyD88 positive and negative cancers ($p = 0.8777$ and 0.1348, respectively). Therefore miR-21 and miR-146a appear to be inversely linked to MyD88 in ovarian cancer. The absence of MyD88 mRNA alteration in the MyD88 negative group suggests that both miR-21 and miR-146a are targeting MyD88 at the post-transcriptional level.

TLR4 and MyD88 expression in a cohort of responders and non-responders

MyD88 mRNA was upregulated 4.9 fold in a cohort of non-responders compared to responders ($p<0.05$). Similarly, TLR4

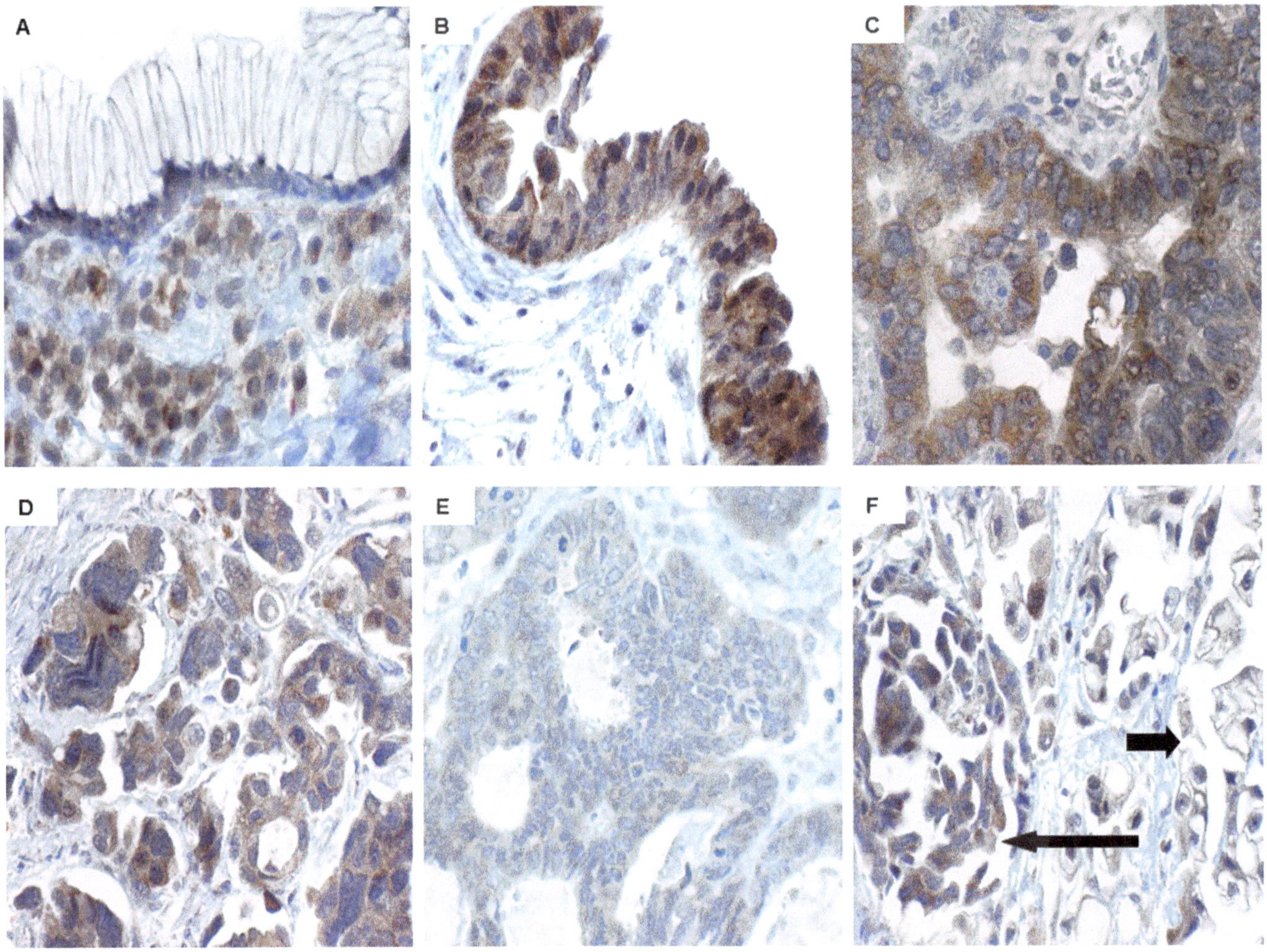

Figure 3. MyD88 expression pattern. A, negative benign mucinous cystadenoma, with positive stromal inflammatory cells (20x). B, positive borderline serous tumour (20x). C, positive low-grade serous carcinoma (40x). D, positive high-grade serous carcinoma (40x). E, negative endometrioid carcinoma (20x). F, positive serous carcinoma (long arrow) with component of negative clear cell carcinoma (short arrow) (40x).

Table 2. Characterisation of TLR4 & MyD88 expression in ovarian cancer.

Malignant Tumours	TLR4 Positive†	TLR4 Negative†	MyD88 Positive†	MyD88 Negative†
Patients (n = 85)	62	23	40	45
Mean age (y) ±SD	60±13	57±15	61±12	56±15
FIGO stage‡				
I	8 (11%)	10 (13%)	3 (4%)	13 (18%)
II	2 (3%)	3 (4%)	2 (3%)	3 (4%)
III	25 (33%)	21 (28%)	27 (38%)	19 (26%)
IV	4 (5%)	2 (3%)	5 (7%)	1 (1%)
Grade of Differentiation				
1	1 (33%)*	2 (67%)	0	3 (100%)
2	13 (65%)	7 (35%)	12 (60%)	8 (40%)
3	17 (45%)	21 (55%)	18 (47%)	20 (53%)

Abbreviations: SD, standard deviation; FIGO, Federation International of Gynecology & Obstetrics.
†TLR4, MyD88 expression by immunohistochemistry (score >4 = positive).
‡Simplified FIGO staging.
*% of each grade.

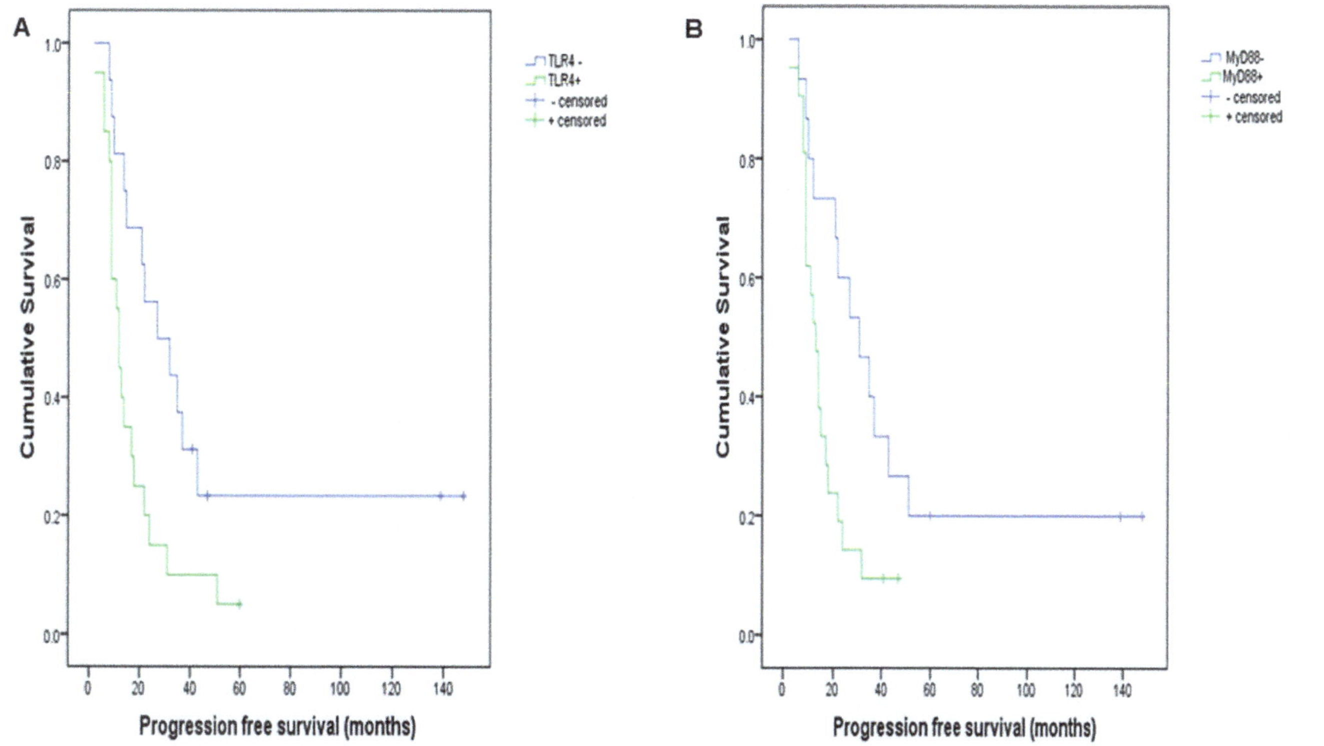

Figure 4. TLR4/MyD88 and progression-free survival (Kaplan-Meier curves; median survival shown in months). TLR4 (A) or MyD88 (B) negative cases had significantly better PFS (15 & 18 months longer; $p<0.05$).

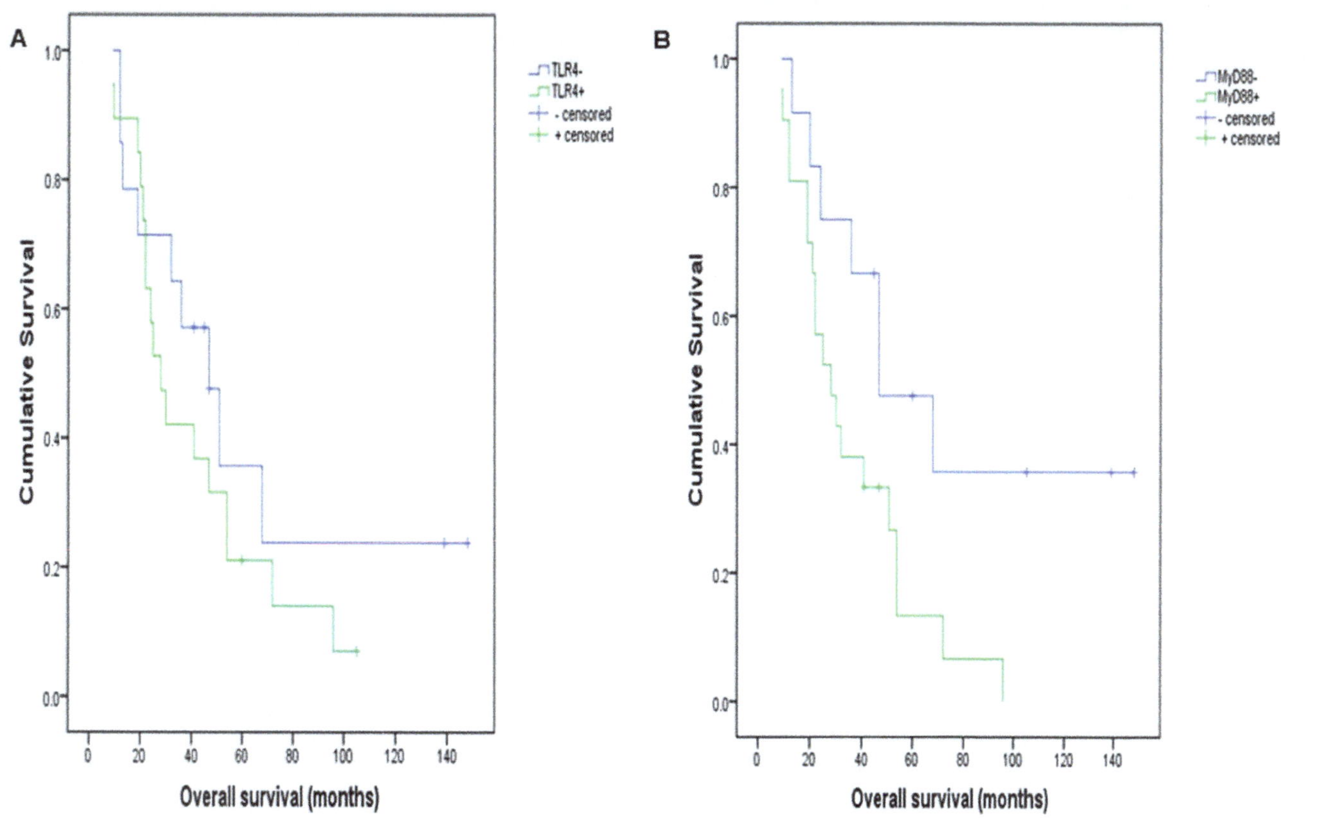

Figure 5. TLR4/MyD88 and overall survival (Kaplan-Meier curves; median survival shown in months). Survival was longer in MyD88 (B) negative cases (by 19 months; $p<0.05$). The difference in survival associated with TLR4 (A) is not significant ($p>0.5$).

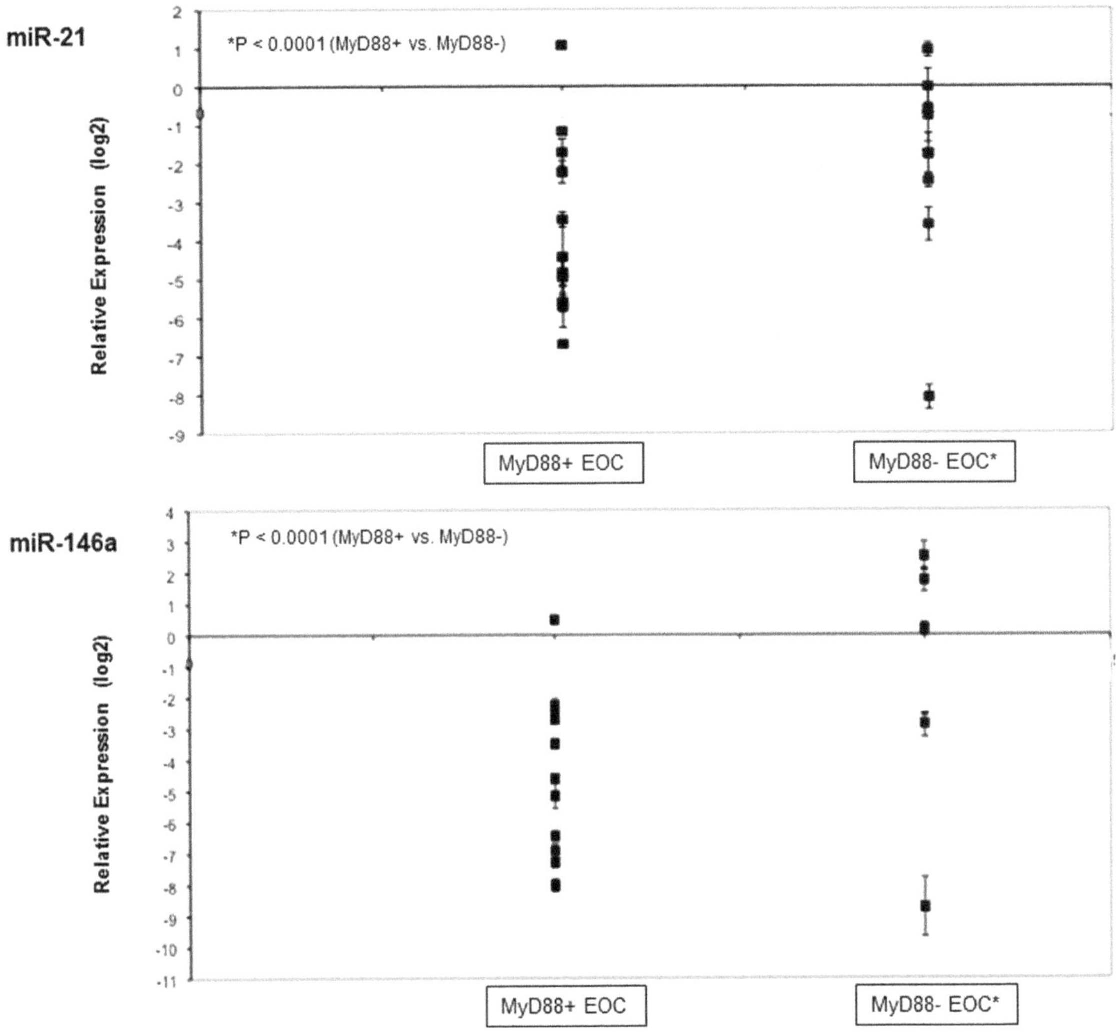

Figure 6. MiR-21 & miR-146a expression in the test series. Scatter plots showing relative microRNA expression with standard deviation (fold changes calculated via the $2^{-\Delta\Delta Ct}$ method). 20 EOC cases (serous carcinomas) grouped as MyD88+ or MyD88- based on protein expression; data shown relative to each group. Average expression of miR-21 & miR-146a increased in MyD88 negative EOC ($p<0.05$).

mRNA was upregulated 3.4 fold in this cohort ($p<0.05$). All patients analysed here had advanced serous papillary adenocarcinomas and received carboplatin and paclitaxel as first line chemotherapy following optimal debulking surgery.

Gene and miRNA expression in cell lines

Significant changes in TLR4 mRNA expression were observed between chemosensitive and chemoresistant cells, although the degree of change was variable (Figure 8A). A2780cis cells showed a 24.1 fold increase in TLR4 compared to A2780. In contrast there was an 18.8 fold decrease in TLR4 in the chemoresistant IGROV-1CDDP cells relative to IGROV-1. KB-8-5-11 cells showed the smallest change from their parent line with only a 1.6 fold increase in TLR4.

Increased MyD88 mRNA expression was observed in all chemoresistant cancer cell lines; these changes were small but statistically significant (Figure 8B). There was a 2.6 fold increase in MyD88 in A2780cis cells compared to MyD88-negative A2780 cells. IGROV-1CDDP cells showed a 1.6 fold increase in MyD88 relative to the chemosensitive IGROV-1 cells. Similar to the TLR4 data, the change in MyD88 expression in KB-8-5-11 cells from the chemosensitive KB-3-1 parent line was the smallest with only a 1.4 fold increase in MyD88.

Variable changes in the levels of miR-21 were observed between chemosensitive and chemoresistant cells (Figure 9A). A2780cis cells showed a 1.5 fold decrease in miR-21 compared to A2780, however this change was not statistically significant ($p = 0.5958$). A 2 fold increase in miR-21 was detected in the chemoresistant IGROV-1CDDP cells relative to IGROV-1. KB-8-5-11 cells showed a 2.9 fold decrease in miR-21 compared to their parent (chemosensitive) line.

Similar to miR-21, changes in miR-146a levels between chemosensitive and chemoresistant cancer cells were variable (Figure 9B). There was a 6.5 fold increase in miR-146a in A2780cis cells compared to MyD88-negative A2780 cells. IGROV-1CDDP cells showed a 1.2 fold increase in MyD88 relative to the chemosensitive IGROV-1 cells, however this change was not statistically significant ($p = 0.4557$). A 2.5 fold reduction in miR-146a was detected in KB-8-5-11 cells compared to their chemosensitive (KB-3-1) parent line.

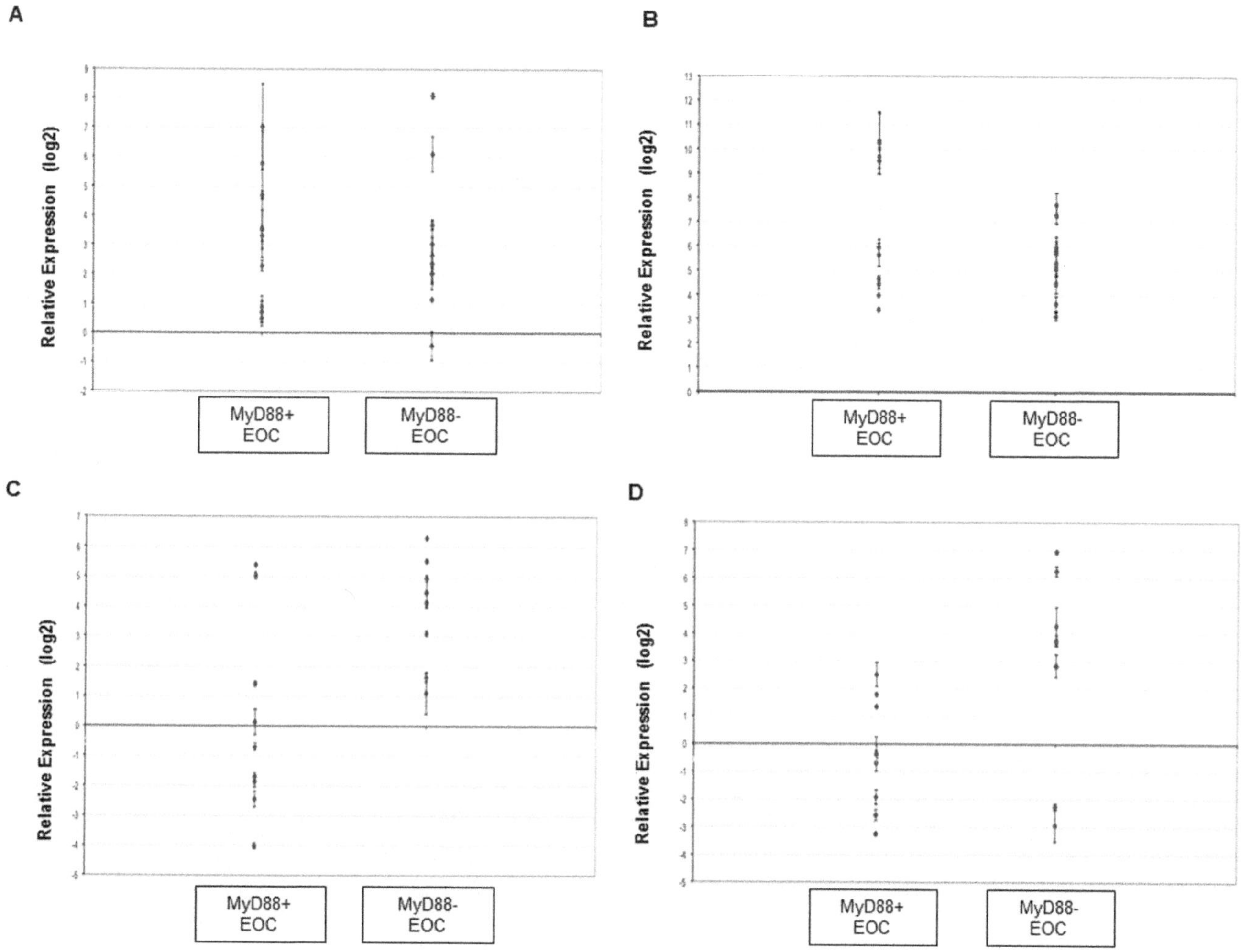

Figure 7. TLR4/MyD88 mRNA and miR-21 & miR-146a expression. Scatter plots showing relative gene and microRNA expression with standard deviation (fold changes calculated via the $2^{-\Delta\Delta Ct}$ method). 22 EOC cases (serous carcinomas) grouped as MyD88+ or MyD88- based on protein expression; data shown relative to each group. A & B, TLR4 & MyD88 mRNA statistically unchanged between MyD88 positive & MyD88 negative groups ($p>0.05$); C & D, levels of both miR-21 & miR-146a up-regulated in MyD88 negative EOC ($p<0.05$).

Reduced TLR4 expression results in increased chemosensitivity of ovarian cancer cells

To functionally evaluate the role of the TLR4/MyD88 pathway on the chemosensitivity of ovarian cancer cells the chemoresistant ovarian cancer cell line SKOV-3 was transfected with siRNA specifically targeting MyD88 or TLR4. After 72 hrs MyD88 was significant decreased at both the mRNA (Figure 10A) and protein (Figure 10B) level in the cells transfected with siMyD88. However, the loss of MyD88 expression had no effect on the chemosensitivity of the cells (Figure 10C). Significant reductions in the expression of TLR4 at the mRNA (Figure 10A) and protein (Figure 10B) level was also observed in cells 72 hrs after transfection. However, the reduced level of TLR4 expression significantly affected the response of the SKOV-3 towards paclitaxel (Figure 10C). There was a 27.1% decrease in cell viability in siTLR4 transfected paclitaxel treated cells compared to untransfected paclitaxel treated cells and a 19.6% decrease when compared to siNeg transfected cells. Thus, the silencing of TLR4 generated a more chemosensitive phenotype in the SKOV-3 ovarian cancer cells.

Embryonal carcinoma cells show reduced MyD88 expression following differentiation

Data from a large-scale microarray experiment (M Gallagher, unpublished data) involving embryonal carcinoma cancer stem cells (NTera2 and 2102Ep) was interrogated for differential TLR4-signalling gene expression, which indicated that MyD88 expression was high in undifferentiated NTera2 cells and decreased rapidly upon differentiation in retinoic acid (RA). To validate microarray data, undifferentiated and differentiated NTera2 and 2102Ep samples were assessed for MyD88 gene and protein expression. As TLR4 was hypothesised to regulate MyD88 in these cells, the expression of TLR4 was also assessed despite constitutive expression in the array studies. Down-regulation of MyD88 upon differentiation of pluripotent NTera2 cells was confirmed across multiple time courses (Figure 11A). TLR4 was constitutively expressed, validating array data. In contrast, the expression of TLR4 and MyD88 was unaltered in nullipotent 2102Ep cells treated with RA (Figure 11A). These alterations were mirrored at protein level (Figure 11B,C). MyD88 protein expression was significantly reduced following differentiation of NTera2 cells (MyD88-), whereas no significant change was

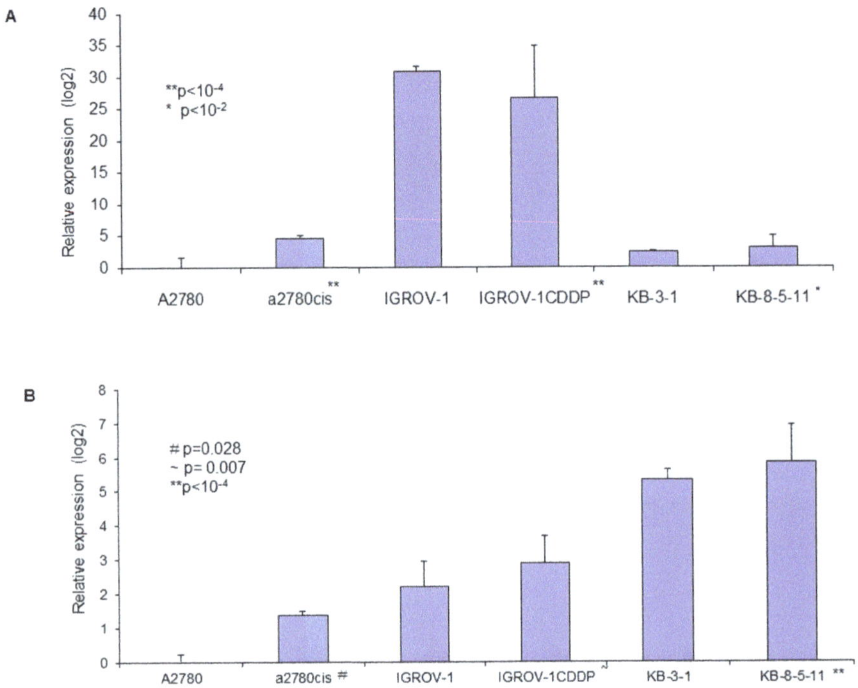

Figure 8. Changes in TLR4 (A) and MyD88 (B) mRNA expression between chemosensitive and chemoresistant cancer cells. Data are expressed as fold change in expression with respect to A2780 cancer cells (with standard deviation).

observed in TLR4 staining (Figure 11B). In contrast 2102Ep cells, both undifferentiated and treated with retinoic acid, were TLR4+, MyD88+ (Figure 11C). In terms of associated microRNA alterations, our group has previously demonstrated that while miR-21 is unaltered in either cell line in response to RA, miR-146a is up-regulated during differentiation of NTera2 cells but unchanged in 2102Ep cells [29]. This suggests that, similar to EOC, miR-146a is inversely linked to MyD88 in differentiated embryonal carcinoma cancer stem cells.

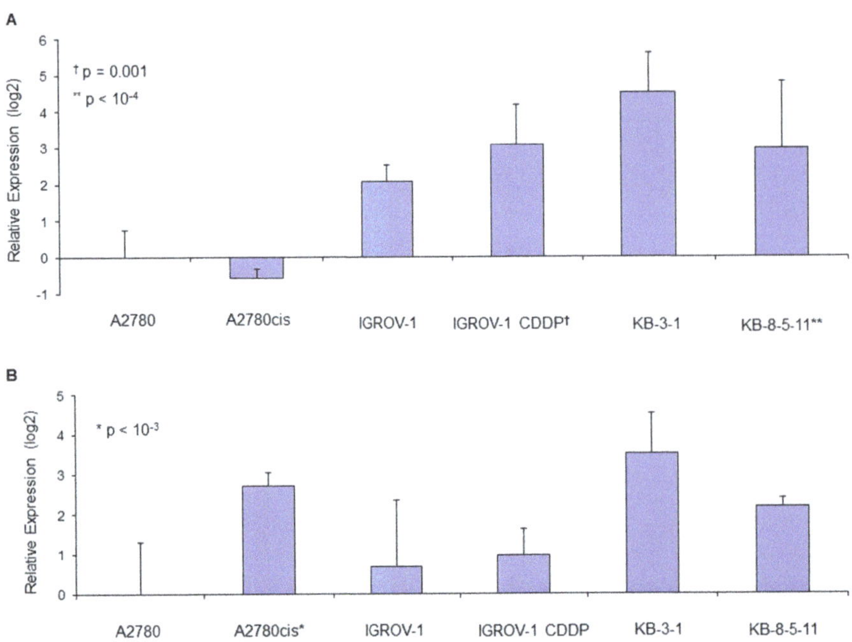

Figure 9. miR-21 (A) and miR-146a (B) expression in chemosensitive and chemoresistant cancer cells. Data are expressed as fold change in expression with respect to A2780 cancer cells (with standard deviation).

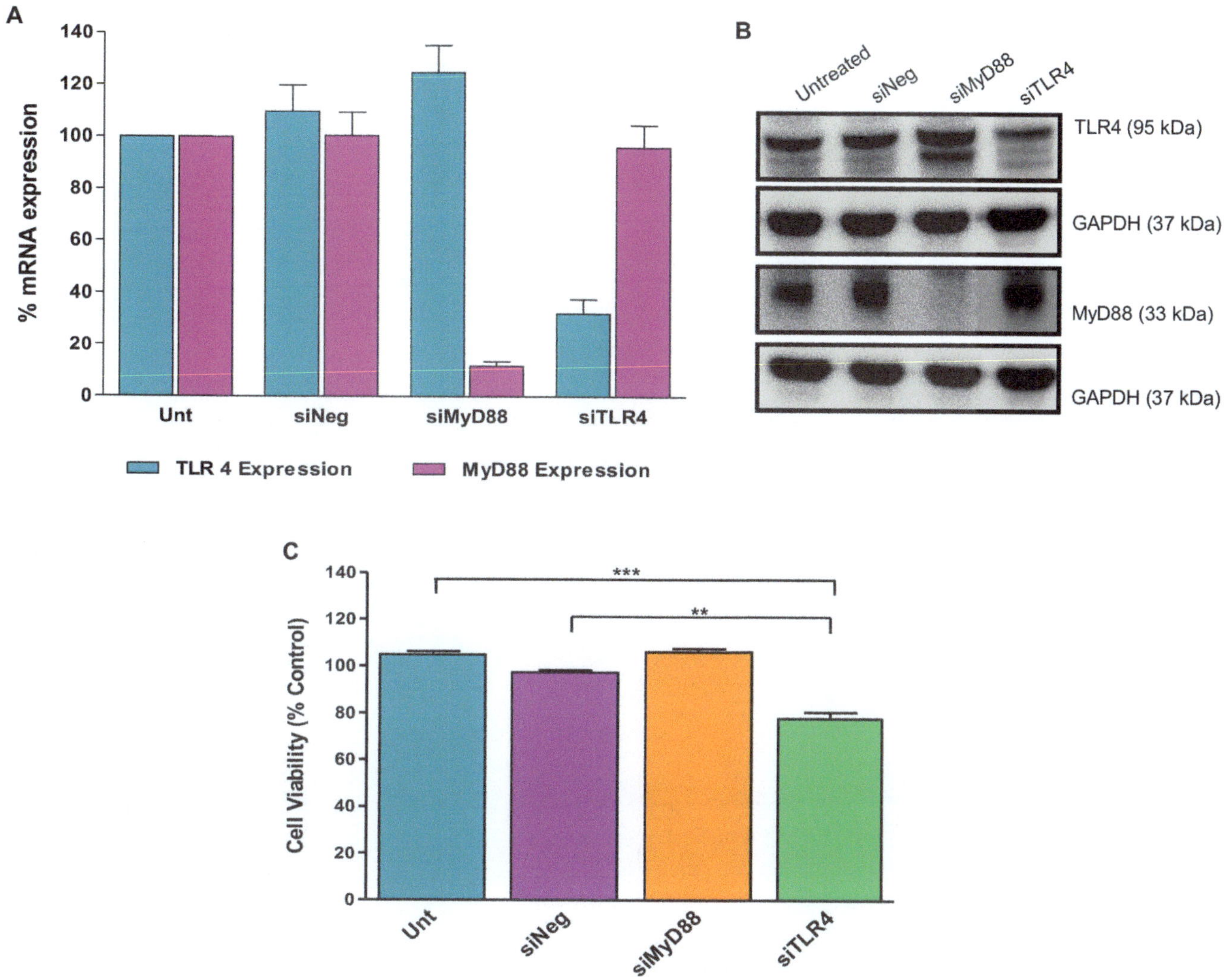

Figure 10. The effect of silencing MyD88 and TLR4 mRNA on the chemoresponsive properties of SKOV-3 cells. SKOV-3 cells were left untransfected (Unt), transfected with negative control siRNA (siNeg), MyD88 targeting siRNA (siMyD88) or TLR4 targeting siRNA (siTLR4). The transfected cells were incubated for 72 hrs before either harvesting for mRNA analysis (A), for protein analysis (B) or treatment with paclitaxel (C). (A) MyD88 and TLR4 mRNA expression levels were evaluated by TaqMan RT-PCR. MyD88 and TLR4 mRNA expression was normalised to that of an endogenous control, B2M, and calibrated to that of untreated cells to establish the relative percentage of mRNA expression (n = 3, mean +SD). (B) MyD88 and TLR4 mRNA expression levels were evaluated by western blot analysis. GAPDH was used as a loading control. (C) Transfected cells were either left untreated, treated with DMSO (vehicle control) or 3.5 nM of paclitaxel (IC25). 48 hrs post treatment, cell viability was assessed by means of the CCK-8 assay. % cell viability rate was calculated by comparing the absorbance values for the vehicle control to the corresponding paclitaxel treated samples. Results are expressed as mean +SD, n = 3; $*p<0.05$, $**p<0.01$ (un-paired Student's t-test).

Discussion

The characterisation here of TLR4 and MyD88 expression in epithelial ovarian neoplasia has shown that while TLR4 expression of some degree is ubiquitous to all types of ovarian epithelium, including non-dysplastic epithelium, MyD88 is only expressed in neoplastic tissue. Such a restriction of MyD88 to neoplastic ovarian tissue corroborates similar findings recently reported in the literature [24]. However in this study, TLR4/MyD88 co-expression showed a predilection for serous neoplasms in general, particularly borderline and malignant serous tumours, and was expressed in both high- and low-grade serous carcinomas. In contrast TLR4 in the absence of MyD88 was associated with non-malignant tissue, non-serous benign and borderline tumours, a subgroup of serous carcinomas and non-serous carcinomas (MyD88 negative EOC). As TLR4 expression was present in all types of ovarian epithelium, it appears that TLR4 signalling is linked to either malignant serous tumours or non-serous tumours proportional to being MyD88-dependent or -independent.

Chen et al. [21] originally postulated that the ratio of MyD88 positive and negative EOC cells may determine tumour characteristics in terms of progression, chemoresistance and recurrence. This is entirely in keeping with our results illustrating the distribution of MyD88 expression in ovarian neoplasia and associations with patient survivial. MyD88 positive cancers analysed in this study recurred 18 months earlier than MyD88 negative cancers, with a similar reduction in overall survival of 19 months ($p<0.05$). The results of this analysis are in exact concordance with recent reports indicating reductions in disease-free intervals and patient survival with MyD88 positive cancers, ranging from 11–35 month reductions in progression-free survival

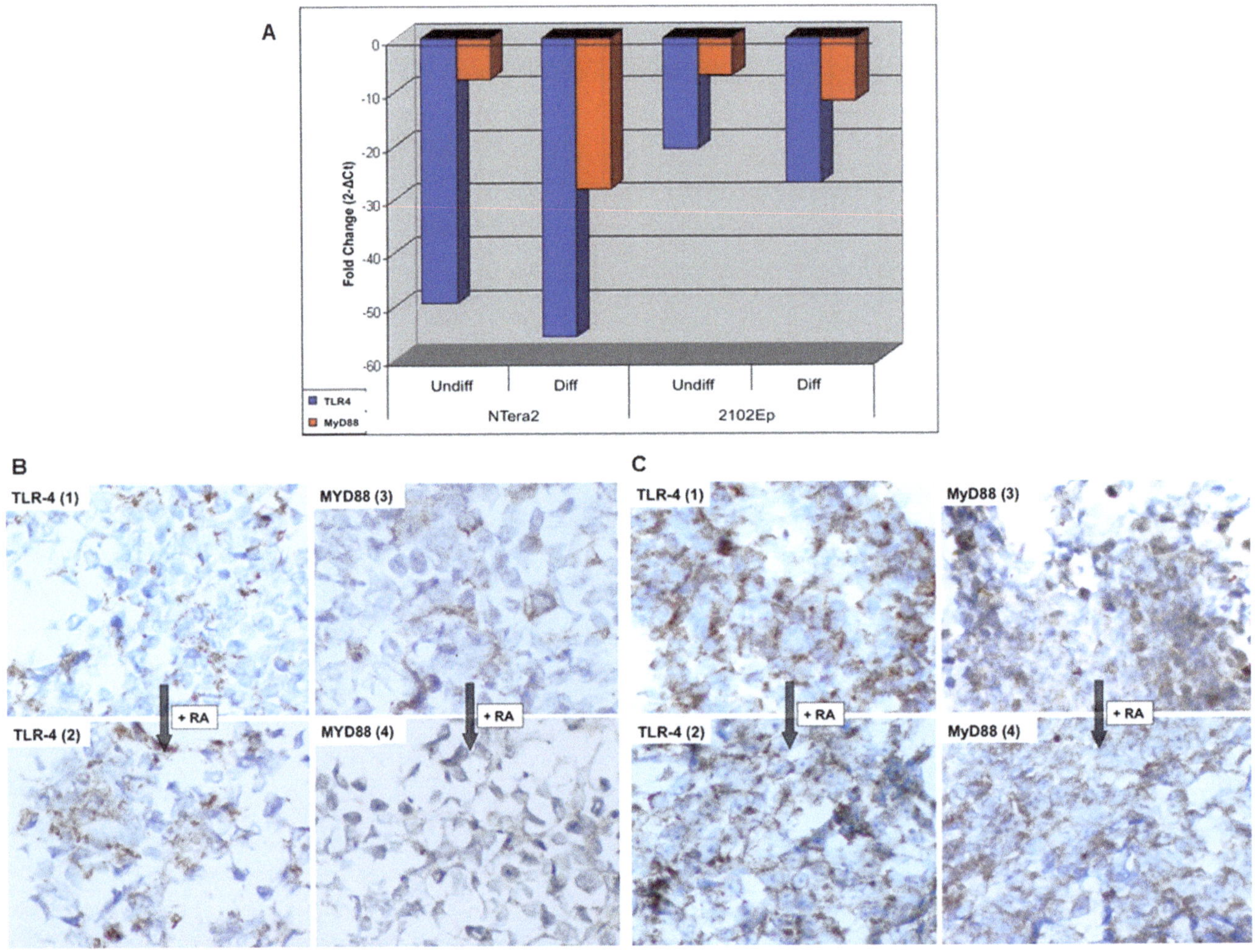

Figure 11. TLR4 and MyD88 expression in undifferentiated and retinoic acid (RA)-differentiated NTera2 and 2102Ep cells. A, qPCR data: MyD88 expression is down-regulated upon NTera2 differentiation, with minimal changes in TLR4; in contrast 2102Ep cells avoid differentiation and maintain both TLR4 & MyD88 expression (fold changes shown are proportional to internal control gene GAPDH and calculated via the $2^{-\Delta\Delta Ct}$ method). **B**, TLR4 and MyD88 protein expression in NTera2 cells: TLR4 staining was unchanged following differentiation (left panel); MyD88 staining in undifferentiated NTera2 cells showed significantly reduced staining after differentiation (right panel) (all 40x). **C**, TLR4 and MyD88 expression in 2102Ep cells: minimal changes in TLR4 (left panel) or MyD88 (right panel) were observed following RA-treatment (all at 40x).

[20,24,27,28] and 26–36 month reductions in overall survival [24,27]. The very large difference in survival that was observed in the test series relative to MyD88 expression is likely due to the small sample size in this cohort, as it is markedly discordant with all previous studies and the validation series examined here.

Furthermore the changes observed in MyD88 expression in embryonal carcinoma (EC) cancer stem cells, one of the best characterized CSC models in use today [30–32], also suggest that MyD88 positive cancer cells are more biologically aggressive than MyD88 negative cells. Undifferentiated stem cell-like populations from malignancies are often sufficient to efficiently regenerate tumours. NTera2 EC cells differentiate *in vivo* to form teratocarcinomas, three germ layer tumours that can arise in the ovary [33]. NTera2 cells are highly-tumourigenic in the undifferentiated state, a property that is greatly reduced or eliminated upon differentiation [32,33]. In contrast, 2102Ep EC cells can avoid differentiation *in vivo* to generate highly aggressive pure embryonal carcinomas [31]. We have shown that while TLR4 is constitutively expressed in EC cells, loss of MyD88 expression is associated with a 'differentiation switch': transition of NTera2 EC cells from their highly-tumourigenic (undifferentiated) to less-tumourigenic (differentiated) states. This change in expression upon differentiation is subtle but highly reproducible, and demonstrates that *ex vivo* manipulation of ovarian CSC differentiation can decrease MyD88 expression. We believe that it supports the hypothesis that EOC MyD88 positive cells may be stem-like due to their MyD88 expression pattern [12,21] and also demonstrates a practical and easily manipulated cancer stem model with relevance to ovarian cancer.

It has recently been reported that miR-21 regulates TLR4 by targeting the tumour suppressor protein PDCD4 [19], whereas miR-146a is NF-κB-dependent [34] and targets and reduces the expression of IRAK-1, IRAK-2 and TRAF-6, which are key MyD88 pathway components [18,35]. Ultimately miR-21 and miR-146a mutually participate in the regulation of TLR4/MyD88 expression, serving as negative regulators of MyD88-dependent TLR4 signalling. The novel analysis of miR-21 and miR-146a expression in this study, based on the categorization of EOC into

MyD88 positive and MyD88 negative, demonstrates that expression of both MyD88 and these microRNAs are linked to ovarian cancer. Subtle but significant alterations in MyD88 mRNA expression were observed between chemosensitive and chemoresistant ovarian and cervical cancer cells. These findings demonstrate that MyD88 expression is linked to miR-21 and miR-146a, and provides further support to previous observations that MyD88 is associated with adverse biological characteristics including resistance to standard platinum and taxane- based chemotherapies, with consequent reduced survival. Examining macro-dissected FFPE sections from responders and non-responders demonstrated significant increases in TLR4 and MyD88 mRNA in non-responders. Knockdown of TLR4 in SKOV-3 ovarian cells recovered chemosensitivity to paclitaxel. Knockdown of MyD88 alone did not. The results suggest that an intact/functioning TLR4/MyD88 pathway is required for the acquisition of the chemoresistant phenotype.

In summary, this data provides additional support to the hypothesis that MyD88 expression is an adverse prognostic factor in ovarian cancer, for which evidence has been mounting in recent studies. Similar to Zhu et al. [24], we have demonstrated a reproducible method of assessing MyD88 status by immunohistochemistry, lending weight to its use as a practical prognostic marker in EOC and which should assist future prospective studies. In addition, MyD88 staining has being optimised for cytological analysis of ascites which could have an important role to play in ovarian cancer treatment, in particular in the neoadjuvant setting. Specific associations with tumour subtype, stage, patient survival, microRNA regulation and cancer stem cell differentiation have been demonstrated.

Materials and Methods

Ethics Statement

Informed consent was obtained from patients. The study was approved the St. James's Hospital/Adelaide and Meath Hospital Dublin, incorporating the National Children's Hospital Research Ethics Committee.

Patient and sample selection

Samples of ovarian tissue from 198 patients who underwent surgery from 1993–2008, in the form of formalin-fixed paraffin-embedded (FFPE) tissue blocks, were accessioned from the archives of St. James's Hospital (SJH), Dublin, Ireland and the Adelaide and Meath Hospital incorporating the National Children's Hospital (AMNCH), Dublin. A test set of 20 malignant tumours (serous adenocarcinomas) was initially selected for TLR4 and MyD88 expression analysis. The subsequent validation series included 50 normal ovaries and 128 neoplasms. The latter include benign serous cystadenomas (n = 5); benign mucinous cystadenomas (n = 5); benign Brenner tumours (n = 5); borderline serous tumours (n = 15); borderline mucinous tumours (n = 13); serous adenocarcinomas (n = 69); mucinous adenocarcinomas (n = 6); clear cell adenocarcinomas (n = 5); endometrioid adenocarcinomas (n = 5). Clinicopathological information was obtained via a retrospective chart review and access to the local laboratory information systems.

Immunohistochemistry

TLR4 and MyD88 antibodies were purchased from Santa Cruz Biotechnology, Inc. (Santa Cruz, CA, USA) at initial concentrations of 200 µg/mL: rabbit polyclonal antibody (RpAb) to TLR4 (clone H-80); RpAb to MyD88 (clone HFL-296). 6 µm sections were cut from each FFPE block and the expression of TLR4 and MyD88 was assessed using the Ventana Benchmark LT DAB system (Ventana Medical Systems, AZ, USA). Standardised protocols were established for each antibody using a high-grade breast (ductal) carcinoma as a positive control, as per the manufacturer's recommendations. Antibody concentrations, initially at 200 µg/mL, were both at 1:30 dilution. Briefly, each protocol included 60-minute standard cell conditioning using CC1 antigen retrieval buffer (Ventana), followed by manual antibody titration and incubation for 32 minutes at 37°C.

Assessment of Immunohistochemical Staining

Initial immunohistochemistry staining for TLR4 (cytoplasmic and membranous) and MyD88 (cytoplasmic) was highly variable, with marked heterogeneity noted within the same sample. This was not geographical but showed distinct and repeated variation between adjacent tumour cells (Figure 12). In an effort to account for this heterogeneity, a novel visual semi-quantification method was employed. This method was developed in order to accurately quantify the expression of TLR4 and MyD88 even in cases with heterogeneous staining, and was derived from similar methods employed in other studies [24,36,37,38]. In addition whole paraffin sections were examined as focal protein expression could potentially be missed in tissue microarrays. Staining was based on immunointensity (II) and immunopositivity (IP). Immunointensity was scored as: 0, negative; 1, weak; 2, moderate; 3, strong (Figure 13). The percentage of immunopositive cells was scored as: 1 (1–10%); 2 (11–40%); 3 (41–70%); 4 (>70%). The product of II and IP produced values ranging from 0 to 12; a cut-off value of >4 determined IHC positivity. Stained slides were assigned random numbers and graded blind by two pathologists.

RNA and miRNA Extraction and Qualitative PCR (qPCR) from FFPE samples

A subset of malignant patient samples (n = 32) was selected for gene and miRNA expression analysis. Tumour cells were isolated from the surrounding stroma using laser capture microdissection (LCM). In brief, 7 µm sections were cut from each FFPE block and following haematoxylin and eosin (H&E) staining for visualisation, tumour epithelial cells were selected and extracted using LCM (Arcturus XT Microdissection Instrument, MDS Analytical Technologies, CA, USA) (Figure 14). cDNA was prepared with the High-Capacity cDNA Archive and TaqMan MicroRNA RT kits according to manufacturers' instructions (Applied Biosystems, CA, USA). For analysis of gene expression individual mRNAs were monitored with the following inventoried TaqMan assays (Applied Biosystems): human GAPDH assay (Hs99999905_m1), human TLR4 assay (Hs00152939_m1) and human MyD88 assay (Hs00182082_m1). For miRNA analysis, individual miRNA TaqMan assays for the endogenous reference RNA RNU6B, miR-21 and miR-146A were done according to the manufacturer's instructions (Applied Biosystems). Amplification and analysis were performed on the ABI Prism 7500 Fast Sequence Detection Systems (Applied Biosystems). All assays were done in triplicate. Changes in expression were calculated by the change in threshold (ΔΔCt) method [39] with GAPDH as the endogenous control for gene expression analysis and RNU6B as the endogenous control for miRNA analysis.

In addition, a cohort of 27 macro-dissected advanced serous cancers were interrogated for TLR4 and MyD88 mRNA expression as described above. All cases were optimally debulked and expression was measured relative to their chemotherapy response status. Chemoresponsive or 'Responders' were defined as patients who had a disease free interval since completion of combination chemotherapy for 12 months or longer. Chemore-

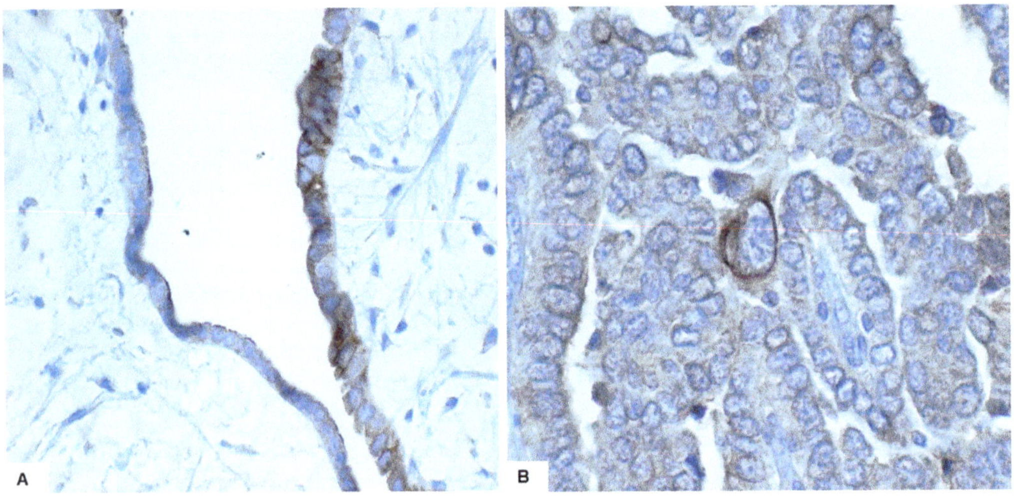

Figure 12. Heterogeneous expression of monoclonal anti-TLR4. A: variable staining observed in adjacent epithelium within a benign serous cystadenoma (20x). B: focal strong staining within a serous carcinoma (40x).

sistant patients, or 'Non-Responders' were defined as patients who experienced a relapse of disease within six months of completing their chemotherapy regimen.

RNA and miRNA Extraction and Qualitative PCR (qPCR) from cell lines

TLR4 and MyD88 gene expression was assessed in epithelial ovarian cancer cells A2780 and IGROV-1, and cervical cancer

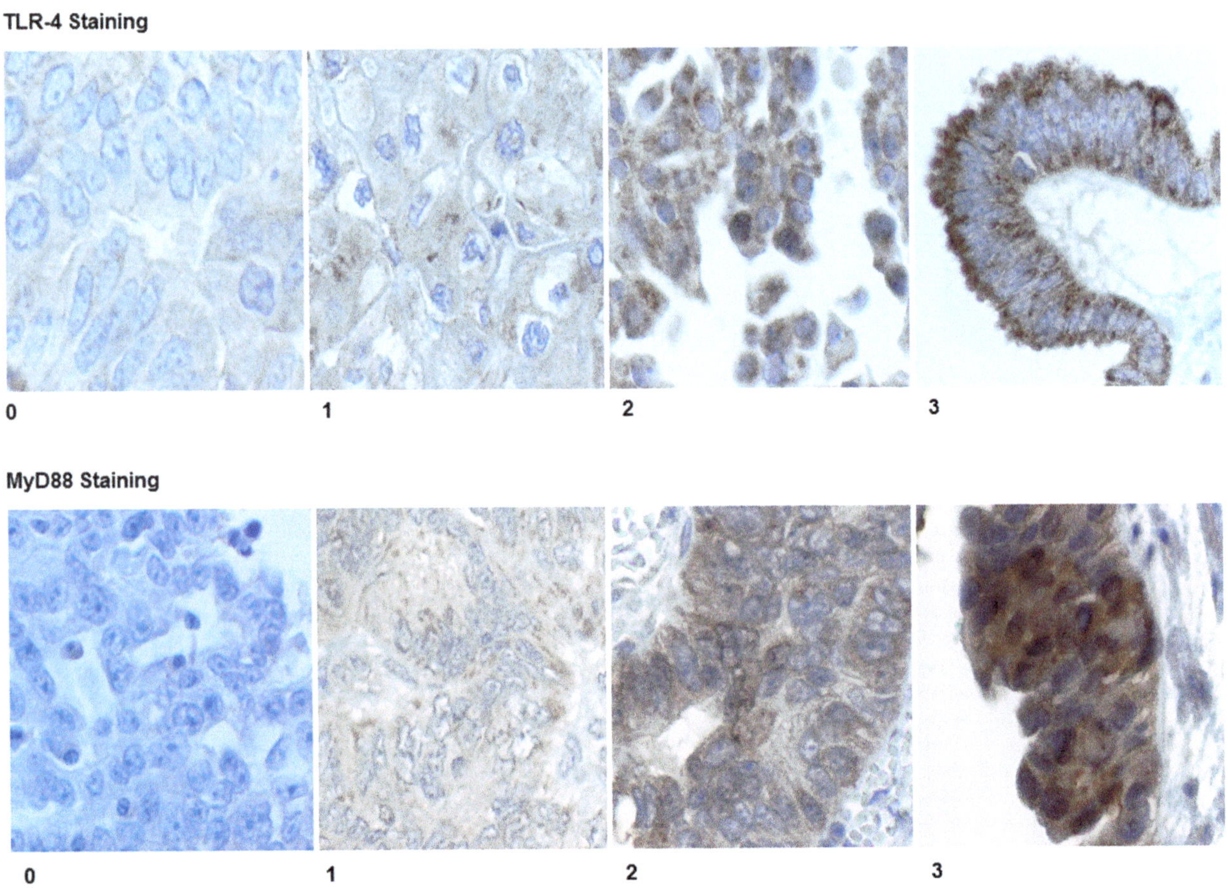

Figure 13. Quantification of immunohistochemical staining of TLR4 and MyD88 (0 = no staining, 1 = weak staining, 2 = moderate staining, 3 = strong staining).

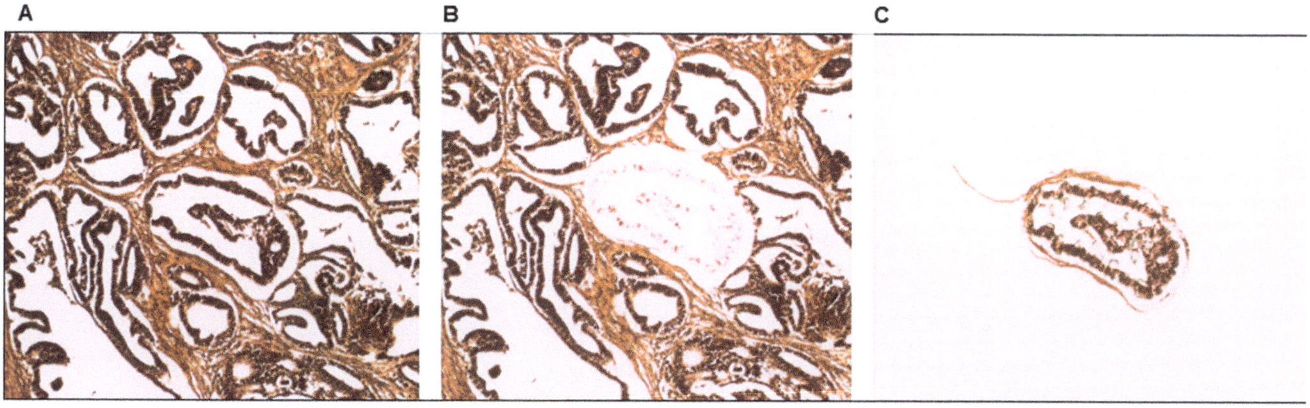

Figure 14. Photomicrographs illustrating the process of laser capture microdissection, including pre-dissection (A), post-dissection with a malignant gland removed from the surrounding stroma (B) and the isolated epithelial sample for genetic analysis (C).

cells KB-3-1, as well as their chemoresistant daughter cells A2780cis (cisplatin-resistant), IGROV-1CDDP [40,41] (cisplatin & paclitaxel-resistant) and KB-8-5-11 [42] (colchicine and paclitaxel-resistant). IGROV-1 and IGROVCDDP cells were grown in antibiotic and chemotherapy-free RPMI (Sigma #R8758) with 10% FCS (Lonza, Belgium). KB-3-1 and its colchicine-resistant variant KB-8-5-11 were grown in DMEM (Sigma #D5671), containing 1% penicillin-streptomycin, 2% L-glutamine and 1% sodium pyruvate with 10% FCS (Lonza). KB-8-5-11 cells were routinely grown with colchicine in the media, and drug was removed for 3 days prior to the start of all experiments. All cell lines were maintained in a humidified atmosphere with 5% CO_2 at 37°C. All cultures were tested routinely and were mycoplasma-free.

Cells (1.25×10^6 cells/10 cm dish) were plated and allowed to attach and grow for 3 days to reach 70–80% confluence. The cells were then trypsinised, washed in 10 mL PBS, centrifuged and the supernatant removed. The cell pellets were stored at −80°C prior to analysis. Total RNA was prepared using a RNeasy Mini Kit (Qiagen, UK) and the mirVANA miRNA Isolation Kit (Applied Biosystems) and expression was assessed as above.

siRNA transfection and validation

The ovarian cancer cell line SKOV-3 was maintained in complete McCoy's media at 37°C in a humidified 5% CO_2 atmosphere. Synthetic siRNAs against mRNA encoding MyD88 (siMyD88) and TLR4 (siTLR4), as well as negative control siRNA (siNeg) were obtained from Ambion. SKOV-3 (2.5×10^4) cells were reverse transfected in 24-well plates with a final concentration of 1 nM siRNA using Lipofectamine RNAiMAX (Invitrogen). The transfected cells were incubated for 72 hrs before either harvesting for mRNA or protein analysis. Total RNA was isolated using the mirVana kit (Ambion). MyD88, TLR4 and B2M mRNA expression levels were evaluated by TaqMan RT-PCR. The data was analysed using the comparative $\Delta\Delta C_T$ method; where MyD88 and TLR4 mRNA expression was normalised to that of B2M and calibrated to that of untreated cells to establish the relative level of mRNA expression. Protein was isolated by cells lysis with RIPA buffer. The lysate samples (30 µg) were then resolved by SDS PAGE electrophoresis and transferred to a PVDF membrane. The membrane was then interrogated with antibodies specific for MyD88 (Cell Signalling), TLR4 (AbCam) or GAPDH (AbCam). GAPDH was used as a loading control.

Drug treatment and cell viability assessment

72 hrs post transfection SKOV-3 cells were either left untreated, treated with DMSO (vehicle control) or 3.5 nM of paclitaxel (IC_{25}). 48 hrs post treatment, cell viability was assessed by means of the CCK-8 assay (Sigma-Aldrich). Cell viability rate was calculated as the percentage of the absorption at 405 nm for each transfection condition, as follows: cell viability (% control) = (mean experimental absorbance/mean vehicle control cell absorbance) ×100.

Embryonal Carcinoma Cell Culture

Pluripotent NTera2 and nullipotent 2102Ep embryonal carcinoma cells were maintained in the undifferentiated state in Dulbecco's Modified Eagle Media (DMEM) supplemented with 10% fetal calf serum (FCS), 5% L-Glutamine and 5% Penicillin-Streptomycin (Lonza, Basel, Switzerland), as per standard protocols. NTera2 cells were passaged via cell scrapping while 2102Ep cells were passaged via trypsinisation. Differentiation (NTera2) or differentiation-resistance mechanisms (2102Ep) were stimulated by the addition of 10 mM retinoic acid (RA) for 3 days. FFPE cell blocks were generated by rinsing and dispersing cell pellets in phosphate buffered saline (PBS) followed by fixation in 10% neutral buffered formalin (NBF) for 2 hours. Cells were then suspended in 1% agarose gel and processed and embedded according to routine laboratory procedures. RNA isolation, cDNA synthesis and TaqMan qPCR was carried out on embryonal carcinoma cell lines as previously described [29], using the TLR4, MyD88 and GAPDH assays listed above.

Statistical analysis

SPSS for Windows, Rel. 16.0 2001. Chicago: SPSS Inc was used for statistical analysis of survival data. Kaplan-Meier survival curves were used; cases where the event had not occurred were censored. Log-rank was used for univariate analysis. Statistical analyses for qPCR used the Student's *t*-test, unpaired for normal distributions of at least three independent experiments. The criterion of statistical significance applied for all analyses was $p < 0.05$. For gene silencing experiments data is expressed as means ± the standard deviation from at least three biological replicates. For all measurements as needed, a Student's t-test was used to assess the statistical significance of treated groups versus vehicle control groups. Student's t-test was performed using the GraphPad Prim version 5 software (GraphPad Software, CA, USA). A statistically significant difference was considered to be present at $p<0.05$.

Author Contributions

Conceived and designed the experiments: CD CS MG MB KC JBOC KH NK C. Murphy PS KOB SP AC B. Ffrench C. Martin DOD BH BS SF AMCC NG TD B. Flood LON OS SOT JOL. Performed the experiments: CD CS MG MB KC JBOC KH NK C. Murphy PS AC C. Martin BS B. Flood. Analyzed the data: CD SOT CS MG MB KC AC B. Flood C. Murphy DOD BH BS SF AMCC B. Ffrench LON OS SOT JOL. Contributed reagents/materials/analysis tools: CD CS MG MB KC JBOC AC B. Ffrench BS SF AMCC NG TD LON OS SOT JOL. Wrote the paper: CD SOT CS MG MB KC JBOC KH NK C.Murphy PS KOB SP AC B. Ffrench C. Martin DOD BH BS SF AMCC NG TD B. Flood LON OS JOL.

References

1. Schwartz PE (2002) Current diagnosis and treatment modalities for ovarian cancer. Cancer Treat Res 107: 99–118.
2. O'Lorcain P, Walsh PM, Comber H (2007) Cumulative cancer mortality risk and potential years of life lost to 64 years of age in Ireland, 1953–2002. Eur J Cancer Prev 16: 167–77.
3. O'Lorcain P, Comber H (2006) Morality predictions for Ireland, 2001–2015: cancers of the breast, ovary, and cervix and Corpus uteri. Int J Gynecol Cancer 16 Suppl 1: 1–10.
4. Lee KR, Tavassoli FA, Prat J, Dietel M, Gersell DJ, et al. (2003) Surface Epithelial-Stromal Tumours. In: Tavassoli FA and Devilee P, editors. World Health Organization Classification of Tumours. Pathology and Genetics of Tumours of the Breast and Female Genital Organs. Lyon: IARC Press. pp. 117–145.
5. Bell DA (2005) Origins and molecular pathology of ovarian cancer. Mod Pathol 18 Suppl 2: S19–32.
6. Marsden DE, Friedlander M, Hacker NF (2000) Current management of epithelial ovarian carcinoma: a review. Semin Surg Oncol 19: 11–9.
7. Armstrong D (2008) Ovaries and fallopian tubes. In: Abeloff MD, Armitage JO, Niederhuber JE, Kastan MB, McKenna WG, editors. Abeloff's Clinical Oncology. 4th ed. Philadelphia: Churcill Livingstone Elsevier. pp. 1827–1850.
8. Piver MS, Wong C (1998) Role of prophylactic surgery for women with genetic predisposition to cancer. Clin Obstet Gynecol 41: 215–24.
9. Stewart JJ, White JT, Yan X, Collins S, Drescher CW, et al. (2006) Proteins associated with Cisplatin resistance in ovarian cancer cells identified by quantitative proteomic technology and integrated with mRNA expression levels. Mol Cell Proteomics 5: 433–43.
10. Beachy PA, Karhadkar SS, Berman DM (2004) Mending and malignancy. Nature 431: 402.
11. Tsan MF (2006) Toll-like receptors, inflammation and cancer. Semin Cancer Biol 16(1): 32–7.
12. Alvero AB, Chen R, Fu HH, Montagna M, Schwartz PE, et al. (2009) Molecular phenotyping of human ovarian cancer stem cells unravels the mechanisms for repair and chemoresistance. Cell Cycle 8: 158–66.
13. O'Neill LA, Bryant CE, Doyle SL (2009) Therapeutic targeting of toll-like receptors for infectious and inflammatory diseases and cancer. Pharmacol Rev 61: 177–97.
14. Conroy H, Marshall NA, Mills KH (2008) TLR ligand suppression or enhancement of Treg cells? A double-edged sword in immunity to tumours. Oncogene 27: 168–80.
15. Zeromski J, Mozer-Lisewska I, Kaczmarek M (2008) Significance of Toll-like Receptors Expression in Tumor Growth and Spreading: A Short Review. Cancer Microenviron 1: 37–42.
16. Baldwin AS Jr (2001) Series introduction: the transcription factor NF-kappaB and human disease. J Clin Invest 107: 3–6.
17. Liew FY, Xu D, Brint EK, O'Neill LA (2005) Negative regulation of toll-like receptor-mediated immune responses. Nat Rev Immunol 5: 446–58.
18. Liston A, Linterman M, Lu MF (2010) MicroRNA in the adaptive immune system, in sickness and in health. J Clin Immunol 30: 339–46.
19. Sheedy FJ, Palsson-McDermott E, Hennessy EJ, Martin C, O'Leary JJ, et al. (2009) Negative regulation of TLR4 via targeting of the proinflammatory tumor suppressor PDCD4 by the microRNA miR-21. Nat Immunol 11: 141–7.
20. Kelly MG, Alvero AB, Chen R, Silasi DA, Abrahams VM, et al. (2006) TLR4 signaling promotes tumor growth and paclitaxel chemoresistance in ovarian cancer. Cancer Res 66: 3859–68.
21. Chen R, Alvero AB, Silasi DA, Steffensen KD, Mor G (2008) Cancers take their Toll—the function and regulation of Toll-like receptors in cancer cells. Oncogene 27: 225–33.
22. Alvero AB, Mor G (2006) MyD88-positive ovarian cancer cells regulate monocyte migration and differentiation. Am J Reprod Immunol 55: 399–400.
23. Szajnik M, Szczepanski MJ, Czystowska M, Elishaev E, Mandapathil M, et al. (2009) TLR4 signaling induced by lipopolysaccharide or paclitaxel regulates tumor survival and chemoresistance in ovarian cancer. Oncogene 28: 4353–63.
24. Zhu Y, Huang JM, Zhang GN, Zha X, Deng BF (2012) Prognostic significance of MyD88 expression by human epithelial ovarian carcinoma cells. J Transl Med 10: 77.
25. Kamsteeg M, Rutherford T, Sapi E, Hanczaruk B, Shahabi S, et al. (2003) Phenoxodiol—an isoflavone analog—induces apoptosis in chemoresistant ovarian cancer cells. Oncogene 22: 2611–20.
26. Pommier Y, Sordet O, Antony S, Hayward RL, Kohn KW (2004) Apoptosis defects and chemotherapy resistance: molecular interaction maps and networks. Oncogene 23: 2934–49.
27. Silasi DA, Alvero AB, Illuzzi J, Kelly M, Chen R, et al. (2006) MyD88 predicts chemoresistance to paclitaxel in epithelial ovarian cancer. Yale J Biol Med 79: 153–63.
28. Szajnik M, Szczepanski M, Czystowska M, Elishaev E, Mandapathil M, et al. (2009) Expression and signaling of Toll-like receptor 4 (TLR4) and MyD88 in ovarian carcinoma cells. J Clin Oncol 27(15S): e16508.
29. Gallagher MF, Flavin RJ, Elbaruni SA, McInerney JK, Smyth PC, et al. (2009) Regulation of microRNA biosynthesis and expression in 2102Ep embryonal carcinoma stem cells is mirrored in ovarian serous adenocarcinoma patients. J Ovarian Res 2: 19.
30. Andrews PW, Damjanov I, Simon D, Banting GS, Carlin C, et al. (1984) Pluripotent embryonal carcinoma clones derived from the human teratocarcinoma cell line Tera-2. Differentiation in vivo and in vitro. Lab Invest 50: 147–62.
31. Andrews PW, Fenderson B, Hakomori S (1987) Human embryonal carcinoma cells and their differentiation in culture. Int J Androl 10: 95–104.
32. Andrews PW (2002) From teratocarcinomas to embryonic stem cells. Philos Trans R Soc Lond B Biol Sci 357: 405–17.
33. Andrews PW, Matin MM, Bahrami AR, Damjanov I, Gokhale P, et al. (2005) Embryonic stem (ES) cells and embryonal carcinoma (EC) cells: opposite sides of the same coin. Biochem Soc Trans 33: 1526–30.
34. Taganov KD, Boldin MP, Baltimore D (2006) NF-kappaB-dependent induction of microRNA miR-146, an inhibitor targeted to signaling proteins of innate immune responses. Proc Natl Acad Sci U S A 103: 12481–6.
35. Bartel DP (2004) MicroRNAs: genomics, biogenesis, mechanism, and function. Cell 116: 281–97.
36. Nisolle M, Gillerot S, Casanas-Roux F, Squifflet J, Berliere M, et al. (1999) Immunohistochemical study of the proliferation index, oestrogen receptors and progesterone receptors A and B in leiomyomata and normal myometrium during the menstrual cycle and under gonadotrophin-releasing hormone agonist therapy. Hum Reprod 14: 2844–50.
37. Geisler S, Lønning PE, Aas T, Johnsen H, Fluge O, et al. (2001) Influence of TP53 gene alterations and c-erbB-2 expression on the response to treatment with doxorubicin in locally advanced breast cancer. Cancer Res 61: 2505–12.
38. Mohsin SK, Weiss H, Havighurst T, Clark GM, Berardo M, et al. (2004) Progesterone receptor by immunohistochemistry and clinical outcome in breast cancer: a validation study. Mod Pathol 17: 1545–54.
39. Livak KJ, Schmittgen TD (2001) Analysis of relative gene expression data using real-time quantitative PCR and the 2(-Delta Delta C(T)) Method. Methods 25: 402–8.
40. Ma J, Maliepaard M, Kolker HJ, Verweij J, Schellens JH (1998) Abrogated energy-dependent uptake of cisplatin in a cisplatin-resistant subline of the human ovarian cancer cell line IGROV-1. Cancer Chemotherapy & Pharmacology 41: 186–192.
41. Stordal B, Hamon M, McEneaney V, Roche S, Gillet JP, et al. (2012) Resistance to paclitaxel in a cisplatin-resistant ovarian cancer cell line is mediated by P-glycoprotein. PLoS One 7:e40717.
42. Shen DW, Fojo A, Chin JE, Roninson IB, Richert N, et al. (1986) Human multidrug-resistant cell lines: increased mdr1 expression can precede gene amplification. Science 232: 643–5.

MicroRNA-7 Inhibits Tumor Metastasis and Reverses Epithelial-Mesenchymal Transition through AKT/ERK1/2 Inactivation by Targeting EGFR in Epithelial Ovarian Cancer

Xingchen Zhou[1,2]⁹, Yuan Hu[1,2]⁹, Lan Dai[1,2], Yunfei Wang[1,2], Jinhua Zhou[1,2], WenWen Wang[1,2], Wen Di[1,2], Lihua Qiu[1,2]*

1 Department of Gynecology and Obstetrics, Renji Hospital, School of Medicine, Shanghai Jiao Tong University, Shanghai, China, **2** Shanghai Key Laboratory of Gynecologic Oncology, Shanghai, China

Abstract

Epidermal growth factor receptor (EGFR) overexpression and activation result in increased proliferation and migration of solid tumors including ovarian cancer. In recent years, mounting evidence indicates that EGFR is a direct and functional target of miR-7. In this study, we found that miR-7 expression was significantly downregulated in highly metastatic epithelial ovarian cancer (EOC) cell lines and metastatic tissues, whereas the expression of, EGFR correlated positively with metastasis in both EOC patients and cell lines. Overexpression of miR-7 markedly suppressed the capacities of cell invasion and migration and resulted in morphological changes from a mesenchymal phenotype to an epithelial-like phenotype in EOC. In addition, overexpression of miR-7 upregulated CK-18 and β-catenin expression and downregulated Vimentin expression, accompanied with EGFR inhibition and AKT/ERK1/2 inactivation. Similar to miR-7 transfection, silencing of EGFR with this siRNA in EOC cells also upregulated CK-18 and β-catenin expression and downregulated Vimentin expression, and decreased phosphorylation of both Akt and ERK1/2, confirming that EGFR is a target of miR-7 in reversing EMT. The pharmacological inhibition of PI3K-AKT and ERK1/2 both significantly enhanced CK-18 and β-catenin expression and suppressed vimentin expression, indicating that AKT and ERK1/2 pathways are required for miR-7 mediating EMT. Finally, the expression of miR-7 and EGFR in primary EOC with matched metastasis tissues was explored. It was showed that miR-7 is inversely correlated with EGFR. Taken together, our results suggested that miR-7 inhibited tumor metastasis and reversed EMT through AKT and ERK1/2 pathway inactivation by reducing EGFR expression in EOC cell lines. Thus, miR-7 might be a potential prognostic marker and therapeutic target for ovarian cancer metastasis intervention.

Editor: Jung Weon Lee, Seoul National University, Korea, Republic Of

Funding: This work was supported by grants from National Natural Science Foundation of China (Grant No. 81072138), Medical-engineering cross project of Shanghai Jiao Tong University (YG2010MS24). The funders had no role in study design, data collection and analysis, decision to publish, or preparation of the manuscript.

Competing Interests: The authors have declared that no competing interests exist.

* E-mail: lilyqiulh@126.com

⁹ These authors contributed equally to this work.

Introduction

Ovarian cancer is the major cause of deaths from gynecologic malignancies and the 5th leading cause of cancer-related deaths among women in the world [1]. According to the national cancer institute (NCI) report, about 22280 new cases will be diagnosed with ovarian cancer in America in 2012, and 15500 patients will die of this disease, and the 5-year survival rate for them is about 30%. It has been speculated that metastasis remains the leading cause of relapse and death from ovarian cancer, and yet the molecular mechanisms associated with acquisition of metastatic ability in human ovarian cancer are poorly understood.

MicroRNAs (miRNAs) are a class of small non-coding RNA of approximately 20–22 nucleotides long that function as post-transcriptional regulators by targeting 3′ untranslated regions (UTR) of mRNAs and causing either inhibition of translation or degradation of mRNA [2]. MiRNAs contribute to diverse cellular processes including proliferation, apoptosis, invasion and morphogenesis [3,4,5]. Moreover, a range of miRNAs have been identified that function as classical oncogenes or tumor suppressor genes [6,7,8]. MiR-7 has been characterized as a tumor suppressor in several human cancers. It targets a number of proto-oncogenes, including insulin-like growth factor-1 receptor (IGF1R) [9] epidermal growth factor receptor (EGFR) [10], p21-activated kinase 1 (Pak1) and associated cdc42 kinase 1 (Ack1) [11]. It's demonstrated that overexpression of miR-7 inhibited schwannoma cell growth both in culture and in xenograft tumor models in vivo, which correlated with downregulation of EGFR, Pak1 and Ack1 [11].

Approximately 70% of epithelial ovarian cancer (EOC) express activated EGFR [12]. EGFR overexpression and activation result in increased proliferation and migration of solid tumors including ovarian cancer [13]. Activation of EGFR tyrosine kinase results in activation of a number of intracellular signals, which culminate in not only cell proliferation but also other processes that are crucial to cancer progression, including cell migration, angiogenesis, metastasis, and epithelial-mesenchymal transition (EMT). These events are mediated through various downstream targets of EGFR (e.g. protein kinase (AKT) and extracellular signal-regulated kinase 1/2 (ERK1/2)) [14,15,16]. Interestingly, it's shown that miR-7 directly targets EGFR mRNA 3′- UTR, and then inhibits expression of its mRNA and protein [17]. Although EGFR signaling is important and well studied with respect to EOC progression, little is known about how miR-7 mediate EGFR signaling to modulate EOC cell metastasis.

In the present study, we identify for the first time that miR-7 plays an important role in EOC metastasis. Furthermore, we show that miR-7 reverses EMT through AKT/ERK1/2 inactivation by targeting EGFR in EOC, which provides a novel insight into the mechanisms underlying metastasis of ovarian cancer.

Materials and Methods

Patients and Ethics

Paired samples of primary epithelial ovarian cancer tissues and metastatic tissues (omentum or peritoneum) were obtained from patients with FIGO stage III-IV advanced EOC who had undergone tumor debulking at Renji Hospital, School of Medicine, Shanghai Jiao Tong University between 2010 and 2012. Among them, 17 paired samples were snap-frozen in liquid nitrogen and stored at −80°C for later RNA extraction, 25 paired samples were Formalin fixed and paraffin embedded. Samples were clinically and pathologically shown to be correctly labeled. The study was approved by the institutional review board of Renji Hospital, School of Medicine, Shanghai Jiao Tong University and written informed consent was obtained from all patients. All clinical investigation was conducted according to the principles expressed in the Declaration of Helsinki.

Materials

MiR-7 plasmid and negative control (NC) were synthesized by Shanghai IBS Company. The sequence of plasmid and NC are as follows: 5′-UGGAAGACUAGUGAUUUUGUUGU-3′; Negative Control: 5′-GAAATCTACTGCGCGTGGAGAC-3′ (IBS company). TaqMan kit (Applied Biosystems) specified for quantification of miRNA was used to assess the expression of miR-7 and U6. EGF receptor Rabbit mAb (# 4267), Phospho-EGF Receptor (Tyr992) Rabbit mAb (#2235), Phospho-p44/42 MAPK (Thr202/Tyr204) Rabbit mAb (#4370), Phospho-Akt (Ser473/Thr308), Rabbit mAb (#4060/#2965), Akt (pan) Rabbit mAb (#4691), LY294002 (PI3K Kinase Inhibitor) (#9901), U0126 (MEK1/2 Inhibitor) (#9903), Vimentin Rabbit mAb (# 5741), and β-catenin rabbit mAb and E-cadherin Rabbit mAb (# 3195) were purchased from Cell Signaling Technology (CST). cytokeratin-18 (CK-18) mAb (T410) pAb (BS1204) was purchased from Bioworld Technology. P44/42 MAPK Rabbit mAb was obtained from Santa Cruz ((sc-33746)). GAPDH mouse mAb was purchased from ABmart (#M20006). 800CW conjugated goat anti-Rabbit IgG((926-32210), highly cross adsorbed and 800CW conjugated goat anti-mouse IgG(926-32211), highly cross adsorbed were purchased from Li-Cor Biosciences. EGFR and control short interfering RNAs (siRNA) were from Sanong Biotech.Has-miR-7-LNA detection probe were purchased from Exiqon (38485-15).

Cell culture

HO-8910pm, HO-8910 cell lines were obtained from the Cell Bank of the Chinese Academy of Sciences (Shanghai, China), CAOV-3, SKOV3, A2780, A2780/DDP, and ES-2 cells were obtained from the ATCC (Manassas, VA). Cells were cultured in Roswell Park Memorial Institute 1640 medium (RPMI-1640) medium (Hyclone) supplemented with 10% fetal bovine serum (Hyclone) and Penicillin/Streptomycin (1:100, Sigma) in a humid atmosphere incubator with 5% CO2 at 37°C. Unless otherwise indicated, cells were grown to 70–80% confluence, then serum-starved overnight in serum-free RPMI-1640 medium prior to treatment.

miRNA and siRNA Transfection

80–90% confluent cells were transfected with human miR-7 plasmid (miR-7) or negative control (NC) and 30–40% confluent cells were transfected with EGFR siRNA or siRNA-NC by Lipofectamine 2000 (Invitrogen) according to the manufacturer's protocol. Total RNA was extracted 24 hours after transfection, and total cell protein were extracted 48 or 72 hours after transfection.

Reverse transcription quantitative real-time PCR

Total RNA was isolated by TRIzol Reagent (Invitrogen). Mature miR-7 was reverse-transcribed with specific RT primers, quantified with a TaqMan probe, and normalized by U6 small nuclear RNA using TaqMan miRNA assays (Applied Biosystems). mRNA expression analysis was conducted by quantitative PCR using SYBR green dye, with relative changes calculated by the ΔΔCt method. Primers used were as follows: GAPDH-F, 5-TGCACCACCAACTGCTTAGC-3; GAPDH-R, 5-GGCATGGACTGTGGTCATGAG-3; EGFR-F, 5-AGCCATGCCCGCATTAGCTC-3; EGFR-R, 5-AAAGGAATGCAACTTCCCAA-3.

Western blotting

Whole cell extracts were prepared as described previously [18] and equal amounts of protein were separated by a 8% or 10% SDS-PAGE and elctrotransferred to a PVDF membrane (Millipore). The membranes were then blocked for 1 hour at room temperature with Li-Cor blocking agent (Li-Cor). With constant shaking, the membranes were incubated with primary antibodies overnight at 4°C followed by incubation for 1 hour with the appropriate secondary antibodies labeled with 800IRdye. Immunoreactivity was detected and quantified with the infrared Odyssey imaging System (Li-Cor).

Migration assays

Cells (8×10^4) were harvested and re-suspended in serum-free RPMI-1640 medium and put into the upper wells of the Boyden chamber (Corning). The medium containing 10% fetal bovine serum was added into the lower chamber. After 8h of incubation, cells remaining on the upper surface of the membranes were removed, cells that had invaded through the 8 μm pore size membrane were fixed, stained, and counted under a microscope at 200 × magnification. The results were averaged among three independent experiments.

Invasion assays

Cells (3×10^4) were placed into the upper chambers coated with 50 μl of Matrigel (1:5 dilution in serum-free medium). Medium supplemented with 10% serum was added to the outer cup. After 24 h of incubation, cells remaining on the upper surface of the

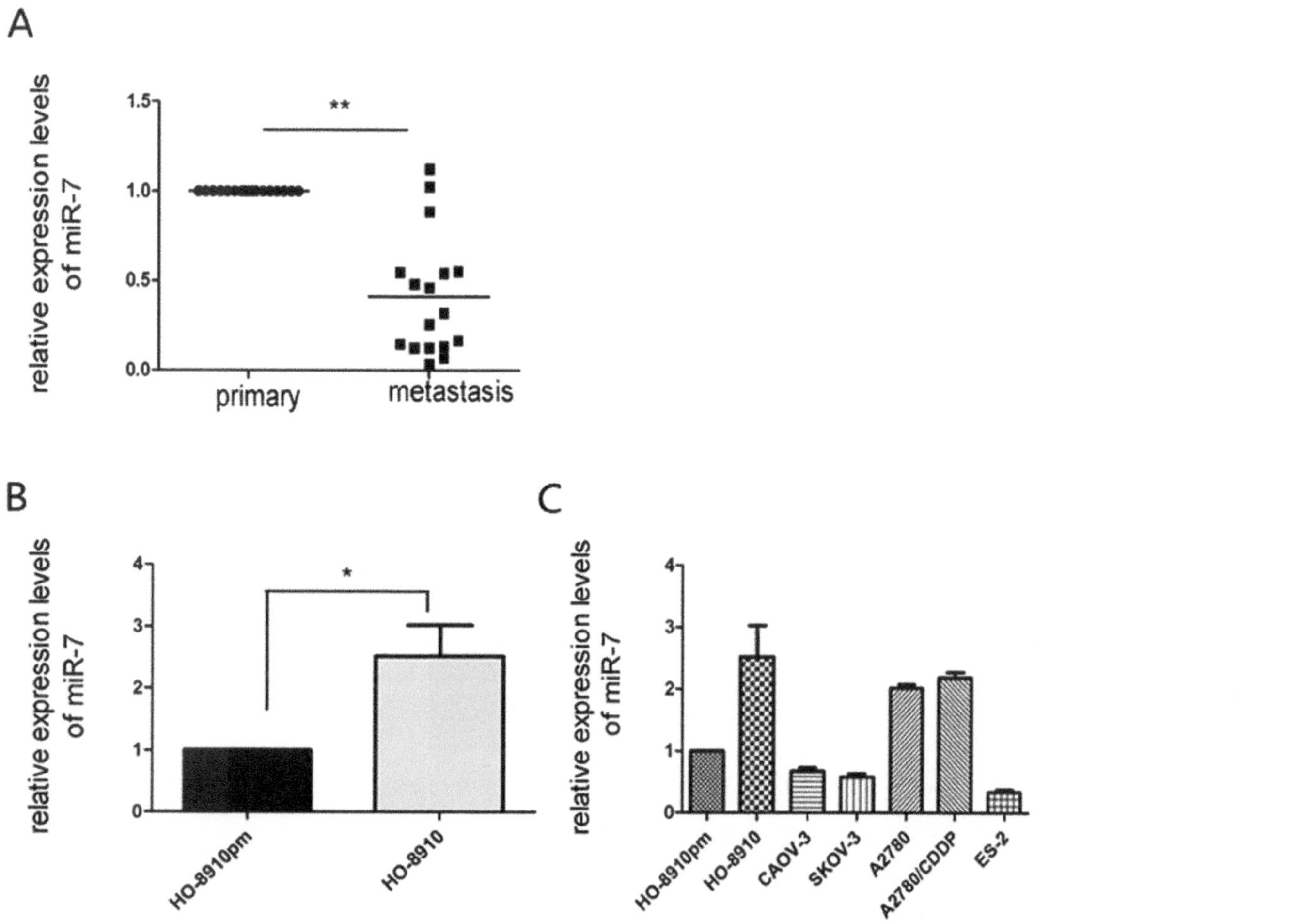

Figure 1. miR-7 expression is inversely correlated with EOC metastasis. (A) The relative expression of miR-7 in 17-paired EOC tissues from omentum or peritoneum metastases and primary EOC tissues was detected by qRT-PCR. The U6 small nuclear RNA was used as an internal control and the fold change was calculated by the ΔΔCt method (B) The expression level of miR-7 in one pair of low and high metastatic EOC cell lines. (C) The expression level of miR-7 in seven EOC cell lines. (*P<0.05. **P<0.01).

membranes were removed, cells that had invaded through the Matrigel and the 8 μm pore size membrane were fixed, stained, and counted under a microscope at 200 × magnification. The results were averaged among three independent experiments.

Immunohistochemistry (IHC) and Chromogenic in situ hybridization(CISH)

Immunohistochemistry (IHC) was performed using the horseradish peroxidase (HRP)-polymer anti-mouse IHC DAB (diaminobenzidine)-based kit (MaxVision, Fuzhou, China), according to the manufacturer protocol. Antigen retrieval was performed using borate buffer (pH = 8), followed by incubation in hydrogen peroxide and additional blocking steps. Antibodies were used at 1:50. The IHC was examined and imaged using an OLYMPUS BX51 microscope (Tokyo, Japan) at 1:200. Positve signals were identified by the intense brown labeling of their cell membranes.

Chromogenic in situ hybridization (CISH) was performed using the Has-miR-7 probe from Exiqon (mercury LNA detection probe 5′ and 3′-DIG (digoxigenin)-labeled). The probe was detected using digoxigenin antibody (Abcam), LSAB2 System-HRP (Dako Denmark A/S, Glostrup, Denmark) and liquid DAB+ Substrate Chromogen System (Dako) according to manufacturer's instruction. The CISH was examined and imaged using an OLYMPUS BX51 microscope (Tokyo, Japan) at 1:200. Positive hybridization signals were identified by the intense brown labeling of their cell cytoplasms.

The results of IHC and CISH were independently scored by two pathologists in a blind manner. The scoring was based on the intensity and extent of staining and was evaluated according to the following histological scoring method. Staining intensity was graded as follows: 0, negative staining; 1, weak staining; 2, moderate staining; 3, strong staining. The mean proportion of staining cells per specimen was determined semi-quantitatively and scored as follows: 0 for staining <1%, 1 for 1–25%, 2 for 26–50%, 3 for 51–75%, and 4 for >75% of the examined cells. The histological score (H-score) for each specimen was computed by the formula: H-score = proportion score×intensity score. A total score of 0–12 was calculated and graded as negative (−, score:0), weak (+, score:1–4), moderate (++, score:5–8) or strong (+++ ,score:9–12).

Statistical analysis

Statistical analysis was performed with the SPSS 12.0 statistical analysis software package. In each in-vitro experiment, a

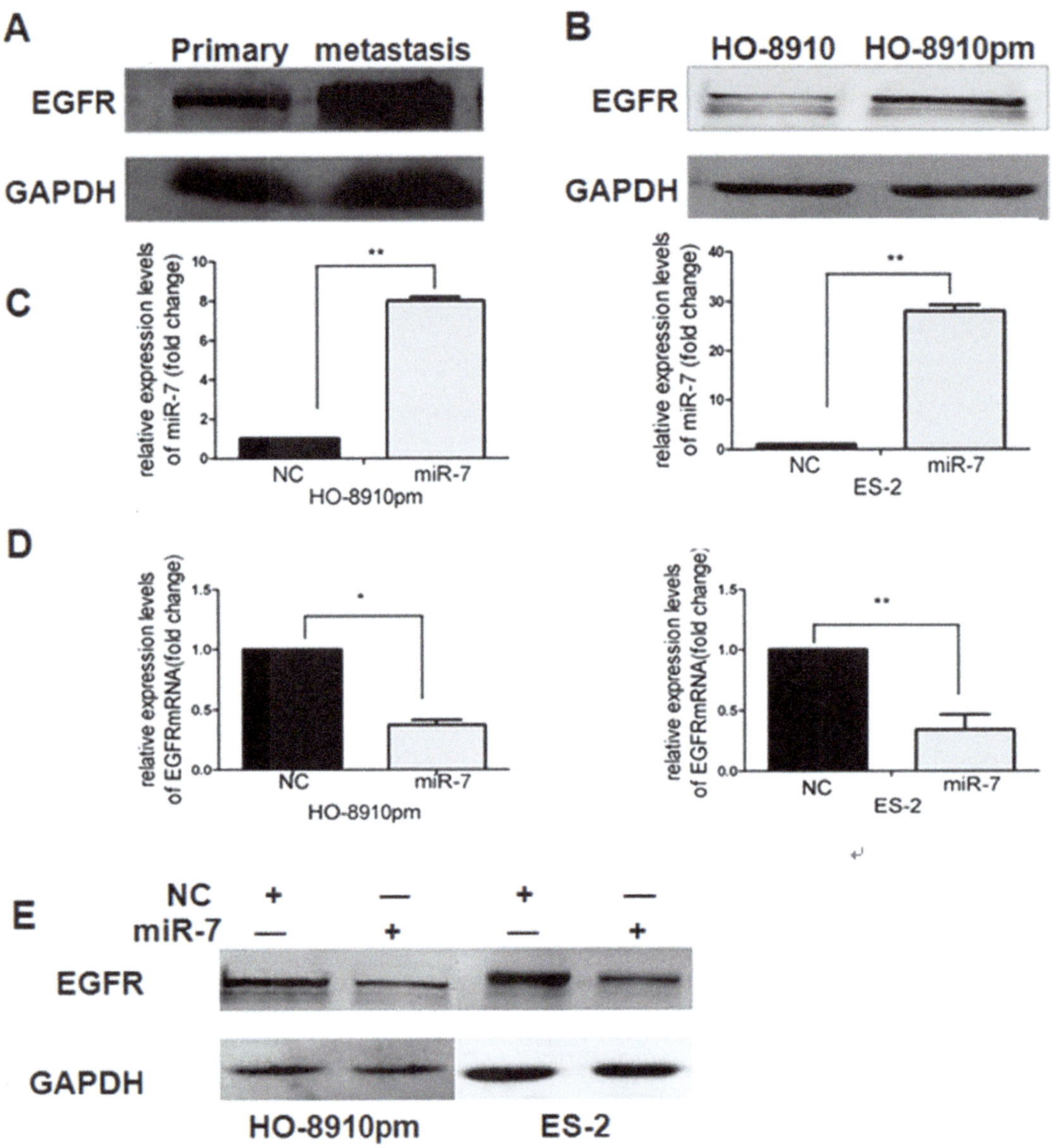

Figure 2. miR-7 downregulates EGFR in EOC cells. (A) The protein expression of EGFR in 17-paired EOC tissues from omentum or peritoneum metastases and primary EOC tissues was examined by western blot. (B) The protein expression of EGFR in HO-8910 and HO-8910pm cell lines was examined by western blotting. (C) The expression level of miR-7 in HO-8910pm and ES-2 cells transfected with miR-7 or NC was analyzed by qRT-PCR. (D) The expression level of EGFR mRNA in HO-8910pm and ES-2 cells transfected with miR-7 or NC was analyzed by qRT-PCR. (E) The expression of EGFR protein was analyzed by western blotting in HO-8910pm and ES-2 cells transfected with miR-7 or NC, Glyceraldehyde 3-phosphate dehydrogenase (GAPDH) was used as an internal control. (*$P<0.05$. **$P<0.01$).

minimum of three wells/dishes was used and similar results were obtained. Each experiment was repeated a minimum of three times, the mean value of the repetitions was calculated and this value was used in the statistical analysis. Experimental data are expressed as means with standard deviation (SD). The differences between groups were evaluated using Student's t test when comparing only two groups or analyzed by one-way ANOVA with post hoc test when more than two groups were compared. The correlation between EGFR and miR-7 was analyzed using Spearman's rank test. The results of IHC and CISH were analyzed using Wilcoxon test. Differences were considered statistically significant at $P<0.05$, *$P<0.05$ and **$P<0.01$.

Results

miR-7 expression is inversely correlated with EOC metastasis

To explore the expression and significance of miR-7 in EOC metastasis, we detected miR-7 expression in 17-paired metastatic EOC tissues and primary EOC tissues. Quantitative real-time PCR (qRT-PCR) showed that tissues from omentum or peritoneum metastases expressed lower levels of miR-7 compared with primary EOC tissues, indicating an inverse relationship between the expression of miR-7 and the metastatic status of EOC tissues (Figure 1A). Furthermore, we selected HO-8910 and its highly metastatic clone HO-8910pm. HO-8910pm was established and

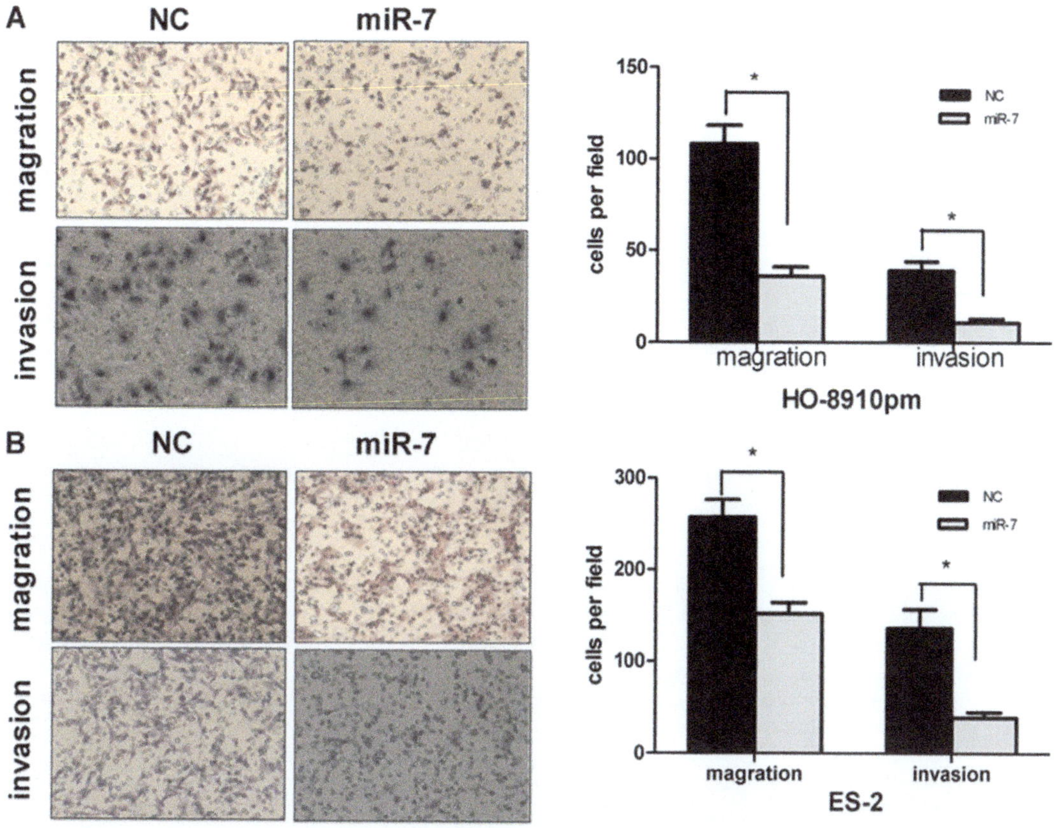

Figure 3. miR-7 suppresses EOC cell invasion and migration in vitro. (A) Transwell migration and invasion assays using HO-8910pm cells transfected with miR-7 or negative control (NC). Representative images are shown on the left, and the quantification of 6 randomly selected fields is shown on the right. (B) Transwell migration and invasion assays using ES-2 cells transfected with miR-7 or NC. Representative images are shown on the left, and the quantification of 6 randomly selected fields is shown on the right. The values shown are expressed as the means ± SD. (*P< 0.05.**P<0.01).

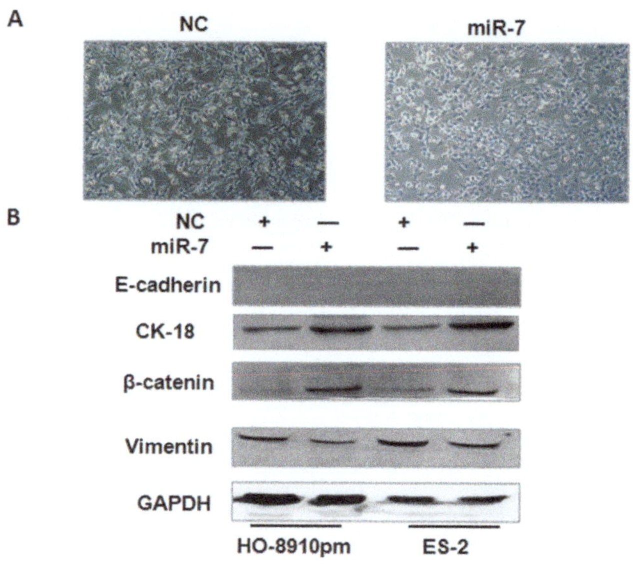

Figure 4. Overexpression of miR-7 reverses EMT in EOC cell. (A) Phase-contrast images of ES-2 cells infected with the miR-7 or NC. (B) The protein expression of E-cadherin, CK-18, β-catenin and Vimentin in HO-8910pm and ES-2 cells transfected with miR-7 or NC were examined by western blotting, GAPDH was used as an internal control. (*P<0.05. **P<0.01).

characterized in Cell Bank, Chinese Academy of Sciences [19,20,21]. We found that miR-7 expression was significantly decreased in highly metastatic clone HO-8910pm compared with HO-8910 (Figure 1B). Taken together, our results suggest that down-regulation of miR-7 is correlated with increased EOC metastasis and that miR-7 might suppress EOC progression. To determine the optimal cell lines for further study, we measured the expression of miR-7 in seven EOC cell lines (HO-8910pm, HO-8910, A2780, A2780/DDP, SKOV-3, CAOV-3 and ES-2). Our data showed that the expression of miR-7 was lowest in ES-2 cell line (P<0.05) (Figure 1C), which is another EOC cell with highly metastatic potential. Therefore, we choose HO-8910PM and ES-2 to study the mechanisms of miR-7 inhibiting metastasis in EOC in the following experiments.

miR-7 downregulates EGFR in EOC cells

To detect the underlying mechanism by which miR-7 inhibit EOC invasion and metastasis, we searched for miR-7 targets using such as TargetScan and Pictar. That identified 181 candidate target genes including EGFR. It's demonstrated that miR-7 downregulates EGFR expression by directly targeting EGFR mRNA 3′-UTR [17]. We were particularly interested in EGFR because of its positive roles in cancer cell migration and invasion and its overexpression in EOC. We further investigated the expression and significance of EGFR in EOC metastasis by detecting EGFR protein expression in 17-paired metastatic EOC

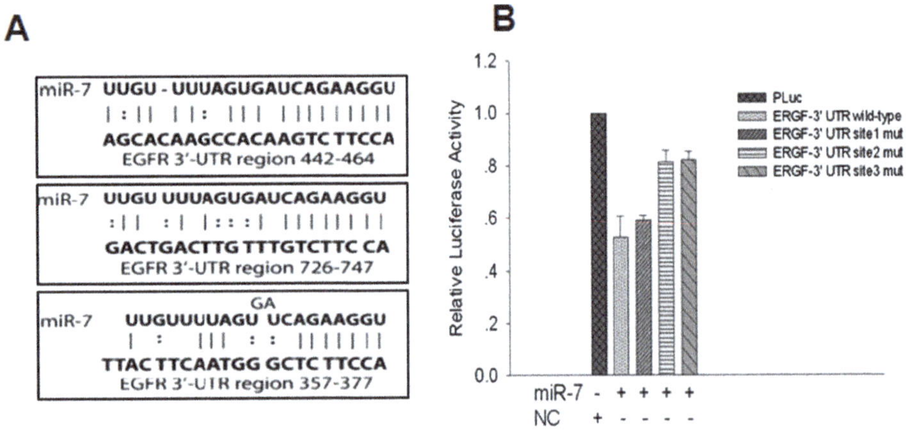

Figure 5. miR-7 downregulate EGFR by interaction with 3′UTR. (A) Diagram of EGFR 3′UTR reporter construct. (B) The wild type or mutant reporter plasmids were cotransfected with miR-7 or NC in ES-2. (*P<0.05. **P<0.01).

tissues and primary EOC tissues. Western blotting analysis showed that tissues from omentum or peritoneum metastases expressed higher levels of EGFR compared with primary EOC tissues, indicating a positive correlation between the expression of EGFR and the metastatic status of EOC tissues (Figure 2A, Figure S1A). Meanwhile, we also detected EGFR protein expression by western blotting in both HO-8910 and HO-8910pm cells. We found that EGFR expression was significantly increased in highly metastatic clone HO-8910pm compared with HO-8910 (Figure 2B, Figure S1B). Taken together, our results suggest that EGFR expression is positively correlated with EOC metastasis and that EGFR might promote EOC progression.

To make sure the roles of miR-7 in regulation of EGFR expression in EOC cells, both HO-8910pm and ES-2 cells were transfected with miR-7 plasmid or miR-NC. qRT-PCR showed that miR-7 expression was significantly increased (Figure 2C) whereas EGFR mRNA expression was significantly decreased (Figure 2D) after miR-7 transfection in both cell lines. Furthermore, Western blotting analysis indicated that EGFR protein expression was significantly decreased after miR-7 transfection in both HO-8910pm and ES-2 cells (Figure 2E, Figure S1C). Our results suggest that miR-7 downregulates EGFR in EOC.

miR-7 suppresses EOC cell invasion and migration in vitro

To investigate whether miR-7 regulates cell invasion and migration in EOC, both HO-8910pm and ES-2 cells were transfected with miR-7 plasmid or miR-NC. Transwell migration and invasion assays were then performed. We found that transfection with miR-7 significantly suppressed the invasion of both HO-8910pm cells (Figure 3A) and ES-2 cells (Figure 3B).

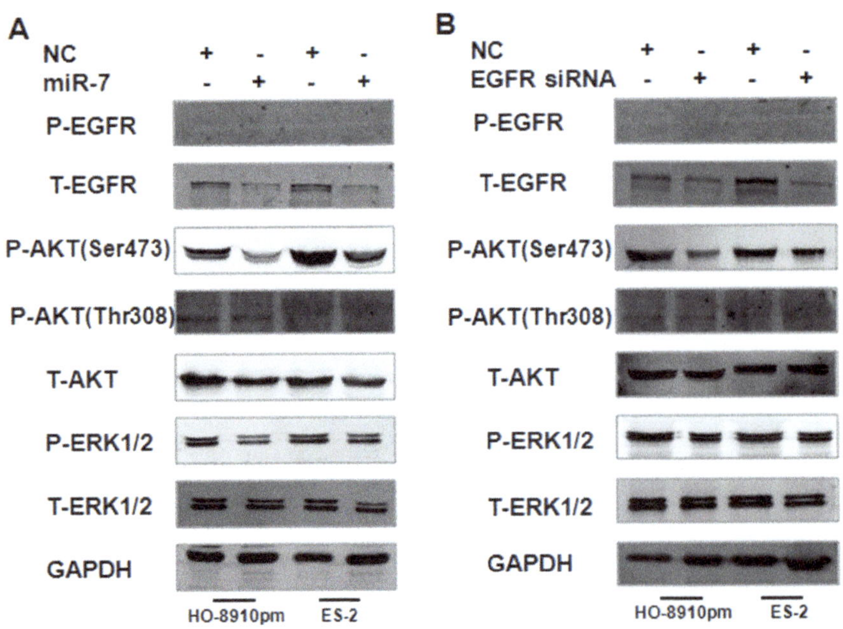

Figure 6. miR-7 suppresses AKT and ERK1/2 pathway activation dependent of its EGFR inhibition in EOC cells. (A) HO-8910pm and ES-2 cells were transfected with miR-7 or NC, EGFR, AKT and ERK1/2 phosphorylation were analyzed by western blotting. (B) HO-8910pm and ES-2 cells were transfected with EGFR siRNA or NC, EGFR, AKT and ERK1/2 phosphorylation were analyzed by western blotting. (*P<0.05. **P<0.01).

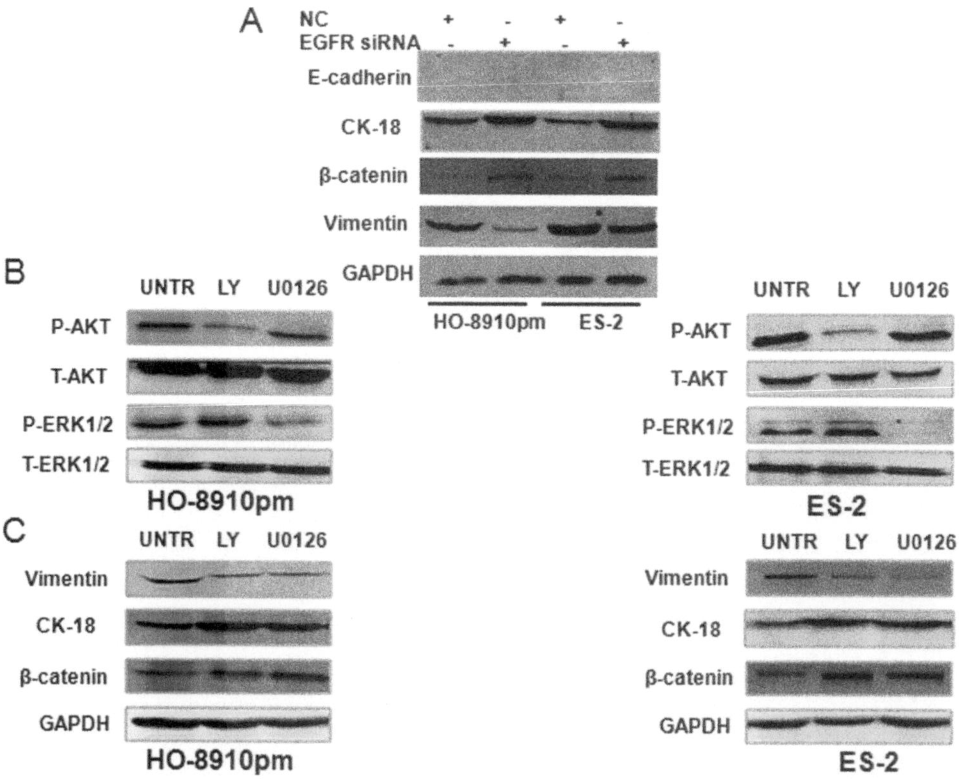

Figure 7. miR-7 reverses EMT through EGFR/AKT and EGFR/ERK1/2 pathway. (A) HO-8910pm and ES-2 cells were transfected with EGFR siRNA or NC, the protein expression of E-cadherin, CK-18, β-catenin and vimentin were explored by western blotting. (B) HO-8910pm and ES-2 cells were treated with LY294002 (20 umol/l) or U0126 (10 umol/l), AKT and ERK1/2 phosphorylation were analyzed by western blotting. (C) HO-8910pm and ES-2 cells were treated with LY294002 (20 umol/l) or U0126 (10 umol/l), the protein expression of CK-18, β-catenin and vimentin were explored by western blotting. GAPDH was used as an internal control (*P<0.05. **P<0.01).

Similarly, migration capacity was also significantly down-regulated in both HO-8910pm-miR-7 cells and ES-2-miR-7 cells versus HO-8910pm-NC cells and ES-2-NC cells (Figure 3A, Figure 3B). These results indicate that miR-7 participates in the regulation of cell migration and invasion in EOC.

Overexpression of miR-7 reverses EMT in EOC cell

In EOC cells, we observed that miR-7 transfection resulted in morphological changes from an elongated, spindle-shaped, mesenchymal phenotype to a more rounded, epithelial-like phenotype, with cells aggregating in groups (Figure 4A). These changes represent the reverse processes of EMT, which is an important reason for epithelial cancer to gain the ability of invasion and metastasis. Furthermore, we examined the protein expression of the epithelial markers E-cadherin, CK-18 and β-catenin, as well as the mesenchymal marker vimentin by Western blotting. Although there were no E-cadherin expression in both cell lines even after miR-7 transfection, CK-18 and β-catenin expression dramatically increased, whereas vimentin expression decreased in both HO-8910pm and ES-2 cells after miR-7 transfection (Figure 4B, Figure S2). Our data suggest that overexpression of miR-7 reverses EMT in EOC cell lines.

Luciferase reporter assays

To understand the molecular mechanism by which miR-7 suppress EOC invasion and metastasis, we used different computational methods to search for miR-7 targets, such as Targetsan and pictar. These methods found 181 possible candidate genes. We were particularly interested in EGFR because of its positive roles in cancer cell invasion. Analysis of the 3′-UTR

Table 1. miR-7 expression in EOC tissues and matched metastases.

	miR-7 expression level				
	(-)	(+)	(++)	(+++)	P-values
EOC	2/25	6/25	12/25	5/25	-
Metastasis	14/25	6/25	0/25	0/25	<0.05

H-score = proportion score×intensity score. A total score of 0–12 was calculated and graded as negative (−, score:0), weak (+, score:1–4), moderate (++, score:5–8) or strong (+++, score:9–12).

Table 2. EGFR expression in EOC tissues and matched metastases.

	EGFR expression level				
	(−)	(+)	(++)	(+++)	P-values
EOC	4/25	15/25	5/25	1/25	-
metastasis	2/25	9/25	10/25	4/25	<0.05

H-score = proportion score × intensity score. A total score of 0–12 was calculated and graded as negative (−, score:0), weak (+, score:1–4), moderate (++, score:5–8) or strong (+++, score:9–12).

sequence of EGFR indentified three possible binding sites for miR-7. To determine whether EGFR is direct target of miR-7, we constructed its 3′-UTR fragments, in which wild-type and mutant binding sites were inserted into the region immediatedly downstream of the reporter gene (Figure 5A), luciferase reporter assays showed that miR-7 transfection caused a remarkable decrease in luciferase activity which contained wild-type 3′-UTR fragments binding sites (Figure 5B).

miR-7 suppresses AKT and ERK1/2 pathway activation dependent of its EGFR inhibition in EOC cells

Previous studies showed that EGFR regulates AKT and ERK1/2 activity in ovarian cancer [15,22]. Because miR-7 can post-transcriptionally inhibit the expression of EGFR, we hypothesized that miR-7 regulates AKT and ERK1/2 pathway activation. To investigate the effect of miR-7 on AKT and ERK1/2, we transfected HO-8910pm and ES-2 cells with miR-7 plasmid or miR-NC, and then examined phosphorylation of AKT and ERK1/2 by western blotting. Transfection with miR-7 suppressed phosphorylation of AKT at Ser473 and ERK1/2 at Thr202/Tyr204, however, miR-7 did not significantly alter AKT phosphorylation at Thr308 (Figure 6A). Since the activation of EGFR is playing major role in the metastasis of many cancers, we also detected its phosphorylation status after miR-7 transfection in HO-8910pm and ES-2 cells. However, in our studies, there was no EGFR phosphorylation pre and post miR-7 transfection, whereas miR-7 transfection did inhibit total EGFR protein expression (Figure 6A, Figure S3 (A-C)). As evidence that miR-7 has many target genes, we sought to determine whether miR-7 mediated AKT and ERK1/2 pathway activation is dependent of its EGFR inhibition. HO-8910pm and ES-2 cells were transfected with EGFR siRNA or the negative control. We showed that silencing of EGFR with this siRNA in ovarian cancer cells decreased phosphorylation of AKT at Ser473 and ERK1/2 at Thr202/Tyr204 on Western Blotting, but there was no significant change in phosphorylation of AKT at Thr308 (Figure 6B, Figure S3 (D-E)).

miR-7 reverses EMT through EGFR/AKT and EGFR/ERK1/2 pathway

To determine whether the EGFR/ AKT and EGFR/ERK1/2 signaling pathways were involved in the reversal of EMT by miR-7, we transfected EGFR siRNA into HO-8910pm and ES-2 cells and then explore the protein expression of E-cadherin, CK-18, β-catenin and vimentin by western blotting. We found that there was no E-cadherin expression pre and post EGFR siRNA transfection in both cell lines, however, CK-18 and β-catenin expression dramatically increased, whereas vimentin expression decreased in both HO-8910pm and ES-2 cells after EGFR siRNA transfection (Figure 7A, Figure S4 (A-C)). Then we used the PI3K/AKT inhibitor LY294002 and the ERK1/2 inhibitor U0126 to specifically block the Akt and the ERK1/2 pathways, respectively. As expected, the PI3K/AKT inhibitor LY294002 inhibited AKT phosphorylation, while ERK1/2 inhibitor U 0126 inhibited ERK1/2 phosphorylation in HO-8910pm and ES-2 cells (Figure 7B, FigureS4 (D-G)). Further, both the AKT and ERK1/2 inhibitors enhanced CK-18 and β-catenin expression and suppressed vimentin expression in HO-8910pm and ES-2 cells (Figure 7C and Figure S4 (H-M)). Our data demonstrated the involvement of the EGFR/ AKT and EGFR/ERK1/2 pathways in the miR-7 reversed EMT in ovarian cancer cells.

miR-7 and EGFR are inversely expressed in EOC primary and metastasis tissues

We used CISH and IHC to detect the expression of miR-7 and EGFR in the same type of tissue. We determined whether miR-7 expression was associated with EGFR expression in EOC tissuses. The tissue contained 25 pairs of primary EOC tissues and their matched metastatic tissues. The CISH analysis showed an overt reduction of miR-7 in the metastatic tissues compared with their corresponding primary EOC tissues (Figure 8A, Table 1). By contrast, IHC results revealed that EGFR expression was higher in metastatic tissues than in primary EOC tissues (Figure 8B, Table 2). Furthermore, statistical analysis showed that EGFR expression was inversely correlated with miR-7 expression (Table 3).

Discussion

miRNAs have emerged as critical regulators of carcinogenesis and malignant progression of cancer by targeting oncogenes and tumor suppressor genes [23,24]. It has been implicated that miR-7 inhibits tumor invasion and metastasis in glioblastoma, schwannoma, lung cancer, breast cancer and many other cancers [25,26,27]. In the present study, we investigated the biological role of miR-7 in human EOC metastasis. We found that miR-7 was down-regulated in metastatic epithelial ovarian cancer (EOC) tissues compared with primary EOC tissues. miR-7 expression was also significantly decreased in highly metastatic clone HO-8910pm compared with HO-8910. Furthermore, we showed that the expression of miR-7 was lowest in ES-2 cell line, which is another EOC cell with highly metastatic potential among seven EOC cell lines (HO-8910pm, HO-8910, A2780, A2780/DDP, SKOV-3, CAOV-3 and ES-2). Therefore, our findings indicated that miR-7 expression is inversely correlated with EOC metastasis.

Interestingly, each miRNA can potentially regulate hundreds of genes at post-transcriptional levels by binding to the specific sequences in the target mRNA molecules based on 'imperfect complementarity'. It has been shown that overexpression of miR-7 inhibited tumor invasion and metastasis by targeting insulin-like growth factor-1 receptor (IGF-1R) in gastric cancer [9]. miR-7 has

Table 3. Correlation between the expression of EGFR protein and miR-7 in 25 pairs of EOC and their matched metastases.

EGFR	miR-7				n	P-values	Spearman's	
	(−)	(+)	(++)	(+++)			P	R
(−)	1	5	0	0	50	<0.05	<0.01	−0.3199
(+)	8	1	11	4	–	–	–	–
(++)	7	4	1	1	–	–	–	–
(+++)	5	2	0	0	–	–	–	–

H-score = proportion score×intensity score. A total score of 0–12 was calculated and graded as negative (−, score:0), weak (+, score:1–4), moderate (++, score:5–8) or strong (+++, score:9–12).

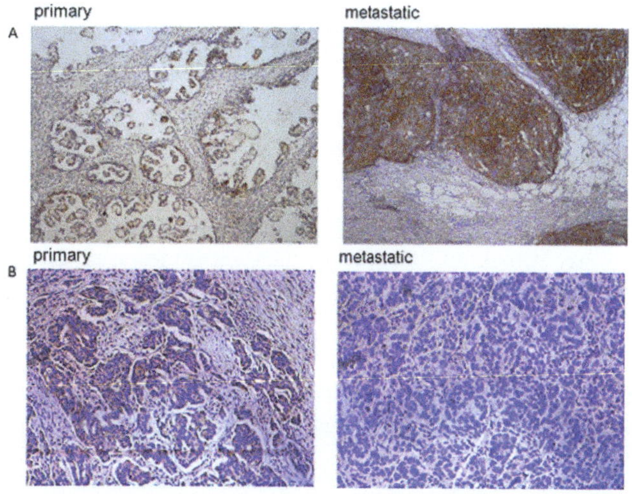

Figure 8. miR-7 and EGFR are inersely expressed in EOC tissues. (A) Expression of miR-7 in primary EOC and its matched metastatic tissue by CISH. (B) Expression of EGFR in primary EOC and its matched metastatic tissue by IHC. (*P<0.05. **P<0.01).

also been reported to target FAK in breast cancer cells [28]. In recent years, mounting evidence indicates that EGFR is a direct and functional target of miR-7 [10,17]. Receptor tyrosine kinase of the EGFR family regulates essential cellular functions, including proliferation, survival, migration, and differentiation. Published data demonstrates that EGFR plays an important role in tumor progression [12,27]. In this study, we found that tissues from omentum or peritoneum metastases expressed higher levels of EGFR compared with primary EOC tissues. Meanwhile, we found that EGFR was upregulated in highly metastatic clone HO-8910pm compared with HO-8910. These results suggest that EGFR is closely related to ovarian cancer metastasis. Our previous studies also showed that EGFR overexpression and activation result in increased metastasis of human ovarian cancer cells [18,29]. However, no study is performed to determine whether miR-7 targets EGFR to modulate the behavior of EOC metastasis. Here, we showed that both EGFR mRNA and EGFR protein expression was significantly decreased after miR-7 transfection in EOC cell lines. We subsequently identified that both invasion and migration capacity were significantly down-regulated after miR-7 transfection in EOC in vitro. Our present experimental results confirmed for the first time that miR-7 suppressed EOC cell invasion and migration. Taken together, our results indicate that miR-7 suppresses cell invasion and migration at least in part, through direct targeting of EGFR in EOC.

EMT refers to a biological process that the epithelial cells transform into mesenchymal cells through the specific program, which plays an important role in embryonic development, chronic inflammation, organize rebuilding, cancer metastasis and a variety of fibrosis disease [30,31,32]. Epithelial cells undergoing EMT towards a more mesenchymal phenotype involves decreased expression of epithelial markers (E-cadherin, β-catenin, CK-18) and increased expression of mesenchymal markers (N-cadherin, vimentin) [31,33,34]. They become more invasive by expressing proteases that allow them to pass through the underlying basement membrane and migrate, both being critical steps in the multi-step process of metastasis. It has been reported that some miRNAs such as miR-200, miR-429 and miR-141 can promote or suppress cancer metastasis and invasion by regulating EMT [35,36]. Recent study showed that miR-155 is upregulated during TGFβ-induced EMT [37,38]. In the present study, we observed that overexpression of miR-7 induced morphological changes from an elongated, spindle-shaped, mesenchymal phenotype to a more rounded, epithelial-like phenotype, with cells aggregating in groups in EOC cells. Although there were no E-cadherin expression in both HO-8910pm and ES-2 cell lines even after miR-7 transfection, epithelial markers CK-18 and β-catenin expression were dramatically increased but mesenchymal marker vimentin expression was decreased after miR-7 transfection. Our data suggest that miR-7 plays important roles in reversing EMT and inhibiting EOC metastasis.

Our work with EGFR pathway in ovarian cancer [18,29,39] led us to investigate whether the EGFR and its downstream signaling pathways were involved in the reversal of EMT by miR-7. The EGFR exerts its function in the cellular environment mainly, if not exclusively, via its tyrosine. Existing data indicated that the effects of EGFR signaling on cell migration and invasion are mediated by PI3K/AKT and ERK1/2 signaling pathways in EOC [15,40,41,42]. It has been shown that antagonism of miR-21 reversed EMT, accompanied with PTEN up-regulation and AKT/ERK1/2 inactivation. The inhibitors of PI3K-AKT and ERK1/2 pathways, LY294002 and U0126 significantly suppressed EMT, indicating that AKT and ERK1/2 pathways are required for miR-21 mediating EMT in breast cancer [27]. In the present study, we have demonstrated that miR-7 suppressed both AKT and ERK1/2 phosphorylation in EOC cells. Meanwhile, overexpression of miR-7 resulted in the reduced expression of total EGFR protein without any change in the phosphorylation state of EGFR. Therefore, we sought to further show the effects of miR-7 on both Akt and ERK1/2 activation were via EGFR inhibition. To address this, we determined the effects on both Akt and ERK1/2 phosphorylation of transfecting the same ovarian cancer cell lines with an EGFR siRNA. Similar to miR-7 transfection, silencing of EGFR with this siRNA blocked phosphorylation of both Akt and ERK1/2, which support the contention that miR-7 decreased both Akt and ERK1/2 activation dependent of its effects on EGFR inhibition. Our results indicate that miR-7 exerted its effects in human ovarian cancer cells via the inactivation of the EGFR/AKT and EGFR/ERK1/2 signaling pathway. The activation of PI3K/AKT signaling has been found to stimulate Snail and Slug expression via GSK-3b/β-catenin signaling and to subsequently promote EMT in different cellular contexts [43,44]. Recent study showed that Gab2 overexpression, via activation of the PI3K-ZEB1 pathway, promotes characteristics of EMT in ovarian cancer cells [45]. More recently it has been demonstrated that EGF induces serous borderline ovarian tumors cell migration and invasion by activating EMT, which involves the activation of the ERK1/2 and PI3K/Akt pathways and, subsequently, Snail, Slug and ZEB1 expression [22]. Here, we observed that silencing of EGFR increased CK-18 and β-cadherin expression and decreased vimentin expression, which confirmed that EGFR is a target of miR-7 in reversing EMT. Furthermore, inhibition of both AKT and ERK1/2 signaling results in upregulation of CK-18 and β-catenin expression and downregulation of vimentin expression in EOC cells. Taken together, our data first demonstrated the involvement of the EGFR/ AKT and EGFR/ERK1/2 pathways in the miR-7 reversed EMT in ovarian cancer cells.

In summary, our results demonstrated that miR-7 expression was inversely correlated with EOC metastasis. Further, miR-7 reversed EMT through AKT and ERK1/2 pathway inactivation by reducing EGFR expression in HO-8910pm and ES-2 cell lines. Thus, miR-7 might be a potential prognostic marker and therapeutic target for ovarian cancer metastasis intervention.

Supporting Information

Figure S1 The quantitative analysis of Western blot images in fig.2. (A) The protein expression of EGFR in 17-paired EOC tissues from omentum or peritoneum metastases and primary EOC tissues was examined by western blot. (B) The protein expression of EGFR in HO-8910 and HO-8910pm cell lines was examined by western blotting. (C) The expression of EGFR protein was analyzed by western blotting in HO-8910pm and ES-2 cells transfected with miR-7 or NC.

Figure S2 The quantitative analysis of Western blot images in fig.4. (A) The protein expression of CK-18 in HO-8910pm and ES-2 cells transfected with miR-7 or NC. (B) The protein expression of β-catenin in HO-8910pm and ES-2 cells transfected with miR-7 or NC. (C) The protein expression of Vimentin in HO-8910pm and ES-2 cells transfected with miR-7 or NC.

Figure S3 The quantitative analysis of Western blot images in fig.6. HO-8910pm and ES-2 cells were transfected with EGFRsiRNA or miR-7. (A/D) T-EGFR were analyzed by western blotting. (B/E) P-AKT were analyzed by western blotting. (C/F) P- ERK1/2 were analyzed by western blotting. (*P<0.05. **P<0.01).

Figure S4 The quantitative analysis of Western blot images in fig.7. HO-8910pm and ES-2 cells were transfected with EGFR siRNA or NC, the protein expression of CK-18(A), β-catenin (B) and vimentin (C) were explored by western blotting. HO-8910pm and ES-2 cells were treated with LY294002 (20 umol/l) or U0126 (10 umol/l), AKT (D/F) and ERK1/2 (E/G) phosphorylation were analyzed by western blotting. HO-8910pm and ES-2 cells were treated with LY294002 (20 umol/l) or U0126 (10 umol/l), the protein expression of vimentin (H/K), CK-18 (I/L) and β-catenin (J/M) were explored by western blotting. GAPDH was used as an internal control(*P<0.05. **P< 0.01).

Author Contributions

Conceived and designed the experiments: LQ WD. Performed the experiments: XZ YH WW. Analyzed the data: YH JZ. Contributed reagents/materials/analysis tools: YW LD. Wrote the paper: XZ.

References

1. Jemal A, Bray F, Center MM, Ferlay J, Ward E, et al. (2011) Global cancer statistics. CA: A Cancer Journal for Clinicians 61: 69–90.
2. Garzon R, Calin GA, Croce CM (2009) MicroRNAs in Cancer. Annual Review of Medicine 60: 167–179.
3. Shi L, Cheng Z, Zhang J, Li R, Zhao P, et al. (2008) hsa-mir-181a and hsa-mir-181b function as tumor suppressors in human glioma cells. Brain Research 1236: 185–193.
4. Liu WG, Chao T, Peng X, Yuan J, Ma Z, et al. (2009) Identification of differentially expressed microRNAs by microarray: a possible role for microRNAs gene in medulloblastomas. Chinese Medical Journal.
5. Wu Z-s, Wu Q, Wang C-q, Wang X-n, Wang Y, et al. (2010) MiR-339-5p inhibits breast cancer cell migration and invasion in vitro and may be a potential biomarker for breast cancer prognosis. BMC Cancer 10: 542.

6. Sampson VB, Rong NH, Han J, Yang Q, Aris V, et al. (2007) MicroRNA let-7a down-regulates MYC and reverts MYC-induced growth in Burkitt lymphoma cells. Cancer Res 67: 9762–9770.
7. Liang S, He L, Zhao X, Miao Y, Gu Y, et al. (2011) MicroRNA let-7f inhibits tumor invasion and metastasis by targeting MYH9 in human gastric cancer. PLoS One 6: e18409.
8. Yang K, Handorean AM, Iczkowski KA (2009) MicroRNAs 373 and 520c are downregulated in prostate cancer, suppress CD44 translation and enhance invasion of prostate cancer cells in vitro. Int J Clin Exp Pathol 2: 361–369.
9. Zhao X, Dou W, He L, Liang S, Tie J, et al. (2012) MicroRNA-7 functions as an anti-metastatic microRNA in gastric cancer by targeting insulin-like growth factor-1 receptor. Oncogene.
10. Kefas B, Godlewski J, Comeau L, Li Y, Abounader R, et al. (2008) microRNA-7 inhibits the epidermal growth factor receptor and the Akt pathway and is down-regulated in glioblastoma. Cancer Res 68: 3566–3572.
11. Saydam O, Senol O, Wurdinger T, Mizrak A, Ozdener GB, et al. (2011) miRNA-7 attenuation in Schwannoma tumors stimulates growth by upregulating three oncogenic signaling pathways. Cancer Res 71: 852–861.
12. Nicholson RI, Gee JM, Harper ME (2001) EGFR and cancer prognosis. Eur J Cancer 37 Suppl 4: S9–15.
13. Maihle NJ, Baron AT, Barrette BA, Boardman CH, Christensen TA, et al. (2002) EGF/ErbB receptor family in ovarian cancer. Cancer Treat Res 107: 247–258.
14. Chang ZG, Wei JM, Qin CF, Hao K, Tian XD, et al. (2012) Suppression of the epidermal growth factor receptor inhibits epithelial-mesenchymal transition in human pancreatic cancer PANC-1 cells. Dig Dis Sci 57: 1181–1189.
15. Loganathan S, Kandala PK, Gupta P, Srivastava SK (2012) Inhibition of EGFR-AKT Axis Results in the Suppression of Ovarian Tumors In Vitro and in Preclinical Mouse Model. PLoS One 7: e43577.
16. Gan Y, Shi C, Inge L, Hibner M, Balducci J, et al. (2010) Differential roles of ERK and Akt pathways in regulation of EGFR-mediated signaling and motility in prostate cancer cells. Oncogene 29: 4947–4958.
17. Webster RJ, Giles KM, Price KJ, Zhang PM, Mattick JS, et al. (2009) Regulation of epidermal growth factor receptor signaling in human cancer cells by microRNA-7. J Biol Chem 284: 5731–5741.
18. Qiu L, Zhou C, Sun Y, Di W, Scheffler E, et al. (2006) Crosstalk between EGFR and TrkB enhances ovarian cancer cell migration and proliferation. Int J Oncol 29: 1003–1011.
19. Zou W, Yang H, Hou X, Zhang W, Chen B, et al. (2007) Inhibition of CD147 gene expression via RNA interference reduces tumor cell invasion, tumorigenicity and increases chemosensitivity to paclitaxel in HO-8910pm cells. Cancer Lett 248: 211–218.
20. Zhang S, Lin QD, Di W (2006) Suppression of human ovarian carcinoma metastasis by the metastasis-suppressor gene, BRMS1. Int J Gynecol Cancer 16: 522–531.
21. Shenhua X, Lijuan Q, Hanzhou N, Xinghao N, Chihong Z, et al. (1999) Establishment of a highly metastatic human ovarian cancer cell line (HO-8910PM) and its characterization. J Exp Clin Cancer Res 18: 233–239.
22. Cheng JC, Auersperg N, Leung PC (2012) EGF-induced EMT and invasiveness in serous borderline ovarian tumor cells: a possible step in the transition to low-grade serous carcinoma cells? PLoS One 7: e34071.
23. Clop A, Marcq F, Takeda H, Pirottin D, Tordoir X, et al. (2006) A mutation creating a potential illegitimate microRNA target site in the myostatin gene affects muscularity in sheep. Nat Genet 38: 813–818.
24. Ji J, Shi J, Budhu A, Yu Z, Forgues M, et al. (2009) MicroRNA expression, survival, and response to interferon in liver cancer. N Engl J Med 361: 1437–1447.
25. Lee RC, Feinbaum RL, Ambros V (1993) The C. elegans heterochronic gene lin-4 encodes small RNAs with antisense complementarity to lin-14. Cell 75: 843–854.
26. Lagos-Quintana M, Rauhut R, Meyer J, Borkhardt A, Tuschl T (2003) New microRNAs from mouse and human. RNA 9: 175–179.
27. Han M, Liu M, Wang Y, Chen X, Xu J, et al. (2012) Antagonism of miR-21 reverses epithelial-mesenchymal transition and cancer stem cell phenotype through AKT/ERK1/2 inactivation by targeting PTEN. PLoS One 7: e39520.
28. Kong X, Li G, Yuan Y, He Y, Wu X, et al. (2012) MicroRNA-7 inhibits epithelial-to-mesenchymal transition and metastasis of breast cancer cells via targeting FAK expression. PLoS One 7: e41523.
29. Zhou C, Qiu L, Sun Y, Healey S, Wanebo H, et al. (2006) Inhibition of EGFR/PI3K/AKT cell survival pathway promotes TSA's effect on cell death and migration in human ovarian cancer cells. Int J Oncol 29: 269–278.
30. Thiery JP (2002) Epithelial–mesenchymal transitions in tumour progression. Nature Reviews Cancer 2: 442–454.
31. Thiery JP, Sleeman JP (2006) Complex networks orchestrate epithelial-mesenchymal transitions. Nat Rev Mol Cell Biol 7: 131–142.
32. Thiery JP, Acloque H, Huang RY, Nieto MA (2009) Epithelial-mesenchymal transitions in development and disease. Cell 139: 871–890.
33. Grossmann TN, Yeh JT, Bowman BR, Chu Q, Moellering RE, et al. (2012) Inhibition of oncogenic Wnt signaling through direct targeting of beta-catenin. Proc Natl Acad Sci U S A.
34. Hassan MQ, Maeda Y, Taipaleenmaki H, Zhang W, Jafferji M, et al. (2012) miR-218 Directs a Wnt Signaling Circuit to Promote Differentiation of Osteoblasts and Osteomimicry of Metastatic Cancer Cells. J Biol Chem.
35. Gregory PA, Bert AG, Paterson EL, Barry SC, Tsykin A, et al. (2008) The miR-200 family and miR-205 regulate epithelial to mesenchymal transition by targeting ZEB1 and SIP1. Nature Cell Biology 10: 593–601.
36. Li Y, VandenBoom TG, Wang Z, Kong D, Ali S, et al. (2010) miR-146a Suppresses Invasion of Pancreatic Cancer Cells. Cancer Research 70: 1486–1495.
37. Kong W, Yang H, He L, Zhao JJ, Coppola D, et al. (2008) MicroRNA-155 is regulated by the transforming growth factor beta/Smad pathway and contributes to epithelial cell plasticity by targeting RhoA. Mol Cell Biol 28: 6773–6784.
38. Gebeshuber CA, Zatloukal K, Martinez J (2009) miR-29a suppresses tristetraprolin, which is a regulator of epithelial polarity and metastasis. EMBO Rep 10: 400–405.
39. Qiu L, Di W, Jiang Q, Scheffler E, Derby S, et al. (2005) Targeted inhibition of transient activation of the EGFR-mediated cell survival pathway enhances paclitaxel-induced ovarian cancer cell death. Int J Oncol 27: 1441–1448.
40. Konishi H, Takagi A, Kurita A, Kaneda N, Matsuzaki T (2012) PEGylated liposome IHL-305 markedly improved the survival of ovarian cancer peritoneal metastasis in mouse. BMC Cancer 12: 462.
41. Wittinger M, Vanhara P, El-Gazzar A, Savarese-Brenner B, Pils D, et al. (2011) hVps37A Status affects prognosis and cetuximab sensitivity in ovarian cancer. Clin Cancer Res 17: 7816–7827.
42. Ji C, Cao C, Lu S, Kivlin R, Amaral A, et al. (2008) Curcumin attenuates EGF-induced AQP3 up-regulation and cell migration in human ovarian cancer cells. Cancer Chemother Pharmacol 62: 857–865.
43. Saegusa M, Hashimura M, Kuwata T, Okayasu I (2009) Requirement of the Akt/beta-catenin pathway for uterine carcinosarcoma genesis, modulating E-cadherin expression through the transactivation of slug. Am J Pathol 174: 2107–2115.
44. Ivanova L, Butt MJ, Matsell DG (2008) Mesenchymal transition in kidney collecting duct epithelial cells. Am J Physiol Renal Physiol 294: F1238–1248.
45. Wang Y, Sheng Q, Spillman MA, Behbakht K, Gu H (2012) Gab2 regulates the migratory behaviors and E-cadherin expression via activation of the PI3K pathway in ovarian cancer cells. Oncogene 31: 2512–2520.

4

Overexpression of piRNA Pathway Genes in Epithelial Ovarian Cancer

Shu Ly Lim[1], Carmela Ricciardelli[2], Martin K. Oehler[2], Izza M. D. De Arao Tan[2], Darryl Russell[2], Frank Grützner[1]*

1 Robinson Research Institute, School of Molecular and Biomedical Sciences, University of Adelaide, Adelaide, SA, Australia, **2** Discipline of Obstetrics and Gynaecology, Robinson Research Institute, University of Adelaide, Adelaide, SA, Australia

Abstract

The importance of the Piwi-interacting RNA (piRNA) pathway for germ cell maintenance, genome integrity, DNA methylation and retrotransposon control raises possible roles of this pathway in cancer. Indeed aberrant expression of human PIWI orthologs and *Maelstrom* has been observed in various cancers. In this study we explored the expression and function of piRNA pathway genes in human ovarian cancer, based on our recent work, which showed widespread expression of piRNA pathway genes in the mammalian. Our work shows that *PIWIL1* and *MAEL* expression is significantly increased in malignant EOC (n = 25) compared to benign tumor tissues (n = 19) and normal ovarian tissue (n = 8). The expression of *PIWIL3* is lower in malignant and benign tissues when compared to normal ovary. Sequencing of *PIWIL1* transcript revealed that in many tumors deletion of exon 17 leads to the introduction of a premature stop codon in the PIWI domain, likely due to a splicing error. *In situ* hybridization on tumor sections revealed that *L1*, *PIWIL1*, *2* and *MAEL* are specifically expressed in epithelial cells (cancerous cells) of EOC. Furthermore, *PIWIL2* and *MAEL* are co-expressed in the stromal cells adjacent to tumor cells. Since *PIWIL1* and *MAEL* are up regulated in malignant EOC and expressed in the epithelial cells, we investigated if these two genes affect invasiveness of ovarian cancer cell lines that do not normally express these genes. *PIWIL1* and *MAEL* were transiently over expressed in the ovarian cancer cell line SKOV3, followed by real-time measurements of cell invasiveness. Surprisingly both *PIWIL1* and *MAEL* over expression decreased the invasiveness of SKOV3 cells. Our findings support a growing body of evidence that shows that genes in this pathway are upregulated in cancer. In ovarian cancer we show for the first time that *Piwil1* transcript may often be abnormal result in non functional product. In contrast to what has been observed in other cell types, we found that *PIWIL1* and *MAEL* have a repressive effect on cell invasiveness.

Editor: Rajeev Samant, University of Alabama at Birmingham, United States of America

Funding: This study was funded by the University of Adelaide. F.G. is supported by an ARC (Australian Research Council) fellowship. The funders had no role in study design, data collection and analysis, decision to publish, or preparation of the manuscript.

Competing Interests: The authors have declared that no competing interests exist.

* E-mail: frank.grutzner@adelaide.edu.au

Introduction

Ovarian cancer is the most lethal gynaecological cancer, and the fifth leading cause of cancer-related death among women in the Western World [1]. The five-year relative survival rate for women with ovarian cancer is only around 40% [1]. Ovarian cancers are heterogeneous tumors which exhibit distinct morphological characteristics, genetic mutations and origins. There are three major types of ovarian cancer - epithelial, germ cell and sex cord stromal tumors. Ovarian germ cell tumors and sex cord stromal tumors comprise 10% of ovarian cancers, and are derived from primitive ovarian germ cells or mesenchymal cells in the sex-cord derived tissue of the ovary, respectively [2]. EOCs account for more than 90% of ovarian malignancies. Based on histology EOCs are classified into four main subtypes (serous, mucinous, endometroid and clear cell carcinomas) with over 70% of the cases diagnosed as serous carcinomas (SCs) [3].

Alterations of the epigenetic landscape such as global DNA hypomethylation and gene specific DNA hypermethylation are frequently reported in cancer cells [4]. Global DNA hypomethylation largely affects the intergenic and intronic regions of the genome, especially repeat sequences and transposable elements (TEs), which account for about 55% of the human genome [5], including 17% *L1* repeats [6]. In somatic cells, DNA methylation of TEs is crucial to prevent their expression which can jeopardise integrity of the genome. During germ cell development, there is a transient period of global DNA hypomethylation which results in temporary activation of TEs [7].

The piRNA pathway is evolutionarily highly conserved in metazoa and consists of 21–26 nt piRNAs which bind PIWI proteins to mediate posttranslational control of TE expression and play a role in epigenetic changes (such as DNA methylation) via interaction with other proteins (such as MAEL or HP1) [8,9]. In mammals there are several *Piwi like* (*Piwil*) genes (three in mice, four in humans). Expression of *Piwil* genes and piRNA pathway associated genes has been demonstrated at various stages of germ cell development in particular in testis. *Piwil1* (*Miwi*) has previously been identified as a gene exclusively expressed in mouse testis and essential for spermatogenesis [10]. More recently expression of *Piwil1* has also been demonstrated in mouse and human ovary [11]. Mutation of *Piwil2*, *Piwil4* and *Mael* in mouse leads to similar phenotypes including elimination of TE DNA methylation and male sterility [8]. There is now growing evidence of piRNA activity also in the mammalian ovary, however knock out experiments of piRNA pathway gene in mice so far has only led to male sterility [12–14].

There is mounting evidence of piRNA pathway activity in various cancers. Expression of *PIWIL1* and *PIWIL2* has been found in a wide range of human cancers such as stomach, breast, gastrointestinal tract and endometrium [15–18] and recently also in ovarian carcinoma [19]. Increased expression of *PIWIL1* is associated with enhanced tumor growth [20] increased tumor grades [21], poor diagnostic outcomes [22] and mortality [23]. *PIWIL2* is widely expressed in early-stage breast and cervical cancers and pre-cancerous stem cells involved in tumorigenesis [18]. The expression pattern of *PIWIL3* and *4* has only been studied in colon cancers [24]. *Maelstrom* (*MAEL*) is a known testis cancer gene [25].

Our finding of expression in ovarian somatic cells [11] together with decreased DNA methylation at *L1* promoter region associated with the progression of cervical and uterus cancers [26] and poor prognosis in ovarian carcinomas [27] led us to investigate whether piRNA pathway genes could play a role in EOCs. In this study, we investigated the expression of *PIWIL1–4* and *MAEL* in 25 EOC, 19 benign tumor samples, and 8 normal ovarian tissues. We found significantly elevated expression of *PIWIL1* and *MAEL* in EOC compared to benign and normal ovarian tissues. However, *PIWIL1* transcripts in EOC may not be functional due to deletions identified in the PIWI domain of this transcript. Furthermore, overexpression of *PIWIL1* and *MAEL* suggests a role of these genes in reducing ovarian cancer cells invasiveness *in vitro*.

Materials and Methods

Tissues

Total RNAs from human testis and pre-menopause ovarian tissues were purchased from Stratagene (USA). Malignant, benign and normal ovarian tissues (Table 1 and Table S3) were collected with informed written consent of the patient and approval by the Ethics Committee of the Royal Adelaide Hospital, Adelaide, South Australia.

Cell lines

Human ovarian cancer cell lines SKOV3 and OVCAR3 were purchased from American Type Culture Collection (ATCC, USA) while OVCAR5 was obtained from Dr. Thomas Hamilton (Fox Chase Cancer Center, Philadelphia, PA) Johnson et al Cancer Res 57: 850–856 1997. Cell lines were maintained in RPMI 1640 medium supplemented with L-glutamine (2 mM), Penicillin-streptomycin (100 U/ml, 100μg/ml) (Sigma). SKOV3 and OVCAR3 cells were supplemented with 5% FBS (Invitrogen) whilst OVCAR5 cells were supplemented with 10% FBS and 7.5 μg/ml insulin. All cell lines were maintained at 37°C in a humid chamber with 5% CO_2.

RNA isolation and cDNA synthesis

RNA was isolated from tissues and cell lines using TRIzol reagent (Invitrogen) following the manufacturer's instructions. RNA was resuspended in nuclease free water, and stored at -80°C. RNA was treated with DNase I (New England Biolabs) before reverse transcription. 1μg of RNA was used to obtain cDNA using the Super Script III First-strand Synthesis System (Invitrogen) following the manufacturer's protocol. Briefly, RNA was incubated with 1μl of 50 μM oligo(dT)$_{20}$ and 1μl of 10 mM dNTPs for 10 mins at 65°C. After incubation, 4μl of 5x RT buffer, 2μl of dithiothreitol (DTT, 0.1 M), 1μl of RNaseOUT (40 U/μl) and 1μl of Super Script III RT enzyme (200 U/μl) were added and incubated for 50 mins at 50°C. The reaction was terminated at 85°C for 5 mins. cDNAs were stored at −20°C.

Gene expression analyses

RT-PCR was performed to determine the level of mRNA for the five piRNA pathway genes (Table S1) and beta actin (*ACTB*) in 52 patient samples and 3 ovarian cancer cell lines. Each 25μl reaction contained 200 ng of cDNA, 5μl of 5x Go Taq Green Master Mix (Promega), 1μl of 5 mM dNTP solution (Roche), 0.5μl of each primer (20 pmol/μl) and 0.5μl Taq DNA polymerase. The PCR conditions were the same for all genes, except the annealing temperature (Table S1), and were as follows: initial denaturation at 95°C for 2 mins, 95°C for 30 secs, annealing at gene specific temperature for 30 secs (Table S1), extension at 72 °C for 1 min, 32 cycles. PCR of *ACTB* control was performed with 27 cycles, followed by 5 mins of final extension at 72 °C. The PCR products were visualized on a 1.5% agarose gel stained with ethidium bromide. Band intensity was measured (Quantity One program, Version 4, Bio-Rad), and the relative intensity of each gene was normalized to that of *ACTB*. PCR products were confirmed by sequencing (Big Dye Terminator v3.1 cycle sequencing kit, Applied Biosystems). RT–PCR was performed in triplicate for each primer pair.

Statistical analyses of gene expression

Data are presented as median relative expression (first quartile to third quartile). The transcript level of each gene was normalized against *ACTB*. Kolmogorov-Smirnov and Shapiro-Wilk tests suggested that the expression level of each gene from all of the 52 samples is not normally distributed. Thus, a Kruskal-Wallis test, which uses a non-parametric method, was used to compare the gene expression from malignant, benign and normal groups. The Spearman's correlation test was performed to investigate the correlation between a patient's age and consequent gene expression. R-value closer to 1 indicates a stronger positive correlation, whereas an R-value closer to -1 shows a stronger negative correlation. In the Kruskal-Wallis and Spearman's tests, a P-value of <0.05 was considered statistically significant.

Table 1. Age and cancer stage of EOC, benign tumors and normal ovaries.

Tissue	n	Median of patient age in years (range)	Cancer stage
Serous carcinomas	25	60 (37–75)	See Table S3
Benign ovarian lesions	19	60 (36–88)	-
Normal ovaries	8	48 (44–76)	-

RNA *in situ* hybridization

Probes were labelled with digoxigenin-11-UTP (Roche Diagnostics) according to the manufacturer's protocol. Formalin-fixed paraffin-embedded tissue sections were deparaffinised in xylene and subsequently washed in graded ethanol. All solutions were prepared in diethylpyrocarbonate (DEPC)-treated H_2O to inactivate RNase activity. mRNA-bound nucleoproteins were removed by proteinase K incubation (1.2µg/ml) (Roche Diagnostics) for 30 mins at 37 °C. Slides were washed with 1x PBS and acetylated (1 M triethanolamin/0.178% HCl/0.25% acetic anhydride). Slides were prehybridised at 65°C for 2 hrs with prehybridization buffer (50% deionized formamide/2x SSC/1x Denhardt's solution/0.005 M phosphate buffer/10% dextran sulphate/1 mg/ml yeast total RNA/1 mg/ml salmon sperm DNA) and hybridised with about 200 ng of cRNA probe in prehybridization buffer overnight at 50°C in a humid chamber. Slides were washed in 2x SSC, 1x SSC, 0.5x SSC and 0.1x SSC for 15 mins each at 50°C. To remove unbound cRNA probes, the tissue was subjected to RNase A (150µg/ml) digestion for 30 mins at 37°C. Specifically bound cRNA probes were detected using an anti-DIG antibody coupled to alkaline phosphatase with nitrobluetetrazolium chloride/X-phosphate-5-bromo-4-chloro-3-indolylphosphate (NBT/BCIP) (Roche Diagnostics) as chromogenic substrate.

Cloning and construct preparation for invasion analyses

The *MAEL* (CCDS1257) and *PIWIL1* (CCDS9268) cDNA sequences were obtained from the NCBI CCDS database. Full-length cDNA sequence was amplified using the Expand High Fidelity PCR system (Roche) according to the manufacturer's protocol and cloned into a pcDNA3.1 mammalian expression vector. Plasmid DNAs including pcDNA 3.1 (Invitrogen) or pEGFP-N1 empty vectors (Clontech) were transfected into SKOV3 cells using Lipofectamine LTX (Invitrogen) following the manufacturer's instruction. SKOV3 cells were selected due to their endogenous *L1* expression levels and the fact that they showed no piRNA pathway gene expression (Fig. 1C). For each transfection, 8×10^4 SKOV3 cells were seeded onto a 24-well plate 14 hrs before transfection and were cultured in RPMI 1640/5% FBS without Penicillin-streptomycin. Plasmid DNA (500 ng) was diluted in 100µl of Opti-MEM medium (Invitrogen) and incubated with 0.5µl Plus reagent (Invitrogen) and 2µl Lipofectamine LTX (Invitrogen) for 30 mins before being added into each well. After 6 hrs, the cell culture medium was replaced with new RPMI 1640/5% FBS medium and cells were incubated for 24 hrs at 37°C, 5% CO_2 before harvesting for *in vitro* invasion analyses. The transfection of pEGFP-N1 empty vectors into SKOV3 cells allowed the transfection efficiency to be measured, as successfully transfected cells expressed the GFP protein. The pEGFP-N1 vector was subjected to the same growth and transfection conditions as outlined above, to determine the transfection efficiency which was approximately 70% after 24 hrs.

In vitro invasion analyses with xCelligence

Cell invasion was tested with real-time invasion assay monitoring using CIM devices and the xCelligence DP system (Roche Diagnostics) [28]. Briefly, 4 hrs before the invasion assay, a CIM plate (Roche) was coated with 1:20 diluted Growth factor reduced Matrigel basement membrane matrix (~450µg/ml) (BD Biosciences). Then 40,000 cells, untransfected or transfected with empty vector (Ev) or *MAEL* or *PIWIL1* vectors, were seeded into each coated well. Cell activity was followed over a time period of 72 hrs by measuring the impedance signal in the CIM plate. The cell activity was recorded every minute in the first 12 hrs and every 5 mins for the following 12 hrs. Then from 24 hrs onwards until the end of the experiment, cell activity was recorded every 30 mins. In each CIM plate, triplicates of each group were performed to obtain the mean and standard deviation. The experiment was repeated three times.

PIWIL1 transcript sequencing

The PIWI domain of *PIWIL1* transcript was PCR amplified and products of different size were cloned into pGEM-T Easy vector (Promega). A total of 30 positive colonies from different PCR bands were selected from each ligation reaction and plasmid DNAs were purified using standard alkaline lysis methods (Qiagen) [29]. 200 ng of plasmid DNA were sequenced (Big Dye Terminator v3.1 Cycle Sequencing Kit, Applied Biosystems) using SP6 and T7 universal primers.

Results

Expression of piRNA pathway genes is increased in malignant EOC compared to benign tumors or normal ovarian tissues

piRNA pathway genes are consistently expressed in the mammalian ovary [11]. In order to investigate a possible role of this pathway in EOC, we performed semi-quantitative RT-PCR to investigate the expression of *PIWIL1*, *PIWIL2*, *PIWIL3*, *PIWIL4* and *MAEL* in advanced stage serous EOC (n = 25), benign ovarian tumors (n = 19) and normal ovarian tissue (n = 8) (Table 1, Table S3 and Fig. 1A, B). Semi quantitative analysis revealed that the relative expression levels of *PIWIL1* and *MAEL* were significantly higher in malignant EOC compared to benign and normal tissues (Fig. 2A, B). The relative expression levels of *PIWIL2* and *PIWIL4* in malignant groups were not significantly different to that in benign or normal ovarian tissues (Fig. 2C, D). However, the expression of *PIWIL2* and *PIWIL4* are significantly lower in benign tumors compared to normal ovarian tissue, suggesting an alteration of gene expression during the progression of EOC. The relative expression of *PIWIL3* is different to other *PIWIL* genes such that the expression of this gene is significantly higher in the normal ovary when compared to both malignant and benign tissues (Fig. 2E). Furthermore, the relative expression of *PIWIL3* in normal ovary is positively correlated with patient age in the normal ovary tissues (n = 8) (r = 0.750, P = 0.05) (Table 2). In contrast to *PIWIL3*, *PIWIL1* expression is negatively correlated with the age of patients (r = −0.737, P = 0.037). *PIWIL1* is expressed in growing follicles in pre-menopausal ovaries, but in this study half of the ovaries tested were from women less than 50 years old and likely to be premenopausal.

L1 and piRNA pathway genes are over expressed in EOC cells

To analyse the expression pattern of piRNA pathway genes and *L1* in EOC, RNA *in situ* hybridization was performed in malignant EOC (n = 5) and benign ovarian tumors (n = 2) (Table 3, Fig. S1). We found strong expression of *L1* in the epithelial cells but *L1* was absent in the stromal cells in all samples (Fig. 3A, E). Also we noted that the expression of *L1* is variable in different patients (Fig. 3A). Strong expression of *PIWIL1* was found in the epithelial cells in all EOC tissues (Fig. 3B, F) while *MAEL* and *PIWIL2* showed strong expression in the epithelial cells and stromal cells of all EOC examined (Fig. 3C, G and D, H respectively).

Multiple *PIWIL1* transcript variants exist in malignant EOC

PCR amplification of the PIWI domain from EOC cDNAs produced two distinct bands compared to cDNAs from normal

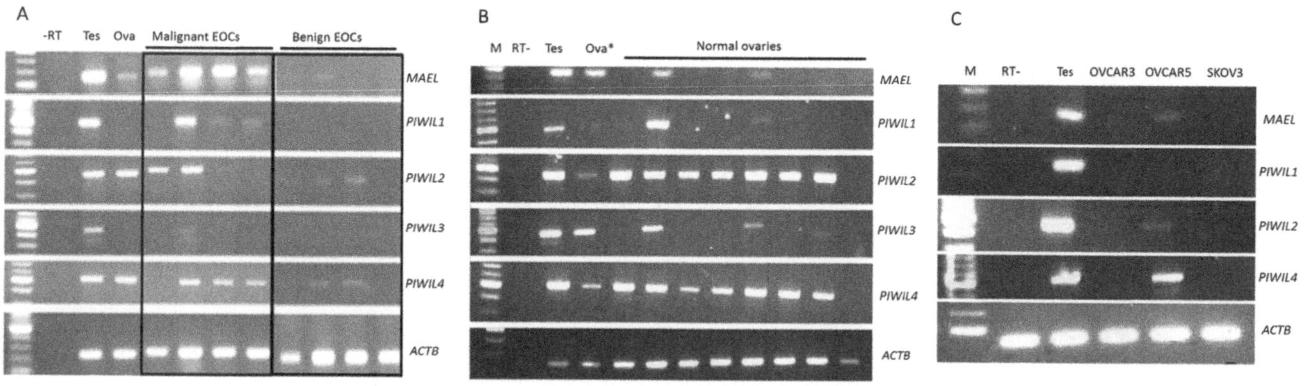

Figure 1. piRNA pathway gene expression in human normal ovaries and ovarian cancers. RT-PCR analyses of *PIWIL1-4* and *MAEL* expression in (A) malignant EOC, benign ovarian cancers (B) normal ovaries and (C) ovarian cancer cell lines. This is a representation of 4 out of 25 malignant EOC and 19 benign ovarian cancer tissues. Increased expression of *PIWIL1, 2, 4* and *MAEL*, but not *PIWIL3*, are found in malignant cancers compared to benign tumors. All normal ovaries show *PIWIL2* and *PIWIL4* expression but only some have *PIWIL1, 3* and *MAEL* expression. No endogenous *PIWIL1, 2, 4* and *MAEL* expression is detected in OVCAR3 and SKOV3 cells. Ova* indicates tissue from a 20-year old pre-menopausal ovary while other ovaries are from individuals aged 44–76 years old.

testis or ovary (Fig. 4), suggesting the presence of multiple *PIWIL1* transcript variants in malignant EOC. PCR products from testis and malignant EOC were extracted, cloned and sequenced. Multiple alignments of clone sequences showed many changes within the PIWI domain at the nucleotide level when compared to the testis and published *PIWIL1* cDNA sequence. Single base pair changes have been identified in *PIWIL1* transcripts of malignant EOCs (Table S2). In addition, most of these clones have exon deletion and unspliced introns which introduce premature stop codons. Importantly a 75-nt deletion which comprised the entire exon 17 was found in most of the sequenced clones in 5 out of 28 EOC patients (Fig. 4B). Furthermore, some clones showed partial splicing of introns 15 and 16 (Fig. 4B) such that 17 bp and 20 bp from the 5′ end of intron 15 and 16, respectively, are unspliced. In order to confirm that the mutations are due to splicing, genomic DNA of tumor samples were isolated and sequenced at the corresponding region. No mutations were identified between exons 15–18 (where the splicing errors occurred) in the genomic *PIWIL1* sequence (Fig. S2). In order to predict if the above post-transcriptional alterations affect PIWIL1 function, sequences were translated and compared to the control (testis cDNA) and published peptide sequence (AAC97371.2). Loss of the entire exon 17 (73-nt deletion) in 11 clones introduced a premature stop codon in the PIWI domain (Fig. S3). Similarly, stop codons were found in clones that have unspliced introns (not shown).

Over expression of piRNA pathway genes reduces invasiveness *in vitro*

In order to investigate the possible role of piRNA pathway genes in cancer progression, full-length *PIWIL1* or *MAEL* transcripts were cloned and transfected transiently into the ovarian cancer cell line SKOV3 and assayed for invasiveness after 24 hrs of transfection. RT-PCR was performed to validate the insertion of plasmids into these cells. RT-PCR confirmed *GFP*, *PIWIL1* or *MAEL* over expression (Fig. S4A). Expression of *MAEL* and *PIWIL1* constructs remained high in the transfected cells 50 hr post-transfection (Fig. S4A). *MAEL*, *PIWIL1* and empty vector (Ev) transfected cells and untransfected SKOV3 cells were applied to the xCELLigence system to investigate their effect on cell invasiveness [30]. Surprisingly, the invasiveness of *MAEL* and *PIWIL1* transfected cells was lower compared to untransfected or empty vector cells (Fig. 5). Cell invasiveness from each group started to reach a plateau after 30 hrs, thus only cell activity of the first 30 hrs is shown. Our results suggest that overexpression of *PIWIL1* and *MAEL* have a repressive effect on SKOV3 cell invasiveness.

Discussion

The piRNA pathway is important for TE silencing, epigenetic regulation and stem cell self-renewal in a wide range of organisms [31,32]. Global DNA hypomethylation and TE derepression, such as *L1*, is a common feature of cancer genomes [33,34] in humans *PIWIL1* and *2* overexpression has been observed in tumors from various tissues [15–18,21–23]. However, it is still unclear whether piRNA pathway genes are differentially expressed in ovarian cancer or have a role in ovarian tumor progression. We examined the expression of piRNA pathway genes *PIWIL1–4*, *MAEL* and *L1* in malignant EOC, benign tumors and normal ovary tissues, and also investigated possible roles of *PIWIL1* and *MAEL* in ovarian cancer cell lines.

Expression of *PIWIL1–2* has been investigated in various cancerous tissues [15–18,21,23,35], but not *MAEL*, *PIWIL3* and *PIWIL4*. Although the expression of *PIWIL2* and *4* appeared high in tumor samples this was not significant, likely due to the fact that *PIWIL2* and *PIWIL4* were strongly expressed in normal ovarian tissues (Fig. 1B) and their expression among malignant tissues is highly variable. The expression of *PIWIL1* and *MAEL* however is significantly increased in malignant EOC when compared to benign tumors. *PIWIL1* and *MAEL*, but not *PIWIL2* and *4*, were significantly up regulated when compared to normal ovaries. In contrast to *PIWIL2* and *4* that are expressed in all normal ovarian tissues examined, the expression of *PIWIL1* and *MAEL* is found only in a subset of normal ovarian tissues from patients who were less than 50 years old. In normal ovary, *PIWIL1* and *MAEL* are expressed in the cumulus cells of growing follicles in human [11]. The normal ovarian tissues tested are from individuals aged 44–76 years old, and half of these samples were derived from individuals less than 50 years old. Thus, the variable expression of *PIWIL1* and *MAEL* in the normal ovaries could be explained by the difference in abundance of growing follicles, which express piRNA pathway genes across the samples.

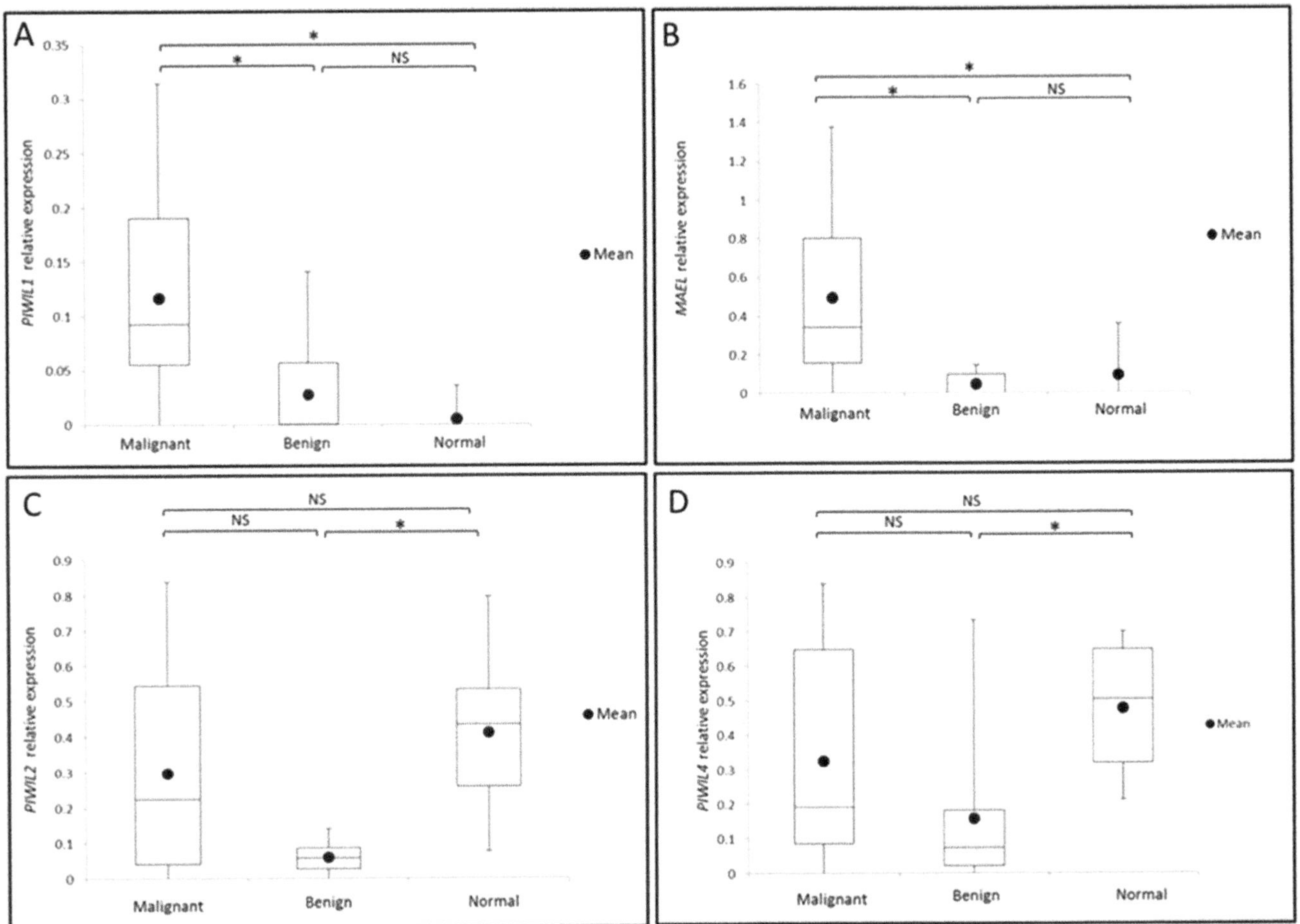

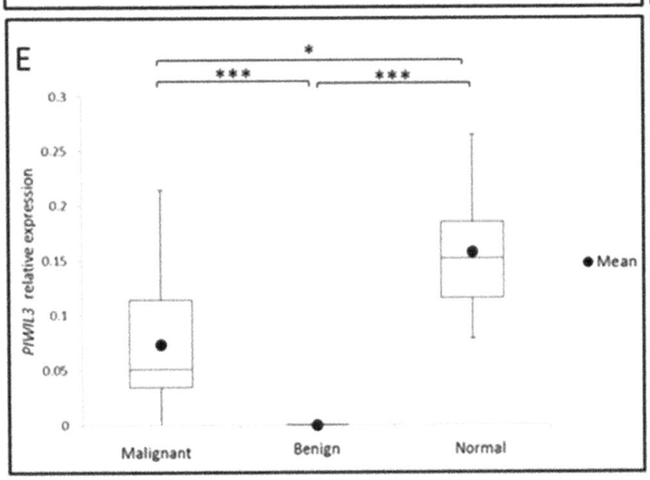

F

Compared group	Genes	P value	
Malignant/ benign	*MAEL*	0.001	*
	PIWIL1	0.002	*
	PIWIL2	0.126	NS
	PIWIL3	<0.001	***
	PIWIL4	0.155	NS
Malignant/ normal	*MAEL*	0.003	*
	PIWIL1	0.001	***
	PIWIL2	0.236	NS
	PIWIL3	0.004	*
	PIWIL4	0.150	NS
Benign/ normal	*MAEL*	0.657	NS
	PIWIL1	0.029	*
	PIWIL2	0.001	*
	PIWIL3	<0.001	***
	PIWIL4	0.019	*

Figure 2. Box plot representing the expression of piRNA pathway genes in malignant EOC, benign ovarian cancer tissues and normal ovaries. Semi-quantitative RT-PCR analysis of mRNA expression (relative to *ACTB*) of (A) *PIWIL1*, (B) *MAEL*, (C) *PIWIL2*, (D) *PIWIL4* and (E) *PIWIL3*. (F) P-value of each comparison group. Malignant EOC (n = 25), benign ovarian cancer tissues (n = 19) and normal ovaries (n = 8). Kruskal-Wallis Test was performed to compare the gene expression level between two groups. Filled dot indicates mean of each group. * indicates $0.001<P<0.05$; *** indicates $P<0.001$; NS, not significant.

MAEL is known as a cancer/testis gene as it is expressed in testis and a number of cancer cell lines [36]. Here we identified for the first time the increased expression of *MAEL* in malignant EOC and benign ovarian tumors. Similar to PIWI, MAEL is essential to ensure proper germline stem cell differentiation in *Drosophila* and other vertebrates [37]. Overexpression of piRNA pathway genes in EOC may indicate that some stem cell characteristics are present in tumor cells or that the piRNA pathway has been activated for example by activity of retrotransposons. Expression of these genes may also be a signature of the presence of ovarian cancer stem cells [38].

Table 2. Correlation between age of patients and piRNA pathway gene expression.

Genes	R-value (M, n = 25)	P-value (M, n = 25)	R-value (B, n = 19)	P-value (B, n = 19)	R-value (N, n = 8)	P-value (B, n = 19)
PIWIL1	−0.376	0.064	−0.194	0.426	−0.737	**0.037***
PIWIL2	−0.080	0.702	−0.442	0.058	0.491	0.217
PIWIL3	−0.082	0.695	0.595	**0.009***	0.75	0.05
PIWIL4	−0.249	0.231	−0.376	0.113	0	1.0
MAEL	−0.087	0.678	0.251	0.457	−0.220	0.601

Spearman's correlation test; M = malignant; B = benign; N = normal; negative value = negative correlation; positive value = positive correlation; P <0.05 and * indicates the correlation between the age of patients and piRNA pathway gene expression is significant. The R-value closer to ± 1 indicates the stronger correlation.

The expression of piRNA pathway genes in normal ovary and certain types of EOC may provide a new perspective on the origin of ovarian cancer. Somatic cells of the maturing follicle may come in contact with the ovarian surface epithelium during ovulation or may be present in the inclusion cyst which is thought to play a role in the origin of epithelial ovarian cancer [3] although the presence of inclusion cysts seems to not per se increase the risk of developing ovarian cancer [39]. Hypomethylation of the *L1* promoter region is correlated with increased *L1* mRNA expression, in malignant breast cancer tissues and cell lines [40,41]. The expression of *PIWIL* genes and *MAEL* in both normal ovary and malignant EOC correlate with increased expression of repeat elements and raises the possibility that the piRNA pathway may have been triggered by TE expression. However, we noticed that *L1* expression was absent in earlier stage malignant tumors (n = 6) but consistently present at all stage 3c tumor samples. This provides some circumstantial evidence that the activation of piRNA pathway genes may precede *L1* expression during tumor progression. This is consistent with work in other tumors that correlate *L1* expression with cancer progression [42]. *Maelstrom* knock out results in decreased DNA methylation in gonads, but not in somatic tissue. In gonads this leads to a dramatic increase in

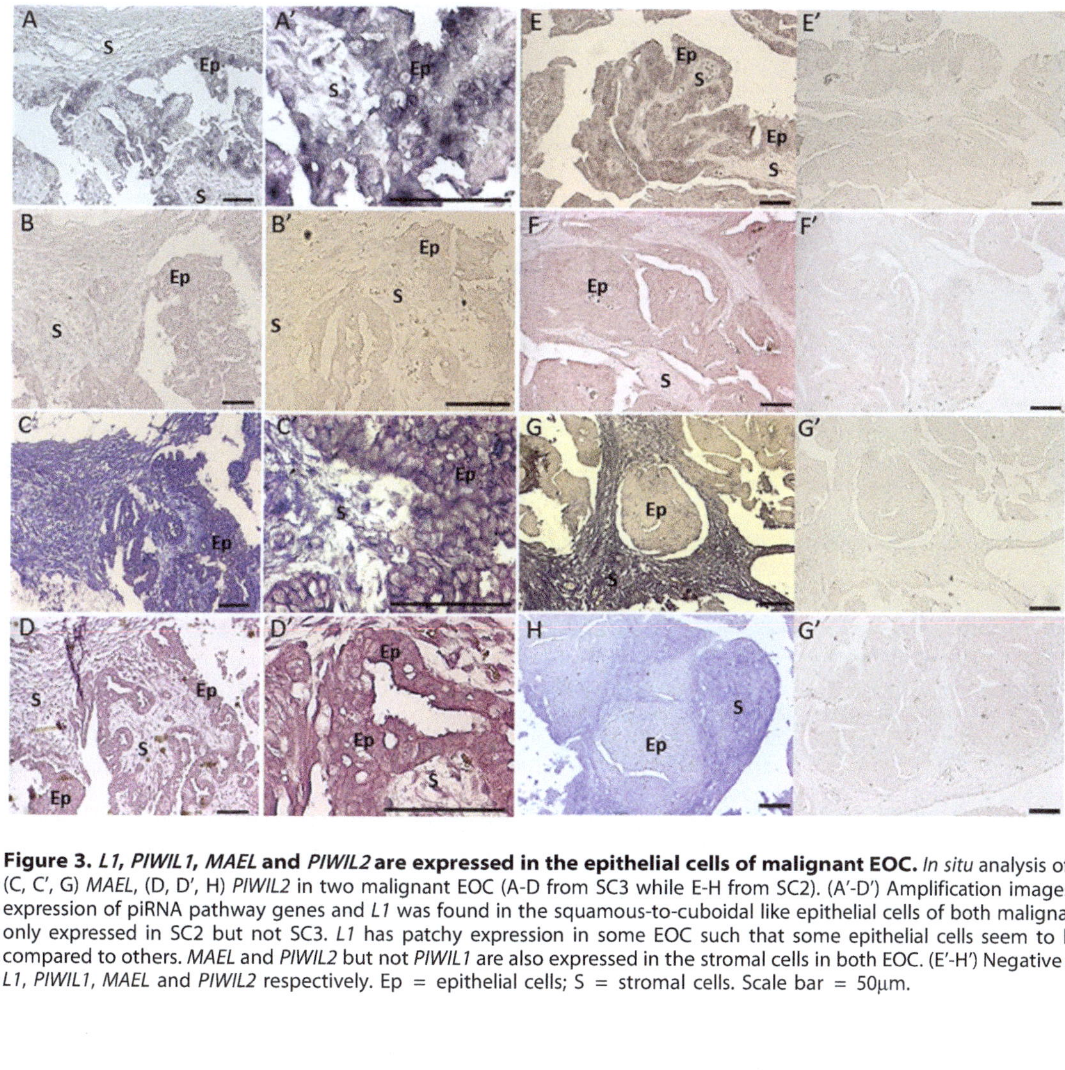

Figure 3. *L1*, *PIWIL1*, *MAEL* and *PIWIL2* are expressed in the epithelial cells of malignant EOC. *In situ* analysis of (A, A', E) *L1*, (B, B', F) *PIWIL1*, (C, C', G) *MAEL*, (D, D', H) *PIWIL2* in two malignant EOC (A-D from SC3 while E-H from SC2). (A'-D') Amplification images of A-D respectively. Strong expression of piRNA pathway genes and *L1* was found in the squamous-to-cuboidal like epithelial cells of both malignant EOC except *PIWIL1* which only expressed in SC2 but not SC3. *L1* has patchy expression in some EOC such that some epithelial cells seem to have stronger *L1* expression compared to others. *MAEL* and *PIWIL2* but not *PIWIL1* are also expressed in the stromal cells in both EOC. (E'-H') Negative controls with sense probe of *L1*, *PIWIL1*, *MAEL* and *PIWIL2* respectively. Ep = epithelial cells; S = stromal cells. Scale bar = 50µm.

Table 3. Expression trends of piRNA pathway genes and *L1* in the EOC after *in situ* hybridisation.

Patient	Gene	Epithelial cells	Stromal cells
SC1	*MAEL*	weak	strong
	PIWIL2	weak	strong
	PIWIL1	strong	-
	L1	strong	-
SC2	*MAEL*	weak	strong
	PIWIL2	weak	strong
	PIWIL1	weak	-
	L1	strong	-
SC3	*MAEL*	strong	strong
	PIWIL2	strong	strong
	PIWIL1	-	-
	L1	strong	weak
SC4	*MAEL*	-	-
	PIWIL2	strong	-
	PIWIL1	strong	-
	L1	strong	-
SC5	*MAEL*	weak	weak
	PIWIL2	weak	-
	PIWIL1	weak	-
	L1	weak	-
BSC1	*MAEL*	weak	weak
	PIWIL2	weak	weak
	PIWIL1	-	-
	L1	-	-
BSC2	*MAEL*	weak	-
	PIWIL2	weak	-
	PIWIL1	-	-
	L1	-	-

"-": undetectable expression.

transposable element expression in the germ cells [43]. Our observation of *MAEL* overexpression in the absence of detectable *L1* expression in early stage tumor samples raises the possibility that non-functional *MAEL* may play a role in decreasing DNA methylation promoting subsequent *L1* expression.

Although *PIWIL1* transcript level was significantly increased in malignant EOC compared to benign and normal tissues, cloning and sequencing of these transcripts suggested that these transcripts may produce aberrant and non-functional PIWIL1 protein. Multiple mutations were found in *PIWIL1* transcripts including unspliced introns, loss of exons as well as single base pair changes. Single base pair changes maybe a result of RNA editing [44]. Among thirty clones of *PIWIL1* transcripts from malignant tissues, one third of these clones have A to G (I) substitution. In addition, most of these clones have exon deletion and unspliced introns which introduced premature stop codons (Table 2). The presence of premature stop codons suggests that although *PIWIL1* expression is high in malignant tissues, the corresponding protein (if any) maybe truncated and non-functional. Such defects in pre-mRNA splicing have been found in liver cancer and have been implicated in its progression [45].

In situ analyses revealed that *L1*, *PIWIL1*, *PIWIL2* and *MAEL* are strongly expressed in the epithelial cells. Surprisingly we also found evidence for *PIWIL2* and *MAEL* expression in the stromal cells in malignant EOC. It is unclear at this point if these are epithelial cells invading stromal tissue or individual stromal cells expressing these genes. Several lines of evidence have demonstrated that alteration of gene expression in stromal cells may create a microenvironment which facilitates tumor growth, playing a role in cancer progression [46–48]. For example, changes of gene expression in the stromal cells surrounding colon cancer cells have been shown to produce matrix metalloproteinases (MMPs) which increase tumor invasion capacity *in vitro* and *in vivo* [47,49].

There are a number of ways in which genes associated with the piRNA pathway can play a role in genome regulation and it has been suggested that activity of these genes can have effects on methylation and expression of TEs as well as genome instability. In addition, PIWI proteins can mediate, activating or repressing effects on chromatin via interaction with heterochromatin protein 1 or polycomb group proteins. Despite this experimental evidence elucidating the role of *PIWIL1* and *MAEL* in cancer is difficult as differing effects are observed. Recent studies suggest that *PIWIL1* maybe a marker for cancer cell proliferation as it is co-expressed

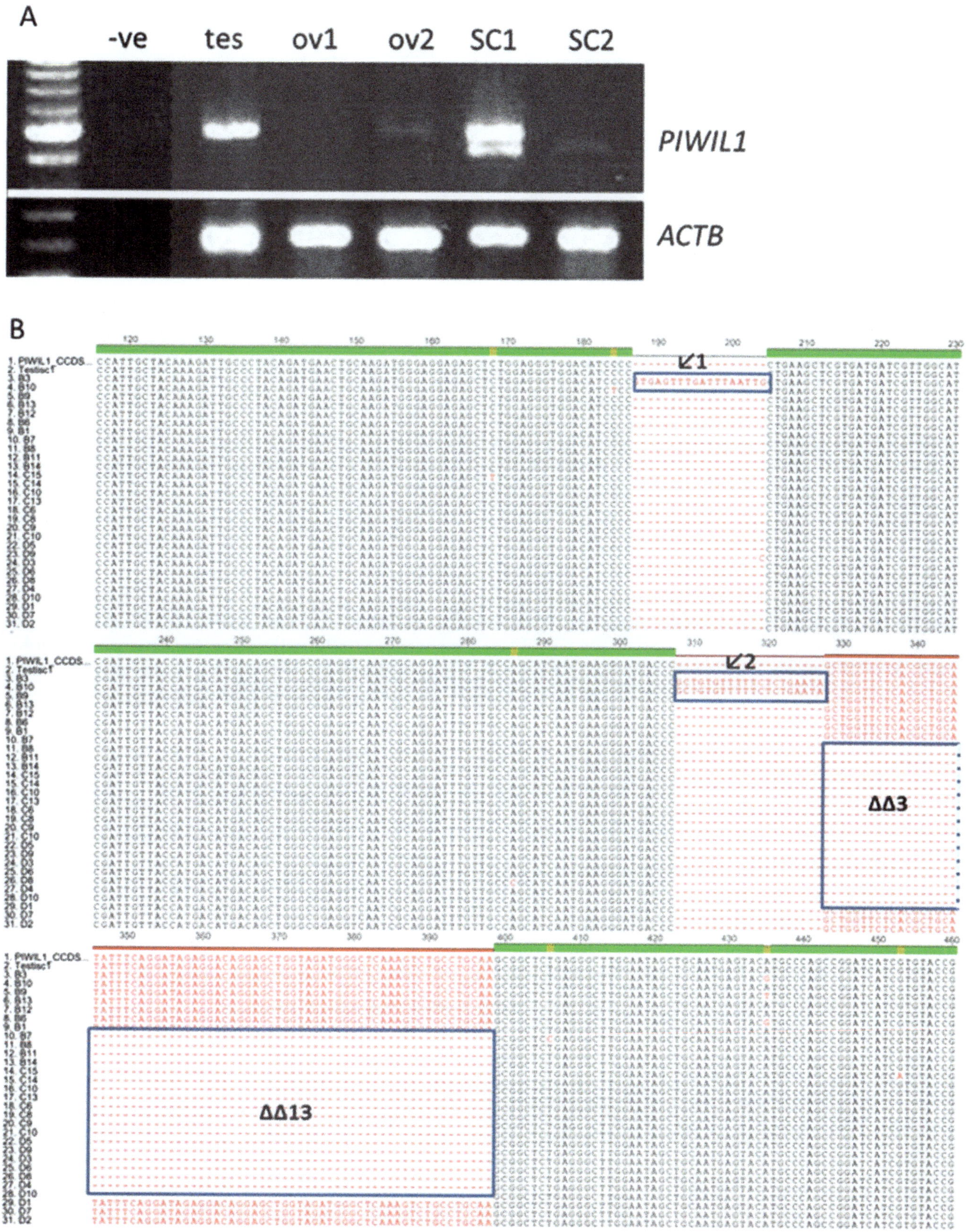

Figure 4. *PIWIL1* transcript variants in EOC. (A) *PIWIL1* expression in control tissues (human testis, normal ovary (ov) 1, 2) and EOC tissue SC1 and 2. In the positive control, a 500 bp band was amplified, but in malignant SC1, two bands were obtained. (B) cDNA multiple alignment (partial) showing that most of the clones have a deletion of exon 17 (ΔΔ3) and 3 clones have partial splicing of intron 15 and 16 (↙1, ↙2). PIWIL1_ccds: published cDNA of *PIWIL1* (CCDS9268); Testis C1: testis transcript clone 1; B1–3, B6, B9–B14, C6, C8, C9, C10–C15, D1–D10: clones with *PIWIL1* transcripts.

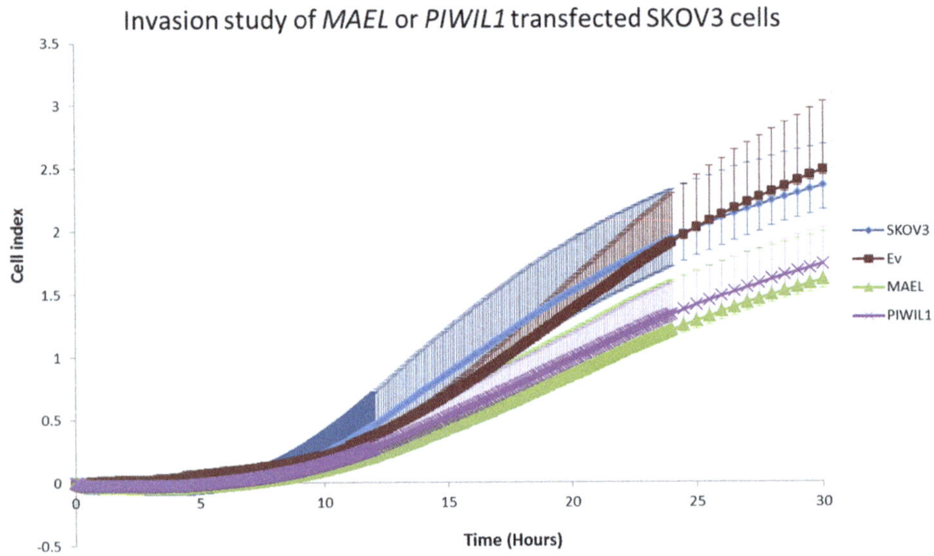

Figure 5. Invasion assay of *MAEL* or *PIWIL1* transfected SKOV3 cells. *PIWIL1* and *MAEL* transfected cells have lower invasiveness compared to untransfected cells and *Ev* transfected cells. In each experiment, each group was performed in triplicate and this experiment was repeated three times. This is a combined data plot of three independent experiments for all groups. Error bars represent standard deviation. *WT* indicates untransfected SKOV3 cells; empty vector (Ev), *MAEL* and *PIWIL1* indicate cells transfected with *MAEL* or *PIWIL1* vectors. *None* indicates well without cells.

with KI67 [16], a reliable proliferating cell marker [50]. In addition, studies in a *Drosophila* brain tumor model suggested that inactivation of *Piwi* suppressed tumor growth and thus *Piwi* may promote cancer progression in this system [51]. This is further supported by slowed tumor growth after knockdown of *PIWIL1* in lung cancer cell lines [52]. Recently several other studies investigated the effect of *PIWI* and *MAEL* overexpression on tumor progression. Liu et al observed increased expression of the *Maelstrom* gene in hepatocellular cancer (HCC). When overexpressed, *MAEL* led to increased growth, migration and invasiveness in HCC cell lines [53]. Liang et al. showed in another study, that stable overexpression of *Piwil2* in mouse embryonic fibroblasts increased proliferation and invasiveness [54]. However, in humans over expression of *PIWIL1* did not increase cell growth but caused programmed cell death in myeloid leukaemia KG1 cells, suggesting that PIWIL1 may prevent tumor development in these cells [55]. Our results in SKOV3 cells support those findings. Together this suggests that MAEL may undergo different roles depending on cell type and differentiation status. Given that these results were obtained in different cell types and tested in different assays and species it is difficult to reconcile the divergent results. One possible pathway that may shed some light on this is the AKT-GSK3b-Snail pathway. Recent work showed that *MAEL* overexpression triggers EMT via the AKT-GSK3b-SNAIL pathway. It has been suggested that activation of AKT will lead to degradation of SNAIL ultimately leading to EMT and increased invasiveness. However in SKOV3 cells *SNAIL* overexpression has been reported to increase invasiveness [56]. The decrease of invasiveness after *MAEL* overexpression observed in the present study could be due to a reduction in SNAIL activity by MAEL.

Conclusions

Increasing evidence of piRNA pathway activity in various cancers raises questions about a role of this pathway in the origin and progression of these malignancies. As reported in this study, over expression of piRNA pathway genes and *L1* elements in malignant ovarian cancer suggest a role of this pathway in EOC. Expression of *PIWIL1* and *MAEL* is significantly up regulated in malignant EOC when compared to benign lesions and normal ovaries. *In situ* analyses revealed that *L1*, *PIWIL1*, *PIWIL2* and *MAEL* are strongly expressed in the cancerous cells but surprisingly *MAEL* and *PIWIL2* expression was also found in the stromal cells lining tumor tissues, suggesting a change in cell composition or identity in the tissue surrounding the cancer cells. Identification of aberrant *PIWIL1* transcript revealed that non-functional PIWIL1 proteins may be produced. In contrast to other cell systems, *in vitro* real-time invasion assay showed that over expression of piRNA pathway components such as *PIWIL1* and *MAEL* has a repressive effect on ovarian cancer cell invasiveness. Together, these results highlight the complexity in which the piRNA pathway may influence tumor progression and warrant further work to better understand the role of the piRNA pathway in the origin and progression of ovarian cancer.

Supporting Information

Figure S1 Expression of piRNA pathway genes and *L1* in malignant EOC. (A) *MAEL* antisense from SC2 which shows strong expression in stromal cells (+++) compared to epithelial cells which have weak expression. (B) *L1* expression in SC3. Epithelial cells have patchy strong expression of *L1* while low expression was observed in the stromal cells. +++ strong expression; + weak expression. (A'–B') Negative controls with a sense probe of *MAEL* and *L1* respectively. Scale bar = 50µm

Figure S2 No mutations found in the genomic *PIWIL1* sequence in serous carcinoma 1. SC1 gDNA was aligned with published *PIWIL1* gDNA (ENSG00000125207) sequence from exon 15 to exon 18. All exon sequences and partial intron sequences were shown. Green bar indicates 100% conservation between the aligned sequences.

Figure S3 ***PIWIL1*** **transcript variants encoded premature stop codon.** (A) 19 clones with exon 17 (ΔΔ13) deletions, 3 clones with unspliced introns and 1 clone with a single base change resulted in the introduction of premature stop codons. PIWIL1_ccds9268: published PIWIL1 peptide sequence (AAC97371.2); Testis C1: translated testis clone 1; B1-3, B6, B9-B14, C6, C8, C9, C10-C15, D1-D10: clones with PIWIL1 translated sequence. * inside the boxes in panel A indicates premature stop codon.

Figure S4 Expression of ***PIWIL1*** **and** ***MAEL*** **is maintained in transfected cells throughout the invasion study.** (A) RT-PCR showing the expression of *GFP, MAEL* and *PIWIL1* in transfected cells (left panel) at the start of invasion study (24 hrs post-transfection) and (right panel) the end of invasion study (74 hrs after transfection). The expression of *GFP, MAEL* or *PIWIL1* can only be detected in specific vector transfected cells but not empty vector transfected or wildtype cells. (B) A high number of GFP positive cells were still observed after 74 hrs of transfection. Scale bar = 10μm.

Acknowledgments

We thank Dr. Tasman Daish and Dr. Enkhjargal Tsend-Ayush (University of Adelaide) for experimental advice, Dr. Briony Forbes (University of Adelaide) for providing the pcDNA3.1 vectors and Dr. Peter McCarthy (University of Adelaide) for providing the pEGFP-N1 vector, Miss Noor Alia Lokman for organising the patient tissues. F.G. is an Australian Research Council Research Fellow.

Author Contributions

Conceived and designed the experiments: FG SLL. Performed the experiments: SLL. Analyzed the data: SLL IMDDAT DR MKO CR FG. Contributed reagents/materials/analysis tools: MKO CR. Wrote the paper: SLL FG.

References

1. Anttonen M, Ketola I, Parviainen H, Pusa AK, Heikinheimo M (2003) FOG-2 and GATA-4 Are coexpressed in the mouse ovary and can modulate mullerian-inhibiting substance expression. Biol Reprod 68: 1333–1340.
2. Jemal A, Siegel R, Ward E, Hao Y, Xu J, et al. (2008) Cancer statistics, 2008. CA Cancer J Clin 58: 71–96.
3. Ricciardelli C, Oehler MK (2009) Diverse molecular pathways in ovarian cancer and their clinical significance. Maturitas 62: 270–275.
4. Feinberg AP, Vogelstein B (1983) Hypomethylation distinguishes genes of some human cancers from their normal counterparts. Nature 301: 89–92.
5. Lander ES, Linton LM, Birren B, Nusbaum C, Zody MC, et al. (2001) Initial sequencing and analysis of the human genome. Nature 409: 860–921.
6. Cordaux R, Batzer MA (2009) The impact of retrotransposons on human genome evolution. Nature reviews Genetics 10: 691–703.
7. Smallwood SA, Kelsey G (2012) De novo DNA methylation: a germ cell perspective. Trends Genet 28: 33–42.
8. Aravin AA, Bourc'his D (2008) Small RNA guides for de novo DNA methylation in mammalian germ cells. Genes & development 22: 970–975.
9. Sarot E, Payen-Groschene G, Bucheton A, Pelisson A (2004) Evidence for a piwi-dependent RNA silencing of the gypsy endogenous retrovirus by the Drosophila melanogaster flamenco gene. Genetics 166: 1313–1321.
10. Deng W, Lin H (2002) miwi, a murine homolog of piwi, encodes a cytoplasmic protein essential for spermatogenesis. Dev Cell 2: 819–830.
11. Lim SL, Tsend-Ayush E, Kortschak RD, Jacob R, Ricciardelli C, et al. (2013) Conservation and Expression of piRNA Pathway Genes in Male and Female Adult Gonad of Amniotes. Biol Reprod.
12. Kuramochi-Miyagawa S, Watanabe T, Gotoh K, Totoki Y, Toyoda A, et al. (2008) DNA methylation of retrotransposon genes is regulated by Piwi family members MILI and MIWI2 in murine fetal testes. Genes Dev 22: 908–917.
13. Zhang D, Xiong H, Shan J, Xia X, Trudeau VL (2008) Functional insight into Maelstrom in the germline piRNA pathway: a unique domain homologous to the DnaQ-H 3′-5′ exonuclease, its lineage-specific expansion/loss and evolutionarily active site switch. Biol Direct 3: 48.
14. Aravin AA, Sachidanandam R, Girard A, Fejes-Toth K, Hannon GJ (2007) Developmentally regulated piRNA clusters implicate MILI in transposon control. Science 316: 744–747.
15. Qiao D, Zeeman AM, Deng W, Looijenga LH, Lin H (2002) Molecular characterization of hiwi, a human member of the piwi gene family whose overexpression is correlated to seminomas. Oncogene 21: 3988–3999.
16. Liu X, Sun Y, Guo J, Ma H, Li J, et al. (2006) Expression of hiwi gene in human gastric cancer was associated with proliferation of cancer cells. International journal of cancer Journal international du cancer 118: 1922–1929.
17. Liu JJ, Shen R, Chen L, Ye Y, He G, et al. (2010) Piwil2 is expressed in various stages of breast cancers and has the potential to be used as a novel biomarker. International journal of clinical and experimental pathology 3: 328–337.
18. Lee JH, Engel W, Nayernia K (2006) Stem cell protein Piwil2 modulates expression of murine spermatogonial stem cell expressed genes. Molecular reproduction and development 73: 173–179.
19. Chen C, Liu J, Xu G (2013) Overexpression of PIWI proteins in human stage III epithelial ovarian cancer with lymph node metastasis. Cancer Biomark 13: 315–321.
20. Janic A, Mendizabal L, Llamazares S, Rossell D, Gonzalez C (2010) Ectopic expression of germline genes drives malignant brain tumor growth in Drosophila. Science 330: 1824–1827.
21. Sun G, Wang Y, Sun L, Luo H, Liu N, et al. (2011) Clinical significance of Hiwi gene expression in gliomas. Brain research 1373: 183–188.
22. Grochola LF, Greither T, Taubert H, Moller P, Knippschild U, et al. (2008) The stem cell-associated Hiwi gene in human adenocarcinoma of the pancreas: expression and risk of tumour-related death. British journal of cancer 99: 1083–1088.
23. Taubert H, Greither T, Kaushal D, Wurl P, Bache M, et al. (2007) Expression of the stem cell self-renewal gene Hiwi and risk of tumour-related death in patients with soft-tissue sarcoma. Oncogene 26: 1098–1100.
24. Li L, Yu C, Gao H, Li Y (2010) Argonaute proteins: potential biomarkers for human colon cancer. BMC cancer 10: 38.
25. Xiao L, Wang Y, Zhou Y, Sun Y, Sun W, et al. (2010) Identification of a novel human cancer/testis gene MAEL that is regulated by DNA methylation. Mol Biol Rep 37: 2355–2360.
26. Shuangshoti S, Hourpai N, Pumsuk U, Mutirangura A (2007) Line-1 hypomethylation in multistage carcinogenesis of the uterine cervix. Asian Pacific journal of cancer prevention: APJCP 8: 307–309.
27. Iramaneerat K, Rattanatunyong P, Khemapech N, Triratanachat S, Mutirangura A (2011) HERV-K hypomethylation in ovarian clear cell carcinoma is associated with a poor prognosis and platinum resistance. International journal of gynecological cancer: official journal of the International Gynecological Cancer Society 21: 51–57.
28. Xi B, Yu N, Wang X, Xu X, Abassi YA (2008) The application of cell-based label-free technology in drug discovery. Biotechnology journal 3: 484–495.
29. Wolf CR, Hayward IP, Lawrie SS, Buckton K, McIntyre MA, et al. (1987) Cellular heterogeneity and drug resistance in two ovarian adenocarcinoma cell lines derived from a single patient. Int J Cancer 39: 695–702.
30. Eisenberg MC, Kim Y, Li R, Ackerman WE, Kniss DA, et al. (2011) Mechanistic modeling of the effects of myoferlin on tumor cell invasion. Proceedings of the National Academy of Sciences of the United States of America.
31. Cox DN, Chao A, Baker J, Chang L, Qiao D, et al. (1998) A novel class of evolutionarily conserved genes defined by piwi are essential for stem cell self-renewal. Genes & development 12: 3715–3727.
32. Siomi MC, Sato K, Pezic D, Aravin AA (2011) PIWI-interacting small RNAs: the vanguard of genome defence. Nature reviews Molecular cell biology 12: 246–258.
33. Roman-Gomez J, Jimenez-Velasco A, Agirre X, Cervantes F, Sanchez J, et al. (2005) Promoter hypomethylation of the LINE-1 retrotransposable elements activates sense/antisense transcription and marks the progression of chronic myeloid leukemia. Oncogene 24: 7213–7223.

34. Piskareva O, Lackington W, Lemass D, Hendrick C, Doolan P, et al. (2011) The human L1 element: a potential biomarker in cancer prognosis, current status and future directions. Current molecular medicine 11: 286–303.
35. Grochola LF, Greither T, Taubert H, Moller P, Knippschild U, et al. (2008) The stem cell-associated Hiwi gene in human adenocarcinoma of the pancreas: expression and risk of tumour-related death. Br J Cancer 99: 1083–1088.
36. Xiao L, Wang Y, Zhou Y, Sun Y, Sun W, et al. (2010) Identification of a novel human cancer/testis gene MAEL that is regulated by DNA methylation. Molecular biology reports 37: 2355–2360.
37. Pek JW, Lim AK, Kai T (2009) Drosophila maelstrom ensures proper germline stem cell lineage differentiation by repressing microRNA-7. Dev Cell 17: 417–424.
38. Foster R, Buckanovich RJ, Rueda BR (2013) Ovarian cancer stem cells: working towards the root of stemness. Cancer Lett 338: 147–157.
39. Sharma A, Apostolidou S, Burnell M, Campbell S, Habib M, et al. (2012) Risk of epithelial ovarian cancer in asymptomatic women with ultrasound-detected ovarian masses: a prospective cohort study within the UK collaborative trial of ovarian cancer screening (UKCTOCS). Ultrasound Obstet Gynecol 40: 338–344.
40. Alves G, Tatro A, Fanning T (1996) Differential methylation of human LINE-1 retrotransposons in malignant cells. Gene 176: 39–44.
41. Asch HL, Eliacin E, Fanning TG, Connolly JL, Bratthauer G, et al. (1996) Comparative expression of the LINE-1 p40 protein in human breast carcinomas and normal breast tissues. Oncol Res 8: 239–247.
42. Gualtieri A, Andreola F, Sciamanna I, Sinibaldi-Vallebona P, Serafino A, et al. (2013) Increased expression and copy number amplification of LINE-1 and SINE B1 retrotransposable elements in murine mammary carcinoma progression. Oncotarget 4: 1882–1893.
43. Soper SF, van der Heijden GW, Hardiman TC, Goodheart M, Martin SL, et al. (2008) Mouse maelstrom, a component of nuage, is essential for spermatogenesis and transposon repression in meiosis. Dev Cell 15: 285–297.
44. Bass BL (2002) RNA editing by adenosine deaminases that act on RNA. Annu Rev Biochem 71: 817–846.
45. Berasain C, Goni S, Castillo J, Latasa MU, Prieto J, et al. (2010) Impairment of pre-mRNA splicing in liver disease: mechanisms and consequences. World J Gastroenterol 16: 3091–3102.
46. Stahtea XN, Roussidis AE, Kanakis I, Tzanakakis GN, Chalkiadakis G, et al. (2007) Imatinib inhibits colorectal cancer cell growth and suppresses stromal-induced growth stimulation, MT1-MMP expression and pro-MMP2 activation. Int J Cancer 121: 2808–2814.
47. Gilles C, Polette M, Piette J, Munaut C, Thompson EW, et al. (1996) High level of MT-MMP expression is associated with invasiveness of cervical cancer cells. Int J Cancer 65: 209–213.
48. Cirri P, Chiarugi P (2011) Cancer associated fibroblasts: the dark side of the coin. Am J Cancer Res 1: 482–497.
49. Okada A, Bellocq JP, Rouyer N, Chenard MP, Rio MC, et al. (1995) Membrane-type matrix metalloproteinase (MT-MMP) gene is expressed in stromal cells of human colon, breast, and head and neck carcinomas. Proc Natl Acad Sci U S A 92: 2730–2734.
50. Brown DC, Gatter KC (2002) Ki67 protein: the immaculate deception? Histopathology 40: 2–11.
51. Janic A, Mendizabal L, Llamazares S, Rossell D, Gonzalez C (2010) Ectopic expression of germline genes drives malignant brain tumor growth in Drosophila. Science 330: 1824–1827.
52. Liang D, Dong M, Hu LJ, Fang ZH, Xu X, et al. (2013) Hiwi knockdown inhibits the growth of lung cancer in nude mice. Asian Pac J Cancer Prev 14: 1067–1072.
53. Liu L, Dai Y, Chen J, Zeng T, Li Y, et al. (2014) Maelstrom promotes hepatocellular carcinoma metastasis by inducing epithelial-mesenchymal transition by way of Akt/GSK-3beta/Snail signaling. Hepatology 59: 531–543.
54. Shahali M, Kabir-Salmani M, Nayernia K, Soleimanpour-Lichaei HR, Vasei M, et al. (2013) A novel in vitro model for cancer stem cell culture using ectopically expressed piwil2 stable cell line. Cell J 15: 250–257.
55. Sharma AK, Nelson MC, Brandt JE, Wessman M, Mahmud N, et al. (2001) Human CD34(+) stem cells express the hiwi gene, a human homologue of the Drosophila gene piwi. Blood 97: 426–434.
56. Lu ZY, Dong R, Li D, Li WB, Xu FQ, et al. (2012) SNAI1 overexpression induces stemness and promotes ovarian cancer cell invasion and metastasis. Oncol Rep 27: 1587–1591.

Label-Free LC-MS^e in Tissue and Serum Reveals Protein Networks Underlying Differences between Benign and Malignant Serous Ovarian Tumors

Wouter Wegdam[1]*, Carmen A. Argmann[2], Gertjan Kramer[3], Johannes P. Vissers[4], Marrije R. Buist[1], Gemma G. Kenter[1], Johannes M. F. G. Aerts[3], Danielle Meijer[1], Perry D. Moerland[5]

1 Department of Gynecology, Academic Medical Center, University of Amsterdam, Amsterdam, the Netherlands, **2** Department of Genetics and Genomic Sciences, Icahn Institute for Genomics and Multiscale Biology, Icahn School of Medicine at Mount Sinai, New York, New York, United States of America, **3** Clinical Proteomics Group, Department of Medical Biochemistry, Academic Medical Center, University of Amsterdam, Amsterdam, the Netherlands, **4** Waters Corporation MS Technologies Center, Manchester, United Kingdom, **5** Bioinformatics Laboratory, Department of Clinical Epidemiology, Biostatistics and Bioinformatics, Academic Medical Center, University of Amsterdam, Amsterdam, the Netherlands

Abstract

Purpose: To identify proteins and (molecular/biological) pathways associated with differences between benign and malignant epithelial ovarian tumors.

Experimental Procedures: Serum of six patients with a serous adenocarcinoma of the ovary was collected before treatment, with a control group consisting of six matched patients with a serous cystadenoma. In addition to the serum, homogeneous regions of cells exhibiting uniform histology were isolated from benign and cancerous tissue by laser microdissection. We subsequently employed label-free liquid chromatography tandem mass spectrometry (LC-MS^e) to identify proteins in these serum and tissues samples. Analyses of differential expression between samples were performed using Bioconductor packages and in-house scripts in the statistical software package R. Hierarchical clustering and pathway enrichment analyses were performed, as well as network enrichment and interactome analysis using MetaCore.

Results: In total, we identified 20 and 71 proteins that were significantly differentially expressed between benign and malignant serum and tissue samples, respectively. The differentially expressed protein sets in serum and tissue largely differed with only 2 proteins in common. MetaCore network analysis, however inferred GCR-alpha and Sp1 as common transcriptional regulators. Interactome analysis highlighted 14-3-3 zeta/delta, 14-3-3 beta/alpha, Alpha-actinin 4, HSP60, and PCBP1 as critical proteins in the tumor proteome signature based on their relative overconnectivity. The data have been deposited to the ProteomeXchange with identifier PXD001084.

Discussion: Our analysis identified proteins with both novel and previously known associations to ovarian cancer biology. Despite the small overlap between differentially expressed protein sets in serum and tissue, APOA1 and Serotransferrin were significantly lower expressed in both serum and cancer tissue samples, suggesting a tissue-derived effect in serum. Pathway and subsequent interactome analysis also highlighted common regulators in serum and tissue samples, suggesting a yet unknown role for PCBP1 in ovarian cancer pathophysiology.

Editor: Rossella Rota, Ospedale Pediatrico Bambino Gesu', Italy

Funding: The study was funded by the Academic Medical Center, University of Amsterdam. Co-author Johannes P. Vissers is employed by Waters Corporation (MS Technologies Center, Manchester, United Kingdom). Waters Corporation provided support in the form of salary for author Johannes P. Vissers. The specific role of this author is articulated in the 'author contributions' section. Both funders, Academic Medical Center and Waters Corporation, had no role in study design, data collection and analysis, decision to publish, or preparation of the manuscript.

Competing Interests: Johannes P. Vissers is employed by Waters Corporation. The methods described in the manuscript make use of the following Waters Corporation marketed products: a nanoAcquity system, a Synapt G2 MS mass spectrometer, ProteinLynx GlobalSERVER (PLGS) v2.5, Mass Prep Quantitation standard, and RapiGest SF. This does not alter the authors' adherence to all the PLOS ONE policies on sharing data and materials.

* Email: W.Wegdam@amc.uva.nl

Introduction

Epithelial ovarian cancer is the leading cause of gynecologic cancer deaths in the Western world [1]. Approximately 70% of epithelial ovarian cancers are detected at an advanced stage. Although about 80% of the patients have complete remission of the disease after treatment with extensive debulking surgery and chemotherapy, the recurrence rate is very high. Currently, there are no curative treatment options for patients with recurrent disease and the 5-year survival rate is less than 30% [1]. In order to improve upon this poor survival rate many studies have tried to identify more sensitive early detection markers and methods for discriminating between different pelvic masses [2,3]. A large number of these studies used various mass-spectrometric methods to search for new markers in patient material such as serum [4]. The OVA1 test, which has been approved by the Food and Drug Administration (FDA) in 2009, was one of the first multimarker diagnostic tests that resulted from this type of research [5]. However, when Moore et al. [6] evaluated several of these biomarkers alone and in combination with CA 125 in prediagnostically collected sera from women in the Prostate, Lung, Colorectal and Ovarian Cancer Screening trial the addition of these biomarkers to CA125 did not improve sensitivity for preclinical diagnosis. Other strategies involve a combination of known serum biomarkers such as Human Epididymal secretory protein 4 (HE4) and CA125 in a discriminatory algorithm such as ROMA (Risk of Ovarian Malignancy Algorithm) [7]. Most of the biomarkers being investigated or used in the clinic today are serum-based proteins, which are logical targets both for use as biomarkers for screening and diagnosis, as well as potential drug targets. However, most of the recently found biomarkers in serum or plasma are acute phase proteins that are not specific for one type of cancer or disease [8]. In fact, only a few FDA approved cancer markers in current clinical use are tumor-derived proteins (e.g., prostate-specific antigen, carcinoembryonic antigen), and are present in serum at very low concentrations (1-10 ng/mL) only [9]. In this study we have tried to overcome the problematic aspecific aspects of blood-based protein markers by aiming to identify proteins differentially expressed between tumor tissue samples of patients with a serous adenocarcinoma of the ovaries versus a benign serous tumor. In tumor tissue the potential marker proteins are present at much higher concentrations, which could facilitate protein identification. By comparing the protein content of tumor tissue with that of serum samples, we aimed to detect or infer reliable tumor-produced serum biomarkers. Directly studying tumor tissue, even though it enhances the probability of finding tumor-derived markers, is challenging nevertheless. Accurate analysis of tumors is often hampered by within-tumor heterogeneity, for example due to the presence of contaminating stroma cells, necrosis or infiltrating lymphocytes [10]. Laser microdissection minimizes this problem via the rapid and reliable isolation of a specific cell population or type from a tissue section under direct microscopic visualization [11,12].

Using laser microdissection we obtained homogenous tumor samples that were subsequently measured with a mass spectrometric approach called LC-MS^e. LC-MS^e differs from traditional data-dependent acquisition (DDA) modes in that all precursor and fragment ions are measured by alternating the collision energy between a low (precursor ions) and elevated (fragment ions) profile without selection of ions. Thus LC-MS^e is able to identify and quantify more peptides in complex samples using a single dimension reversed phase ultra-high pressure liquid chromatography (UPLC) separation, than DDA on quadrupole time-of-flight instruments (QTOF) [13,14].

The primary objective of the present study was to identify differentially expressed proteins in tissue and serum, comparing benign and malignant serous ovarian tumors. After initial protein identification we performed extensive pathway and network analyses in order to find differences in the underlying protein pathways associated with benign and malignant ovarian tumors.

Experimental Procedures

Patients and Ethics Statement

After written informed consent was obtained, serum and tissue samples were prospectively collected from patients admitted at the Academic Medical Center (AMC) for treatment of an ovarian tumor. The study was performed in agreement with the Helsinki Declaration and approved by the Ethical Committee at the Academic Medical Center, University of Amsterdam. For serum analysis, we included 6 patients that were newly diagnosed with non-familial invasive serous epithelial ovarian carcinoma, stage IIIB or higher based on FIGO (Fédération Internationale de Gynécologie Obstétrique) criteria, and 6 patients with benign serous cystadenomas. For 4 of the 6 patients with benign disease and 3 of the 6 with a malignant tumor, also tissue was available. To increase sample size for the tissue comparison, we included two additional patients with benign disease and two additional patients with a malignant tumor. Both in serum and tissue, the two groups were matched for age, body mass index (BMI), menopausal status and sample-storage duration. Clinicopathological data are listed in Table 1. All samples were collected using a strict protocol. Blood was collected from all patients by the same operator, at least two hours after the patient's last meal, and left to clot for 30 minutes. After centrifugation (at 1750×g) serum was immediately frozen and stored at -80°C. Samples used for these experiments were only thawed once.

Laser microdissection and protein isolation

During surgery tumor tissue was collected, snap frozen in liquid nitrogen, and stored at −80°C within 30 minutes of surgery. From these samples 10 μm cryostat sections were prepared. One section was stained with hematoxylin and examined microscopically in order to detect tissue areas of interest for microdissection. Corresponding consecutive tissue sections were mounted on a microscope slide coated with a membrane (polyethylene naphtalate (PEN) Zeiss/Palm, Bernried, Germany) and stored at −80°C. Comparison of stained and unstained tissue sections revealed that hematoxylin staining had no influence on the quantitative protein measurements and identification using LC-MS^e.

Tissue areas were cut using a Veritas Microdissection System (Arcturus Molecular Devices, CA, USA), as described earlier [15]. Slides were stained for 1 minute with hematoxylin. Dissected cancer samples contained at least 90% cancer cells (Figure 1). Using microdissection, the samples from benign cystadenomas were enriched for 75%–90% epithelial cells.

We obtained 100,000 cells from each sample. Cells were denatured in 20 μl 0,1% RapiGest detergent solution (Waters Corp., Milford, MA) and heated at 80°C for 15 minutes. After centrifugation at 1750×g for 10 min, the supernatants were collected. Several tests were performed to determine optimal lysis conditions. Protein concentrations were measured using a Bicinchoninic Acid (BCA) solution (Sigma-Aldrich Chemie GmbH, Schnelldorf, Germany) and 4% CuSO4. The average protein concentration obtained from 100.000 cells was 1 mg/ml.

Sample preparation for LC-MS analysis

Serum samples were diluted in 50 mM ammoniumhydrogencarbonate (Fluka), 1% RapiGest SF (Waters Corp., Milford, MA) to ~10 μg/μl total protein concentration. Laser dissected tissue samples were lysed in 50 mM ammoniumhydrogencarbonate, 0.1% RapiGest SF, prior to protein determination by BCA-assay (Thermo-Scientific) according to the manufacturer's protocol. Subsequently serum samples were denatured at 80°C for 15 min and tissue samples at 95°C for 10 min prior to reduction of

Table 1. Patients characteristics.

	Serum		Tissue	
	Malignant	*Benign*	*Malignant*	*Benign*
Patients	6	6	5	6
Age (mean, SD)	53 (16.5)	57 (7.2)	51 (15.2)	56 (9.8)
BMI (mean, SD)	25 (4.9)	25 (5.1)	23 (3.3)	26 (4.8)
Pre-menopausal	3	1	2	2
Post-menopausal	3	5	3	4
CA125 kU/L (median, range)	6946 (113–14100)	12 (7–26)	2651 (113–7737)	70 (7–376)
Differentiation grade				
2	1		1	
3	5		4	
Figo Stage				
III	5		5	
IV	1			

Clinicopathological characteristics of the patient groups. SD: standard deviation.

disulfide bridges 5 mM dithiorthreitol at 60°C for 30 min. Free sulfhydryl groups were alkylated by addition of 15 mM iodoaceteamide and incubation at ambient temperature for 30 min. in the dark. Samples were digested overnight by addition of 0.3 activity units/µg total protein content of sequencing grade modified trypsin (Promega, Madison WI) and incubation overnight at 37°C. Following digestion the acid-labile detergent was hydrolyzed by incubation in the presence of 0.5% trifluoroaceticacid (Biosolve, the Netherlands) at 37°C for 45 min and removal of immiscible debris by centrifugation at 20.000×g for 10 min, collecting the supernatant. Prior to analyses, serum digest samples were diluted with aqueous 0.1% formic acid solution (Biosolve, the Netherlands) to ~0.5 µg/µl total protein concentration. Subsequently both serum digest and tissue digest samples were mixed 1:1 with a Mass Prep Quantitation standard (Waters, Milford MA) for quantitation purposes (mix with either 100 fmol/µl Enolase or Alcohol dehydrogenase 1 from *S. cerevisiae* for tissue samples or 250 fmol/µl ClpB from *Escherichia coli* for serum samples).

LC-MS analysis

0.5 µg of total protein was loaded onto a Nano-Acquity system (Waters Corporation) equipped with a Bridged Ethyl Hybrid C18 1.7 µm, 15-cm×150-µm analytical reversed phase column (Waters Corporation) and operated at a column flow rate of 1 µl/min. All samples were measured in triplicate. Apart from the column dimension and flow rate, all other gradient conditions were as detailed earlier [14]. Analysis of tryptic peptides was performed using a Synapt G2 quadrupole time of flight mass spectrometer (Waters Corporation, Manchester, UK) with the operating and experimental conditions as previously described [14]. Accurate mass precursor and fragment ion LC-MS data were collected in data-independent MS^e mode of acquisition. This method alternates the energy applied to the collision cell of the mass spectrometer between a low and elevated energy state [16,17]. Briefly, the low energy portion of the obtained data sets is typically used for quantification of the proteins, whereas the combined low and elevated energy information are utilized for identification purposes. In both modes of acquisition, mass spectral information was obtained from *m/z* 50 to 1990 at a resolving power of at least 10,000 full width half maximum.

Data processing and protein identification

Continuum LC-MS^e data were processed and searched using ProteinLynx Globalserver version 2.5 (PLGS 2.5, Waters Corporation). Protein identifications were obtained with the embedded ion accounting algorithm [18] of the software and searching the

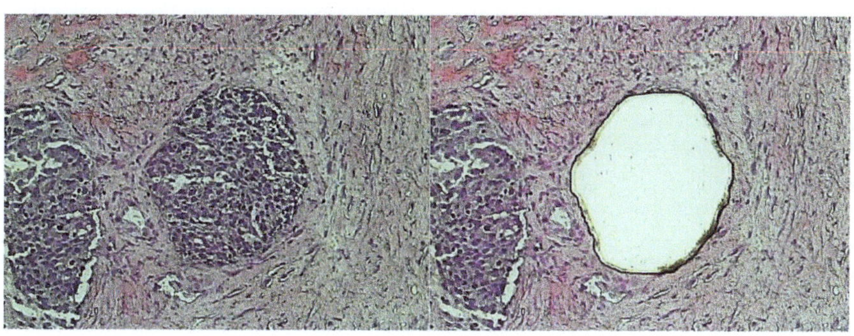

Figure 1. Laser capture microdissection of tumor tissue. A 10 µm hematoxylin stained cryostat section of a serous adenocarcinoma of the ovaries. The picture on the left is prior to microdissection, on right the same slide after microdissection is shown.

human SwissProt entries of the UniProt database (release 13.2) that was modified to include N-terminal processing of proteins using the protein maturation device software [19] and to which enolase and alcohol dehydrogenase 1 of *S. cerevisiae* or ClpB from *Escherichia coli* were appended as the internal standard to provide the ability to address technical variation and to accommodate concentration determinations [13]. The search tolerances were set to automatic, typically 10 ppm for precursor and 25 ppm for product ions, cysteine carbamidomethylation specified as a fixed modification and N-terminal acetylation, deamidation of asparagine and glutamine and oxidation of methionine as variable modifications. Estimation of false positive identification rates was performed by searches in a shuffled version of the UniProt human protein database generated in PGLS 2.5. Robust criteria were applied for quantification, including the identification of minimally three and seven product ion matches per peptide and protein, respectively. In addition, at least two peptides per protein had to be identified and the identification had to occur in at least two independent patient serum or tissue samples. Protein false positive identification rate, taking into account the criteria mentioned above, was less than one percent. Label free quantitation of proteins was based on the sum of the signal intensities of the three most abundant peptides of a protein, divided by the sum of the signal intensities of the three most abundant peptides of the internal standard, times the amount in fmol of standard injected on the column. This gives an estimation of the molar amount of each protein injected on the column. PLGS 2.5 determines the molar amount (the amount in ng is determined using the molecular weight in the database) for each protein based on the ratio of its three most abundant peptides (HI3) determined in each individual experiment [13]. These measured amounts were used for proteins that met the criteria for identification indicated above in order to calculate the average concentration of each protein in g/L using the dilution factor of the samples. Protein identity and quantitative data were exported as a comma separated value file for further statistical and pathway analysis. The mass spectrometry proteomics data have been deposited to the ProteomeXchange consortium (http://proteomecentral.proteomexchange.org) [20] via the PRIDE partner repository with the dataset identifier PXD001084. A list of filenames deposited in ProteomeXchange and their corresponding sample annotation can be found in the supporting information section (Table S1, worksheet 'Filenames').

Statistical analyses

Statistical analyses were performed using Bioconductor packages and in-house scripts in the statistical software package R [21]. Serum and tissue data were analyzed separately. Missing values in the raw quantitative data were imputed with the minimum value measured for the sample in which the missing value occurred. Data were scale normalized to the same mean intensity across samples; resulting values were then log2-transformed with an offset of 1 in order to stabilize their variance. The array Quality Metrics R package was used to assess whether all MS samples were of good quality. The tissue samples were measured in two separate batches; quality control clearly showed the presence of a pronounced batch effect in the normalized data. Tissue data were made comparable across batches by fitting a linear model, including both batches and regular conditions, and removing the component due to the batch effects (function 'removeBatchEffect' from the R package limma). After normalization and batch correction (tissue study), the technical replicate samples for each patient were highly similar. A more detailed description of the quality control analysis is given in Text S1. The technical replicates of the batch corrected data were averaged and resulting data was used for hierarchical clustering analyses. For benign tissue sample 4 only two technical replicates were used for data analyses due to technical problems with the third measurement.

For each identified protein a linear model was fit on the normalized data containing the two conditions (benign and malignant) as explanatory variable; for the tissue study a batch factor was also included in the linear model. A consensus between-replicate correlation was estimated for the technical replicates (function 'duplicateCorrelation' from the R package limma) and included in the linear model fit. Differentially expressed proteins between benign and malignant tumors were detected using a moderated t-test. P-values were adjusted for multiple-testing using the Benjamini-Hochberg false discovery rate [22]. Proteins were considered to be significantly differentially expressed between the two conditions with an adjusted $p\text{-value}<0.05$, and a fold change ≤ -1.4 or ≥ 1.4. Moreover, the protein had to be present before imputation in at least 50% of the samples in at least one of the two conditions.

Hierarchical clustering and enrichment analyses

Two-dimensional clustering (Pearson correlation, average linkage) was performed on protein expression values using the function 'heatmap.2' from the R package gplots [23]. The Cytoscape plugin "ClueGO" v2.0.2 was used for protein set enrichment analysis by uploading the list of proteins with their UniProt IDs and using a custom background reference set consisting of all proteins detected in the experiment. [24,25]. For exploratory pathway enrichment analyses a less stringent cutoff, using an unadjusted p-value less than 0.05 was used. Lists of serum or tumor proteins differentially expressed between malignant and benign cases were submitted for protein set enrichment analysis according to the gene ontology (GO) biological process domain. Within ClueGO we used the 'compare lists' feature and compared protein set enrichment (one-sided hypergeometric test) for the differentially expressed serum and tumor proteomes simultaneously. The edges of the resulting ClueGO network are based on kappa statistics and reflect the relationships between the GO terms (network nodes) based on the similarity of their associated proteins.

Protein accession numbers and their corresponding fold changes were imported into the web-based integrative software MetaCore (v 6.8 build 30387; Thomson Reuters, St. Joseph, MI) for network analysis [26]. MetaCore analysis was used for network enrichment and interactome analysis using the differentially expressed proteins (unadjusted $p\text{-value}<0.05$) in either the serum or tissue samples of benign versus malignant samples with the background reference set consisting of all proteins detected in the experiment. Relative connectivity of proteins inside a set (intra-connectivity) and between a set and the global interactome (inter-connectivity) were calculated using MetaCore protein interaction database. A ranking of importance was given by using a "knowledge-based" analysis that considers the differentially expressed proteins in the context of their known interactors in complex protein and molecular networks.

Results

Hierarchical clustering of serum and tissue proteome

In total, we identified 84 proteins in serum and 209 in tissue, which were present in at least 50% of the samples in at least one of the conditions (benign or malignant) (Table S1). Of those proteins 20 and 71 were significantly differentially expressed between benign and malignant disease in serum and tissue samples, respectively (Figure 2). Only 16 proteins were detected in both

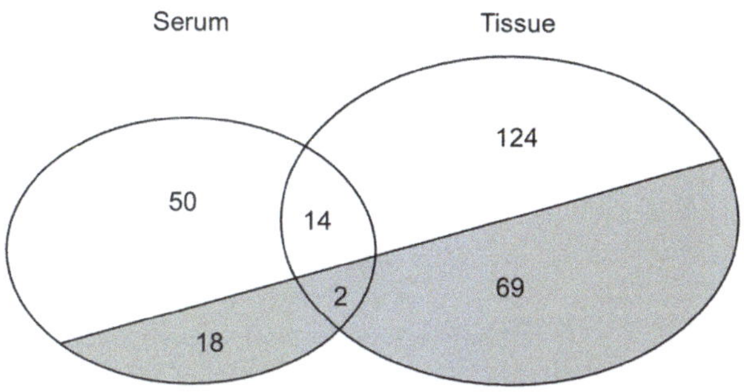

Figure 2. Venn diagram of the detected proteins. We detected a total of 84 proteins in serum and 209 in tissue, present in at least 50% of the samples in at least one of the conditions (benign or malignant). The grey area represents the proteins with an adjusted p-value of <0.05 when comparing benign with malignant.

serum and tissue samples (highlighted in yellow in Table S1). Of these, only two proteins had an adjusted p-value of <0.05, Apolipoprotein A-I and Serotransferrin.

Hierarchical cluster analysis was used to group serum and tumor samples according to the similarity of their expression profiles. Clustering the 84 and 209 proteins detected in serum and tumor samples respectively, could perfectly separate the benign and the malignant tumors (Figure 3). This illustrates that malignancy was the strongest signal in this dataset and that the benign and malignant samples constitute well-defined groups that could reveal differences in underlying biology between the processes leading to malignancy. This result also supported our methodology in which we minimized heterogeneity by going through detailed patient and sample selection and by micro-dissecting the tumor tissue.

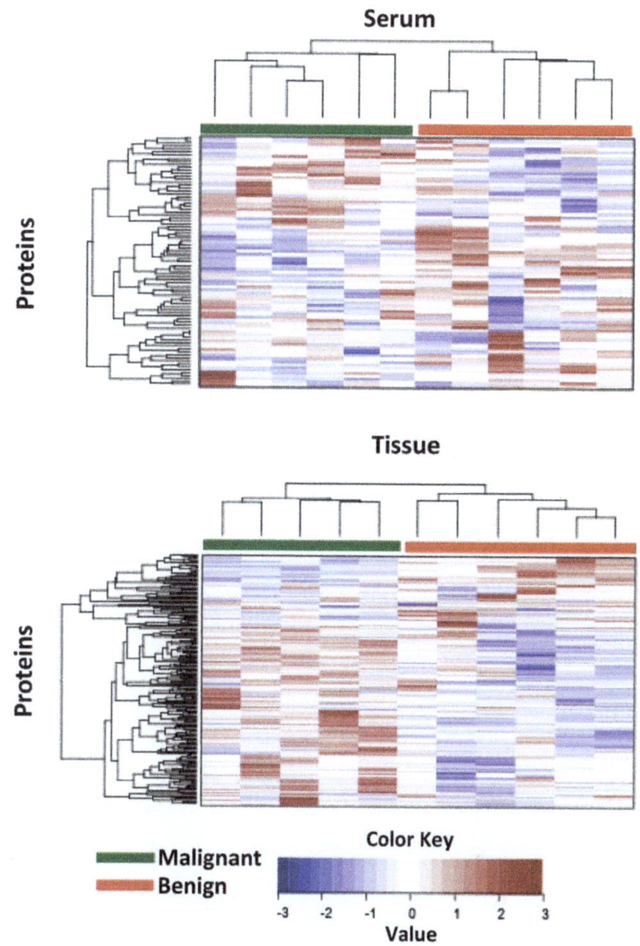

Figure 3. Unsupervised hierarchical clustering. Unsupervised hierarchical clustering was performed of the 84 and 209 proteins detected in serum and tumor tissue samples, respectively. The key color bar indicates standardized protein expression levels (dark red indicates relatively higher expression; dark blue indicates relatively lower expression).

Biological functions and networks enriched in serum and tumor signatures between malignant and benign samples

To explore and compare the biological processes that contribute to changes of the serum and tumor proteome during ovarian cancer development, a protein set biological enrichment analysis was performed on the differentially expressed protein signatures derived from the serum and tissue comparisons. The serum proteome signature was significantly enriched in categories associated with immune function and lipoprotein metabolism. In contrast, the tumor proteome signature was significantly enriched in categories associated with glucose metabolism and the unfolded protein response (Figure 4; Bonferroni corrected p-value<0.05). Interestingly, there is little overlap in the biological processes enriched in serum and tissue signatures. The proteins associated with these protein sets and the relevant statistics are summarized in Table S2.

Key transcriptional regulatory networks in ovarian cancer

We subjected the lists of differentially expressed serum and tissue proteins to the transcriptional regulation network algorithm in MetaCore. This was used to infer potentially important transcription factors in the carcinogenic process. Summaries of the top scoring transcriptional regulatory networks and the key associated transcription factors in respectively serum and tissue are shown in Table S3. The most significant transcriptional regulatory network in serum was GCR-alpha (glucocorticoid receptor alpha) signaling. Eleven proteins that are upstream or downstream of GCR-alpha signaling were found differentially expressed in the serum of patients with a serous adenocarcinoma of the ovaries compared to patients with a serous cystadenoma. The pathways linked to GCR-alpha signaling may explain regulation of the acute inflammatory response that was seen altered in the cancer patients. In the tumor tissue, GCR-alpha was also highlighted in the top scoring transcriptional networks although associated with pathways related to cellular localization and protein folding (Table S3). Figure 5A summarizes, which proteins in our dataset are potentially regulated by GCR-alpha. Interestingly, despite the limited overlap in terms of differentially expressed proteins (Figure 2) and significantly enriched biological processes (Figure 4), two GCR-alpha target proteins, ApoA-1 and Serotransferrin, were present in the signatures of both the serum and the tumor proteome (Figure 5A). These results suggest that the serum cancer proteome could be used to detect changes in GCR-alpha tumor associated processes.

Sp1 was associated with the third top scoring transcriptional network in tumor tissue (Table S3) after the well-known cancer-related transcription factor c-Myc and also CREB-1 that was recently found to be associated with OVCA cell line platinum sensitivity and overall survival [27]. Sp1 was also associated with the top scoring transcriptional networks in the cancerous serum

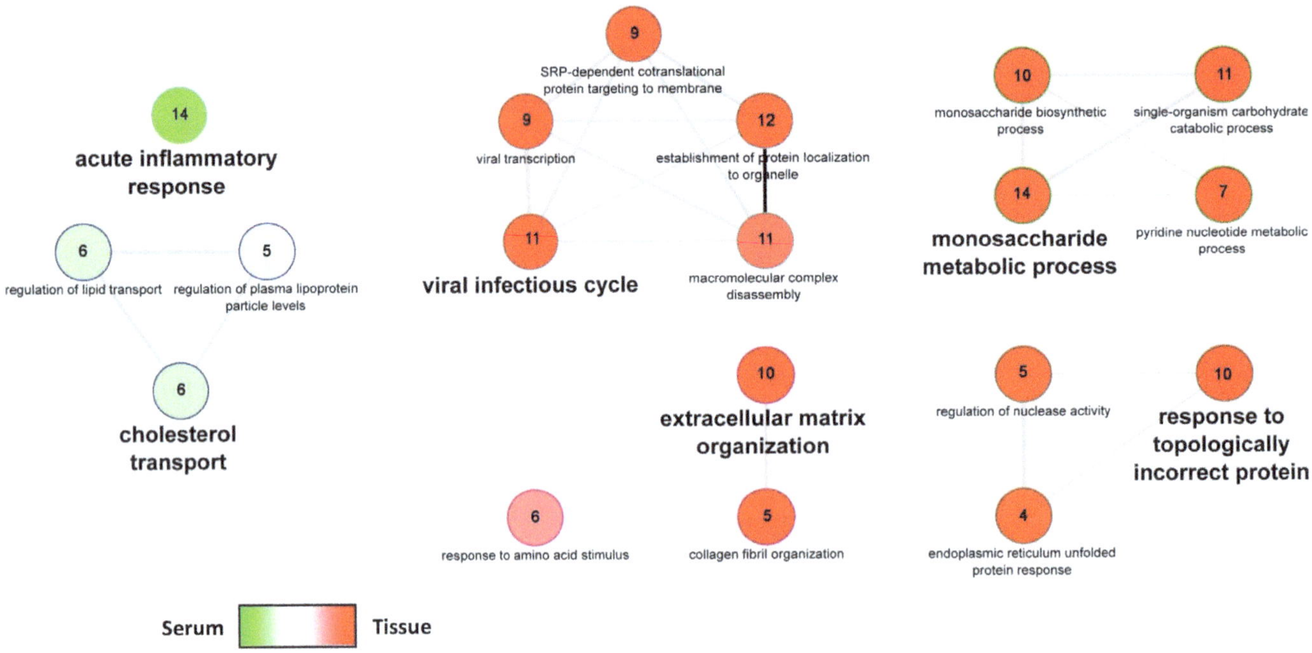

Figure 4. Protein set enrichment analysis using the Cytoscape plugin 'ClueGO'. In the network, only significantly enriched categories (p-value<0.05, Bonferroni corrected) are shown. The node color represents the commonality of members of either the differentially expressed serum or tumor proteome list. Dark red highlights categories that are specific to the tissue proteome signature while dark green represents biological processes that are specific to the serum proteome signature. The number of proteins associated with each GO category are indicated within the corresponding node. The edges of the resulting ClueGO network are based on kappa statistics and reflect the relationships between the GO terms (network nodes) based on the similarity of their associated proteins. The complete results and relevant statistics are summarized in Table S2.

signature. In total, 32 proteins associated with the Sp1 transcriptional pathway were differentially expressed between benign and malignant tissue samples (Figure 5B). Biological processes associated with Sp1 included several pathways related to lipid metabolism such as regulation of cholesterol and sterol transport, and acute-phase response and response to endogenous stimulus. This suggests that this transcriptional regulator might be an important contributor to the metabolic reprogramming that occurs within the tumor as highlighted by our ontology analysis (Figure 4).

Overlap between candidate key-regulatory transcription factors in serum and tumor tissue as highlighted by the transcriptional regulatory network analysis was far greater than at the individual protein level. Nine of the top-20 significantly associated transcription factors in serum were also found in the top-20 of tumor tissue, among them well known cancer-associated transcription factors such as p53 and c-Jun.

Key proteins differentially expressed between benign and malignant ovarian tumors

In an attempt to move beyond transcriptional regulation and find other regulatory proteins that are statistically significantly "overconnected" within our proteomics signatures, we subjected the list of differentially expressed proteins in ovarian tumor samples to "interactome analysis by protein function". This helps in prioritizing potentially relevant individual proteins or hubs. Table 2 summarizes the results of the interactome analysis. Only five proteins were found to be significantly over-connected in the tumor proteome signature namely, PCBP1, 14-3-3 zeta, 14-3-3 beta, alpha actinin-4, and HSP60 (CH60/HSPD-1). These proteins were significantly upregulated in malignant tumors and have all been linked to cancer previously and all but one, PCBP1, specifically to ovarian cancer.

To further investigate the role of PCBP1 in ovarian cancer, we retrieved the transcriptional profiles of an independent ovarian cancer dataset containing 30 tumors of low malignant potential and 60 serous ovarian cancer tumor samples [28] available at Gene Expression Omnibus (http://www.ncbi.nlm.nih.gov/geo/; accession no. GSE12172). Compared to low malignant potential tumors, there was a significant increase in PCBP1 gene expression in malignant ovarian tumors (Figure 6). Furthermore, OncoPrints from the cBioportal for Cancer Genomics (http://www.cbioportal.org) showed that about 10% of all serous malignant ovarian tumors had an altered PCBP1 mRNA expression (data not shown) [29]. The combined observations of elevated protein expression of PCBP1, with the computational analysis highlighting over-representation of PCBP1 protein interactions in this study, as well as the elevated gene expression in a microarray dataset, are suggestive of a role of PCBP1 in ovarian tumor biology, a previously unreported finding.

Discussion

In order to identify proteins and pathways underlying the differences between benign and malignant ovarian tumors, we performed a comparative proteomic analysis of ovarian tumor tissue and serum, from a limited number of patients using a combination of LC-MS^{e} label-free mass-spectrometry and extensive bioinformatics analyses. Our control group consisted of patients with a benign ovarian tumor instead of healthy women. Therefore, the proteins differentially expressed in our study are more likely to be ovarian tumor-specific instead of reflecting a more general response to disease. We further enhanced robustness

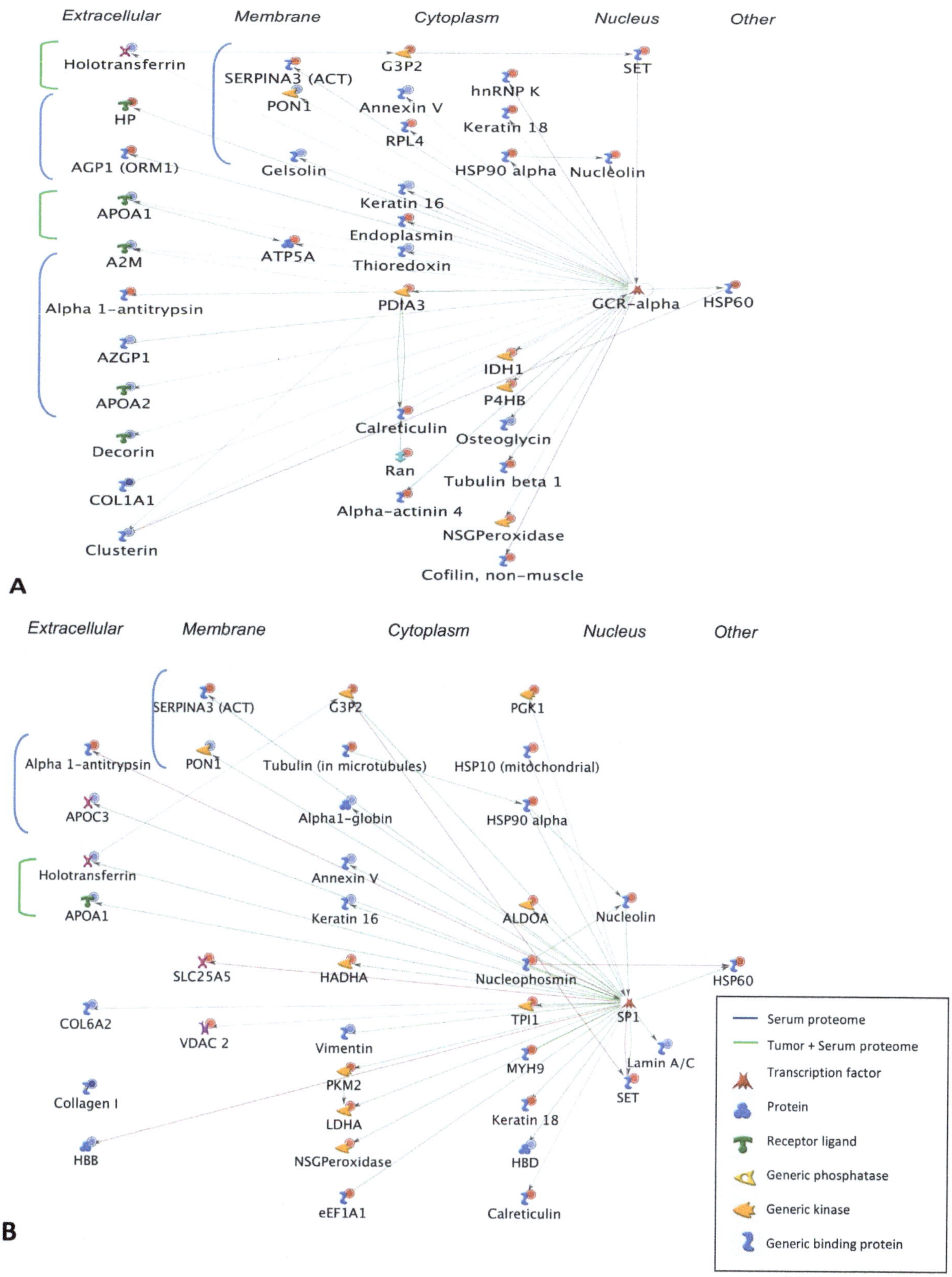

Figure 5. Proteins in the serum and tumor datasets that are potentially associated with GCR-alpha (A) and SP1 (B) pathways. The proteins marked in blue were found in the serum dataset, those marked in green in both tumor and serum. Unmarked proteins are specific for the tumor signature (except GCR-alpha and SP1). Proteins are ordered according to their position within the cell (extracellular, membrane bound, cytoplasmic or nucleic). Individual proteins are represented as nodes, the different shapes of the nodes represent the functional class of the proteins. The arrowheads indicate the direction of the interaction, the color of the lines between nodes describes activation (green), inhibition (red), and unspecified (black) interactions. The small circles on top of the protein symbols indicate up-regulation (red) or down-regulation (blue).

Table 2. Interactions by protein function.

Protein	Actual	n	R	N	Expected	Ratio	p-value	z-score
PCBP-1	11	108	13	296	4.743	2.319	0.000402	3.68
Alpha-actinin 4	14	108	19	296	6.932	2.019	0.000754	3.476
HSP60	17	108	27	296	9.851	1.726	0.003122	2.993
14-3-3 beta/alpha	34	108	56	296	20.43	1.664	3.71E-05	4.176
14-3-3 zeta/delta	55	108	97	296	35.39	1.554	5.33E-07	5.035

Interactions by protein function based on the connectivity with the tumor tissue signatures and with proteins from the human proteome MetaCore database. The proteins were considered over-connected when the number of observed interactions exceeded the number of expected interactions. Actual: number of network objects in the signature which interact with the chosen object; n: number of network objects in the signature; R: number of network objects in the background list which interact with the chosen object; N: total number of protein-based objects in the background list; Expected: mean of hypergeometric distribution. Ratio: connectivity ratio (Actual/Expected); z-score: (Actual-Expected)/(standard deviation); p-value: probability to have the value of Actual or higher (lower for negative z-score) by chance under null hypothesis of no over- or under-connectivity.

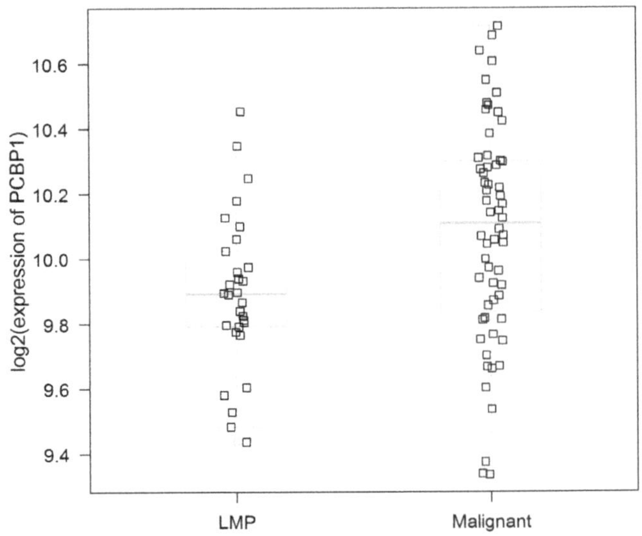

Figure 6. PCBP1 expression in serous ovarian cancer. Expression of PCBP1 (probeset 208620_at) in serous tumors of low malignant potential (LMP) versus malignant serous ovarian tumors [28]. PCBP1 was significantly up-regulated (p = 0.003, Welch's t-test) in malignant tumors. Squares represent the individual samples used in the microarray experiment. Boxplots are overlaid with the lower and upper ends of a box indicating the 25th and 75th percentiles, respectively. The solid black line inside a box indicates the median.

of our results by using well matched patient groups and by reducing within-tumor heterogeneity via the use of laser micro-dissected tumor tissue lysates. In addition we used strict experimental protocols, extensive quality control and state-of-the-art bioinformatics analyses to control for false positive results.

Our study revealed a large number of changes in protein expression in serum and tissue from patients suffering from benign and malignant ovarian tumors. Some proteins were already known to play a role in ovarian cancer, others are new candidates, which may provide new insights into the etiology of the disease or act as potential new disease markers. For a large subset of proteins identified in this study, literature searches confirmed their role in ovarian cancer. For example, Dieplinger et. al. also measured decreased plasma concentrations of Afamin and APOA4 in patients with ovarian cancer, with APOA4 adding independent diagnostic information to CA125 and age for differentiating ovarian cancer from benign and healthy samples [30]. The observed reduction in serum of PON1, that usually mediates enzymatic protection against oxidative stress, may lead to increasing DNA damage and consequently to malignant transformation. It has been suggested before, that SNPs reducing PON1 activity may be associated with an increased risk of epithelial ovarian cancer [31]. In addition, we found a significant decrease of APOA1 in serum of ovarian cancer patients as has been shown before in various studies [32,33] and in tissue. To our knowledge this significant decrease in tumor tissue samples has not been described yet. The altered serum signature, which is also enriched for other proteins involved in cholesterol and lipid metabolism, suggests that an alteration of these pathways may be beneficial for the cancer cells.

Although substantial efforts have been devoted to detect new serum biomarkers for ovarian cancer, we are the first to describe proteomic analysis in both serum and tissue. This approach may lead to detection of serum proteins directly derived from the tumor, which can give new insights in the pathways active in benign and malignant disease. Only 16 proteins were identified in both serum and tissue, however, with only Apolipoprotein A-I and Serotransferrin being significantly differentially expressed in both. This limited overlap is probably due to the fact that we only detect abundant proteins in both serum and tissue and that abundant tissue proteins have a different concentration in serum and vice versa. Some of the detected proteins are also compartment specific, and therefore only detectable in serum or tissue.

In order to see whether there might be similarities in significantly enriched processes or altered transcription factors within the serum and tissue datasets we performed enrichment analyses using MetaCore. This analysis revealed that 9 out of the top-20 transcription factors associated with key transcriptional regulatory networks in serum were also found in the top-20 of tumor tissue. These results indicate that although the detected proteins only overlap to a limited extent between the 2 datasets, the detected tumor cancer proteome is reflected by the serum proteome at the molecular subnetwork level. This approach may provide another strategy for biomarker discovery.

Amongst others Sp1 and GCR-alpha were detected as potential key transcription factors of the key transcriptional regulatory networks underlying the proteomic signatures in both tissue and serum. The protein encoded by the Sp1 gene is a zinc finger transcription factor that binds to GC-rich motifs of many promoters. It is involved in many cellular processes, including cell differentiation, cell growth, apoptosis, immune response, response to DNA damage, and chromatin remodeling [34]. Post-translational modifications such as phosphorylation, acetylation, glycosylation, and proteolytic processing significantly affect the activity of this protein, which can be an activator or a repressor. Sp1 has been suggested to be responsible for many features of ovarian cancer cells like oncogenic transformation and epithelial to mesenchymal transition for example through activation of KLF8 [35]. Expression of Sp1 is frequently increased in human epithelial ovarian cancers and inhibitors of Sp1-dependent transcription both in vitro and in tumor xenografts have been suggested as interesting candidates for treatment [36].

Receptors for glucocorticoids, like GCR-alpha, are present in tumor cells of almost 90% of ovarian cancer cells and mRNA of GCR-alpha was detected in a wide range of ovarian cancer cell lines [37]. In vitro studies suggests that glucocorticoids may have an adverse effect on outcome in several cancers, including ovarian [38]. However, other investigators have reported favorable effects of GCs in vitro [39]. A study in GCR-positive patients gave no evidence that GCR expression had any prognostic value nor was there any evidence of poorer survival in a small subset of GCR-positive patients who received GC treatment [40]. A recent study has discovered a role for the glucocorticoid receptor within the SLIT glycoprotein ligand and their ROBO receptor pathway. This pathway plays a fundamental role in mammalian development by promoting apoptosis and repulsing aberrant cell migration. SLIT/ROBO expression could be increased by reducing the expression of the glucocorticoid receptor using siRNA. Their findings indicate that in the post-ovulatory phase a role of cortisol may be to temporarily inhibit SLIT/ROBO expression to facilitate regeneration of the ovarian surface epithelium. Therefore this pathway may be a target to develop strategies to manipulate the SLIT/ROBO system in ovarian cancer [41].

Interactome analysis revealed 5 proteins that were significantly overconnected in our tumor tissue signature, meaning they had more connections within the tumor signature than expected by chance and thus are potentially highly relevant in tumor pathophysiology. Two of those, 14-3-3 beta/alpha and 14-3-3 zeta/delta, are members of the 14-3-3 protein family which have been described in previous studies to promote cell survival through suppression of apoptosis [42]. Due to its upregulation in a variety of human tumors and its involvement in cancer progression and treatment resistance, 14-3-3 zeta is currently undergoing extensive investigation as a novel therapeutic target [43].

The other overconnected proteins were actinin-4, HSP60, and PCBP1. Actinin-4 is an isoform of non-muscular-actinin, which enhances cell motility by bundling the actin cytoskeleton [44]. Implications of actinin-4 have been demonstrated in some human malignancies including ovarian cancer. Yamamoto *et al.* have demonstrated high actinin-4 protein expression in 57% of the primary ovarian carcinomas [45,46]. High expression was associated with serous histology, high histological grade, and poor patient outcome.

Heat shock proteins (HSPs), like HSP60, are important players in protein homeostasis and cell and tissue physiology, as well as in protection against stressors [47]. HSPs intervene not only in protein folding, refolding, trafficking and degradation but also in the regulation of cell growth and differentiation, apoptosis and cell-to-cell crosstalk, inflammation, and tissue repair [47,48]. The importance of HSPs has come into focus in the past few years because it has been realized that they can be pathogenic factors in a variety of conditions. Among these pathologies there are various forms of cancer, in which the proteins are normal but work in favor of the tumor rather than protect the patient [49]. In these conditions, HSPs enhance tumor cell survival and growth by inhibiting apoptosis and the anti-tumor immune response, or by promoting neoangiogenesis [50]. In our study, several of the HSPs had altered expression. Besides the overconnected HSP60, six HSP family members were found to be upregulated in the malignant tissue samples, further highlighting their importance in ovarian cancer biology.

The fifth overconnected protein, PCBP1, was originally discovered as an RNA-binding protein, which participates in mRNA processing at multiple steps. Subsequent studies showed that PCBP1 possesses multiple functions in transcription, splicing, and translation. The protein is capable of switching among its various functions depending upon its state of phosphorylation as well as its cellular localization, and can therefore act as a corepressor and a coactivator in response to different environmental signals [51]. In the cBioPortal database, almost all neighboring genes connected to PCBP1 have altered expression in more than 20% of the serous ovarian cancer samples (data not shown) providing further evidence of a critical role for PCBP1 in the pathophysiological processes underlying malignant ovarian tumors. Importantly, we further implicated PCBP1 within ovarian tumor biology by the fact that the network built in MetaCore using the 5 overconnected proteins as seed notes and their nearest neighbors, generated a network highly interconnecting all 5 seed nodes. The results of this network analysis also revealed an interesting connection to the androgen receptor-signaling pathway (Figure 7). As PCBP1 has been previously found to regulate the androgen receptor in androgen-responsive cells, like the prostate cancer LNCaP cells [52], this connection might be underlying the function of PCBP1 in ovarian tumor biology as well. Overall this network analysis, which attempts to reconstruct the biological mechanism underlying the proteomics profile, provides further mechanistic insights for future validation as well as potential targets of intervention.

In summary, by quantifying protein expression in serum and tissue we found proteins differentially expressed between benign and malignant samples. These included proteins previously identified to play a role in ovarian cancer, but also candidates

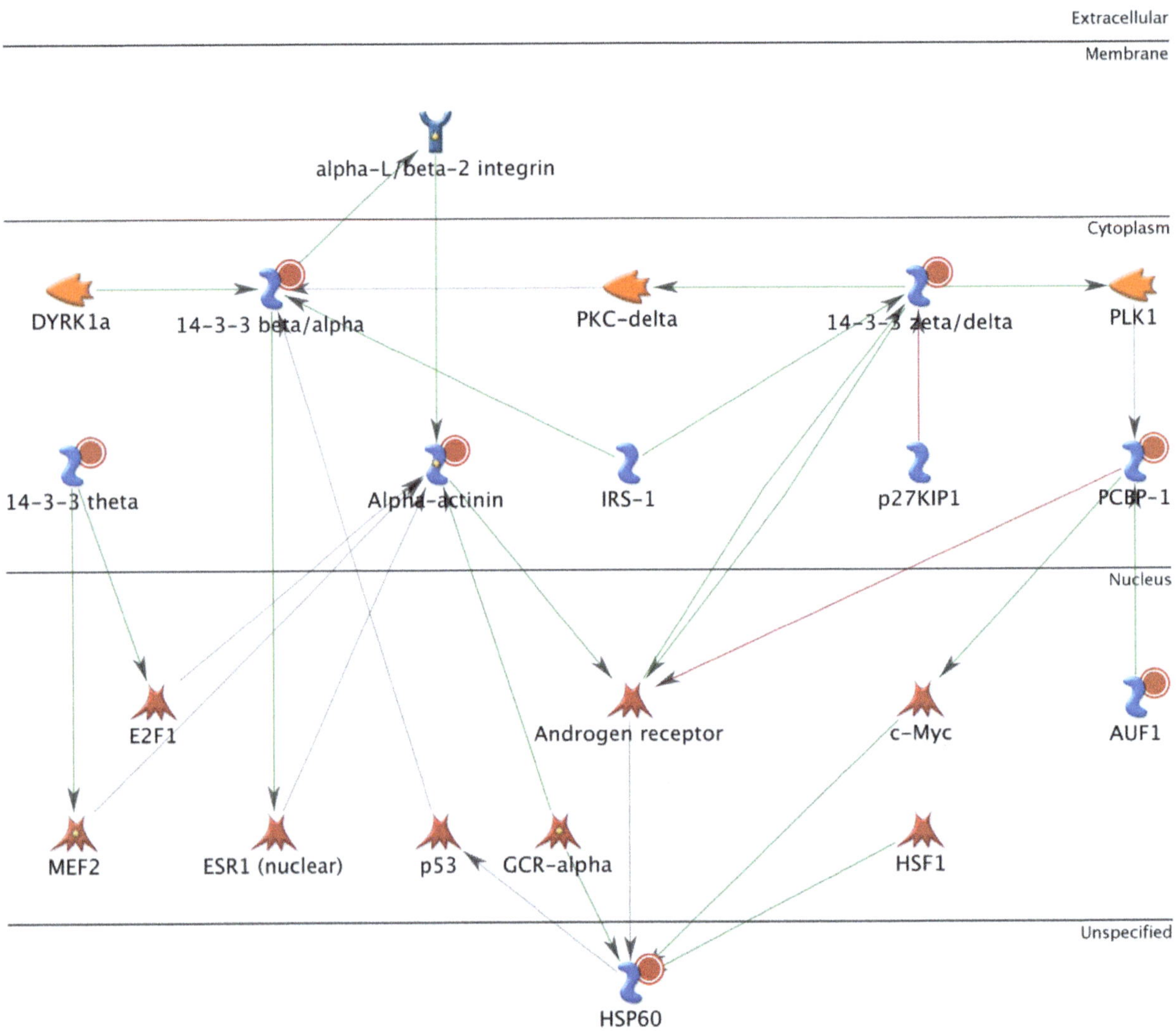

Figure 7. Interactions between overconnected proteins in tumor tissue. A network built in MetaCore using the 5 overconnected proteins, PCBP-1, Alpha-actinin 4, HSP60, 14-3-3 beta/alpha and 14-3-3 zeta/delta as seed nodes yielded a highly interconnected network amongst the seed nodes and implicated a role for androgen receptor signaling.

that had not been implicated in the disease process before. We observed not only a significant decrease in serum APOAI and Serotransferrin, as previously reported, but provide evidence for decreased expression in the tumor site as well. Although the serum and tissue signatures had only 16 proteins in common, we highlighted common transcription factors potentially relevant for changes in both the serum and tumor proteome through in-silico analyses. Important roles are suggested for GCR-alpha and Sp1. In addition, our results implicate an as yet unknown role for PCBP1 in ovarian cancer. We hypothesize that the protein network including PCBP1 contributes to the malignant properties of ovarian tumors, possibly through regulation of the androgen receptor. Further experiments are warranted to unravel the precise mechanism of PCBP1 in ovarian cancer.

Supporting Information

Table S1 List of proteins identified in serum and tissue of ovarian cancer vs. benign patients. List of file names as reported in ProteomeXchange with the corresponding sample annotation in worksheet named 'Filenames'. List of all the measured samples with a complete list of protein identifications in worksheet named 'Raw data' together with separate worksheets containing the filtered data named 'Serum (filtered)' and 'Tissue (filtered)'. Detailed information on the annotation of the proteins and the outcome of the differential expression analysis is provided.

Table S2 Protein set enrichment analysis using the Cytoscape plugin "ClueGO". The proteins associated with significant GO categories are displayed as well as the p-value associated with the GO term. The first four categories are mostly specific to the serum proteome signature while the other categories represent biological processes that are mainly specific to the tissue proteome signature.

Table S3 Serum and tissue transcriptional regulation network list. The column 'GO processes' states the different biological processes associated with the network. The total number

of objects in the network is indicated in the 'Total nodes' column. The p-values represent the probability of intersection between the experimental signature and the prebuilt content in MetaCore. The column 'zScore' gives the level of saturation of the networks taking into account the size of the database, the number of objects in the subnetwork and the number of objects in the signature used to construct the network. The higher the z-score the more saturated a subnetwork is. The transcriptional regulation networks are ranked according to p-value.
(XLS)

Text S1 Batch effect and batch correction for the tissue samples.
(DOC)

Acknowledgments

The Department of Pathology of the Academic Medical Center is kindly acknowledged for their assistance with the laser microdissection experiments. Dr. Richard R. Sprenger for initial technical support of the project.

Author Contributions

Conceived and designed the experiments: WW DM PDM MRB JMFGA GGK. Performed the experiments: WW DM GGK. Analyzed the data: PDM CAA WW DM. Contributed reagents/materials/analysis tools: JMFGA. Wrote the paper: WW DM CAA PDM. Provided technical support during the mass-spectrometry measurements, but did not have any additional role in the study design, data collection and analysis, decision to publish, or preparation of the manuscript: JPV.

References

1. Jemal A, Siegel R, Xu J, Ward E (2010) Cancer statistics, 2010. CA Cancer J Clin 60: 277–300.
2. Zhang Z, Bast RC, Yu Y, Li J, Sokoll LJ, et al. (2004) Three biomarkers identified from serum proteomic analysis for the detection of early stage ovarian cancer. Cancer Res 64: 5882–5890.
3. Rai AJ, Zhang Z, Rosenzweig J, Shih I-MI, Pham T, et al. (2002) Proteomic approaches to tumor marker discovery. ArchPatholLab Med 126: 1518–1526.
4. Skates SJ, Horick N, Yu Y, Xu F-J, Berchuck A, et al. (2004) Preoperative sensitivity and specificity for early-stage ovarian cancer when combining cancer antigen CA-125II, CA 15-3, CA 72-4, and macrophage colony-stimulating factor using mixtures of multivariate normal distributions. J Clin Oncol 22: 4059–4066.
5. Ueland FR, Desimone CP, Seamon LG, Miller RA, Goodrich S, et al. (2011) Effectiveness of a multivariate index assay in the preoperative assessment of ovarian tumors. Obstet Gynecol 117: 1289–1297.
6. Moore LE, Pfeiffer RM, Zhang Z, Lu KH, Fung ET, et al. (2012) Proteomic biomarkers in combination with CA 125 for detection of epithelial ovarian cancer using prediagnostic serum samples from the Prostate, Lung, Colorectal, and Ovarian (PLCO) Cancer Screening Trial. Cancer 118: 91–100.
7. Moore RG, Jabre-Raughley M, Brown AK, Robison KM, Miller MC, et al. (2010) Comparison of a novel multiple marker assay vs the Risk of Malignancy Index for the prediction of epithelial ovarian cancer in patients with a pelvic mass. Am J Obstet Gynecol 203: 228.e1–6.
8. Füzéry AK, Levin J, Chan MM, Chan DW (2013) Translation of proteomic biomarkers into FDA approved cancer diagnostics: issues and challenges. Clin Proteomics 10: 13.
9. Ludwig JA, Weinstein JN (2005) Biomarkers in cancer staging, prognosis and treatment selection. Nat Rev Cancer 5: 845–856.
10. Xu BJ (2010) Combining laser capture microdissection and proteomics: methodologies and clinical applications. Proteomics Clin Appl 4: 116–123.
11. Espina V, Wulfkuhle JD, Calvert VS, VanMeter A, Zhou W, et al. (2006) Laser-capture microdissection. Nat Protoc 1: 586–603.
12. Lawrie LC, Curran S (2005) Laser capture microdissection and colorectal cancer proteomics. Methods Mol Biol 293: 245–253.
13. Silva JC, Gorenstein M V, Li G-Z, Vissers JPC, Geromanos SJ (2006) Absolute quantification of proteins by LCMSE: a virtue of parallel MS acquisition. Mol Cell Proteomics 5: 144–156.
14. Vissers JPC, Langridge JI, Aerts JMFG (2007) Analysis and quantification of diagnostic serum markers and protein signatures for Gaucher disease. Mol Cell Proteomics 6: 755–766.
15. Wegdam W, Moerland PD, Meijer D, de Jong SM, Hoefsloot HCJ, et al. (2012) A critical assessment of SELDI-TOF-MS for biomarker discovery in serum and tissue of patients with an ovarian mass. Proteome Sci 10: 45.
16. Geromanos SJ, Vissers JPC, Silva JC, Dorschel CA, Li G-Z, et al. (2009) The detection, correlation, and comparison of peptide precursor and product ions from data independent LC-MS with data dependant LC-MS/MS. Proteomics 9: 1683–1695.
17. Silva JC, Denny R, Dorschel CA, Gorenstein M, Kass IJ, et al. (2005) Quantitative proteomic analysis by accurate mass retention time pairs. Anal Chem 77: 2187–2200.
18. Li G-Z, Vissers JPC, Silva JC, Golick D, Gorenstein M V, et al. (2009) Database searching and accounting of multiplexed precursor and product ion spectra from the data independent analysis of simple and complex peptide mixtures. Proteomics 9: 1696–1719.
19. Martens L, Vandekerckhove J, Gevaert K (2005) DBToolkit: processing protein databases for peptide-centric proteomics. Bioinformatics 21: 3584–3585.
20. Vizcaíno JA, Deutsch EW, Wang R, Csordas A, Reisinger F, et al. (2014) ProteomeXchange provides globally coordinated proteomics data submission and dissemination. Nat Biotechnol 32: 223–226.
21. Gentleman RC, Carey VJ, Bates DM, Bolstad B, Dettling M, et al. (2004) Bioconductor: open software development for computational biology and bioinformatics. Genome Biol 5: R80.
22. Benjamini Y, Hochberg Y (1995) Controlling the false discovery rate: a practical and powerful approach to multiple testing. J R Stat Soc Series B: 289–300.
23. Warnes GR, Bolker B, Bonebakker L, Gentleman R, Huber W, et al. (2013) Various R programming tools for plotting data. Available: http://cran.r-project.org/web/packages/gplots/gplots.pdf.
24. Bindea G, Mlecnik B, Hackl H, Charoentong P, Tosolini M, et al. (2009) ClueGO: a Cytoscape plug-in to decipher functionally grouped gene ontology and pathway annotation networks. Bioinformatics 25: 1091–1093.
25. Smoot ME, Ono K, Ruscheinski J, Wang P-L, Ideker T (2011) Cytoscape 2.8: new features for data integration and network visualization. Bioinformatics 27: 431–432.
26. Bessarabova M, Ishkin A, JeBailey L, Nikolskaya T, Nikolsky Y (2012) Knowledge-based analysis of proteomics data. BMC Bioinformatics 13 Suppl 1: S13.
27. Bicaku E, Xiong Y, Marchion DC, Chon HS, Stickles XB, et al. (2012) In vitro analysis of ovarian cancer response to cisplatin, carboplatin, and paclitaxel identifies common pathways that are also associated with overall patient survival. Br J Cancer 106: 1967–1975.
28. Anglesio MS, Arnold JM, George J, Tinker A V, Tothill R, et al. (2008) Mutation of ERBB2 provides a novel alternative mechanism for the ubiquitous activation of RAS-MAPK in ovarian serous low malignant potential tumors. Mol Cancer Res 6: 1678–1690.
29. Cerami E, Gao J, Dogrusoz U, Gross BE, Sumer SO, et al. (2012) The cBio cancer genomics portal: an open platform for exploring multidimensional cancer genomics data. Cancer Discov 2: 401–404.
30. Dieplinger H, Ankerst DP, Burges A, Lenhard M, Lingenhel A, et al. (2009) Afamin and apolipoprotein A-IV: novel protein markers for ovarian cancer. Cancer Epidemiol Biomarkers Prev 18: 1127–1133.
31. Lurie G, Wilkens LR, Thompson PJ, McDuffie KE, Carney ME, et al. (2008) Genetic polymorphisms in the Paraoxonase 1 gene and risk of ovarian epithelial carcinoma. Cancer Epidemiol Biomarkers Prev 17: 2070–2077.
32. Melvin JC, Seth D, Holmberg L, Garmo H, Hammar N, et al. (2012) Lipid profiles and risk of breast and ovarian cancer in the Swedish AMORIS study. Cancer Epidemiol Biomarkers Prev 21: 1381–1384.
33. Clarke CH, Yip C, Badgwell D, Fung ET, Coombes KR, et al. (2011) Proteomic biomarkers apolipoprotein A1, truncated transthyretin and connective tissue activating protein III enhance the sensitivity of CA125 for detecting early stage epithelial ovarian cancer. Gynecol Oncol 122: 548–553.
34. Li L, Davie JR (2010) The role of Sp1 and Sp3 in normal and cancer cell biology. Ann Anat 192: 275–283.
35. Wang X, Urvalek AM, Liu J, Zhao J (2008) Activation of KLF8 transcription by focal adhesion kinase in human ovarian epithelial and cancer cells. J Biol Chem 283: 13934–13942.
36. Previdi S, Malek A, Albertini V, Riva C, Capella C, et al. (2010) Inhibition of Sp1-dependent transcription and antitumor activity of the new aureolic acid analogues mithramycin SDK and SK in human ovarian cancer xenografts. Gynecol Oncol 118: 182–188.
37. Gubbay O, Guo W, Rae MT, Niven D, Langdon SP, et al. (2005) Inflammation-associated gene expression is altered between normal human ovarian surface epithelial cells and cell lines derived from ovarian adenocarcinomas. Br J Cancer 92: 1927–1933.
38. Runnebaum IB, Brüning A (2005) Glucocorticoids inhibit cell death in ovarian cancer and up-regulate caspase inhibitor cIAP2. Clin Cancer Res 11: 6325–6332.
39. Yano A, Fujii Y, Iwai A, Kageyama Y, Kihara K (2006) Glucocorticoids suppress tumor angiogenesis and in vivo growth of prostate cancer cells. Clin Cancer Res 12: 3003–3009.
40. Woenckhaus J, Franke FE, Hackethal A, Von Georgi R, Münstedt K (2006) Glucocorticosteroid receptors in ovarian carcinomas. Oncol Rep 15: 1137–1140.
41. Dickinson RE, Fegan KS, Ren X, Hillier SG, Duncan WC (2011) Glucocorticoid regulation of SLIT/ROBO tumour suppressor genes in the ovarian surface epithelium and ovarian cancer cells. PLoS One 6: e27792.

42. Zhao J, Meyerkord CL, Du Y, Khuri FR, Fu H (2011) 14-3-3 proteins as potential therapeutic targets. Semin Cell Dev Biol 22: 705–712.
43. He Y, Wu X, Liu X, Yan G, Xu C (2010) LC-MS/MS analysis of ovarian cancer metastasis-related proteins using a nude mouse model: 14-3-3 zeta as a candidate biomarker. J Proteome Res 9: 6180–6190.
44. Honda K, Yamada T, Endo R, Ino Y, Gotoh M, et al. (1998) Actinin-4, a novel actin-bundling protein associated with cell motility and cancer invasion. J Cell Biol 140: 1383–1393.
45. Yamamoto S, Tsuda H, Honda K, Kita T, Takano M, et al. (2007) Actinin-4 expression in ovarian cancer: a novel prognostic indicator independent of clinical stage and histological type. Mod Pathol 20: 1278–1285.
46. Yamamoto S, Tsuda H, Honda K, Onozato K, Takano M, et al. (2009) Actinin-4 gene amplification in ovarian cancer: a candidate oncogene associated with poor patient prognosis and tumor chemoresistance. Mod Pathol 22: 499–507.
47. Macario AJL, Conway de Macario E (2005) Sick chaperones, cellular stress, and disease. N Engl J Med 353: 1489–1501.
48. Ciocca DR, Calderwood SK (2005) Heat shock proteins in cancer: diagnostic, prognostic, predictive, and treatment implications. Cell Stress Chaperones 10: 86–103.
49. Cappello F, Marino Gammazza A, Palumbo Piccionello A, Campanella C, Pace A, et al. (2014) Hsp60 chaperonopathies and chaperonotherapy: targets and agents. Expert Opin Ther Targets 18: 185–208.
50. Barazi HO, Zhou L, Templeton NS, Krutzsch HC, Roberts DD (2002) Identification of heat shock protein 60 as a molecular mediator of alpha 3 beta 1 integrin activation. Cancer Res 62: 1541–1548.
51. O'Malley BW, Kumar R (2009) Nuclear receptor coregulators in cancer biology. Cancer Res 69: 8217–8222.
52. Cloke B, Shah K, Kaneda H, Lavery S, Trew G, et al. (2010) The poly(c)-binding protein-1 regulates expression of the androgen receptor. Endocrinology 151: 3954–3964.

6

Gene Expression Profiling Reveals Epithelial Mesenchymal Transition (EMT) Genes Can Selectively Differentiate Eribulin Sensitive Breast Cancer Cells

Zoltán Dezső, Judith Oestreicher¤, Amy Weaver, Stephanie Santiago, Sergei Agoulnik, Jesse Chow, Yoshiya Oda, Yasuhiro Funahashi*

Biomarkers and Personalized Medicine Core Function Unit, Eisai Product Creation Systems, Eisai Inc., Andover, Massachusetts, United States of America

Abstract

Objectives: Eribulin mesylate is a synthetic macrocyclic ketone analog of the marine sponge natural product halichondrin B. Eribulin is a mechanistically unique inhibitor of microtubule dynamics. In this study, we investigated whether selective signal pathways were associated with eribulin activity compared to paclitaxel, which stabilizes microtubules, based on gene expression profiling of cell line panels of breast, endometrial, and ovarian cancer in vitro.

Results: We determined the sets of genes that were differentially altered between eribulin and paclitaxel treatment in breast, endometrial, and ovarian cancer cell line panels. Our unsupervised clustering analyses revealed that expression profiles of gene sets altered with treatments were correlated with the in vitro antiproliferative activities of the drugs. Several tubulin isotypes had significantly lower expression in cell lines treated with eribulin compared to paclitaxel. Pathway enrichment analyses of gene sets revealed that the common pathways altered between treatments in the 3 cancer panels were related to cytoskeleton remodeling and cell cycle regulation. The epithelial-mesenchymal transition (EMT) pathway was enriched in genes with significantly altered expression between the two drugs for breast and endometrial cancers, but not for ovarian cancer. Expression of genes from the EMT pathway correlated with eribulin sensitivity in breast cancer and with paclitaxel sensitivity in endometrial cancer. Alteration of expression profiles of EMT genes between sensitive and resistant cell lines allowed us to predict drug sensitivity for breast and endometrial cancers.

Conclusion: Gene expression analysis showed that gene sets that were altered between eribulin and paclitaxel correlated with drug in vitro antiproliferative activities in breast and endometrial cancer cell line panels. Among the panels, breast cancer provided the strongest differentiation between eribulin and paclitaxel sensitivities based on gene expression. In addition, EMT genes were predictive of eribulin sensitivity in the breast and endometrial cancer panels.

Editor: Surinder K. Batra, University of Nebraska Medical Center, United States of America

Funding: The funding for the work was from the research and development budget of Eisai Inc.. The funders had no role in study design, data collection and analysis, decision to publish, or preparation of the manuscript.

Competing Interests: The authors have read the journal's policy and have the following conflicts. All authors were employed by Eisai Inc., the funder of this study. Eribulin is an Eisai product. There are no further patents, products in development or marketed products to declare. This does not alter their adherence to all the PLOS ONE policies on sharing data and materials, as detailed online in the guide for authors.

* Email: Yasuhiro_Funahashi@eisai.com

¤ Current address: Infinity Pharmaceuticals, Cambridge, Massachusetts, United States of America

Introduction

Eribulin mesylate (eribulin) is a synthetic macrocyclic ketone analog of the marine sponge natural product halichondrin B and an inhibitor of microtubule dynamics [1], [2]. Eribulin inhibits microtubule dynamics through a novel mechanism relative to other tubulin-targeting agents, including the taxanes and vinca alkaloids, by specifically binding with high affinity to the plus ends of microtubules and thereby suppressing microtubule dynamics and leading to inhibition of microtubule growth in the absence of effects on microtubule shortening at microtubule plus ends, and formation of nonproductive tubulin aggregates [3], [2]. This results in G2-M cell-cycle arrest, disruption of normal mitotic spindles, and induction of apoptosis. Eribulin (as Halaven) has been approved in a number of countries worldwide for the treatment of certain patients with advanced breast cancer. In breast cancer, the use of taxanes and anthracyclines is often effective early on, although resistance to these agents commonly limits their potential at late-line settings [4], and as a result the prognosis for metastatic breast cancer remains poor. Knowledge of eribulin's unique interactions with microtubules compared to other tubulin-binding drugs has generated interest in the possibility that eribulin may have a unique spectrum of anticancer activities and may provide new treatment options for patients who are resistant to other tubulin binding agents. In this study we have focused on comparing eribulin to paclitaxel, a taxane widely used for breast cancer and gynecological cancers such as ovarian and endometrial cancers, which stabilizes microtubule polymers leading to mitotic arrest and apoptosis [5], [6]. Several studies have identified gene mutations and expression patterns associated with paclitaxel resistance, with some of the biomarkers predictive of such resistance including beta-tubulin mutations [7]–[9], overexpression of beta-3-tubulin [10], overexpression of the microtubule-associated protein stathmin [11], upregulation of ErbB2 [12], and mutation of p53 [13], [14]. Although numerous studies have focused on paclitaxel resistance, molecular biomarkers for predicting efficacy of eribulin, or the relative benefit of eribulin compared with paclitaxel, have not yet been reported.

In this study our goal was to investigate whether selective pathways were associated with eribulin activity compared to paclitaxel and to find potential biomarkers predictive of eribulin sensitivity or resistance when compared to paclitaxel. We performed gene expression profiling of breast, ovarian, and endometrial cancer cell line panels treated with eribulin and paclitaxel. In addition, we measured in vitro anti proliferative activities (IC_{50}) for both eribulin and paclitaxel for the same cell line panels. High throughput expression profiles combined with in vitro proliferation data represents an unbiased approach that enables us to identify multiple components of pathways with altered expression that may be selectively activated by eribulin compared to paclitaxel and that may contribute to cellular susceptibility to the drugs. Furthermore, the inclusion of 3 cancer panels in our analyses allowed us to compare the altered pathway profiles identified for each cancer type. Our first approach was to identify genes with significantly changed expression between the two compounds for each cancer panel and perform functional pathway analyses. Next, gene sets and affected signaling pathways were correlated with in vitro antiproliferative data to investigate if any of the differentially affected pathways were associated with drug resistance. Finally, we confirmed our main findings in the breast cancer panel by qPCR.

Methods

In vitro antiproliferative activity

In vitro antiproliferative activities (IC_{50}) were determined in 27 breast, 19 endometrial, and 21 ovarian cancer cell lines treated with eribulin and paclitaxel. Three hours after plating, serial dilutions of tested compounds were added. Each experiment was performed in triplicate. Mean IC_{50} values and 95% confidence intervals (CI) were calculated based on IC_{50} values generated from separate sigmoidal curves representing the growth inhibition activity versus eribulin and paclitaxel concentrations in 3 independent experiments. Statistical analyses were performed using GraphPad Prism version 5.02 (GraphPad Software, San Diego, CA). IC_{50} values for all 3 cancer panels are included in Table S1.

Gene expression profiling (Affymetrix)

We performed gene expression analysis of 27 breast, 19 endometrial, and 21 ovarian cancer cell lines treated with eribulin or paclitaxel for 24 hours at concentrations of $10\times IC_{50}$. Total RNA was extracted using RNeasy Mini kit (Qiagen) and was used to prepare biotinylated fragmented cRNA for analysis on Human Genome U133 plus 2.0 arrays (Affymetrix). Three technical replicates were included for eribulin, paclitaxel, and untreated cell lines. Arrays were processed according to the GeneChip Expression Analysis Technical Manual (Affymetrix). Each gene chip was analyzed using Affymetrix Microarray Analysis Suite version 5.0 to obtain raw data. Genes with average expression <100 were considered not expressed and excluded from the analysis. Gene expression data from these studies are available at the GEO public repository website (accession number GSE50832).

Quantitative (q)PCR analysis

We extracted genes from the "Development Regulation of epithelial-to-mesenchymal transition (EMT)" pathway from the knowledge base of the commercially available Metacore. There were 36 out of 92 genes expressed in breast cancer cell lines based on the Affymetrix array (intensity >100). Effects of eribulin and paclitaxel on the expression profiles of these 36 genes from the EMT pathways and 8 tubulin isotypes was confirmed in the breast cancer panel by qPCR using Custom TaqMan Low Density Cards (TLDA) with ABI7900HT (Life Technologies) instruments. The 27 breast cancer cell lines were treated with eribulin and paclitaxel for 24 hours at concentrations of $10\times IC_{50}$. Three technical replicates were included for eribulin, paclitaxel, and untreated cell lines. We calculated ΔCT values for sample-to-sample normalization based on the average CT values of 4 endogenous controls (GAPDH, GUSB, HPRT1, PPIA). Statistical analysis and clustering were performed on ΔCT values. Fold changes were calculated after $2^{-\Delta CT}$ transformation into linear space. The ΔCT values for the 2 treatments in the 3 cancer panels are included in Table S2. The clustering result of the EMT pathway was based on the spearman distance metric.

To investigate long-term effects of compounds on expression of EMT-related genes, five breast cancer cells (HCC1806, BT474, HCC38, HCC70 and AU565) were incubated in the presence of eribulin at $1\times IC_{50}$ for 7 days. All treatments were done in triplicates. Total RNA was isolated using the RNeasy Mini kit (Qiagen, Valencia, CA, USA). Reverse transcription was carried out using the High Capacity cDNA Reverse Transcription kit (Life Technologies, Grand Island, NY, USA). Gene expression was measured with Taqman probes on Custom TaqMan Low Density Cards (TLDA) using ABI7900 (Applied Biosystems, Life Technologies). We calculated ΔCT values for sample-to-sample normalization based on the CT values of ACTB endogenous control (Table S4).

Statistical and pathway analysis of gene expression

Gene expressions were analyzed using Expressionist software (Genedata) and R statistical software [15]. After data normalization log2 ratios were calculated for both treatments normalized to control. To identify genes significantly altered between treatments we applied paired t-tests between the log transformed expression ratios of the treated cell lines for each cancer cell line panel separately. Genes with fold change (FC) >1.5 between treatments for at least one cell line and p value <0.01 based on the paired t-test were considered significantly altered between treatments (Table S3). Pathway analysis of significantly altered genes was performed using Metacore commercial software. Pathways were considered significant based on $p<0.05$ false discovery rate (FDR) adjusted threshold for multiple comparison correction. Cell lines were clustered based on their gene expression profiles by unsupervised hierarchical clustering, where the distance metric was the Pearson distance and both the "ward" and "average" linkage criteria was used. We picked in each case the algorithm which gave the highest average silhouette (using the "cluster" library in R), a measure characterizing how tightly the data are grouped in the clusters. In order to be able to perform statistical tests between the drug sensitivity of the cell line clusters we considered only results where the clusters contained at least three cell lines with associated IC_{50} data. The best clustering was retained and the top two and three clusters in the hierarchical tree were correlated with in vitro antiproliferative activity. A t-test was applied to identify significant differences between the cell line clusters.

Predictions of drug sensitivity based on signature genes

We tested the predictive power of the EMT pathway genes based on the elastic net regression method [18]. This method is suited for cases where the number of features (genes) is greater than the number of samples and some of the features are highly correlated. The algorithm combines two penalty terms to strike a balance between the need to generate a sparse model, but at the same time retaining groups of correlated genes. We used this method because the number of genes was larger than the number of samples, and because the genes were extracted from the same pathway we expected a high correlation among the expression profiles. We used the "glmnet" package [16] in R, where the regression model is built based on two parameters (α, λ). The first parameter (α) controls the relative strength of the two penalty terms ($\alpha = 0$ and 1 corresponds to the ridge and lasso regression, respectively). The second parameter (λ) controls the overall strength of the penalties [17]. We performed a leave-one-out cross validation to evaluate the prediction power of the gene sets. To predict the sensitivity of the left out sample we generated a sequence of 100 values of α between 0 and 1 and for each α value a λ was chosen to minimize the mean square error based on a 10 fold cross-validation of the training data (total number of sample minus one). For this step, 100 values of λ were tested based on the sequence generated by the default setting in the "glmnet" package. The α and λ pair which had the smallest mean square error was retained for prediction. The performance of each model was evaluated using the Pearson correlation coefficient between the predicted values and the measured IC_{50} values.

Results

Comparison of gene signatures and correlation with drug sensitivity

Our goal was to identify selective signaling pathways associated with eribulin compared to paclitaxel in the 3 cell line panels based on the gene expression profiling. We started the analysis by identifying the genes differentially altered between treatments with eribulin and paclitaxel. We performed a paired t-test for each cancer panel and calculated fold changes for each cell line separately between the two treatments. After applying a threshold on p values and fold-changes ($p<0.01$ and $FC>1.5$), we defined the gene signatures consisting of 91, 159, and 327 genes for ovarian, endometrial, and breast cancer cell lines, respectively (Figure 1, Table S3). A large fraction of the genes were unique: 78% of genes from signatures were unique to breast, 57% to endometrial and 60% to ovarian cancer. There was only a small overlap (18 genes). The gene signatures also showed differences in the direction of alteration between the drugs in the three cancer panel. We compared the number of genes up- or down-regulated in at least one cell line ($FC>1.5$) between treatments and found that in breast and endometrial cancers the majority of signature genes were up-regulated for eribulin treatment as compared to paclitaxel (76% and 56% in breast and endometrial cancer, respectively). On the other hand, in ovarian cancer the majority of signature genes were down-regulated for eribulin treatment compared to paclitaxel (74% of genes). Next we performed unsupervised clustering based on the gene sets in all three cancer panels for both treatments. We identified two distinct clusters based on eribulin expression profile and three clusters based on paclitaxel expression profiles in breast cancer (Figure 2). We found that the drug treated expression profiles for breast cancer correlated with sensitivity for both compounds ($p = 0.004$ for eribulin and $p = 0.06$ for paclitaxel; Table 1 and Figure 2). We considered the top two or three clusters in each case and reported the best p value. The choice of hierarchical clustering algorithm was determined based on the silhouette average, a measure which characterizes how tightly the data are grouped in the clusters (Material and Methods). For ovarian cancer we found no significant correlation of expression with drug sensitivity, and for endometrial cancer we found significant correlation only with the paclitaxel signature ($p = 0.006$, Table 1). Because breast cancer expression showed the most significant association with eribulin sensitivity, in the next part of the analysis we investigated in more detail the clustering results. We identified the most resistant clusters for eribulin (HCC1500, HCC1419, UACC893, HCC2218, UAC812) and paclitaxel (HCC1143, HCC2218, HCC1954, BT20, HCC70, UACC812), both characterized by distinct expression profiles (Figures 2A and 2B, indicated with red boxes) and significantly higher IC_{50} values from the rest of the cell lines ($p = 0.004$ and $p = 0.06$, respectively). The two resistant clusters shared two common cell lines (HCC2218 and UACC812) and had several unique ones. These cell lines were predicted based on the drug treated expression profile patterns to be uniquely resistant to one or the other compound. To compare the sensitivity of the cell lines to the two compounds we examined the scatter plot of the IC_{50} values of eribulin and paclitaxel. The scatter plot (Figure 2C) shows a weak correlation (correlation = 0.19, not significant) that means differences between antiproliferative activity between eribulin and paclitaxel in breast cancer panel, because there are several cell lines located off-diagonal in the top-left (most sensitive to eribulin as compared to paclitaxel) or bottom-right (most sensitive to paclitaxel as compared to eribulin) corner of the plot. These cell lines had the most difference in drug sensitivity between the two drugs. The clustering results predicted that HCC1500, HCC1419 and UACC893 are resistant to eribulin but not to paclitaxel. Indeed, two of the cell lines (Figure 2C, red) are the top two cell lines most resistant to eribulin compared to paclitaxel based on the scatter plot. We note that for the cell line UACC893 we could not determine the IC_{50} values because of slow cell growth issues in the in vitro proliferation assay. Similarly, three of four cell lines (HCC1954, HCC70, BT20) predicted by the clustering results are among the top most resistant to paclitaxel compared to eribulin (yellow) based on the IC_{50} scatter plot. The remaining cell line (HCC1143) appears to be resistant both to paclitaxel and eribulin. Although it was not part of the eribulin resistant cluster, the cell line shows similarity in gene expression profile (up-regulation) to the resistant cluster (Figure 2A). These results showed that in the breast cancer panel, drug resistant cell lines were characterized by distinct expression profiles which can differentiate eribulin and paclitaxel antiproliferative activity.

Functional analysis of gene signatures

The gene signatures in the cancer panels were quite unique; nevertheless, there was a small overlap of 18 genes. Interestingly a large fraction of the overlapping genes were tubulins (11 out of 18). These tubulins were down-regulated under eribulin treatment as compared to paclitaxel in most cell lines across all 3 cancer types. The significant differences in tubulin expression levels were confirmed by qPCR in the breast cancer panel. Based on the qPCR analysis, 4 tubulins (TUBA1B, TUBA4A, TUBB, TUBB4B) had significantly decreased expression under eribulin treatment compared to control (based on paired t-test, Table 2). In contrast, 7 of 8 tubulins (TUBA1B, TUBA1C, TUBA4A, TUBB2A, TUBB3, TUBB4B, TUBB6) had significant increases in expression under paclitaxel treatment compared to control. There was a large variation in fold-changes for the individual cell lines, but all 4 tubulins with significant changes under eribulin treatment had >1.5 fold changed decreases in expression in at

Table 1. Correlation of gene signatures with in vitro antiproliferative data.

Gene signatures	Breast cancer (p values)		Ovarian cancer (p values)		Endometrial cancer (p values)	
Eribulin signature	0.004		NS		NS	
Paclitaxel signature	0.06		NS		0.006	
EMT pathway	**Clustering**	**Prediction**	**Clustering**	**Prediction**	**Clustering**	**Prediction**
Eribulin (EMT)	0.06 (0.05)*	0.03	NS	NS	NS	0.04
Paclitaxel (EMT)	NS	NS	NS	NS	0.006	0.02

We performed unsupervised hierarchical clustering based on gene signatures for the 3 cancer panels. Significant ($p<0.05$) or marginally significant ($p<0.1$) p values are listed for the cell line panels where we identified clusters of cell lines with different sensitivities. For the EMT pathway we tested the predictive power of the expression profiles based on the elastic net regression model. The predicted and measured values (IC_{50}) were correlated based on the Pearson correlation coefficient. In cases where significant correlations existed, p values are listed. Significance of EMT pathway clustering was confirmed for breast cancer by qPCR ($p=0.05$). *confirmed by TLDA (NS indicates not significant p values>0.1).

least 11 cell lines in breast cancer. Similarly, 6 of 7 tubulins with significant changes had increases in expression of >1.5 fold in at least 7 cell lines under paclitaxel treatment when compared to control. All the tubulins tested by qPCR were significantly down-regulated under eribulin treatment when compared to paclitaxel ($p<0.001$ for all tubulins except TUBB6, $p<0.05$, Table 2). We found that reduced expression of 4 tubulins (TUBA1C, TUBA4A, TUBB3, TUBB6) significantly correlated with eribulin sensitivity ($p<0.05$), and that of one tubulin had a weak correlation (TUBB, $p<0.1$). Only one tubulin (TUBB2A) had significant correlation with paclitaxel sensitivity ($p<0.05$) and several (TUBA4A and TUBA1B) showed marginal significances ($p<0.1$, Table 2).

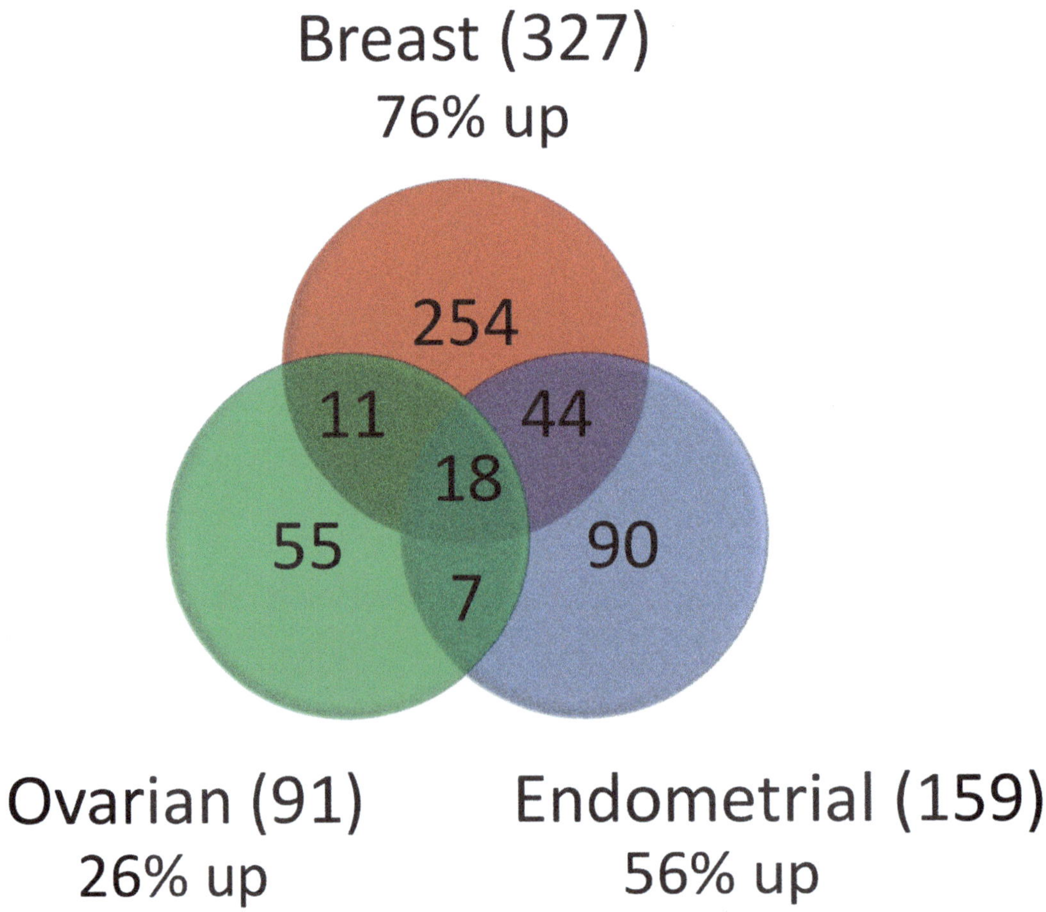

Figure 1. Overlap among gene signatures for the 3 cancer panels. We identified sets of genes with significantly altered gene expression profiles between eribulin and paclitaxel treatments for breast, ovarian, and endometrial cancer. The signature consisted of 327, 91, and 159 genes for breast, ovarian, and endometrial cancer, respectively. The percentage of genes having higher expression in cell lines treated with eribulin compared to paclitaxel is 76%, 56%, and 26% for breast, endometrial, and ovarian cancer, respectively.

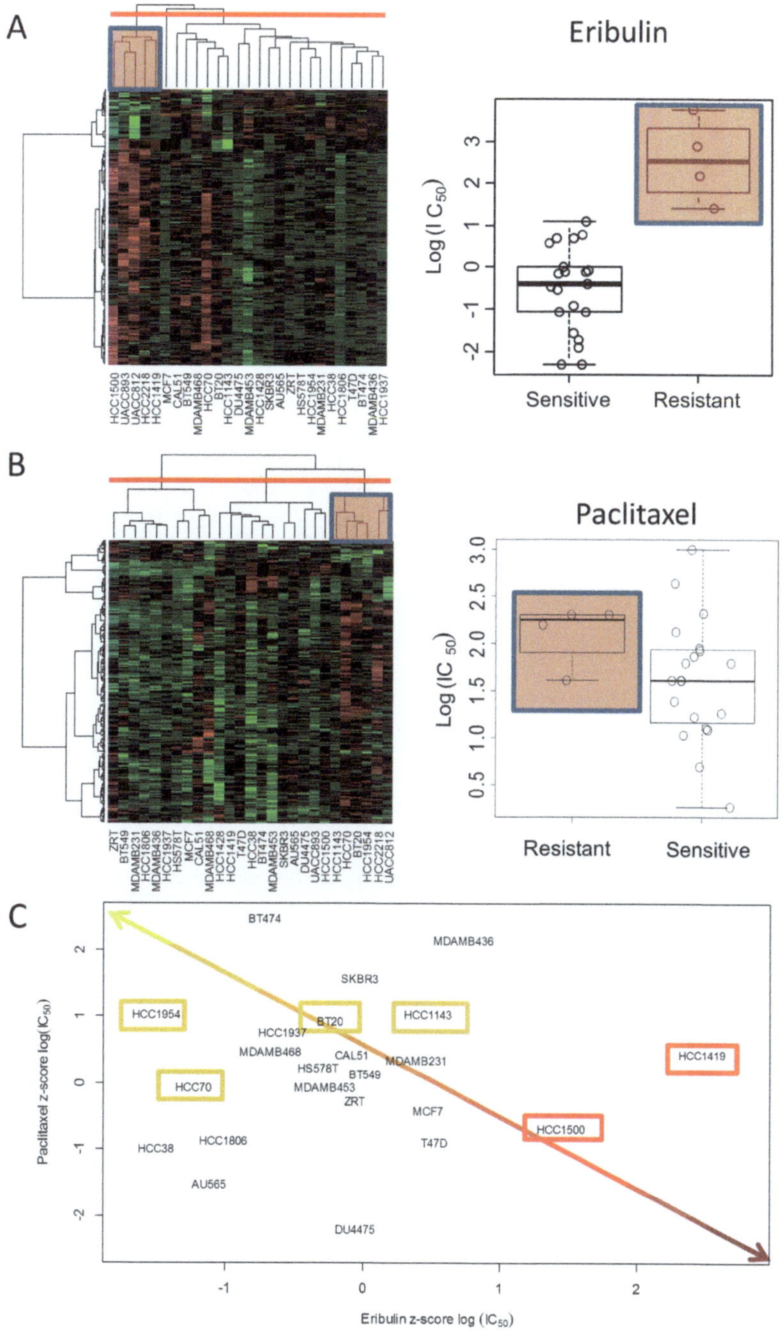

Figure 2. Correlation of expression profiles with drug sensitivity. A) Correlation of eribulin signature with drug sensitivity. Hierarchical clustering of eribulin expression signature identified two clusters of cell lines with significantly different sensitivity to eribulin ($p = 0.004$). The red box indicates the eribulin resistant cluster. B) Correlation of paclitaxel signature with drug sensitivity. Hierarchical clustering of paclitaxel expression signature identified cluster with differences of paclitaxel sensitivity ($p = 0.06$). The red box indicates the most paclitaxel resistant cell line cluster. C) Scatter plot of eribulin and paclitaxel sensitivity. Cell lines located in the upper left corner are the most resistant to paclitaxel as compared to eribulin, and cell lines located at the lower right corner are the most resistant to eribulin as compared to paclitaxel. Yellow and red boxes indicate the cell lines identified based on expression profiles as uniquely resistant to paclitaxel and eribulin, respectively.

The correlative analysis of the signature gene sets with altered expression between treatments indicated a significant correlation with drug sensitivity for breast and endometrial but not for ovarian cancer (Table 1). We investigated the functional role of the genes differentiating eribulin from paclitaxel based on gene expression by performing pathway enrichment analysis using the commercially available Metacore software. The three genes sets were used for enrichment analysis and a significance threshold of $p < 0.05$ was applied with the FDR adjustment. Table 3 shows the significantly enriched pathways grouped as common and unique for the different cancer panels. There were several common pathways for the 3 cancer types: cytoskeleton remodeling related pathways (neurofilaments and keratin filaments), and the role of Nek in the cell cycle regulation pathway. Breast and endometrial cancers

Table 2. Correlation of tubulin expression with drug sensitivity and fold changes between drug treatments.

	Eribulin		Paclitaxel		Eribulin vs control	Paclitaxel vs control	Paclitaxel vs Eribulin
Tubulin	pv	cor	pv	cor	Fold change	Fold change	Fold change
TUBA1B	NS	0.16	0.07	−0.38	0.75 (p<0.001)	1.17 (p<0.05)	1.87 (p<0.001)
TUBA1C	0.01	0.49	NS	−0.16	NS	1.31 (p<0.01)	1.61 (p<0.001)
TUBA4A	0.007	0.52	0.08	−0.36	0.84 (p<0.01)	1.64 (p<0.001)	2.42 (p<0.001)
TUBB	0.08	0.36	NS	−0.23	0.7 (p<0.001)	NS	1.65 (p<0.001)
TUBB2A	NS	−0.01	0.04	−0.44	NS	1.76 (p<0.001)	1.81 (p<0.001)
TUBB3	0.04	0.42	NS	−0.17	NS	1.68 (p<0.001)	1.67 (p<0.001)
TUBB4B	NS	0.06	NS	−0.2	0.78 (p<0.001)	1.39 (p<0.001)	2.1 (p<0.001)
TUBB6	0.02	0.48	NS	−0.03	NS	1.34 (p<0.01)	1.42 (p<0.05)

Correlations were calculated based on the Pearson correlation, and p values between treatment and controls are based on paired t-test (NS indicates a not significant p value>0.1).

were uniquely enriched in two EMT related pathways ("Dependence of TGF beta independent induction of EMT via RhoA, PI3K and ILK" and "Development regulation of epithelial-to-mesenchymal transition") and a cell adhesion pathway related to cell migration ("Cell adhesion chemokines and adhesion"). There was only one pathway uniquely enriched for endometrial and ovarian cancer ("Cell adhesion gap junction"). There were several unique pathways enriched for each cancer panel: 5 unique pathways significantly enriched for both breast and ovarian cancer and two unique pathways for endometrial cancer (Table 3). Most unique pathways were related to specific processes in cytoskeleton remodeling, cell cycle and immune response (Table 3). Additional pathways included regulation of eNOS pathway enriched for breast cancer, transcriptional role of AP1 for endometrial cancer, activin A signal regulation, and development of beta-adrenergic receptor transactivation of EGFR enriched for ovarian cancer.

The analysis revealed that two EMT related pathways were commonly enriched for breast and endometrial cancer. Interestingly these were the two cancer panels which had gene signatures with significant correlation with eribulin and/or paclitaxel sensitivity. We tested the hypothesis that EMT pathway being common in these two cancer types may be a selective pathway associated with drug sensitivity. To investigate the expression profile in more detail we extracted the list of genes from the "Development regulation of epithelial-to-mesenchymal transition" pathway. Out of the 91 genes 36, 33, and 41 genes were expressed in breast, ovarian, and endometrial cancer, respectively. First, we applied hierarchical clustering based on these genes for breast cancer and analyzed the sensitivity between two groups which were divided by hierarchical clustering. EMT pathway expression correlated with eribulin ($p = 0.06$; Table 1, Figure 3), but not with paclitaxel sensitivity (Table 1). For ovarian cancer there was no correlation between EMT gene expression and drug sensitivity. Lastly, EMT pathway expression had a significant correlation with paclitaxel sensitivity in endometrial cancer ($p = 0.006$). Next we tested if the differentiation of EMT gene expression profile between resistant and sensitive cell lines would enable us to predict drug sensitivity. The predictive power of the EMT expression profile was evaluated by applying the elastic net approach [18] with leave-one-out cross validation (See Materials and Methods). The predicted and measured drug sensitivity (IC_{50} value) had significant correlation in breast cancer ($p = 0.03$) and in endometrial cancer ($p = 0.04$) with eribulin sensitivity. The predicted drug sensitivity was also significant for paclitaxel in endometrial cancer ($p = 0.02$). On the other hand, there was no significant prediction power for ovarian cancer based on EMT expression profile. The predictions are in agreement with the unsupervised clustering results, suggesting that the separation observed in the EMT expression profile between sensitive and resistant cell lines in breast and endometrial cancer can be used to predict drug sensitivity. The agreement between these two different computational approaches also suggests the robustness of these findings. Although we have not found significant separation between eribulin sensitive and resistant cell lines based on the clustering of EMT expression profile in endometrial cancer, the genes from EMT pathway still had significant predictive power of eribulin sensitivity. This may be due to the fact that in this case the best predictive model in elastic net includes a relatively small number of genes from the EMT pathway as opposed to the clustering which is based on all genes expressed in EMT (7 genes from EMT are included in the model to predict eribulin sensitivity in endometrial cancer compared to 13 and 21 genes included in the models to predict paclitaxel sensitivity in endometrial cancer and eribulin sensitivity in breast cancer, respectively).

Table 3. Pathway enrichment analysis of the three gene signatures altered between eribulin and paclitaxel treatments.

Breast cancer	Endometrial cancer	Ovarian cancer
Cytoskeleton remodeling (3.5×10^{-7}, 1.6×10^{-3}, 9.3×10^{-4})		
Cell cycle: Role of Nek in cell cycle regulation (1.5×10^{-4}, 4.7×10^{-4}, 5.9×10^{-8})		
Cytoskeleton remodeling: Neurofilaments (1.3×10^{-4}, 1.6×10^{-5}, 1.2×10^{-6})		
Cytoskeleton remodeling: Keratin filaments (7.5×10^{-4}, 1×10^{-4}, 1.8×10^{-4})		
Development of TGF beta dependent induction of EMT via RhoA, PI3K and ILK (6.7×10^{-6}, 2.2×10^{-3})		
Development regulation of epithelial-to-mesenchymal transition (EMT) (2.5×10^{-5}, 1.3×10^{-3})		
Cell adhesion Chemokines and adhesion (4.1×10^{-5}, 1.4×10^{-3})		
	Cell adhesion gap junction (1.5×10^{-4}, 5.8×10^{-4})	
Cytoskeleton remodeling_Integrin outside-in signaling (1.5×10^{-5})	Immune response_IL-1 signaling pathway (2.6×10^{-4})	Immune response_Human NKG2D signaling (1.4×10^{-3})
Cytoskeleton remodeling_TGF, WNT and cytoskeletal remodeling (3.8×10^{-5})	Transcription_Role of AP-1 in regulation of cellular metabolism (1.5×10^{-3})	Immune response_Murine NKG2 signaling (1.5×10^{-3})
Cell cycle_Spindle assembly and chromosome separation (6.4×10^{-5})		Cytoskeleton remodeling_Reverse signaling by ephrin B (1.7×10^{-3})
Muscle contraction_Regulation of eNOS activity in endothelial cells (1.1×10^{-4})		Development_Beta-adrenergic receptors transactivation of EGFR (2×10^{-3})
Immune response_ETV3 on CSF1-promoted macrophage differentiation (3×10^{-4})		Signal transduction_Activin A signaling regulation (2.2×10^{-3})

The EMT genes expressed in breast cancer (36 genes) were included in a custom TLDA assay to confirm our results. Based on the higher sensitivity TLDA assay, both EMT correlation with eribulin sensitivity ($p = 0.05$) and the significant alteration of EMT expression between eribulin and paclitaxel sensitivity was confirmed. We found that 9 genes from the EMT pathway had significantly higher expression ($p<0.05$) under eribulin treatment when compared to paclitaxel, supporting our results from the microarray data (Figure 4B). These 9 genes had a large variation across the cell line panels, but they were mostly up-regulated and the fold-changes were larger than 1.5 for at least 3 cell lines. Eleven genes had significantly higher expression under eribulin

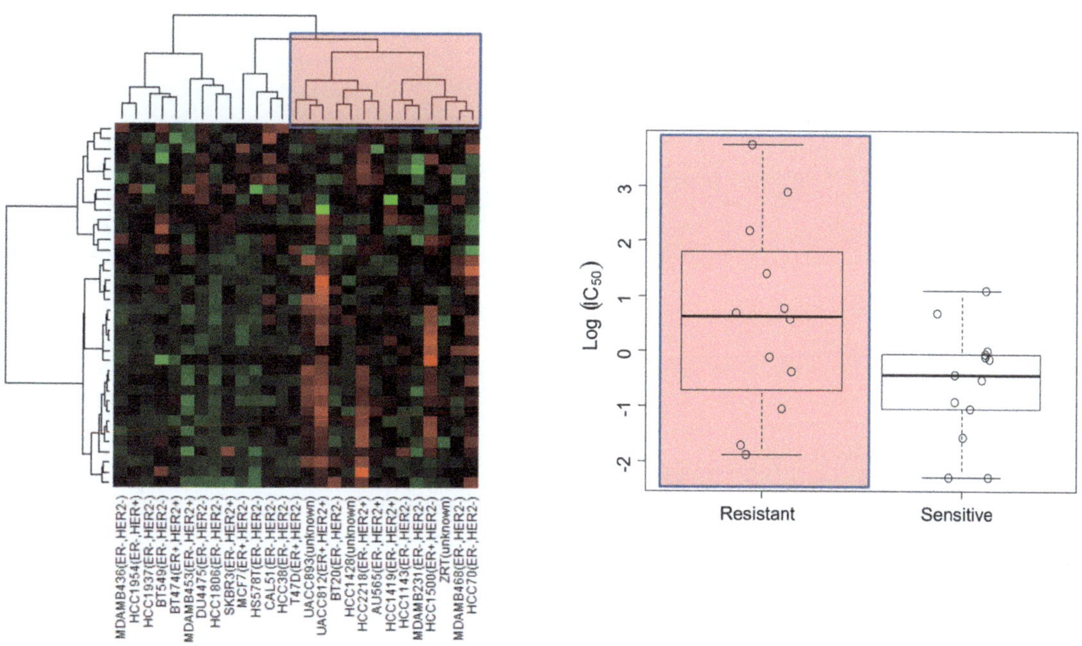

Figure 3. The EMT expression profile correlates with eribulin sensitivity. Unsupervised hierarchical clustering defined groups of breast cancer cell lines with altered expression under eribulin treatment (left panel). The cell lines consisting of many upregulated EMT genes are more resistant to eribulin treatment (right panel, $p = 0.06$). The ER and HER2 status of cell lines are indicated in the parenthesis.

treatment for the resistant cluster when compared to the sensitive cell line cluster (Figure 4C). A detailed investigation of the EMT pathway map revealed that several genes identified as overexpressed under eribulin treatment or overexpressed in the eribulin resistant cell lines were key elements of the epithelial to mesenchymal process (Figure 4A). EMT is mediated by a number of signaling pathways, including TGF-beta, WNT, EGF, and HGF signaling [19]–[22]. Our results indicated a significant alteration of expression in key EMT marker genes such as vimentin and claudin-1 (upregulated under eribulin treatment compared to paclitaxel) and occludin (upregulated in eribulin resistant cell lines). Indeed, overexpression of claudin-1 was shown to induce EMT through activation of slug and zeb1 in human liver cells [23], and to mediate TNF-alpha induced cell migration in human lung carcinoma [24]. Another important gene of the EMT pathway is TGF-beta, which is able to induce the EMT pathway via the SMAD family members [22]. Our map indicates overexpression of both TGF-beta and SMAD2 suggesting a possible mechanism for the activation of the pathway. We found that endothelin-1 was significantly overexpressed under eribulin treatment compared to paclitaxel as well as in the eribulin resistant cell lines. The TGF-beta 1 dependent secretion of endothelin-1 is known to be associated with the induction of the EMT [25]. These findings based on gene expression profiling suggest that EMT pathway response differentiates eribulin from paclitaxel and it is uniquely associated with eribulin sensitivity in breast cancer cell lines.

Discussion

The similarity of the signatures of altered expression profiles for the 3 cancer panels was analyzed based both on gene and pathway levels. Although the gene level overlap was very small (only 18 genes) among the 3 panels, the pathway analysis revealed that several common or functionally closely related pathways were enriched (related mostly to cell cycle, cytoskeleton remodeling, and immune response). Our analysis showed that the tubulins were significantly downregulated under eribulin treatment compared to paclitaxel. The downregulation under eribulin treatment and the upregulation under paclitaxel treatments of several tubulins was validated by qPCR in breast cancer (Table 2). The alteration of expression profiles of cell cycle, cytoskeleton remodeling and immune response pathways under paclitaxel treatment has been reported previously both in vivo and in vitro in ovarian cancer [26], [27], which was consistent with our data including breast and endometrial cancer panel. The upregulation of tubulin expression and changes in expression of cytoskeleton maintenance genes under paclitaxel treatment has also been reported in rat smooth muscle cells [28]. Previous studies indicated that alpha- and beta-tubulin synthesis is auto-regulated by posttranscriptional mechanisms that can alter mRNA levels of tubulins in response in the unassembled tubulin subunit concentration [29]. Based on these findings, the upregulation of tubulin expression by paclitaxel is likely driven by a compensatory mechanism to increase the supplies of tubulin monomers depleted because of the microtubule polymerization, whereas the downregulation of tubulins by eribulin could be explained by the opposite effect of increasing the number of tubulin monomers by inhibiting microtubule polymerization [30]. Although expression profiles of tubulins treated with paclitaxel has been analyzed in vitro before, a comprehensive analysis of tubulin alteration under eribulin treatment and comparison with paclitaxel has not yet been done. Furthermore, our correlation analysis revealed unique sets of tubulins correlating with eribulin sensitivity which could potentially allow us to identify subpopulations with relative benefit to eribulin compared to paclitaxel. These findings need further investigation and validation.

The analysis of expression profiles revealed that the EMT pathway was significantly altered between the two treatments. EMT is a process in which epithelial cells acquire mesenchymal properties and show loss of intercellular cohesion, increased cellular migration, and increased resistance to apoptosis and anticancer agents. In tumor cells, EMT may increase the motility and invasiveness of cancer cells and is thought to play a fundamental role during invasion and metastasis (for example [31], [32]). In previous studies, the EMT signature has been found to correlate in vitro with cisplatin resistance in ovarian cancer [33], [34], and resistance to gemcitabine, 5-FU and cisplatin in pancreatic cancer [35]. Moreover, EMT regulators have been shown to modulate resistance to EGFR inhibitors in bladder cancer [36]. Our findings indicate that in breast cancer, EMT pathway expression correlates with eribulin resistance, but not with paclitaxel resistance. Detailed analysis of the EMT pathway after mapping significantly altered genes based on qPCR revealed that many key elements of the signaling pathway were significantly altered both between eribulin sensitive and resistant cell lines and between treatments with the two compounds. Vimentin, one of the important markers of EMT pathway activation, was significantly upregulated in eribulin resistant cell lines. Several studies have reported overexpression of vimentin as a marker of basal-like breast cancer cells [37], [38]. Furthermore, it has been shown that overexpression of vimentin in the non-invasive MCF7 breast cancer cell line increases invasiveness [39].

In this study, it is not clear if eribulin will cause EMT in resistant cancer cells, because we determined limited gene signature in the EMT pathway a short time after treatment (24 hour). Eribulin caused MET, which is an opposite to EMT, in one of triple negative breast cancer cell line, which has a mesenchymal phenotype [40]. Additionally, we examined the EMT gene expression 7 days after eribulin treatment for 5 selected breast cancer cell lines (Table S4). Thirteen genes out of 48 from EMT pathway showed consistent down-regulation (Table S5) in three cell lines sensitive to eribulin based on EMT expression profiling (Figure 3). This indicates that eribulin may cause MET change in vitro as well in the sensitive cell lines. These pre-clinical findings additionally suggest that based on specific alterations in EMT gene expression we may identify the sub-population of patients with more benefit from eribulin treatment compared to paclitaxel treatment. These patients may be identified by rapidly analyzing the gene signature of EMT pathway after the drug treatment.

Our correlation analysis indicated an interesting interrelatedness of the EMT pathways association with eribulin and paclitaxel sensitivity among the 3 cancer panels. We found that alterations in EMT expression are predictive of eribulin sensitivity in breast cancer and with both eribulin and paclitaxel sensitivity in endometrial cancer. We found no significant correlation in ovarian cancer. These in vitro findings may be related to the similarity of the molecular profiles among some cell lines from the 3 cancer panel. Recently the development of several high content assays provided an opportunity for the comprehensive analysis of the molecular profiles of the breast, endometrial, and ovarian cancers [41]–[43]. Integrated analysis of mRNA expression, DNA copy number, DNA methylation and sequencing data revealed a similarity among the molecular profiles in sub-types of these cancers. The molecular profiling revealed a common molecular signature among basal-like breast cancer, serous ovarian and serous endometrial cancers. This profile was markedly different from the other endometrial and luminal breast cancer types. The

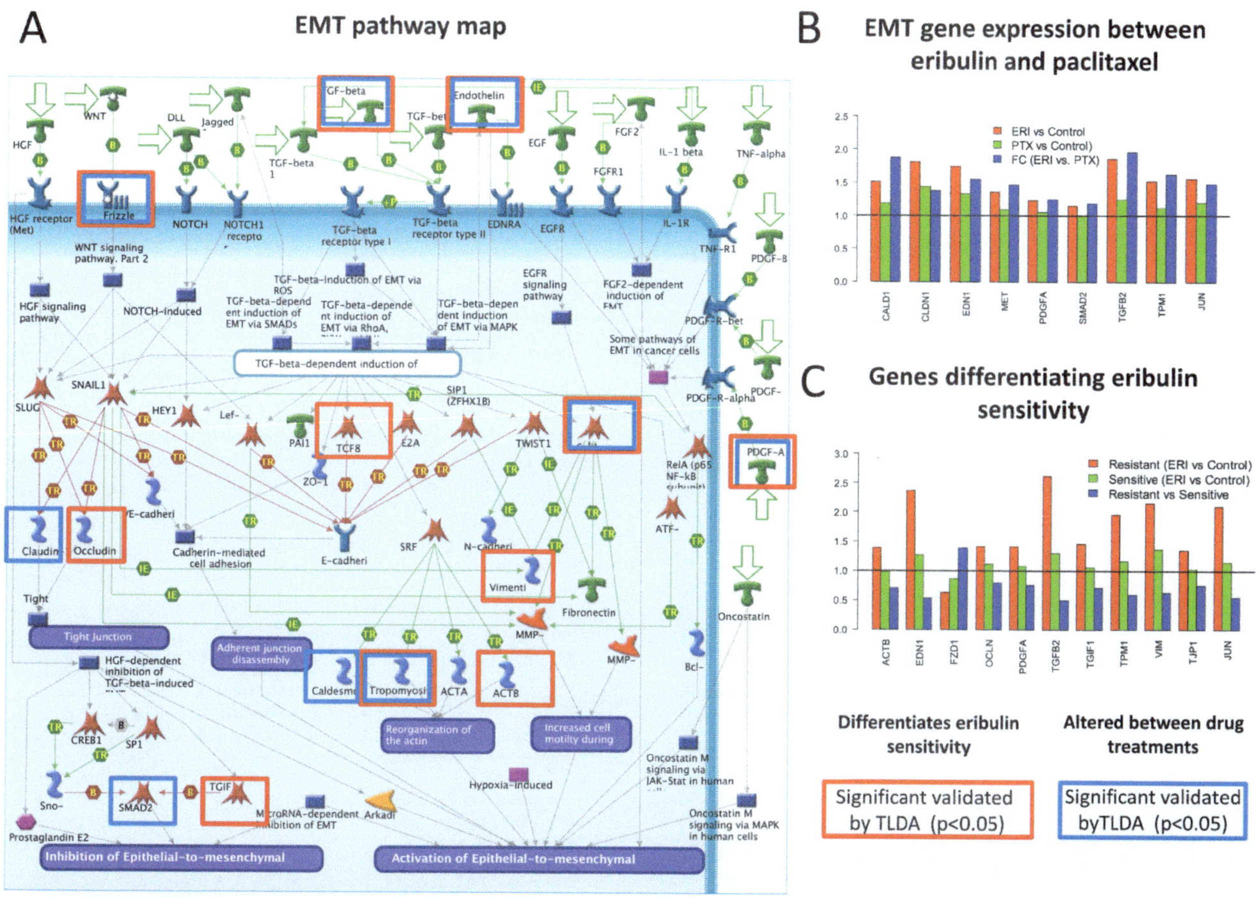

Figure 4. Gene expression profiles of EMT pathway. A) The EMT pathway. The boxes show genes with significantly different expression between eribulin sensitive and resistant cell lines (red) and with significantly different expression between eribulin and paclitaxel treatments (blue). B) EMT gene expression between eribulin and paclitaxel. The plot shows the fold-changes of significantly altered genes between paclitaxel and eribulin (red: eribulin vs. control; green: paclitaxel vs. control; blue: eribulin vs. paclitaxel). C) Genes differentiating eribulin sensitivity. The plot shows the fold-changes of significantly altered genes between eribulin sensitive and resistant cell lines (red: resistant; green: sensitive; blue: resistant vs. sensitive).

mRNA clustering of endometrial cancer defined 3 robust clusters of subtypes called the "mitotic", "hormonal" and "immunoreactive". The hormonal endometrial cancer showed similar molecular profile to the luminal breast cancer which is hormone receptor positive. The finding that both breast and endometrial cancer are related to the sensitivity of the drugs may be related to the fact that the similar molecular profile is driving the sensitivity to treatment and not the cancer type. For example the observation that the breast and endometrial EMT gene signature was predictive of eribulin sensitivity may be related to subtypes of breast and endometrial cancer with common molecular profiles. Indeed we found the highest similarity between endometrial and breast cancer based both on gene and pathway level analysis. Breast cancer signatures shared twice as many genes with endometrial cancer compared to ovarian cancer when the overlapping genes were normalized to the relative sizes of the gene sets. The majority of the genes were upregulated for eribulin treatment compared to paclitaxel for the breast cancer (76%) and endometrial cancer (56%) signatures as opposed to the ovarian cancer signature, where the majority of genes were down regulated (74%). The finding that the EMT signature correlated with paclitaxel sensitivity only for endometrial cancer may be indicative of a cancer subtype with a unique molecular profile. Alternatively, the endometrial cancer subtype resistant to paclitaxel may have similar molecular profiles to some breast or ovarian cancer subtypes not included in the cell line panels.

In summary, the correlative analyses and results of predictions based on the EMT signature in breast and endometrial cancers suggest that EMT pathway genes may serve as biomarkers to predict response to eribulin in breast cancer, and eribulin and paclitaxel in endometrial cancer. Additionally, our findings indicate that the gene signature can separate eribulin resistant subgroups from paclitaxel resistant subgroups in breast cancer panel. We found that tubulin isotopes had significantly lower expression in cell lines treated with eribulin compared to paclitaxel. Lastly, we found that reduced expression of 4 tubulins (TUBA1C, TUBA4A, TUBB3, TUBB6) significantly correlated with eribulin sensitivity and that of one tubulin (TUBB2A) significantly correlated with paclitaxel sensitivity.

Acknowledgments

The authors would like to thank Bruce Littlefield for reviewing and proof reading the manuscript and Juni Matsui, Mamoru Yanagimachi and Tadashi Kadowaki for their comments.

Author Contributions

Conceived and designed the experiments: ZD JO SA JC YO YF. Performed the experiments: JO AW SS SA. Analyzed the data: ZD JO YF. Contributed reagents/materials/analysis tools: JO AW SS SA JC YO. Wrote the paper: ZD.

References

1. Towle MJ, Salvato KA, Budrow J, Wels BF, Kuznetsov G, et al. (2001) In vitro and in vivo anticancer activities of synthetic macrocyclic ketone analogues of halichondrin B. Cancer Res 61: 1013–1021.
2. Jordan MA, Kamath K, Manna T, Okouneva T, Miller HP, et al. (2005) The primary antimitotic mechanism of action of the synthetic halichondrin E7389 is suppression of microtubule growth. Mol Cancer Ther 4: 1086–1095.
3. Smith JA, Wilson L, Azarenko O, Zhu X, Lewis BM, et al. (2010) Eribulin binds at microtubule ends to a single site on tubulin to suppress dynamic instability. Biochemistry 49: 1331–1337.
4. Chien AJ, Moasser MM (2008) Cellular Mechanisms of Resistance to Anthracyclines and Taxanes in Cancer: Intrinsic and Acquired. Semin Oncol 35: S1–S14.
5. Schiff PB, Fant J, Horwitz SB (1979) Promotion of microtubule assembly in vitro by taxol. Nature 277: 665–667.
6. Scatena CD, Stewart ZA, Mays D, Tang LJ, Keefer CJ, et al. (1998) Mitotic phosphorylation of Bcl-2 during normal cell cycle progression and Taxol-induced growth arrest. J Biol Chem 273: 30777–30784.
7. Gonçalves A, Braguer D, Kamath K, Martello L, Briand C, et al. (2001) Resistance to Taxol in lung cancer cells associated with increased microtubule dynamics. Proc Natl Acad Sci U S A 98: 11737–11742.
8. Barlow SB, Gonzalez-Garay ML, Cabral F (2002) Paclitaxel-dependent mutants have severely reduced microtubule assembly and reduced tubulin synthesis. Cell Sci 115: 3469–3478.
9. Hari M, Loganzo F, Annable T, Tan X, Musto S, et al. (2006) Paclitaxel-resistant cells have a mutation in the paclitaxel-binding region of beta-tubulin (Asp26Glu) and less stable microtubules. Mol Cancer Ther 5: 270–278.
10. Mozzetti S, Ferlini C, Concolino P, Filippetti F, Raspaglio G, et al. (2005) Class III beta-tubulin overexpression is a prominent mechanism of paclitaxel resistance in ovarian cancer patients. Clin Cancer Res 11: 298–305.
11. Alli E, Bash-Babula J, Yang JM, Hait WN (2002) Effect of stathmin on the sensitivity to antimicrotubule drugs in human breast cancer. Cancer Res 62: 6864–6869.
12. Yu D (2001) Mechanisms of ErbB2-mediated paclitaxel resistance and trastuzumab-mediated paclitaxel sensitization in ErbB2-overexpressing breast cancers. Semin Oncol 28: 12–17.
13. Wahl AF, Donaldson KL, Fairchild C, Lee FY, Foster SA, et al. (1996) Loss of normal p53 function confers sensitization to Taxol by increasing G2/M arrest and apoptosis. Nat Med 2: 72–79.
14. Zhang CC, Yang JM, White E, Murphy M, Levine A, et al. (1998) The role of MAP4 expression in the sensitivity to paclitaxel and resistance to vinca alkaloids in p53 mutant cells. Oncogene 16: 1617–1624.
15. R Development Core Team (2010) R: A Language and Environment for Statistical Computing. Vienna, Austria: R Foundation for Statistical Computing.
16. Friedman J, Hastie T, Tibshirani R (2008) Sparse inverse covariance estimation with the graphical lasso. Biostatistics 9: 432–441.
17. Friedman J, Hastie T, Tibshirani R (2010) Regularization Paths for Generalized Linear Models via Coordinate Descent. J Stat Softw, 33: 1–22.
18. Zou H, Hastie T (2005) Regularization and variable selection via the elastic net. J Roy Stat Soc B 67: 301–320.
19. Thiery JP, Sleeman JP (2006) Complex networks orchestrate epithelial-mesenchymal transitions. Nat Rev Mol Cell Biol 7: 131–142.
20. Yook JI, Li XY, Ota I, Hu C, Kim HS, et al. (2006) A Wnt-Axin2-GSK3beta cascade regulates Snail1 activity in breast cancer cells. Nat Cell Biol 12: 1398–1406.
21. Lo HW, Hsu SC, Xia W, Cao X, Shih JY, et al. (2007) Epidermal growth factor receptor cooperates with signal transducer and activator of transcription 3 to induce epithelial-mesenchymal transition in cancer cells via up-regulation of TWIST gene expression. Cancer Res 67: 9066–9076.
22. Zavadil J, Bottinger EP (2005) TGF-beta and epithelial-to-mesenchymal transitions. Oncogene 24: 5764–5774.
23. Suh Y, Yoon CH, Kim RK, Lim EJ, Oh YS, et al. (2012) Claudin-1 induces epithelial-mesenchymal transition through activation of the c-Abl-ERK signaling pathway in human liver cells. Oncogene 1: 1–10.
24. Shiozaki A, Bai XH, Shen-Tu G, Moodley S, Takeshita H, et al. (2012) Claudin 1 mediates TNFα-induced gene expression and cell migration in human lung carcinoma cells. PLoS ONE 7: e38049. doi:10.1371/journal.pone.0038049.
25. Jain R, Shaul PW, Borok Z, Willis BC (2007) Endothelin-1 induces alveolar epithelial-mesenchymal transition through endothelin type A receptor-mediated production of TGF-beta1. Am J Respir Cell Mol Biol 37: 38–47.
26. Bani MR, Nicoleti MI, Alkharouf NW, Ghilardi C, Petersen D, et al. (2004) Gene expression correlating with response to paclitaxel in ovarian carcinoma xenografts. Mol Cancer Ther 3: 111–121.
27. L'Espérance S, Bachvarova M, Tetu B, Mes-Masson AM, Bachvarov D (2008) Global gene expression analysis of early response to chemotherapy treatment in ovarian cancer spheroids. BMC Genomics 9: 99. doi:10.1186/1471-2164-9-99.
28. Charles PC, Mapara S, Parker JS, Herrmann RA, Patterson C (2007) Gene Expression Profiling In Rat Smooth Muscle Cells Reveals Novel Regulatory Pathways Modulated by Rapamycin and Paclitaxel. The Internet Journal of Genomics and Proteomics 3: 1. doi:10.5580/1501.
29. Bachurski CJ, Theodorakis NG, Coulson RM, Cleveland DW (1994) An amino-terminal tetrapeptide specifies cotranslational degradation of beta-tubulin but not alpha-tubulin mRNAs. Mol Cell Biol 14: 4076–4086.
30. Stargell LA, Heruth DP, Gaertig J, Gorovsky MA (1992) Drugs Affecting Microtubule Dynamics Increase α-Tubulin mRNA Accumulation via Transcription in Tetrahymena thermophila. Mol Cell Biol 12: 1443–1450.
31. Larue L, Bellacosa A (2005) Epithelial–mesenchymal transition in development and cancer: role of phosphatidylinositol 3′ kinase/AKT pathways. Oncogene 24: 7443–7454.
32. Vallesa AM, Edmea N (2000) Induction and regulation of epithelial–mesenchymal transitions. Biochem Pharmacol 60: 1091–1099.
33. Haslehurst AM, Koti M, Dharsee M, Nuin P, Evans K, et al. (2012) EMT transcription factors snail and slug directly contribute to cisplatin resistance in ovarian cancer BMC Cancer 12: 91. doi:10.1186/1471-2407-12-91.
34. Helleman J, Smid M, Jansen MP, van der Burg ME, Berns EM (2010) Pathway analysis of gene lists associated with platinum-based chemotherapy resistance in ovarian cancer: the big picture. Gynecol Oncol 117: 170–176.
35. Haslehurst AM, Koti M, Dharsee M, Nuin P, Evans K, et al. (2012) EMT transcription factors snail and slug directly contribute to cisplatin resistance in ovarian cancer. BMC Cancer 12: 91. doi:10.1186/1471-2407-12-91.
36. McConkey DJ, Choi W, Marquis L, Martin F, Williams MB, et al. (2009) Role of epithelial-to-mesenchymal transition (EMT) in drug sensitivity and metastasis in bladder cancer. Cancer Metastasis Rev 28: 335–44.
37. Kokkinos MI, Wafai R, Wong MK, Newgreen DF, Thompson EW, et al. (2007) Vimentin and epithelial-mesenchymal transition in human breast cancer–observations in vitro and in vivo. Cells Tissues Organs 185: 191–203.
38. Neve RM, Chin K, Fridlyand J, Yeh J, Baehner FL, et al. (2006) A collection of breast cancer cell lines for the study of functionally distinct cancer subtypes. Cancer Cell 10: 515–527.
39. Hendrix MJ, Seftor EA, Seftor RE, Trevor KT (1997) Experimental co-expression of vimentin and keratin intermediate filaments in human breast cancer cells results in phenotypic interconversion and increased invasive behavior. Am J Pathol 150: 483–495.
40. Yoshida T, Ozawa Y, Kimura T, Sato Y, Kuznetsov G, et al (2014) Eribulin mesilate suppresses experimental metastasis of breast cancer cells by reversing phenotype from epithelial-mesenchymal transition (EMT) to mesenchymal-epithelial transition (MET) states. Br J Cancer 110, 1497–1505.
41. The Cancer Genome Atlas Research Network (2013) Integrated genomic characterization of endometrial carcinoma. Nature 497: 67–73.
42. The Cancer Genome Atlas Research Network (2011) Integrated Genomic Analyses of Ovarian Carcinoma. Nature 474: 609–615.
43. The Cancer Genome Atlas Research Network (2012) Comprehensive molecular portraits of human breast tumours. Nature 490: 61–70.

7

Doxycycline Inducible Kruppel-Like Factor 4 Lentiviral Vector Mediates Mesenchymal to Epithelial Transition in Ovarian Cancer Cells

Zixuan Chen[1,2,4], Yinan Wang[1,2,3], Wen Liu[1,2,3], Guannan Zhao[1,2,5], Suechin Lee[3], Andrea Balogh[3], Yanan Zou[6], Yuqi Guo[5], Zhan Zhang[5], Weiwang Gu[3], Chengyao Li[4]*, Gabor Tigyi[3], Junming Yue[1,2]*

1 Department of Pathology and Laboratory Medicine, University of Tennessee Health Science Center, Memphis, Tennessee, United States of America, **2** Center for Cancer Research, University of Tennessee Health Science Center, Memphis, Tennessee, United States of America, **3** Department of Physiology, University of Tennessee Health Science Center, Memphis, Tennessee, United States of America, **4** Southern Medical University, Guangzhou, P. R. China, **5** The Third Affiliated Hospital, Zhengzhou University, Zhengzhou, P. R. China, **6** The Second Affiliated Hospital of Harbin Medical University, Harbin, P. R. China

Abstract

Ovarian cancer presents therapeutic challenges due to its typically late detection, aggressive metastasis, and therapeutic resistance. The transcription factor Krüppel-like factor 4 (KLF4) has been implicated in human cancers as a tumor suppressor or oncogene, although its role depends greatly on the cellular context. The role of KLF4 in ovarian cancer has not been elucidated in mechanistic detail. In this study, we investigated the role of KLF4 in ovarian cancer cells by transducing the ovarian cancer cell lines SKOV3 and OVCAR3 with a doxycycline-inducible KLF4 lentiviral vector. Overexpression of KLF4 reduced cell proliferation, migration, and invasion. The epithelial cell marker gene E-cadherin was significantly upregulated, whereas the mesenchymal cell marker genes vimentin, twist1and snail2 (slug) were downregulated in both KLF4-expressing SKOV3 and OVCAR3 cells. KLF4 inhibited the transforming growth factor β (TGFβ)-induced epithelial to mesenchymal transition (EMT) in ovarian cancer cells. Taken together, our data demonstrate that KLF4 functions as a tumor suppressor gene in ovarian cancer cells by inhibiting TGFβ-induced EMT.

Editor: Chunming Liu, University of Kentucky, United States of America

Funding: This project was partially supported by National Institute of Health (HL095957, HD061420 to J.Y., and CA092160 to G.T.) and UTHSC startup funding, Western clinic Cancer Center (J.Y.) and Chinese Government (2010CB530204 to C.L., 112102310110 to Y.G., 2011DFA33290 to W.G.). The funders had no role in study design, data collection and analysis, decision to publish, or preparation of the manuscript.

Competing Interests: Junming Yue is a PLOS ONE Editorial Board member. This does not alter the authors' adherence to PLOS ONE Editorial policies and criteria. All authors have no competing interest to declare.

* Email: jyue@uthsc.edu (JY); chengyaoli@hotmail.com (CL)

Introduction

Ovarian cancer has a high mortality rate, reportedly causes 15,000 deaths annually in the US [1]. Although significant improvements have been made in the detection of ovarian cancers in the past decade, more than 20,000 new cases are diagnosed every year [1,2]. The therapeutic options for ovarian cancer are limited because of its resistance to chemo- and radiation therapy leading to frequent recurrences [3,4].

KLF4 has been shown to regulate cell proliferation and differentiation, its role has been extensively investigated in several human cancers by using gain- and loss-of-function approaches. In colon and prostate cancer, KLF4 acts as an oncogene [5,6]. In contrast, it plays a tumor suppressor role in neuroblastoma, lung cancer, gastric cancer, lymphoma, cervical cancer, pancreatic ductal cancer, and hepatocellular carcinoma [7,8,9,10,11,12,13]. In breast cancer, KLF4 can function both as an oncogene [14,15] and a tumor suppressor [16,17,18]. The role of KLF4 in ovarian cancer has not been adequately and mechanistically addressed. A previous study indicates that the expression level of KLF4 was significantly reduced in ovarian cancer compared to normal ovarian epithelium, suggesting that KLF4 might potentially act as a tumor suppressor in ovarian cancer [19].

KLF4 plays a unique role in stem cell reprogramming by facilitating the mesenchymal to epithelial transition (MET) [20]. The cellular phenotypic switch from epithelial to mesenchymal cell transition (EMT) is a fundamental process in tumor metastasis that is a prominent feature of ovarian carcinomas. The MET or EMT leads to the alterations of epithelial and mesenchymal marker gene expression that include snail1 & 2, Zeb 1 &2, Twist, vimentin, E-cadherin [18,21,22]. EMT is regulated by multiple signaling pathways, which include WNT, TGFβ, and Notch. [23,24,25]. Recent studies indicate that miRNAs regulate EMT or MET pathways by targeting epithelial or mesenchymal cell marker genes that include miR-194, miR-203, and miR-200c [22,26]. KLF4 has been shown to regulate EMT in several different cancer cells. In hepatocellular carcinoma, breast, and prostate cancer cells, KLF4 activates the transcription of the epithelial cell marker gene E-cadherin and represses the mesenchymal cell marker gene snail 2(slug) by binding to their respective promoters. KLF4 in these cancers promotes MET and inhibits tumor cell growth [10,24,27].

In the present study, we investigated the role of KLF4 in ovarian cancer cells using a doxycycline (Dox)-dependent KLF4-inducible lentiviral vector (Tet-on) and found that inducible overexpression of KLF4 reduced cell proliferation, migration, and invasion through promoting MET in ovarian cancer cells.

Materials and Methods

Cell culture

The ovarian cancer cell lines SKOV3, OVCAR3 and breast cancer cell line MCF7 were obtained from ATCC and cultured in Dulbecco's Modified Eagle Medium (DMEM) supplemented with 10% FBS (Hyclone; Logan, UT), 100 U/ml penicillin, and 100 μg/ml streptomycin (Invitrogen; Carlsbad, CA). HEK293 FT cells were cultured in DMEM media with 10% FBS, 100 U/ml penicillin, 100 μg/ml streptomycin, 1% glutamine, 1% nonessential amino acid, and geneticin with a final concentration of 1 μg/ml.

Lentiviral vector production

The Dox-inducible KLF4, reverse transactivator (rtTA-M3), and EGFP lentiviral vectors were packaged in HEK293FT cells and produced as described previously [28]. Stable cell lines with overexpression of KLF4- or EGFP- were generated by co-transducing the SKOV3, OVCAR3, and MCF7 cells with the lentiviral vectors KLF4, EGFP with rtTA-M3 and selected with 5 μg/ml puromycin. To induce KLF4 and EGFP expression, Dox was added into normal growth medium as indicated.

Cell colony formation assay

SKOV3, MCF7 and OVCAR3 cells transduced with KLF4 or EGFP overexpression viruses (200 cells/well each) were plated in triplicate into 6-well plates and cultured for 2 weeks. They were then stained with 0.1% crystal violet, and cell colonies were counted as described previously[29].

MTT assay

Cells were plated 8000 per well in 96-well plates and cultured for 24 h. Thereafter, 10 μl of MTT reagent were added to each well and incubated for ~4 h. The reaction was terminated by adding 100 μl detergent reagent; the plates were incubated at 22°C in the dark for 2 h; and then the absorbance was measured at 570 nm wavelength.

Cell migration assay

Transduced cells (3×10^5 cells per well) were seeded in triplicate into 6-well plates and cultured for 24 h. The cell surface was scratched with a pipette tip and washed three times with PBS. Fresh growth medium was added for an additional 24 h. The migration rate was calculated using the following formula: (area of the wound area at 0 h - the wound area at 24 h)/the wound area at 0 h. The transwell migration assay was performed using a modified chamber (BD Falcon, San Jose, CA). These chambers were inserted into a 24-well plate. Cells (3×10^4) in 300 μl serum-free DMEM were added to the upper chamber. The chemoattractant in DMEM was added into the lower chamber of each well and cells were incubated for 24 h. The medium and non-migrated cells in the upper chamber were removed whereas, the migrated cells in the lower side of the membranes were fixed with methanol and stained with crystal violet. Pictures were taken at 10X magnification. Cells in at least three different fields were counted.

Cell invasion assay

SKOV3 and OVCAR3 cells (5×10^5) transduced with EGFP and KLF4 overexpression viruses were seeded in serum-free DMEM onto inserts precoated with Matrigel (BD BioCoat, 24-well Tumor Invasion System (BD BioSciences, San Jose, CA). DMEM containing 10% FBS was added to the bottom chamber of the invasion system as the chemoattractant. After 24 h, the transwell inserts were stained using 4 μg/ml of Calcein AM (Life Technologies, Grand Island, NY) at 37°C for 1 h. The fluorescent intensity was measured using the BioTek Synergy (Winooski, VT) plate reader at excitation and emission wavelengths of 485 nm and 528 nm, respectively.

Soft agar assay

For the bottom agar, 0.6% Noble agar in DMEM containing 10% FBS was added to 6-well plates. Two million cells in DMEM containing 10% FBS and 0.35% Noble agar were added to the bottom agar. Growth medium was then added to the top agar once it had solidified and the cells were fed with fresh growth medium every 5 d, and colonies were counted under a light microscope after 2 weeks.

Immunofluorescent staining

To detect the expression of EMT-associated marker genes, KLF4-expressing and control SKOV3 cells were fixed for 10 min using 4% PFA, washed three times with 0.1% Tween20 in PBS (PBST), and incubated with blocking buffer (5% normal goat serum, 3% bovine serum albumin, and 0.1% Triton-X 100 in PBS) for 1 h. The primary antibodies to E-cadherin, snail2, and vimentin (1:200 dilution, Cell Signaling, Danvers, MA), were incubated with fixed cells overnight. After rinsing three times for 5 min with PBST, Alexa 488 or 594 conjugated goat anti-rabbit (1:200 dilution, Life Technologies) antibodies were added for 1 h at room temperature. Cell nuclei were counterstained with DAPI (Vector Laboratories, Inc.; Burlingame, CA). Images were taken using a Nikon inverted fluorescence microscope.

Chromatin immunoprecipitation (ChIP)

ChIP was performed using the ChIP-IT Express Enzymatic kit (Active Motif, Carlsbad, CA) according to the manufacturer's instructions. Briefly, KLF4-expressing and control SKOV3 cells were cross-linked with 1% formaldehyde for 10 min at room temperature. Cells were harvested and sonicated to shear chromosomal DNA. Immunoprecipitation was performed by binding 10 μg of rabbit anti-KLF4 antibody or IgG (Santa Cruz Inc., Dallas, Texas) to the lysates and incubated at 4°C with rotation overnight. Chromatin complexes were eluted from magnetic beads by reverse-crosslink. Chromatin DNA was purified using the QIAquick PCR Purification Kit (Qiagen, Valencia, CA) and eluted into 40 μl of water. DNA (4 μl) was used for quantitative PCR reaction to detect the presence of E-cadherin promoter. Primers used to detect the promoter of E-cadherin were 5′-TAG AGG GTC ACC GCG TCT AT-3′ (forward) and 5′-TCA CAG GTG CTT TGC AGT TC-3(reverse) as described previously [16].

Western blot

Ovarian and breast cancer cells were collected in RIPA buffer (Thermo Scientific; Rockford, IL) containing 1% Halt Proteinase Inhibitor Cocktail (Thermo Scientific; Rockford, IL). An equal amount of protein (40 μg/lane) was loaded onto 10% SDS-PAGE gels and transferred onto nitrocellulose membranes. The membranes were blocked with 5% non-fat milk for 1 h and incubated

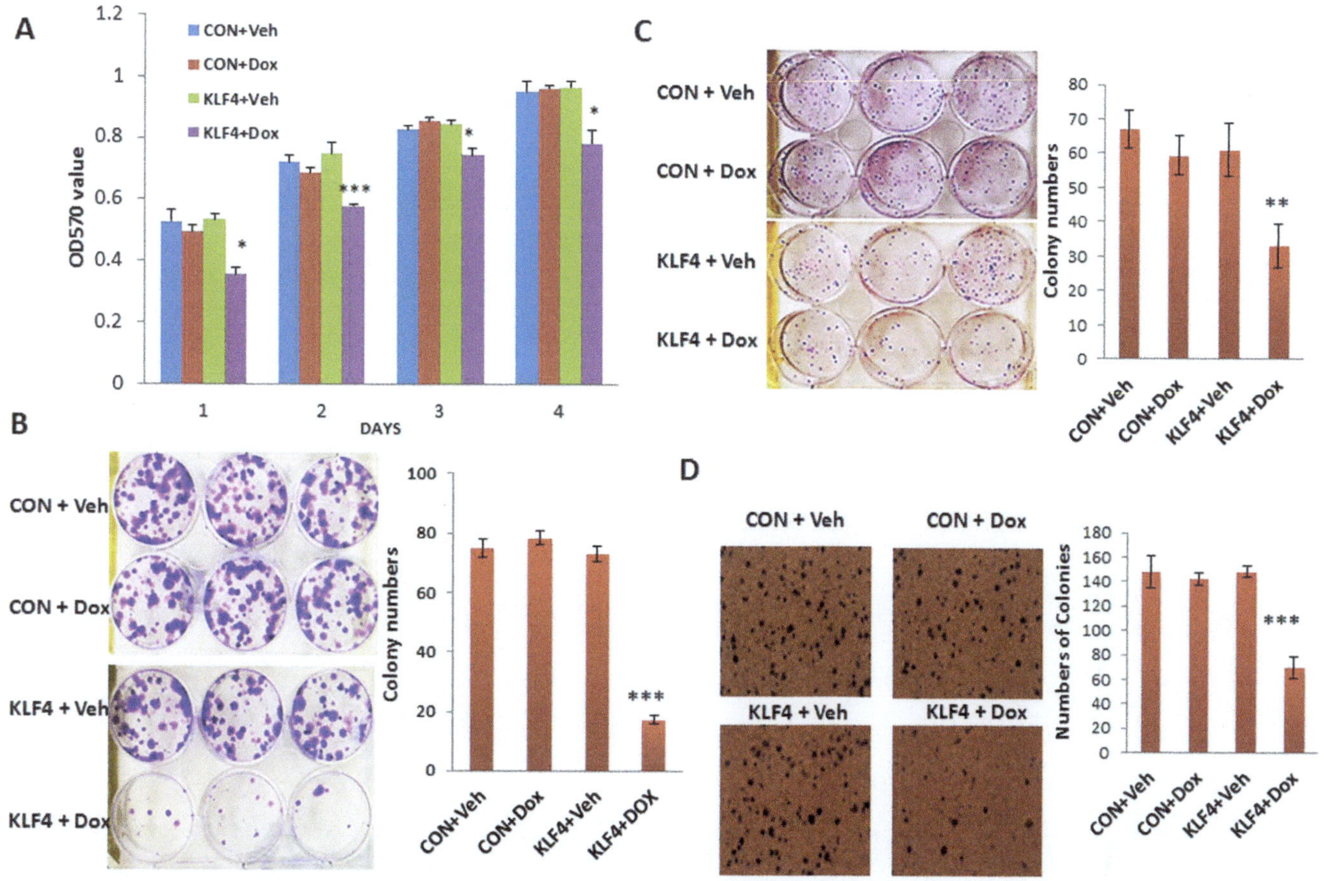

Figure 1. KLF4 inhibits cell proliferation and colony formation. A. Cell proliferation of SKOV3 cells transduced with either EGFP or KLF4 was examined by MTT assay at different time points following Dox treatment. Overexpression of KLF4 significantly reduced cell proliferation compared to that in Dox-treated control cells (*$p<0.05$). **B.** 200 SKOV3 cells transduced with lentiviral KLF4 or EGFP control vectors were seeded into each well of a 6-well plate and cultured for 14 d. Cell colonies were counted following crystal violet staining. The number of colonies in KLF4-overexpressing cells was significantly reduced compared to that in Dox-treated control cells (***$p<0.001$). **C.** The number of colonies in KLF4-overexpressing OVCAR3 cells was significantly reduced compared to that in Dox-treated control cells (**$p<0.01$). **D.** Soft agar colony formation assay was performed in triplicate using SKOV3 cells. Colonies were photographed and counted after 3 weeks. The number of colonies in KLF4-overexpressing cells was significantly reduced compared to that in Dox-treated control cells (***$p<0.001$).

with primary antibodies against KLF4 (Cell Signaling), GAPDH (Sigma; St. Louis, MO), vimentin, E-cadherin, or snail2 (Cell Signaling).

Statistical analysis

Significant differences were determined from two or three independent experiments performed in triplicate and presented as means ± S.D. using Student's *t*-test. $p<0.05$ was considered significant.

Results

Overexpression of KLF4 in ovarian cancer cells using Tet-on system

To determine the role of KLF4 in ovarian cancer cells, we constructed an inducible lentiviral vector, in which the KLF4 gene was driven by tetracycline- (Tet) or a Dox-responsive promoter (TRE-tight). The reverse transcription activator rtTA-M3 was driven by a constitutive human ubiquitous C promoter cloned into a separate lentiviral vector (Figure S1A). KLF4 expression can be activated by rtTA-M3 in the presence of Dox in a dose-dependent manner. An EGFP-inducible lentiviral vector was constructed and served as control. To examine the induced expression of KLF4 and EGFP in the ovarian cancer cell lines SKOV3 and OVCAR3, Dox was added at a final concentration of 1 μg/ml, and the expression of KLF4 and EGFP at different time points was detected by Western blot. Expression of EGFP and KLF4 increased gradually over a 24 h period (Figure S1B). EGFP expression in SKOV3 and OVCAR3 ovarian cancer cells was visualized using fluorescent microcopy 48 h after the addition of Dox (Fig. S2A, B). Dox treatment caused changes in cell morphology of SKOV3 cells. A rounded epithelial cell-like morphology was observed in KLF4-transduced SKOV3 cells compared to flattened multipolar epithelial cell-like shape of EGFP or KLF4 control cells at 48 and 72 h (Fig. S1C and Fig. S2C). However, the morphology in KLF4-transduced OVCAR3 cells was not altered following Dox treatment compared with control cells (data not shown).

KLF4 inhibits cell proliferation and colony formation

To investigate the role of KLF4 in ovarian cancer cell proliferation, the MTT assay was performed in KLF4-transduced SKOV3 and control cells. Following Dox treatment, proliferation in KLF4-overexpressing cells was significantly inhibited compared

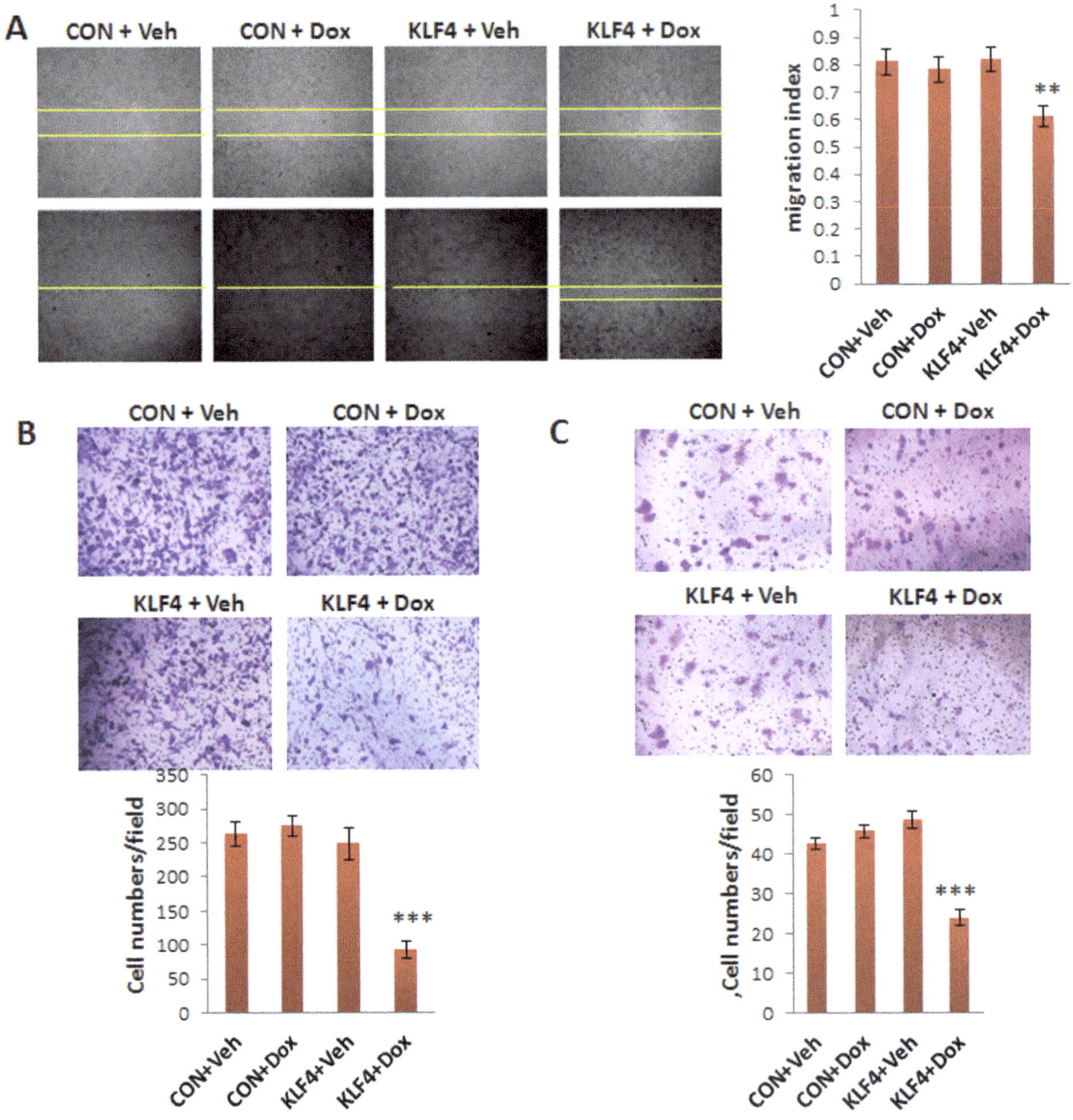

Figure 2. KLF4 reduces cell migration in ovarian cancer cells. A. Wound-healing assay was performed to examine the migration rate of SKOV3 cells transduced with KLF4 and EGFP lentiviral vectors. Photographs were taken at 0 and 24 h following the initial scratch. Migration rates were quantified by measuring three different wound areas. Three separate experiments were performed. Migration rate was significantly reduced in KLF4-overexpressing cells compared to that in Dox-treated controls (**$p<0.01$). **B, C**. Transwell migration assay was performed in SKOV3 and OVCAR3 cells. Overexpression of KLF4 significantly reduced cell migration in SKOV3 (**B**) and OVCAR3 (**C**) cells compared with that in Dox-treated controls (***$p<$ 0.001).

to EGFP or KLF4 (non-Dox) control cells (Figure 1A). We also performed colony formation assays on SKOV3 and OVCAR3 cells transduced with KLF4 and EGFP control vectors. The number of colonies in KLF4-overexpressing cells was significantly reduced compared to EGFP and KLF4 control cells (Figure 1B, C). In addition, soft agar colony formation assays were also performed to determine whether KLF4 affects anchorage-independent cell growth. Similarly, our results indicated that KLF4 inhibits cell proliferation in the semisolid culture media compared to control cells (Figure 1D).

KLF4 reduces cell migration and invasion

One crucial property of invasive cancer cells is their increased mobility. To investigate whether KLF4 affects cell migration in the ovarian cancer cell line SKOV3, wound-healing assay was performed using KLF4-transduced SKOV3 and control cells. As shown in Figure 2A, the cell migration rate was significantly reduced in KLF4-overexpressing cells compared to rates in EGFP- and KLF4-transduced control cells. Cell chemotaxis was examined using the transwell migration assay. As shown in Figure 2B and C, migrated cells were significantly reduced in KLF4-overexpressing

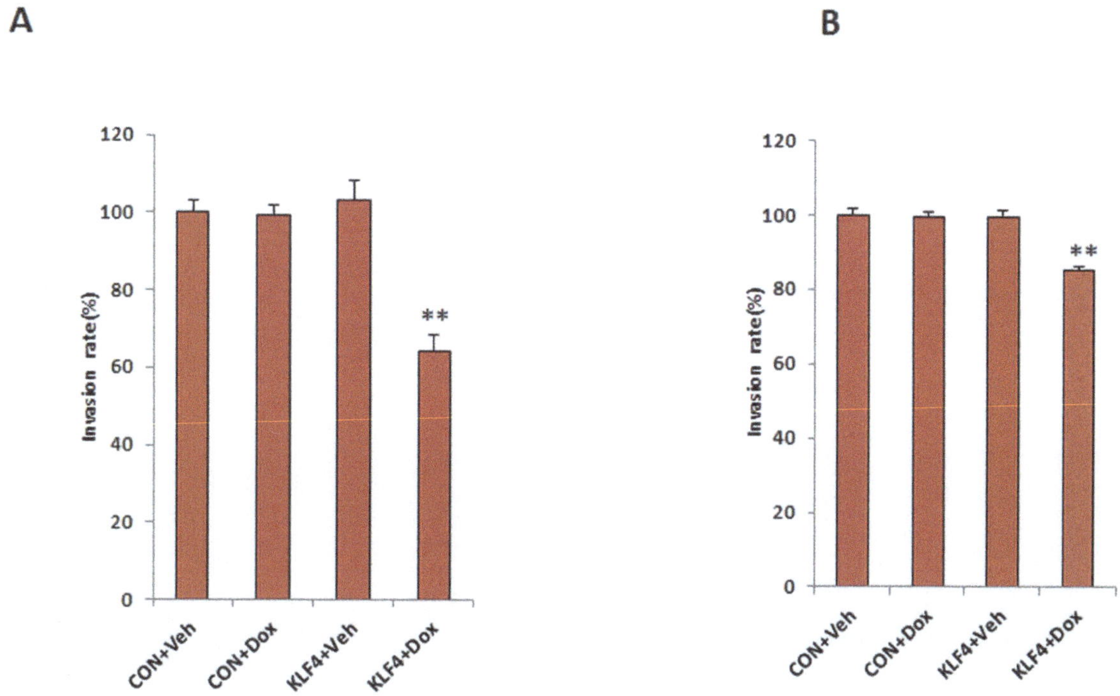

Figure 3. KLF4 reduces ovarian cancer cell invasion. A, B. Cell invasion assay was performed using Matrigel-coated transwell plates for SKOV3 (**A**) and OVCAR3 cells (**B**). The invasion rate was significantly reduced in KLF4-overexpressing cells compared to that in Dox-treated control cells from both SKOV3 and OVCAR3 cells (**$p<0.01$). Data were collected from three separate experiments and analyzed using Student *t*-tests.

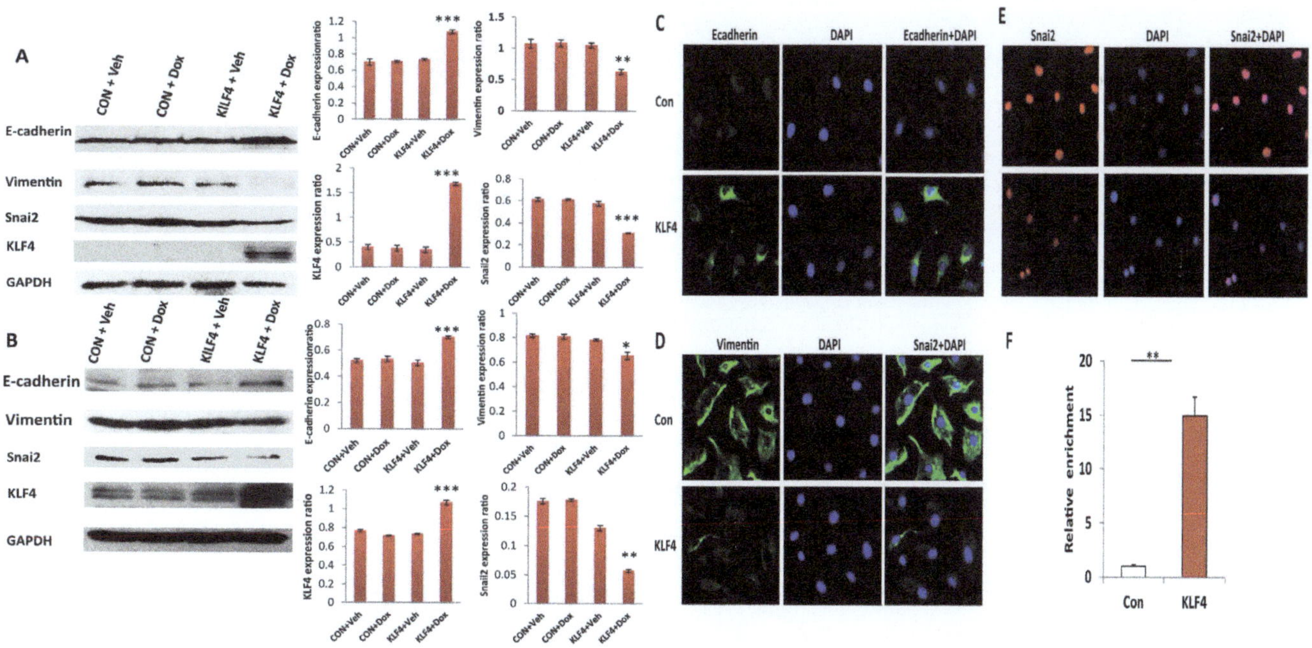

Figure 4. KLF4 promotes mesenchymal-epithelial cell transition. A. B. Western blots were performed in KLF4- and EGFP-transduced SKOV3 (**A**) and OVCAR3 cells (**B**) with or without Dox induction. E-cadherin expression was significantly upregulated (***$p<0.001$), whereas vimentin (**$p<0.01$) and snail2 (***$p<0.001$) were downregulated in KLF4- overexpressing SKOV3 cells compared to control cells (**A**). E-cadherin (**$p<0.01$) was upregulated, whereas vimentin (*$p<0.05$) and snail2 (***$p<0.001$) were downregulated in KLF4-overexpressing OVCAR3 cells compared to Dox-treated control cells (**B**). E-cadherin (**C**) and vimentin (**D**) were immunostained in cellular membranes in KLF4-expressing and control SKOV3 cells. **E.** Snail2 was stained in cell nuclei in KLF4-expressing and control SKOV3 cells. **F.** KLF4 binding to the promoter of E-cadherin in SKOV3 cells was examined by chromatin immunoprecipitation using KLF4 antibody and detected by real-time PCR using E-cadherin-specific primers. The ChIP-enriched DNA levels were normalized to input DNA, followed by subtraction of non-specific binding determined by control IgG (***$p<0.001$).

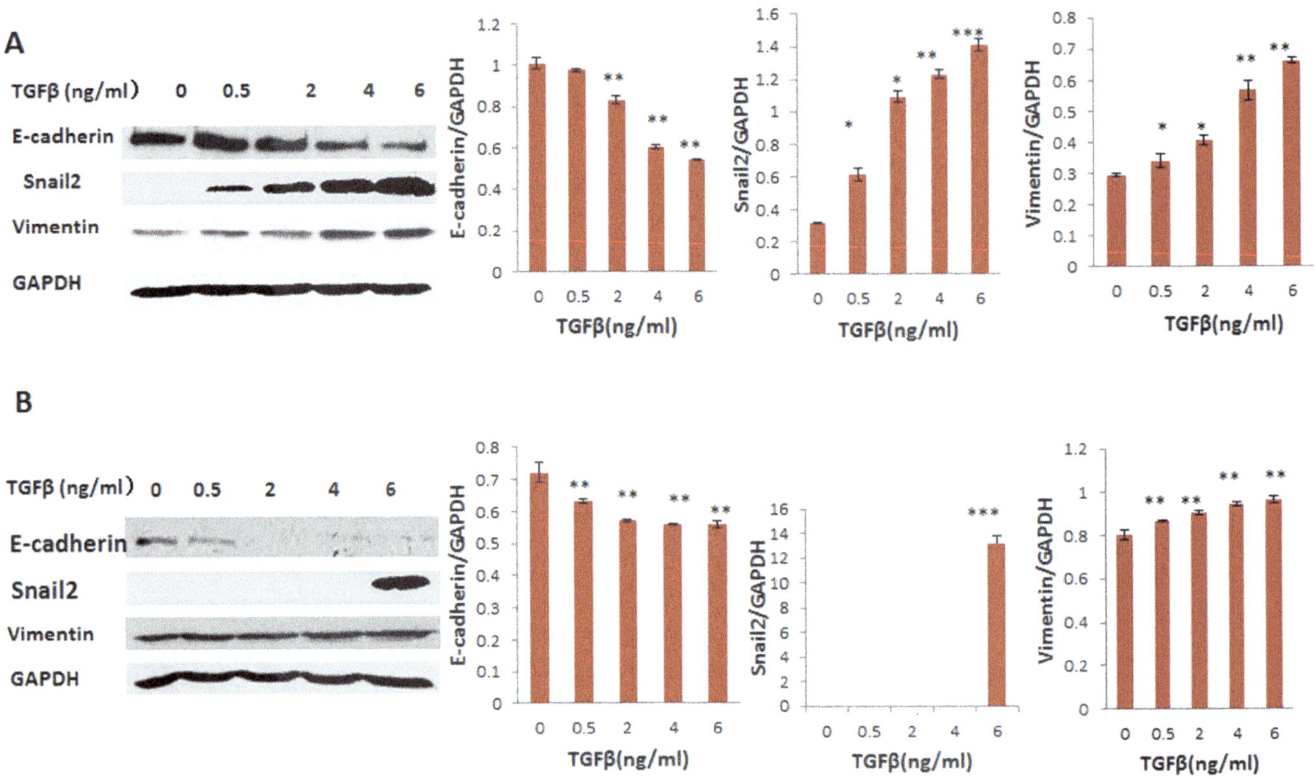

Figure 5. TGFβ promotes EMT in ovarian cancer cells. Human ovarian cancer cell lines SKOV3 (**A**) and OVCAR3 (**B**) were treated with different doses of TGFβ for 48 h. EMT-associated marker genes, including E-cadherin, snail2, and vimentin were examined using Western blot. Significances were determined by comparing TGFβ treated to non-treatment (*$p<0.05$, **$p<0.01$, ***$p<0.001$).

SKOV3 and OVCAR3 cells compared to cells EGFP and KLF4 controls. To examine whether KLF4 affects cell invasion, a cell invasion assay was performed on KLF4-transduced SKOV3 and OVCAR3 cells using Matrigel-coated transwell plates. Overexpression of KLF4 significantly reduced cell invasion compared to that in controls in both cell lines (Figure 3A, B).

KLF4 promotes MET in ovarian cancer cells

To investigate whether KLF4 regulates EMT in ovarian cancer cells, the epithelial cell marker gene E-cadherin and mesenchymal marker genes snail2 and vimentin were examined in KLF4-transduced SKOV3 and OVCAR3 cells using Western blot. The epithelial marker E-cadherin was significantly upregulated, whereas the mesenchymal markers vimentin and snail2 were significantly reduced in KLF4-overexpressing cells compared to EGFP and KLF4 controls (Figure 4A, B). We also performed immunostaining on KLF4-overexpressing and control cells to examine MET markers. Both E-cadherin and vimentin staining were prominent in cellular membranes, whereas snail2 stained the cell nuclei. Similarly to the Western blots, immunostaining showed that E-cadherin expression was upregulated, whereas vimentin and snail2 were downregulated (Figure 4C, D, and E). We also examined the expression of twist1 using realtime RT-PCR in KLF4 transduced SKOV3 cells and found that twist1 was significantly downregulated in KLF4 expressing SKOV3 cells compared with control (Fig. S4). These results support the hypothesis that KLF4 promotes MET in ovarian cancer cells. To further examine whether E-cadherin upregulation was caused by transcriptional activation, we performed chromatin immunoprecipitation in KLF4-expressing and control SKOV3 cells, and the promoter region of E-cadherin was amplified from enriched chromatic DNA by real-time PCR as described previously [16]. KLF4 expression in SKOV3 cells led to an approximately 15-fold enrichment of E-cadherin compared to controls (Figure 4F), indicating that KLF4 binds to the promoter of E-cadherin and activates E-cadherin expression in ovarian cancer cells.

KLF4 inhibits TGFβ-induced EMT in ovarian cancer cells

To examine the mechanism whether KLF4 regulates TGFβ induced EMT in ovarian cancer cells, SKOV3 and OVCAR3 cells were treated with different doses of TGFβ. Expression of the EMT marker proteins E-cadherin, vimentin, and snail2 was examined using Western blot. Our data indicate that TGFβ promoted EMT in ovarian cancer cells by downregulating E-cadherin and upregulating snail2 and vimentin (Figure 5A, B). Furthermore, when we treated KLF4-expressing and control SKOV3 and OVCAR3 cells with increasing doses of TGFβ, KLF4 expression significantly inhibited TGFβ-induced EMT in both cell lines (Figure 6A, B).

Discussion

In this study, we investigated the role of KLF4 in ovarian cancer cells using lentiviral vector mediated inducible expression. Previous studies showed that KLF4 was downregulated in ovarian cancers compared to controls and that KLF4 did not affect cell proliferation but increased the Bcl-2/Bax ratio and inhibited apoptosis [19]. In contrast, we found that KLF4 inhibits the proliferation of SKOV3 cells in colony formation and MTT assays (Fig. 1A, B, and C). The discrepancy may be caused by the low

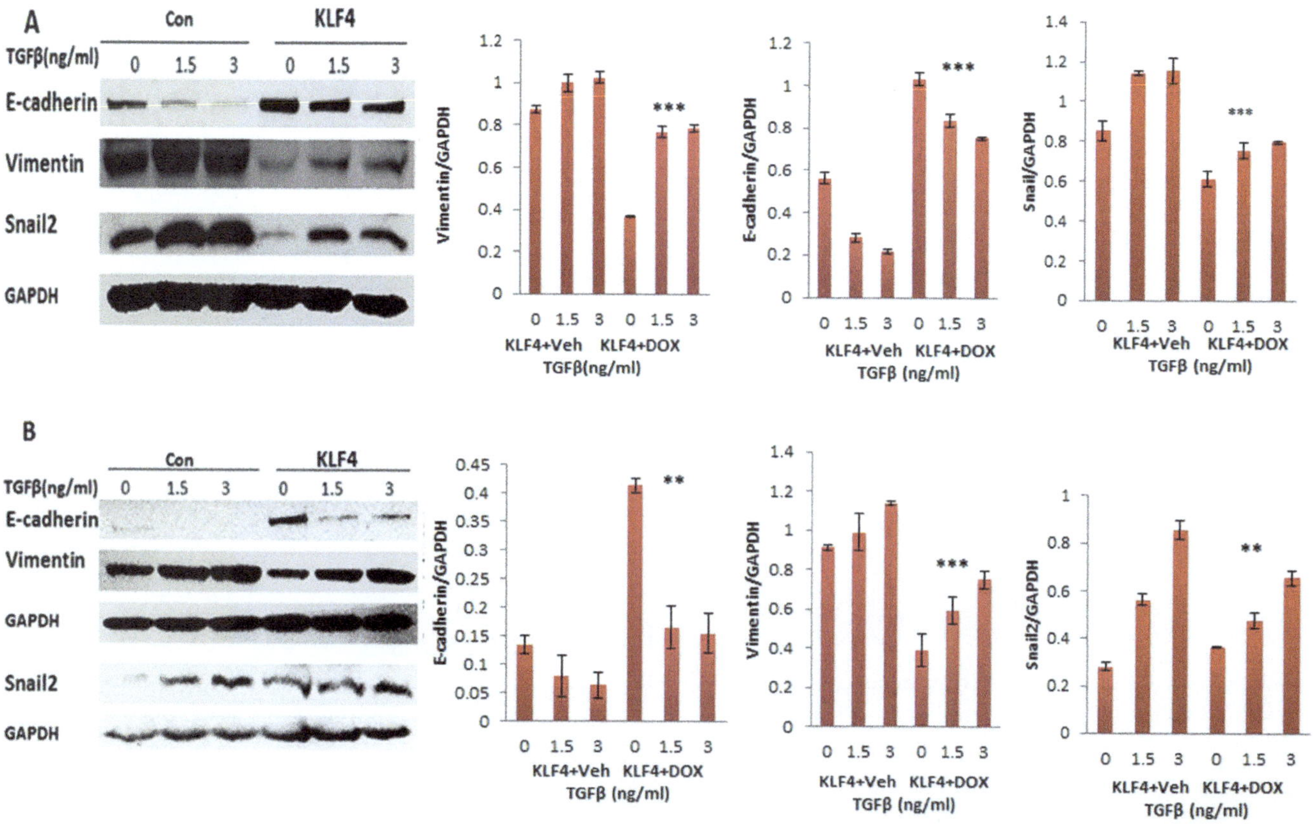

Figure 6. KLF4 inhibits TGFβ-induced EMT in ovarian cancer cells. Ovarian cancer cell lines SKOV3 (**A**) and OVCAR3 (**B**) transduced with lentiviral KLF4 overexpression and control vector were treated with TGFβ for 48 h, and the protein expressions of EMT-associated marker genes E-cadherin, snail2 and vimentin were examined using Western blot. Significant differences were compared between KLF4 expressing and control group (**$p<0.05$, ***$p<0.001$).

transfection efficiency in that study compared to our highly efficient inducible lentiviral transduction. We also found that KLF4 inhibits cell proliferation in OVCAR3 cells (Fig. 1C). Our data demonstrate that KLF4 inhibits cell proliferation, migration, and invasion, hence it functions as a tumor suppressor in both SKOV3 and OVCAR3 cells.

KLF4 can have a dual effect either as an oncogene or a tumor suppressor in breast cancer cells [14,16,18,30]. To compare the actions of KLF4 in MCF7 breast cancer with that in ovarian cancer cells, we performed similar experiments using the same lentiviral Tet-on inducible vector-transduced in MCF7 cells. We found that KLF4 inhibits MCF7 cell proliferation (Fig. S3A). Our finding is similar to the results shown in MCF10A cells by Yori et al. [16]. Yu et al., however, showed that KLF4 functions as an oncogene in MCF7 cells [14], which is opposite to our finding.

The morphology in KLF4 expressing SKOV3 cells in the presence of Dox was clearly altered from control cells without Dox at the different time points (Fig S2C); however, we did not observe obvious morphological alteration in OVCAR3 cells following induction of KLF4 expression. One of reasons causing this phenomenon is that KLF4 also induced cell apoptosis in ovarian cancer cells based on our unpublished data. The morphological differences may be caused by the different responses to KLF4 induced apoptosis in both cell lines. In both SKOV3 and OVCAR3 cells the epithelial cell marker gene E-cadherin was upregulated, and the mesenchymal marker genes vimentin and snail2 were downregulated following induction of KLF4 overexpression (Fig. 4A, B). Altogether, these data suggest that KLF4 primarily promoted MET in ovarian cancer cells. The expression of EMT associated marker genes in ovarian cancer cells are similar to what we observed in MCF7 breast cancer cells, although the endogenous expression of vimentin in MCF7 was not detectable in KLF4-overexpressing or control cells. This may be caused by low endogenous expression level of vimentin in MCF7 cells. Our data support the hypothesis that KLF4 is a key regulator promoting MET and inhibiting EMT in ovarian and breast cancer cells.

Previous studies showed that KLF4 binds to the promoter regions of E-cadherin and snail2, thus can activate the expression of E-cadherin or repress the expression of snail2 in fibroblasts and several cancer cell lines [18,24,27,31]. The expression of epithelial cell marker E-cadherin is required for stem cell reprogramming. KLF4 facilitates the MET process by activating E-cadherin expression [31]. In ovarian cancer cells, we observed a KLF4-dependent upregulation of E-cadherin and a downregulation of vimentin and snail2. Our data indicate that KLF4 transcriptionally binds to the promoters of E-cadherin, thus leading to the activation of E-cadherin expression in ovarian cancer cells.

The EMT or MET is tightly regulated by multiple signaling pathways. Several studies have shown that multiple signaling pathways, including WNT, Notch, NFkB, and TGFβ, are involved in EMT or MET transition in cancers [32,33,34,35]. Previous studies also showed that TGFβ promotes EMT in ovarian cancer cells [36,37]. However, there are no related studies on describing the mechanism how KLF4 is involved in EMT and interacts with those pathways in ovarian cancer cells. Our current studies indicate that KLF4 inhibits TGFβ-induced EMT in both SKOV3 and OVCAR3 cells (Fig. 6A, B), suggesting that KLF4 attenuates the TGFβ induced EMT in ovarian cancers. Therefore, synergistically overexpression of KLF4 and inhibition of TGFβ pathway will provide a novel approach in the developing new therapeutic drugs for the treatment of ovarian cancers.

In summary, this is the first report showing that KLF4 functions as a tumor suppressor by inhibiting cell proliferation, migration and invasion in ovarian cancer cells through attenuating TGFβ-induced EMT.

Supporting Information

Figure S1 Induction of KLF4 expression in ovarian cancer cells using lentiviral Tet-on vector. A. Lentiviral Tet-on vector system. Reverse transactivator (rtTA-M3) was driven by human ubiquitin C (UBC promoter), and EGFP or KLF4 was driven by the Dox inducible promoter TRE-tight. To induce the expression of EGFP or KLF4, Dox is required to activate the Tet promoter following rtTA binding to the Tet-responsive element in the promoter region. **B**. EGFP and KLF4 expressions were induced by Dox in SKOV3 ovarian cancer cells and detected by Western blot. **C**. SKOV3 cells overexpressing KLF4 display rounded epithelial cell-like morphology.

Figure S2 Dox-induced EGFP expression in SKOV3 and OVCAR3 cells. EGFP expressions in SKOV3 (**A**) and OVCAR3 cells (**B**) transduced with EGFP lentiviral vector were visualized under fluorescent microscopy with or without Dox induction. Cell morphologies were examined under light microscopy. **C**. Cell morphologies were imaged at different time points under light microscopy.

Figure S3 KLF4 promotes MET in breast cancer MCF7 cells. A. Colony formation was performed in MCF7 cells transduced with EGFP and KLF4 overexpression lentiviral vectors. The number of colonies in KLF4-overexpressing cells was significantly reduced compared to that in Dox-treated controls (***$p<0.001$). **B**. Western blot analysis of KLF4 (**$p<0.01$), E-cadherin (**$p<0.01$), and snail2 (*$p<0.05$) in MCF7 cells overexpressing KLF4 and EGFP with or without Dox treatment.

Figure S4 KLF4 downregulates twist1 expression in ovarian cancer SKOV3 cells. Twist1 expression in KLF4 expressing SKOV3 and control cells was detected by real time RT-PCR following KLF4 induction for 24 h using 1 ug/ml of doxycycline (*$p<0.05$).

Author Contributions

Conceived and designed the experiments: JY GT. Performed the experiments: ZC YW WL GZ SL AB YZ. Analyzed the data: ZC JY. Contributed reagents/materials/analysis tools: YG ZZ WG CL GT. Contributed to the writing of the manuscript: JY GT.

References

1. Su Z, Graybill WS, Zhu Y (2013) Detection and monitoring of ovarian cancer. Clin Chim Acta 415: 341–345.
2. Lowe KA, Chia VM, Taylor A, O'Malley C, Kelsh M, et al. (2013) An international assessment of ovarian cancer incidence and mortality. Gynecol Oncol 130: 107–114.
3. Yue P, Zhang X, Paladino D, Sengupta B, Ahmad S, et al. (2012) Hyperactive EGF receptor, Jaks and Stat3 signaling promote enhanced colony-forming ability, motility and migration of cisplatin-resistant ovarian cancer cells. Oncogene 31: 2309–2322.
4. Chou JL, Su HY, Chen LY, Liao YP, Hartman-Frey C, et al. (2010) Promoter hypermethylation of FBXO32, a novel TGF-beta/SMAD4 target gene and tumor suppressor, is associated with poor prognosis in human ovarian cancer. Lab Invest 90: 414–425.
5. Leng Z, Tao K, Xia Q, Tan J, Yue Z, et al. (2013) Kruppel-like factor 4 acts as an oncogene in colon cancer stem cell-enriched spheroid cells. PLoS One 8: e56082.
6. Le Magnen C, Bubendorf L, Ruiz C, Zlobec I, Bachmann A, et al. (2013) Klf4 transcription factor is expressed in the cytoplasm of prostate cancer cells. Eur J Cancer 49: 955–963.
7. Mohan N, Ai W, Chakrabarti M, Banik NL, Ray SK (2013) KLF4 overexpression and apigenin treatment down regulated anti-apoptotic Bcl-2 proteins and matrix metalloproteinases to control growth of human malignant neuroblastoma SK-N-DZ and IMR-32 cells. Mol Oncol 7: 464–474.
8. Deng Y, Liu Q, Luo C, Chen S, Li X, et al. (2012) Generation of induced pluripotent stem cells from buffalo (Bubalus bubalis) fetal fibroblasts with buffalo defined factors. Stem Cells Dev 21: 2485–2494.
9. Yang WT, Zheng PS (2012) Kruppel-like factor 4 functions as a tumor suppressor in cervical carcinoma. Cancer 118: 3691–3702.
10. Lin ZS, Chu HC, Yen YC, Lewis BC, Chen YW (2012) Kruppel-like factor 4, a tumor suppressor in hepatocellular carcinoma cells reverts epithelial mesenchymal transition by suppressing slug expression. PLoS One 7: e43593.
11. Zammarchi F, Morelli M, Menicagli M, Di Cristofano C, Zavaglia K, et al. (2011) KLF4 is a novel candidate tumor suppressor gene in pancreatic ductal carcinoma. Am J Pathol 178: 361–372.
12. Zhou Y, Hofstetter WL, He Y, Hu W, Pataer A, et al. (2010) KLF4 inhibition of lung cancer cell invasion by suppression of SPARC expression. Cancer Biol Ther 9: 507–513.
13. Guan H, Xie L, Leithauser F, Flossbach L, Moller P, et al. (2010) KLF4 is a tumor suppressor in B-cell non-Hodgkin lymphoma and in classic Hodgkin lymphoma. Blood 116: 1469–1478.
14. Yu F, Li J, Chen H, Fu J, Ray S, et al. (2011) Kruppel-like factor 4 (KLF4) is required for maintenance of breast cancer stem cells and for cell migration and invasion. Oncogene 30: 2161–2172.
15. Liu Z, Yang H, Luo W, Jiang Q, Mai C, et al. (2013) Loss of cytoplasmic KLF4 expression is correlated with the progression and poor prognosis of nasopharyngeal carcinoma. Histopathology.
16. Yori JL, Seachrist DD, Johnson E, Lozada KL, Abdul-Karim FW, et al. (2011) Kruppel-like factor 4 inhibits tumorigenic progression and metastasis in a mouse model of breast cancer. Neoplasia 13: 601–610.
17. Akaogi K, Nakajima Y, Ito I, Kawasaki S, Oie SH, et al. (2009) KLF4 suppresses estrogen-dependent breast cancer growth by inhibiting the transcriptional activity of ERalpha. Oncogene 28: 2894–2902.
18. Tiwari N, Meyer-Schaller N, Arnold P, Antoniadis H, Pachkov M, et al. (2013) Klf4 is a transcriptional regulator of genes critical for EMT, including Jnk1 (Mapk8). PLoS One 8: e57329.
19. Yoon O, Roh J (2012) Downregulation of KLF4 and the Bcl-2/Bax ratio in advanced epithelial ovarian cancer. Oncol Lett 4: 1033–1036.
20. Brosh R, Assia-Alroy Y, Molchadsky A, Bornstein C, Dekel E, et al. (2013) p53 counteracts reprogramming by inhibiting mesenchymal-to-epithelial transition. Cell Death Differ 20: 312–320.
21. Pinho AV, Rooman I, Real FX (2011) p53-dependent regulation of growth, epithelial-mesenchymal transition and stemness in normal pancreatic epithelial cells. Cell Cycle 10: 1312–1321.
22. Wellner U, Schubert J, Burk UC, Schmalhofer O, Zhu F, et al. (2009) The EMT-activator ZEB1 promotes tumorigenicity by repressing stemness-inhibiting microRNAs. Nat Cell Biol 11: 1487–1495.
23. Miyamoto S, Nakanishi M, Rosenberg DW (2013) Suppression of colon carcinogenesis by targeting Notch signaling. Carcinogenesis.
24. Liu YN, Abou-Kheir W, Yin JJ, Fang L, Hynes P, et al. (2012) Critical and reciprocal regulation of KLF4 and SLUG in transforming growth factor beta-initiated prostate cancer epithelial-mesenchymal transition. Mol Cell Biol 32: 941–953.
25. Hoffmeyer K, Raggioli A, Rudloff S, Anton R, Hierholzer A, et al. (2012) Wnt/beta-catenin signaling regulates telomerase in stem cells and cancer cells. Science 336: 1549–1554.
26. Dong P, Kaneuchi M, Watari H, Hamada J, Sudo S, et al. (2011) MicroRNA-194 inhibits epithelial to mesenchymal transition of endometrial cancer cells by targeting oncogene BMI-1. Mol Cancer 10: 99.
27. Yori JL, Johnson E, Zhou G, Jain MK, Keri RA (2010) Kruppel-like factor 4 inhibits epithelial-to-mesenchymal transition through regulation of E-cadherin gene expression. J Biol Chem 285: 16854–16863.

28. Yue J, Sheng Y, Ren A, Penmatsa S (2010) A miR-21 hairpin structure-based gene knockdown vector. Biochem Biophys Res Commun 394: 667–672.
29. Guo Y, Tian P, Yang C, Liang Z, Li M, et al. (2013) Silencing the Double-Stranded RNA Binding Protein DGCR8 Inhibits Ovarian Cancer Cell Proliferation, Migration, and Invasion. Pharm Res.
30. Yu F, Shi Y, Wang J, Li J, Fan D, et al. (2013) Deficiency of kruppel-like factor KLF4 in mammary tumor cells inhibits tumor growth and pulmonary metastasis and is accompanied by compromised recruitment of myeloid-derived suppressor cells. Int J Cancer.
31. Li R, Liang J, Ni S, Zhou T, Qing X, et al. (2010) A mesenchymal-to-epithelial transition initiates and is required for the nuclear reprogramming of mouse fibroblasts. Cell Stem Cell 7: 51–63.
32. Li Y, Ma J, Qian X, Wu Q, Xia J, et al. (2013) Regulation of EMT by Notch Signaling Pathway in Tumor Progression. Curr Cancer Drug Targets.
33. Ren D, Minami Y, Nishita M (2011) Critical role of Wnt5a-Ror2 signaling in motility and invasiveness of carcinoma cells following Snail-mediated epithelial-mesenchymal transition. Genes Cells 16: 304–315.
34. Reichl P, Haider C, Grubinger M, Mikulits W (2012) TGF-beta in epithelial to mesenchymal transition and metastasis of liver carcinoma. Curr Pharm Des 18: 4135–4147.
35. Radisky DC, Bissell MJ (2007) NF-kappaB links oestrogen receptor signalling and EMT. Nat Cell Biol 9: 361–363.
36. Cheng JC, Auersperg N, Leung PC (2012) TGF-beta induces serous borderline ovarian tumor cell invasion by activating EMT but triggers apoptosis in low-grade serous ovarian carcinoma cells. PLoS One 7: e42436.
37. Zhu Y, Nilsson M, Sundfeldt K (2010) Phenotypic plasticity of the ovarian surface epithelium: TGF-beta 1 induction of epithelial to mesenchymal transition (EMT) in vitro. Endocrinology 151: 5497–5505.

WMAXC: A Weighted Maximum Clique Method for Identifying Condition-Specific Sub-Network

Bayarbaatar Amgalan, Hyunju Lee*

School of Information and Communications, Gwangju Institute of Science and Technology, Gwangju, South Korea

Abstract

Sub-networks can expose complex patterns in an entire bio-molecular network by extracting interactions that depend on temporal or condition-specific contexts. When genes interact with each other during cellular processes, they may form differential co-expression patterns with other genes across different cell states. The identification of condition-specific sub-networks is of great importance in investigating how a living cell adapts to environmental changes. In this work, we propose the weighted MAXimum clique (WMAXC) method to identify a condition-specific sub-network. WMAXC first proposes scoring functions that jointly measure condition-specific changes to both individual genes and gene-gene co-expressions. It then employs a weaker formula of a general maximum clique problem and relates the maximum scored clique of a weighted graph to the optimization of a quadratic objective function under sparsity constraints. We combine a continuous genetic algorithm and a projection procedure to obtain a single optimal sub-network that maximizes the objective function (scoring function) over the standard simplex (sparsity constraints). We applied the WMAXC method to both simulated data and real data sets of ovarian and prostate cancer. Compared with previous methods, WMAXC selected a large fraction of cancer-related genes, which were enriched in cancer-related pathways. The results demonstrated that our method efficiently captured a subset of genes relevant under the investigated condition.

Editor: Frank Emmert-Streib, Queen's University Belfast, United Kingdom

Funding: This work was supported by the Systems biology infrastructure establishment grant provided by Gwangju Institute of Science & Technology in 2014, and by the MSIP (The Ministry of Science, ICT and Future Planning), Korea and Microsoft Research, under IT/SW Creative research program supervised by the NIPA (National IT Industry Promotion Agency) (NIPA-2013-H0503-13-1019). The funders had no role in study design, data collection and analysis, decision to publish, or preparation of the manuscript.

Competing Interests: The authors have declared that no competing interests exist.

* Email: hyunjulee@gist.ac.kr

Introduction

A central problem in network biology is the identification of genes and pathways involved in the same biological processes or physiological conditions. The details of control mechanisms in biological processes can be understood by analyzing interacting neighbors and local patterns. Network structures often have been used to describe these complex bio-molecular pathways and functional modules by representing a whole set of interactions as overlapping sub-networks, each associated with a specific condition [1,2].

Many methods have been developed to construct bio-molecular networks by comparing multiple sets of microarray data under different conditions. Because expressions of different genes in a series of biological conditions influence each other, correlations between genes have been widely used to analyze microarray gene-expression measurements. Waaijenborg and Zwinderman [3] developed a penalized canonical correlation analysis method to extract a subset of variables that capture the common features among genes by maximizing a canonical correlation between expression of genes. Witten and Tibshirani [4] presented some extension formulas to the sparse canonical correlation analysis as a supervised method, which resulted in the identification of linear combinations of sets of variables that are correlated and associated with its outcome.

To fully understand the complex biological processes, the effective integration of diverse sets of data and knowledge is required. Protein-DNA interaction and gene expression data were combined for regulatory network identification [5]. Integrating protein-protein interaction (PPI) data with gene expression data has also been attempted for the identification of biologically meaningful and cancer-related networks in cancer studies [6–9]. The integration increases the accuracy in identifying genes jointly regulated in the same condition. Guo et al. [10] developed an edge-based scoring function for gene-gene co-expression by using both gene expression and PPI data. However, in this method, PPI information is used to define existence of edges in the bio-molecular network so that only gene pairs that are included in the existing PPI network are considered in the scoring function. Lai et al. [11] extended the traditional F-statistic to obtain an expected conditional F-statistic (ECF-statistic), which measures the connectivity between genes. The ECF-statistic was used in a COSINE method [12] to measure gene-gene co-expression from gene expression data. For the use of the PPI information in COSINE, only the number of interactions in a selected sub-network was considered in their scoring function to calculate its sub-network adjust score, instead of using each interaction in the PPI network.

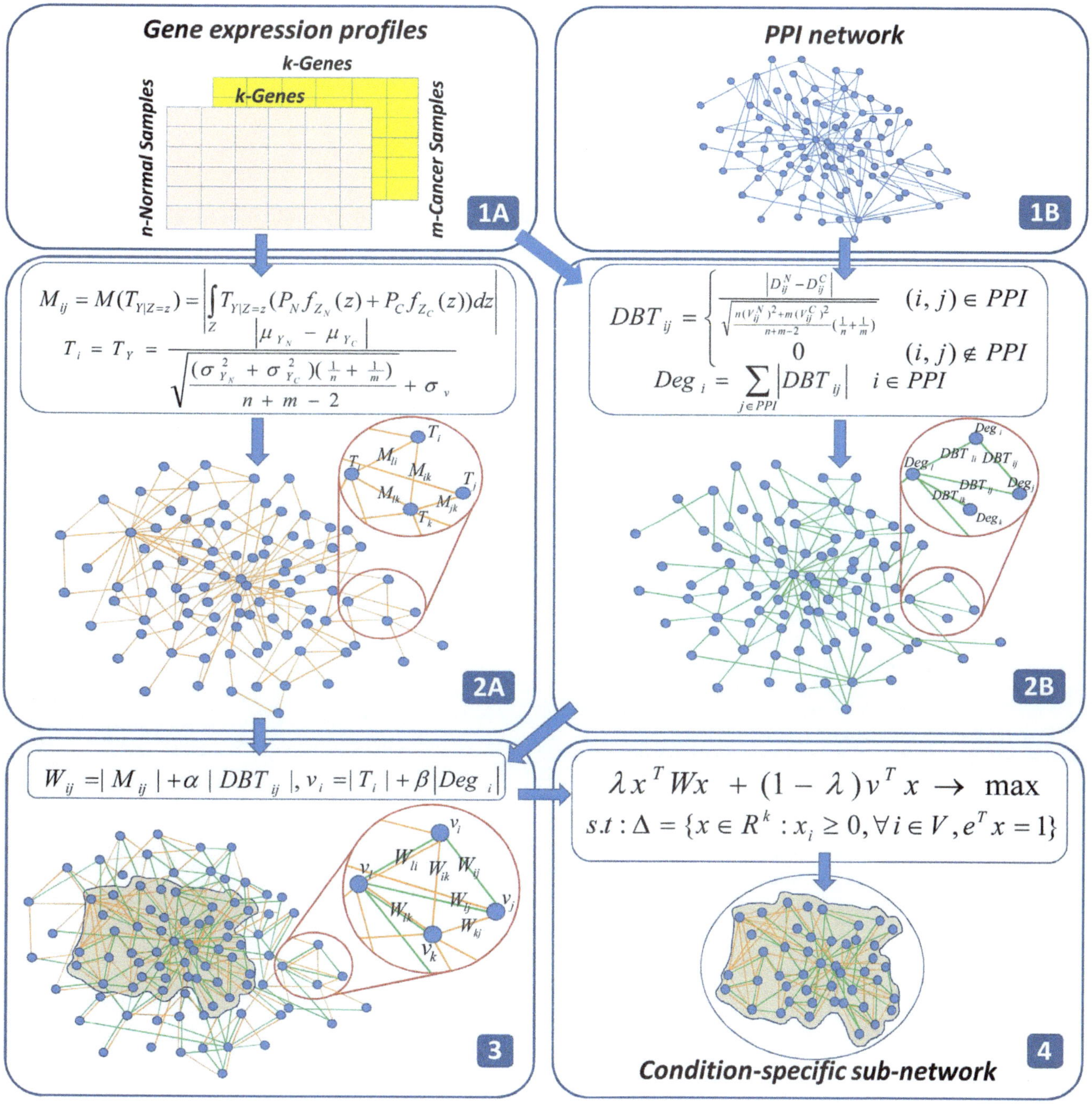

Figure 1. Workflow of WMAXC. (1) Gene expression data consisting of normal and cancer samples (1A) and the PPI network (1B) are used as inputs. (2) We begin by constructing two responsive networks under the investigated condition: In (2A), we use two statistic measurements to construct a bio-molecular network. For each gene, T_i is used to measure activity of gene i (a node score) and for each pair of genes M_{ij} is used to measure connectivity relationship between gene i and gene j (an edge score). In (2B), for each interaction in PPI network, DBT_{ij} is used to measure activity of interaction behavior between gene i and gene j (an edge contribution score from PPI) and for each gene, Deg_i is used to measure the weighted degree of gene i (a node contribution score from PPI) under the condition. (3) We then combine the two responsive networks to construct the background network by assigning node and edge scores to a set of genes. Orange edges represent gene-gene co-expression estimated from only gene expression data and green edges represent activity of interactions in the PPI network. In the process of combining two networks, new edges are included to (2A) although they are not in the existing PPI network. (4) Finally, we solve the constrained optimization problem to obtain the single optimal sub-network.

A mixed integer linear programming model [13] and an integer linear programming approach [14] were developed to identify differentially expressed pathways using both data sets. However, these two integer linear programming approaches have used expression values of individual genes without accounting for correlation or co-expression information, which might be less informative.

Finding a sub-network that maximizes the score of differential expressions of genes and differential co-expression of gene pairs can be formulated as a combinatorial optimization problem. In practice, bio-molecular networks are often large in scale [15]. Hence, it is impossible to exactly solve a large combinatorial optimization problem within a reasonable time. For examples, in the COSINE method [12], a genetic algorithm was used to find a binary vector, in which 1 or 0 represents presence or absence of a gene in the sub-network, and its space complexity is exponential as 2^p, where p is the total number of genes. In the edge-based method [10], a searching procedure based on simulated annealing was used to find the sub-network. It iteratively tests whether the addition or removal of an edge will increase their sub-network adjust score during the annealing process, and its space complexity is also exponential as 2^q, where q is the number of possible edges (edges in the PPI network). Ideker et al. [6] also used the simulated annealing approach; however, it tended to produce a large sub-network that was often difficult to interpret. Although Rajagopalan and Agarwal [16] and Nacu et al. [17] offered several improvements, they were also based on heuristic techniques with combinatorial selection and required the estimation of additional parameters. Various graph theory-based approaches, such as sequential greedy heuristics [18,19], have been presented. These heuristics generate a maximal scoring sub-network through the repeated addition of a vertex into a partial sub-network, or by the repeated deletion of a vertex from a sub-network. In addition to heuristics, several local optimization-based approaches have been presented to extract condition specific sub-networks. A method developed by Wang and Xia [15] was inspired by a KKT condition and was used to iteratively find a local minimum from a predetermined initial solution. A large number of local solutions can be found for the non-convex problem. Depending on the selection of the initial solution, many of them might not be significant under the investigated condition, which may give rise to false positives.

In our work, we reformulate the sub-network identification problem as a constrained optimization problem for continuous variables. It is an approximation of the general combinatorial problem, based on the theorem posed by Motzkin and Straus [20]. To construct a background network under investigated condition, we used two statistical measurements to represent activity of each genes and interaction behaviors of each pair of genes; a modified T-statistic as the differential expression of each gene and a conditional expectation of the modified T-statistic as the differential gene-gene co-expression. In our first experiment, we used the two measurements to construct the background network that represents the weight parameters of the optimization problem. We then employed a continuous genetic algorithm, which has the advantage of being capable of jumping out of local solutions, and used a projection procedure that maximizes our objective function under a sparsity constraint. In the second experiment, we reconstructed the background network by integrating PPI information with the gene expression profiles for each gene pair, and obtained a more robust estimation of the neighbors of each gene in the network. We first tested the performance of our method using simulated data sets, and then applied the method to analyze human ovarian and prostate cancer data sets. The results demonstrated that our method efficiently captures relevant interaction behaviors under the investigated conditions. An overview of the workflow is presented in Figure 1, and more detailed descriptions are given in the Methods section.

Methods

We first describe scoring functions to measure gene expression differences and gene-gene correlations for given two conditions, which generate weight values of nodes and edges in a background network. We then introduce an optimization model to identify the maximal scoring sub-network. Finally, the proposed model is extended to include PPI interactions.

Scoring function of WMAXC

The entire background network is represented as a graph $\mathbb{G}=(\mathbb{V},\mathbb{E})$, where a set of nodes $\mathbb{V}$ represents genes, and a set of edges $\mathbb{E}$ represents the connectivity relationships among these genes. Let $\mathbb{V}$ be a set of k genes. For each gene, n and m denote the numbers of samples in two different conditions, such as normal and cancer. We then have a gene expression data set, given as two matrices with sizes of $n\times k$ and $m\times k$. A modified T-statistic is used as a scoring function to measure the differential expression of each gene. For each node in $\mathbb{V}$, the differential expression value of the corresponding gene Y is computed as

$$T_Y=\frac{\mu_{Y_N}-\mu_{Y_C}}{\sqrt{\frac{(\sigma^2_{Y_N}+\sigma^2_{Y_C})(\frac{1}{n}+\frac{1}{m})}{n+m-2}}+\sigma_v}, \tag{1}$$

where μ_{Y_N}, μ_{Y_C} and σ_{Y_N}, σ_{Y_C} are the sample means and standard deviations of gene Y in the normal and cancer conditions, respectively, and σ_v is a constant chosen to minimize the coefficient of variation of T-statistic [21] (see more descriptions and Figure S1 in File S1).

For each edge in $\mathbb{E}$, the conditional expectation of the modified T-statistic is used to measure differential gene-gene co-expressions across two conditions. To measure the gene-gene correlations for a pair of genes, we assume that samples of genes are jointly normal distributed in a particular condition, such as normal (N) or cancer (C). By the assumption, a bivariate normal distribution of two genes Y and Z in the normal condition is

$$(Y_N,Z_N)\sim\mathcal{N}\left((\mu_{Y_N},\mu_{Z_N}),\begin{pmatrix}\sigma^2_{Y_N} & \rho_N\sigma_{Y_N}\sigma_{Z_N}\\ \rho_N\sigma_{Y_N}\sigma_{Z_N} & \sigma^2_{Z_N}\end{pmatrix}\right).$$

The conditional distribution of Y_N given $Z_N=z$ is

$$Y_N|Z_N=z\sim\mathcal{N}\left(\mu_{Y_N}+\rho_N(z-\mu_{Z_N})\frac{\sigma_{Y_N}}{\sigma_{Z_N}},\sigma^2_{Y_N}(1-\rho^2_N)\right). \tag{2}$$

Similarly, the conditional distribution of Y_C given $Z_C=z$ in the cancer condition is

$$Y_C|Z_C=z\sim\mathcal{N}\left(\mu_{Y_C}+\rho_C(z-\mu_{Z_C})\frac{\sigma_{Y_C}}{\sigma_{Z_C}},\sigma^2_{Y_C}(1-\rho^2_C)\right), \tag{3}$$

where ρ_N and ρ_C are the sample correlations of a pair of genes (Y,Z) in the normal and cancer conditions, respectively. By replacing mean and variance in Equation (1) with the corresponding conditional means and variances from Equations (2) and (3), we obtain a conditional T-statistic as follows.

$$T_{Y|Z=z} = \frac{\mu_{Y_N} + \rho_N(z - \mu_{Z_N})\frac{\sigma_{Y_N}}{\sigma_{Z_N}} - \mu_{Y_C} - \rho_C(z - \mu_{Z_C})\frac{\sigma_{Y_C}}{\sigma_{Z_C}}}{\sqrt{\frac{[\sigma^2_{Y_N}(1-\rho^2_N) + \sigma^2_{Y_C}(1-\rho^2_C)](\frac{1}{n}+\frac{1}{m})}{n+m-2} + \sigma_v}}. \quad (4)$$

For gene Z, let $f_{Z_N}(z) \sim \mathcal{N}(\mu_{Z_N}, \sigma^2_{Z_N})$ and $f_{Z_C}(z) \sim \mathcal{N}(\mu_{Z_C}, \sigma^2_{Z_C})$ be the probability density function of the normal and cancer conditions, respectively. Then, the probability density function of Z is $f_Z(Z) = p_N f_{Z_N}(z) + p_C f_{Z_C}(z)$, where $p_N = \frac{n}{n+m}$ and $p_C = \frac{m}{n+m}$ are the probabilities that a sample is selected from the normal or cancer conditions. By calculating the expectation over all samples of gene Z, we obtain the connectivity relationship between gene Y and gene Z as follows.

$$\begin{aligned} M(T_{Y|Z=z}) &= \int_Z T_{Y|Z} f_Z(z)dz \\ &= \int_Z (p_N T_{Y|Z=z} f_{Z_N}(z) + p_C T_{Y|Z=z} f_{Z_C}(z))dz \end{aligned} \quad (5)$$

As we described above, $T_{Y|Z}$, $f_{Z_N}(z)$ and $f_{Z_C}(z)$ are functions of z so that the integration in Equation (5) can be numerically computed over all samples in the normal and cancer conditions.

In summary, the modified T-statistic is used to measure the differential expression of each gene, and the conditional expectation $M(T_{Y|Z=z})$ is used to measure differential co-expression of each pair of genes across two conditions. Note that we calculated the differential co-expression patterns $M(T_{Y|Z})$ for all pairs of nodes in the background network because the co-expression of two genes might be significant although each gene may not be differentially expressed. In this work, we will use a matrix notation M_{ij} for $M(T_{Y|Z})$ and a vector notation T_i for T_Y, and the matrix M is symmetric, in which its entries represent weights of undirected edges and the entries in the vector T represent weights of nodes in the background network.

Optimization model

A remarkable connection between the maximum clique problem and a certain standard quadratic programming problem was established [20] by providing an alternative proof of a slightly weaker version of the fundamental theorem [22].

Let $\bar{\mathbb{G}} = (\bar{\mathbb{V}}, \bar{\mathbb{E}})$ be an unweighted and undirected graph, and Δ denotes the standard simplex in the k-dimensional Euclidean space $\mathbb{R}^k$, and $\Delta_{\mathbb{S}} = \{x \in \Delta : x_i = 0 \text{ if } i \notin \mathbb{S}\}$ is the face of Δ corresponding to a subset $\mathbb{S} \subseteq \bar{\mathbb{V}}$. A characteristic vector $x^{\mathbb{S}}$ denotes the vector in Δ defined by $x_i^{\mathbb{S}} = 1/\|\mathbb{S}\|$ if $i \in \mathbb{S}$ and $x_i^{\mathbb{S}} = 0$, otherwise. The maximum clique problem can then be formulated as the following quadratic programming problem.

$$\begin{aligned} &f(x) = x^T A_{\bar{\mathbb{G}}} x \rightarrow \max, \\ &\Delta = \{x \in \mathbb{R}^k : x_i \geq 0, \forall i \in \bar{\mathbb{V}}, e^T x = 1\}, \end{aligned} \quad (6)$$

where e^T denotes the transpose of the vector e consisting of unit entries, $A_{\bar{\mathbb{G}}} = (a_{ij})_{i,j \in \bar{\mathbb{V}}}$ is the adjacency matrix (binary matrix) of $\bar{\mathbb{G}}$, and x^* is a global solution of f on Δ. Motzkin et al. [20] proved that the clique number of $\bar{\mathbb{G}}$ is related to $f(x^*)$ in the following formula.

$$\omega(\bar{\mathbb{G}}) = \frac{1}{1-f(x^*)} \geq \frac{1}{1-f(x)}, \forall x \in \Delta, \quad (7)$$

where $\omega(\bar{\mathbb{G}})$ is the size of the maximum clique in $\bar{\mathbb{G}}$. Essentially, they proved that a subset of nodes $\mathbb{S}$ is a maximum clique of $\bar{\mathbb{G}}$ if and only if its characteristic vector $x^{\mathbb{S}}$ is a global solution of f on Δ (for a comprehensive review, see [23]).

Based on the theoretical validation, we reformulate the sub-network identification problem as a continuous optimization problem that is an approximation of the general combinatorial problem and a generalization of the problem in Equation (6). The proposed method relates the densest part (a maximum scored clique) of a weighted graph to the optimization of a quadratic function under sparsity constraints. A weaker formula of the maximum clique problem, the optimization problem for identifying a condition-specific sub-network from a bio-molecular network, can be formulated as follows.

$$\begin{aligned} &\lambda x^T W x + (1 - 1\lambda) v^T x \rightarrow max, \\ &\Delta = \{x \in \mathbb{R}^k : x_i \geq 0, \forall i \in \mathbb{V}, e^T x = 1\}, \end{aligned} \quad (8)$$

where v is a vector in which v_i represents a node score measuring differential expression for gene i, W is a symmetric matrix in which W_{ij} represents an edge score measuring the connectivity strength between gene i and gene j, and λ is a positive parameter to balance and to integrate the two terms of the objective function in Equation (8). A k-dimensional non-negative vector $x = (x_1, x_2, ..., x_k)$, determined by solving our optimization problem, represents the contribution to each gene belonging to the condition specific sub-network. Particularly, x_i indicates whether its corresponding node is contained in a selected sub-network ($x_i > 0$) or not ($x_i = 0$). Since we maximize the interconnectivity of sub-network, a gene i with both a high node confidence score in v and high confidence scores in W_{ij} should be selected in the sub-network and its corresponding x_i should be assigned to have a high contribution score. Therefore, the subset of variables corresponding to the nonzero elements in the optimal solution x^* forms the maximum scored sub-network in the background network. Moreover, the genes that have higher contribution scores are more likely to be related to the phenotype (cancer) being analyzed.

Sub-network identification from gene expression and PPI network data

We extend our model to incorporate the assumption that the significance score of one gene or its interactions in a network depends not only on its own gene expression profile but also on the profiles of its neighbors in the PPI network. Some interactions in the PPI network are activated under the investigated condition while others are not activated. If two genes interact with each other under a particular condition, the expression distance between them might be significantly changed across two conditions (a normal condition and a cancer condition). Based on this assumption, we propose a scoring function called the distance-based T-score to measure the change in gene expression distances across two conditions for each pair of genes in the PPI network. This function is used to test the significance score of each interaction in the PPI network.

As described in the section of scoring function of WMAXC, the gene expression profile data are given as two matrices with sizes of $n \times k$ and $m \times k$. Let $(g^1_{1i}, g^1_{2i}, g^1_{3i}, ..., g^1_{ni})^T$ and $(g^2_{1i}, g^2_{2i}, s^2_{3i}, ..., g^2_{mi})^T$ be the samples of gene i in normal and cancer conditions, respectively, and $\mathbb{PPI}$ denote a set of pair indexes of genes with interactions in the PPI network. For a pair $(i,j)\in\mathbb{PPI}$, let $D_{ij}^N = \frac{1}{n}\sqrt{\sum_{l=1}^{n}(g_{li}^1 - g_{lj}^1)^2}$ and $D_{ij}^C = \frac{1}{m}\sqrt{\sum_{l=1}^{m}(g_{li}^2 - g_{lj}^2)^2}$ be the normalized distances between gene i and gene j in the normal and cancer conditions, respectively. Then, the distance-based T-score, DBT_{ij}, can be formulated as follows.

$$DBT_{ij} = \begin{cases} \dfrac{D_{ij}^N - D_{ij}^C}{\sqrt{\dfrac{n*(V_{ij}^N)^2 + m*(V_{ij}^C)^2}{n+m-2}\left(\dfrac{1}{n}+\dfrac{1}{m}\right)}}, & (i,j)\in\mathbb{PPI} \\ 0, & (i,j)\notin\mathbb{PPI}, \end{cases} \quad (9)$$

where V_{ij}^N and V_{ij}^C are the geometric averages of the standard deviations of samples of gene i and gene j in the normal and cancer conditions, respectively (see more descriptions and Figure S2 in File S1). One of the advantages of using DBT score is that less relevant interactions in the PPI network under the investigated condition can be thinned out. Since both the conditional expectation of the modified T-statistic and the distance-based T-score are estimated from the same population, we reconstruct our background network by integrating the two types of information. To quantify absolute changes of expression under the investigated condition, we transformed T_i, M_{ij}, Deg_i and DBT_{ij} in their absolute values. The weight parameters of the objective function in Equation (8) are then calculated as follows.

$$W_{ij} = |M_{ij}| + \alpha * |DBT_{ij}|, \quad v_i = |T_i| + \beta * Deg_i, \quad (10)$$

where $Deg_i = \sum_j |DBT_{ij}|$ is a weighted degree for gene i in the PPI network, $i,j = 1,2,\ldots,k$ are gene indexes, α and β are positive scaling parameters defining the contribution of PPI information to the condition-specific network. We set $\alpha = \frac{\max_{i,j}\{M_{ij}\}}{\max_{i,j}\{DBT_{ij}\}}$ and $\beta = \frac{\max_i\{T_i\}}{\max_i\{Deg_i\}}$, where α ensures that the maximum of entries in the M matrix is equal to the maximum of entries in the DBT matrix and similar normalization is applied to β.

The PPI network is very sparse; the percentage of interacting protein pairs is only 0.0888% for the ovarian cancer data and 0.1280% for the prostate cancer data. Moreover, some interactions in the existing PPI network might not be significantly activated under the investigated condition. In this case, they might have very small values in DBT_{ij} (near to zero). Therefore, the DBT score matrix becomes more sparse, and only the entries corresponding to significant interactions in the PPI network have observable contributions to the matrix W and the vector v. However, the weight matrix M and the weight vector T are not sparse, because until now we used all differential expression and co-expression values without considering the significance of them. Therefore, genes with non-significant changes and correlations in expression values contribute their weights to W and v. In other words, all non zero entries in W and v can influence the behavior (slope) of the continuous objective function even though their values are not high. The influence in the objective function may lead the solution to a local maximum. To avoid the local convergence, we define two hard thresholds as follows.

$$T_i = \begin{cases} |T_i|, & |T_i| < \mu_v \\ 0, & otherwise, \end{cases} \quad M_{ij} = \begin{cases} |M_{ij}|, & |M_{ij}| < \mu_W \\ 0, & otherwise, \end{cases} \quad (11)$$

where μ_v is the mean value of T, computed as $\mu_v = \frac{1}{k}\sum_{i=1}^{k}|T_i|$, and μ_W is the maximum of $\mu_{W_1}, \mu_{W_2}, \ldots, \mu_{W_k}$, and for each i, $\mu_{W_i} = \frac{1}{k}\sum_{j=1}^{k}|M_{ij}|$.

Estimation of weight parameter λ

A reasonable balance between the quadratic and linear terms of the objective function in Equation (8) is essential for the stability and robustness of the optimization result. Unfortunately, it is difficult to define an objective criterion for biological relevance. Regarding optimization, the term with greater value should be more informative in our task. To achieve the stability of the solution, we compared the magnitudes of edge and node scores in terms of statistical distributions of score values. Because of the restrictions imposed by the sparsity constraint, the sub-network scores are not affected by their size. For both score terms, sub-network scores of different sizes behave similarly, and the majorities of edge and node score values fall in the region around their means. Therefore, the edge and node score values of a randomly selected sub-network have more chances to fall around the mean (distribution plots are given in Figures S3 and S4 in File S1), which allows the possibility of estimating the magnitudes that make the solution more stable. To estimate the magnitudes of the two terms, we used the following procedure: 1) Randomly sample a large number of sub-networks by selecting points on Δ. Each point $x^i\in\Delta$ presents a sub-network, and the edge and node scores of the sub-network are calculated as $x^{i^T}Wx^i$ and v^Tx^i, respectively; 2) Compute the means μ_W and μ_v, standard deviations s_W and s_v of two score terms; 3) The magnitudes of both edge and node score terms are defined as follows: $M_W = \frac{\mu_W}{s_W}$, $M_v = \frac{\mu_v}{s_v}$; and then 4) We set $\lambda = \frac{M_W}{M_W + M_v}$.

Searching for condition specific sub-network

If the matrix $-W$ is positive definite, the objective function in Equation (8) is concave (concave maximization is equivalent to convex minimization), and any local solution can also be the global maximum. Unfortunately, in the WMAXC method, the weight matrix W is generally indefinite. There are a large number of local maxima, each representing a densely connected subgraph. Because of the high complexity of the problem, it is a common practice to solve it using metaheuristics, such as evolutionary algorithms. This study implements a combination of a continuous genetic algorithm [24] and a projection procedure [25–27] to avoid the local maxima and reduce computational costs.

The continuous genetic algorithm is a parallel search procedure commonly used in a high-dimensional global optimization problem. For constrained optimizations, depending on the shape of the constraint and the dimension of the problem, the implementation of a genetic algorithm should be adapted to a particular problem. Because the standard simplex $\Delta\subset\mathbb{R}^k$ is a subspace of the l_∞ ball $[0,1]^k\subset\mathbb{R}^k$ (see Figure S5 in File S1), we first apply the continuous genetic algorithm to maximize the objective function in Equation (8) over $[0,1]^k$ and find a single optimal solution. Let $\hat{x}$ be the global maximum of Equation (8) over $[0,1]^k$. We then project the solution $\hat{x}$ onto Δ in the Euclidean space $\mathbb{R}^k$ using the algorithm [26] to obtain a sparser solution [27]. Since projection of any point onto convex set is unique (see the projection theorem and Figure S6 in File S1) and the Δ is convex, the problem of finding the Euclidean projection of a vector $\hat{x}\in\mathbb{R}^k$ onto Δ can be described by the following convex optimization problem.

$$x^* = \arg\min_{x \in \Delta} \|x - \hat{x}\|^2, \quad (12)$$

where x is a k-dimensional vector used as an optimization variable, and $x^* = (x_1^*, x_2^*, ..., x_k^*)$ is the projection of $\hat{x}$ onto Δ (see File S1). In view of the Lagrangian duality, the optimal solutions of the primal and dual problems are equal to a saddle point. In our task, the optimization variable of the dual problem is simply a scalar. Hence, it is more efficient to solve the dual problem instead of directly solving the primal problem in Equation (12). By considering the well-known result of the projection onto standard simplex [25], the optimal projection x^* is expressed as follows.

$$x_i^* = \begin{cases} \hat{x}_i - \theta, & \hat{x}_i > \theta \\ 0, & otherwise, \end{cases} \quad (13)$$

where the dual optimal point θ^* is given by the root of the following equation:

$$D'(\theta) = \sum_{i=1}^{n} \max\{0, \hat{x}_i - \theta\} - 1 = 0. \quad (14)$$

The root θ^* of Equation (14) can be numerically found using the algorithm from [26] and is used in Equation (13). The solution of Equation (13) represents the optimal solution of the problem in Equation (8). After the procedure is completed, the nodes corresponding to non-zero entries in the solution vector are selected to represent the subset of genes forming the condition-specific sub-network.

Data sets

- Protein-protein interaction data: We used the Human Protein Reference Database released in 2010 [28]. There were 39,240 binary protein-protein interactions involving 9,617 genes. After excluding self-interactions, 37,080 interactions remained.
- Ovarian cancer data: Gene expression data was collected from the TCGA project [29]. It contains 17,814 genes with the expression profiles of 587 cancer samples and 62 normal samples. For the cancer samples, we only considered 332 samples without missing values. For the normal samples, we imputed the missing values in the samples using the Weighted K-Nearest Neighbors method, based on available observations in the samples. For the analysis of ovarian cancer, we considered only the genes that were included in the PPI network, which consists of 8,721 genes and 33,771 interactions.
- Prostate cancer data: Gene expression data was collected from [30] with gene expression omnibus (GEO) accession number GSE3933. It contains the gene expression profiles of 71 cancer samples and 41 normal samples. The gene expression data was initially used in COSINE [12]. In order to compare our results with the results of COSINE using the same data, we used the data set prepared by the authors of COSINE. This data set consists of 5,335 genes with 18,234 interactions in the PPI network.

Results

Simulation studies

We showed the performance of WMAXC on simulated data by comparing it with COSINE [12], because COSINE was initially compared to several other methods, including jActiveModules [6], an edge-based method [10], and a local method [15]. We constructed five simulation data sets from multivariate normal distributions: four case data sets and one reference data set.

Each data set consisted of 1,000 variables (genes) for 50 samples. For each gene i, we draw the mean μ_i and the standard deviation σ_i from the uniform distribution on the observed range of normal data $[-0.5, 0.5]$, and then estimated the correlation coefficient ρ_{ij} for each pair of genes (i,j). Let $\mu = (\mu_1, \mu_2, ..., \mu_{1000})$ denote the mean vector, and $\Sigma = \{\sigma_{ij}\}_{i,j=1,...,1000}$ denote the covariance matrix, where $\sigma_{ij} = \rho_{ij} * \sigma_i * \sigma_j$ is the covariance between gene i and gene j.

We first simulated the reference data from joint normal distribution $N(\mu, \Sigma)$, and the reference data was compared to each of the four case data sets. In each of four case data sets, 200 of 1,000 genes were selected as significant genes. For the particular genes, some shifts in the mean expressions and higher correlations among the genes were assigned to represent significant alterations in expression values. Let $\mathbb{I}$ denote the set of indexes for the significant genes.

$$\hat{\mu}_i = \begin{cases} \mu_i + k, & i \in \mathbb{I} \\ \mu_i, & i \notin \mathbb{I}, \end{cases} \quad \hat{\rho}_i = \begin{cases} \rho_{ij} + r, & i,j \in \mathbb{I} \\ \rho_{ij}, & i,j \notin \mathbb{I}, \end{cases} \quad (15)$$

In each of four case data sets, the expression data was simulated from jointly normal distribution $N(\hat{\mu}, \hat{\Sigma})$, where $\hat{\mu} = (\hat{\mu}_1, \hat{\mu}_2, ..., \hat{\mu}_{1000})$ is the mean vector, and $\hat{\Sigma} = \{\hat{\sigma}_{ij}\}_{i,j=1,...,1000}$ is the covariance matrix and its entries were calculated as $\hat{\sigma}_{ij} = \hat{\rho}_{ij} * \sigma_i * \sigma_j$. For case data 1, $k = 0.6$ and $r = 0.65$ were used in Equation (15), $k = 0.3$ and $r = 0.65$ for case data 2, and $k = 0.6$ and $r = 0.35$ for case data 3, and $k = 0.3$ and $r = 0.35$ for case data 4. Compared to the results of COSINE, WMAXC provided higher accuracy in sub-network size, recall, precision, and F-measure (Table 1). In the simulated data, the sub-network sizes identified by COSINE were smaller than desired, whereas WMAXC identified approximately 200 genes. Regarding the running time, WMAXC was much faster than COSINE; in the analysis on simulated data, it took 10 minutes to convergence, while COSINE took around 30 hours.

Comparison with other methods on real data sets

We applied the WMAXC method on gene expression profiles of two real data sets to identify a cancer type specific sub-network. Then, the performance of WMAXC was compared to other methods, COSINE [12] and BMRF [5].

Comparison on ovarian cancer. To evaluate whether the genes in the identified sub-network are related to ovarian cancer, we used a set of 379 experimentally verified ovarian cancer-related genes from the Dragon Database of Genes [31] as reference genes. Among the 379 genes, 315 were included in the 8,721 genes of our data set. For WMAXC, the initialization parameters of the genetic algorithm were set as follows: the number of iterations $= 60,000$, mutation rate $= 1/(k+1)$ and crossover rate $= 0.5$, where k is the number of optimization variables (the number of genes). We first applied our method using only the gene expression profile data, and then integrated the PPI network with gene expression profiles

Table 1. Comparison on simulated data with COSINE.

methods	WMAXC				COSINE			
Case data	Case 1	Case 2	Case 3	Case 4	Case 1	Case 2	Case 3	Case 4
sub-network size	204	230	219	237	137	178	126	128
λ	0.157	0.215	0.087	0.223	0.61	0.85	0.11	0.39
Recall	1	0.97	1	0.975	0.66	0.685	0.61	0.605
Precision	0.9803	0.8434	0.9132	0.8227	0.9635	0.7696	0.9682	0.9453
F-measure	0.9901	0.9023	0.9546	0.8924	0.7833	0.7248	0.7484	0.7378

Recall, precision and F-measure are defined as follows: Recall (R) = $\frac{TP}{TP+FN}$, Precision (P) = $\frac{TP}{TP+FP}$ and F-measure = $\frac{2PR}{P+R}$, where TP, FP, and FN represent true positive, false positive, and false negative, respectively.

using the Distance Based T-score as described in the Methods section. Performances of the two approaches are shown in Table 2. The fold enrichment of the genes selected among the ovarian cancer-related genes had increased from 1.828 to 2.454 when the PPI network was integrated with the gene expressions, compared to using only the gene expressions. A list of 100 genes with the highest contribution scores to the condition-specific network is given in Table S1 in File S1. Using a CPU with 3.40 GHz and 32 GB RAM, it took 26 hours to search for the maximal scoring sub-network. To test whether the genetic algorithm reached the convergence, we quantified the variations in objective function values for the population in each iteration. For both ovarian and prostate cancer data, the variation was almost zero after running 60,000 iterations, and the minimum values of the objective function became stable in the last 10,000 iterations. This result suggests that the solution had reached convergence.

For the COSINE method, both gene expression profile and PPI data were used. After five different λ's were tried, the λ giving the highest adjusted score of the scoring function was used. As a result, the sub-network with a size of 806 was selected. The fold enrichment was 1.237, and it took around 56 hours with 1,000 iterations. For the BMRF method, both gene expression profile and PPI data were used. In addition, a set of hub genes related to the investigated condition was required as an input. Hence, we collected a set of 209 hub genes from KEGG, consisting of genes included in the ovarian cancer-related pathways, such as ubiquitin, coagulation, and hedgehog signaling pathways. BMRF extracted the sub-network of the size of 916 genes, and the fold enrichment was around 1.75. However, its accuracy was depending on the choice of the set of hub genes; for a set of randomly selected genes, the fold enrichment was decreased to 1.041. Overall, the comparison demonstrated that WMAXC outperformed both the COSINE and BMRF methods on the real data set.

Comparison on prostate cancer. For the method evaluation, 703 genes related to prostate cancer from the Dragon Database of Genes [32] were used as reference genes. Among the 703 genes, 400 were included in our dataset. $\lambda = 0.041$ was used for the WMAXC method, and the initialization parameters of the genetic algorithm were the same as those used in the analysis of the ovarian cancer data. WMAXC extracted a sub-network of the size 539 and a fold enrichment of 2.35. A list of 100 genes with the highest contribution scores to the condition specific network is given in Table S2 in File S1. COSINE selected a relatively smaller network with the size of 243 and a fold enrichment of 1.262 [12]. With a set of hub genes included in the mark signaling pathway from KEGG, BMRF selected the sub-network with the size of 601 genes and a fold enrichment of 2.086. However, for a set of randomly selected genes, the fold enrichment was decreased to 0.98. Performances of methods are summarized in Table S3 in File S1, confirming that WMAXC outperformed the other two methods.

Analysis on real data

Although only 57 out of 643 genes forming the condition-specific sub-network were included in DDOC as shown in Table 2, some ovarian cancer-related genes might not be included in DDOC. Hence, we manually checked whether 20 candidate genes with the highest contribution scores were ovarian cancer-related genes. Among them, 16 genes were known to be related to ovarian cancer by DDOC or the manual literature search (Table S4 in File S1). The remaining four genes are SELL, UBAP2L, TFEB and DPPA4. Although there were no evidences of their involvements in ovarian cancer development, these four genes were highly co-expressed with other ovarian cancer and cancer

Table 2. Performance on ovarian cancer data.

Methods	COSINE	BMRF	WMAXC1	WMAXC2
λ	0.871	-	0.173	0.2715
Selected genes	806	916	567	643
Recovered interactions	275	635	483	2015
Recovered genes	36	58	38	57
Fold enrichment	1.237	1.753	1.828	2.454

WMAXC1 represents the results obtained using only gene expression profile data, whereas the WMAXC2 results were obtained by integrating gene expression profiles and PPI network data. 'Fold enrichment' was used to evaluate the performance of the methods and was calculated as $\frac{\text{'Recovered genes'} * \text{'All genes'}}{\text{'Selected genes'} * \text{'Reference genes'}}$, where 'Selected genes' is the number of selected genes by the method, 'Reference genes' is the number of reference genes from the Ovarian Cancer Dragon Database of genes, 'Recovered genes' is recovered genes by the method among the reference genes, and 'All genes' represents all genes in the entire network. 'Recovered interactions' represents the number of interactions recovered from the PPI network.

related genes in the condition specific network. As shown in Figure 2, they directly shared significant co-expression patterns with 159 neighbors. Surprisingly, 59.1% (94/159) of neighbors of these four genes are ovarian cancer-related genes and 35.8% (57/159) are other cancer-related genes. A list of these genes with their literature evidences is shown in Table S5 in File S1. For only 5% (8/159) of neighbor genes, we cannot find literature evidences showing their relevance to cancer. We further investigated that these four genes were actively involved in the other cancer types and biological phenomenon. L-selectin, SELL, is a member of a family of adhesion receptors that play important roles in lymphocyte-endothelial cell interactions. Resto et al. [33] investigated adhesive interactions between lymphocytes and head and neck cancer cells (HNSCC cells) under shear stress, and the interactions can be mediated by L-selectin. Kuiper et al. [34] investigated that upregulation of the transcription factor TFEB in some particular chromosomal position may play an important role in the regulation of renal cancer progression. Maldonado-Saldivia et al. [35] provided an evidence that DPPA4 is downregulated during fetal germ line progression and this process might be required to facilitate appropriate germ line differentiation. Moreover, it may provide an implication in the development of germ cell cancer in human. Although there was no much evidence of their involvements in ovarian cancer, our results suggest that these genes might be closely related to ovarian cancer progression.

By applying the WMAXC method to the ovarian cancer data, we identified a biologically meaningful sub-network involved in many ovarian cancer related pathways. Measured using Database for Annotation, Visualization and Integrated Discovery (DAVID) [36], 60 pathways were significantly enriched by the KEGG pathway, including the ErbB signaling pathway, the Notch signaling pathway, and the TGF-β signaling pathway (Table S6 in File S1). The epidermal growth factor receptor (EGFR) is a member of the ErbB family of tyrosine kinase receptors. Overexpression of EGFR and its downstream targets are associated with resistance to chemotherapy for ovarian cancer [37]. Ovarian cancer cells, in which Notch3 was frequently amplified and overexpressed, are dependent on the Notch3 signaling pathway for cellular survival and growth. Notch3 expression is also associated with chemo resistance in ovarian high-grade serous carcinoma [38]. The TGF-β signaling pathway is activated in ovarian cancer, and the inhibition of this pathway by a small molecule is a promising strategy in the treatment of ovarian cancer [39].

The sub-network identified using the prostate cancer data included 62 significantly enriched KEGG pathways, including prostate cancer, neurotrophinn signaling, MAPK signaling, Wnt signaling, TGF-β signaling, chemokine signaling pathways, and the regulation of actin cytoskeleton (Table S7 in File S1). For instance, it has been demonstrated that the progression of prostate cancer is affected by changes in the expression of auctocrine neurotrophins [40]. MAPK signaling is shown to be activated in prostate cancer, especially in later stages of the disease [41–43], and it was recently suggested that the MAPK signaling pathway may be a target for prostate cancer therapy, if it is inhibited simultaneously with other pathways, such as PI3K/AKT signaling [44]. The upregulation of some Wnt pathway members was observed in ERG-positive prostate cancers, and it has been shown that knockdown of the ERG gene in VCaP prostate cancer cells causes an activation of cell adhesion and expression changes in Wnt signaling. These findings were validated by gene expression data from both clinical prostate cancer samples and from ERG over-expressing non-transformed prostate epithelial cells [45]. Several studies have shown that changes in the levels of TGF-β pathway components are related to prostate cancer progression and cellular responses [46], [47], and [48]. In addition, chemokine signaling pathways and the regulation of actin cytoskeleton have been studied and experimentally validated to be associated with prostate cancer [15,49].

In summary, the analysis of both simulated and real data provides evidence that the WMAXC method can yield new insights that contribute to a better understanding of diseases.

Discussion

Our main goal was to design an algorithm that reveals a subset of genes closely related to a particular disease. Based on an optimization framework, we proposed an effective method, WMAXC, for identifying a condition-specific sub-network under a particular condition. WMAXC has the following advantages: (1) It extracts the global optimal sub-network that exhibits significant alterations across two phenotypes; WMAXC considers the weighted contributions of both expression difference for each single gene and the differential correlation of each pair of genes. (2) WMAXC effectively integrates diverse sets of data and knowledge to construct the background network under a particular condition. (3) An optimization formulation with strong theoretical validation is used to represent a continuous version of the general combinatorial problem for identifying a condition-specific sub-network. (4) WMAXC considers all nodes and edges at the same time to search a single optimal sub-network. (5) Genetic algorithm and a projection procedure are combined to approximate the

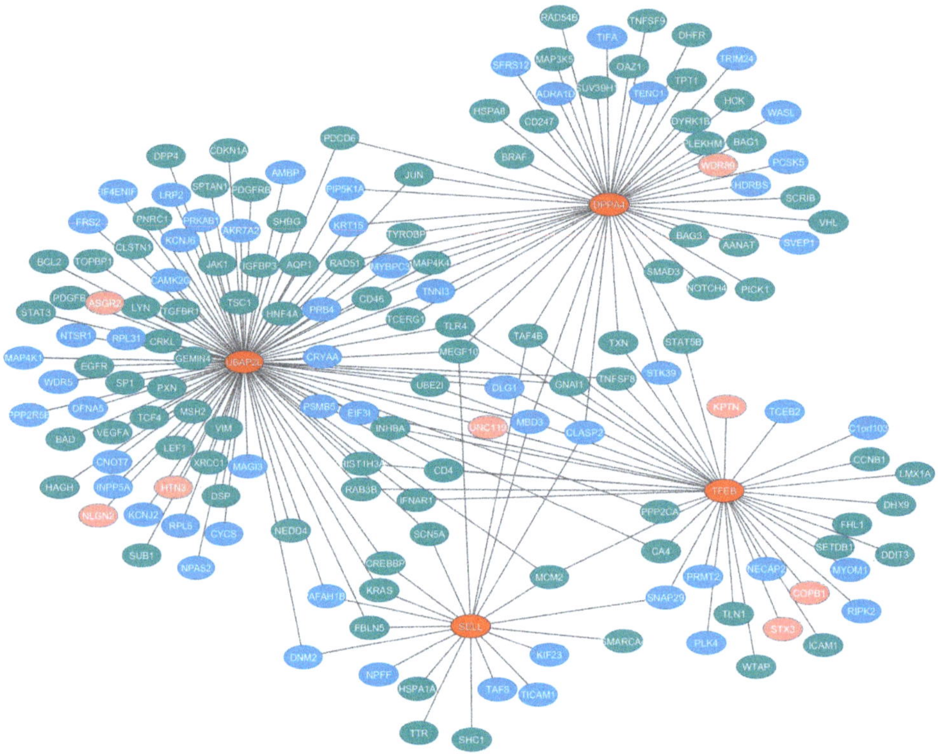

Figure 2. The four candidate genes for ovarian cancer and their neighbor genes in the condition specific network. The four candidate ovarian cancer-related genes are colored in red, ovarian cancer-related genes in green, cancer-related genes in blue and the remaining genes in pink. Edges represent significant co-expressions between genes in the given ovarian cancer.

global solution to our problem. (6) A weight parameter λ is chosen to make the solution stable to the problem, and it is also adaptive to the specific dataset being analyzed.

WMAXC integrates gene expressions and the PPI network, and the positive scaling parameters α and β in Equation (10) are contribution factors of the PPI network in identifying disease-specific genes. We expect that for larger α and β values, the accuracy will increase with a high-quality PPI network, while false positive genes might be included with a low-quality PPI network. In the Results section, we used a high-quality PPI network, and $\alpha = \frac{\max_{i,j}\{M_{ij}\}}{\max_{i,j}\{DBT_{ij}\}} = 26.336$ and $\beta = \frac{\max_i\{T_i\}}{\max_i\{Deg_i\}} = 31.242$ provide a stable performance, and the fold enrichment is relatively high as around 2.45. To show how the performances of the method are affected depending on PPI data quality and scaling parameters, we simulated three PPI data sets with different qualities by randomly removing a fraction of existing edges from the PPI network and randomly adding the same numbers of edges into the PPI network. Then, the simulated PPI data sets were used with three different sets of scaling parameters in our model and corresponding results for each scaling parameter are given in Table 3. For relatively high-quality data sets such as the original PPI and data set-1, the fold enrichment was increased with larger values of α and β. On the other hand, for the low-quality PPI data sets such as data set-3, the fold enrichment was decreased with larger values of α and β.

WMAXC is flexible. It can be simply adapted to directed graphs or even to the integration of gene expression and pathways. For example, instead of using a PPI network, the union of regulatory pathways can be used to represent directed interaction and to compute the DBT score for a pair of genes. In this case, the weight matrix W is non-symmetric, and only slight modifications are required to construct a bio-molecular network from the gene expression profile. The solution to the constrained optimization problem can be approximated by combining the genetic algorithm and the projection procedure.

Table 3. Performances on simulated PPI data with different scaling parameters.

Parameters	Original PPI network	PPI data set-1	PPI data set-2	PPI data set-3
$\alpha=5$, $\beta=6$	2.2704	1.7681	2.0443	1.7569
$\alpha=26.336$, $\beta=31.224$	2.454	2.3092	2.2176	1.615
$\alpha=50$, $\beta=60$	2.4592	2.3843	2.1657	1.5638

For the PPI data set-1, set-2 and set-3, 30%, 50% and 70% of edges from the original data are randomly removed and then the same number of edges are randomly added, respectively. Performances are measured using the fold enrichment, which is described in Table 2.

Supporting Information

File S1 Supplementary material. The combined supporting information file contains multiple supporting Figures, Tables and Descriptions of some fundamental concepts used in the work.

Author Contributions

Conceived and designed the experiments: BA HL. Performed the experiments: BA. Analyzed the data: BA HL. Contributed reagents/materials/analysis tools: HL. Wrote the paper: BA HL.

References

1. Wu X, Jiang R, Zhang M, Li S (2008) Network-based global inference of human disease genes. Mol Syst Biol 4: 189.
2. Barabási A, Gulbahce N, Loscalzo J (2011) Network medicine: a network-based approach to human disease. Nat Rev Genet 12: 56–68.
3. Waaijenborg S, Zwinderman A (2009) Sparse canonical correlation analysis for identifying, connecting and completing gene-expression networks. The American Journal of Pathology 10: 315.
4. Witten D, Tibshirani R (2009) Extensions of sparse canonical correlation analysis with applications to genomic data. Statistical Applications in Genetics and Molecular Biology 8: 28.
5. Chen L, Xuan J, Riggins R, Wang E Y Hoffman, Clarke R (2010) Multilevel support vector regression analysis to identify condition-specific regulatory networks. Bioinformatics 26: 1416–1422.
6. Ideker T, Ozier O, Schwikowski B, Siegel A (2003) Discovering regulatory and signalling circuits in molecular interaction networks. Bioinformatics 18: s233–s240.
7. Chuang H, Lee E, Lee D, Ideker T (2007) Network-based classification of breast cancer metastasis. Molecular Systems biology 3.
8. Chen L, Xuan J, Riggins R, Wang E Y Hoffman, Clarke R (2012) Identifying protein interaction subnetworks by a bagging markov random field-based method. Nucleic Acids Research 41: e42.
9. Taylor I, Linding R, Warde-Farley D, Liu Y, Pesquita C, et al. (2009) Dynamic modularity in protein interaction networks predicts breast cancer outcome. Nature Biotechnology 27: 199–204.
10. Guo Z, Li Y, Gong X, Yao C, Ma W, et al. (2007) Edge-based scoring and searching method for identifying condition-responsive protein-protein interaction sub-network. Bioinformatics 23: 2121–2128.
11. Lai Y, Wu B, Chen L, Zhao H (2004) A statistical method for identifying differential gene-gene coexpression patterns. Bioinformatics 20: 3146–3155.
12. Ma H, Schadt E, Kaplan L, Zhao H (2011) Condition-specific sub-network identification using a global optimization method. Bioinformatics 27: 1290–1298.
13. Qiu YQ, Zhang S, Zhang XS, Chen L Identifying differentially expressed pathways via a mixed integer linear programming model. IET Systems Biology 3: 475–486.
14. Backes C, Rurainski A, Klau W, et al. (2011) An integer linear programming approach for finding deregulated subgraphs in regulatory networks. Nucleic Acids Research 40: e43.
15. Wang Q, Symes A, Kane C, Freeman A, Nariculam J, et al. (2010) A novel role for wnt/ca^{2+} signaling in actin cytoskeleton remodeling and cell motility in prostate cancer. PLoS ONE: e10456.
16. Rajagopalan D, Agarwal P (2005) Inferring pathways from gene lists using a literature-derived network of biological relationships. Bioinformatics 21: 788–793.
17. Nacu S, Critchley-Thorne R, Lee P, Holmes S (2007) Gene expression network analysis and applications to immunology. Bioinformatics 23: 850–858.
18. Breitling R, Amtmann A, Herzyk P (2004) Graph-based iterative group analysis enhances microarray interpretation. BMC Bioinformatics 5.
19. Ulitsky I, Karp R, R S (2008) Detecting disease-specific dysregulated pathways via analysis of clinical expression profiles. In Proceedings of Research in Computational Molecular Biology 4955: 347–359.
20. Motzkin S, Straus G (1965) Maxima for graphs and a new proof of a theorem of turan. Canadian Journal of Mathematics 17: 533–540.
21. Tusher V, Tibshirani R, Chu G (2001) Significance analysis of microarrays applied to the ionizing radiation response. PNAS 98: 5116–5121.
22. Turan P (1941) On an extremal problem in graph theory. Mat Fiz Lapok 48: 435–452.
23. Du D, Pardalos P (1999) Handbook of combinatorial optimization.
24. Haupt R, Haupt S (2004) Chapter 3: The continuous genetic algorithm. Book, Practical Genetic Algorithms Second Edition: 51–66.
25. Michelot C (1986) A finite algorithm for finding the projection of a point onto the canonical simplex of $\mathbb{R}^n$. Journal of Optimization Theory and Applications 50: 195–200.
26. Songsiri J (2011) Projection onto an l_1-norm ball with application to identification of sparse au-toregressive models. Asian Symposium on Automatic Control Vietnam.
27. Kyrillidis A, Becker S, Cevher V, Koch C (2013) Sparse projections onto the simplex. 30th International Conference on Machine Learning (ICML) 28: 235–243.
28. Prasad T, Goel R, Kandasamy K, Keerthikumar S, Kumar S, et al. (2009) Human protein reference database. Nucleic Acids Research 37: D767–D772.
29. Atlas TCG The results published here are in whole or part based upon data generated by the cancer genome atlas pilot project established by the nci and nhgri. information about tcga and the investigators and institutions who constitute the tcga research network can be found at http://cancergenome.nih.gov. Data accessed 20 July 2011 .
30. Lapointe J, Li C, Higgins J, van de Rijn M, Bair E, et al. (2004) Gene expression profiling identifies clinically relevant subtypes of prostate cancer. PNAS 101: 811–816.
31. Kaur M, Radovanovic A, Essack M, Schaefer U, Maqungo M, et al. (2008) Ddpc: Database for exploration of functional context of genes implicated in ovarian cancer. Nucleic Acids Research 37: D820–D823.
32. Maqungo M, Kaur M, Kwofie S, Radovanovic A, Schaefer U, et al. (2011) Ddpc: Dragon database of genes associated with prostate cancer. Nucleic Acids Research 39: D980–D985.
33. Resto VD, Burdick M, Dagia N, McCammon S, Fennewald S (2008) L-selectin-mediated lymphocyte-cancer cell interactions under low fluid shear conditions. The Journal of Biological Chemistry 283: 15816–15824.
34. Kuiper R, Schepens M, Thijssen J, van Asseldonk M, van den Berg E, et al. (2003) Upregulation of the transcription factor tfeb in t(6;11) (p21;q13)-positive renal cell carcinomas due to promoter substitution. Human Molecular Genetics 12: 1661–1669.
35. Maldonado-Saldivia J, van den Bergen J, Krouskos M, Gilchrist M, Lee C, et al. (2007) Dppa2 and dppa4 are closely linked sap motif genes restricted to pluripotent cells and the germ line. Stem Cells 25: 19–28.
36. Huang D, Sherman B, Lempicki R (2008) Systematic and integrative analysis of large gene lists using david bioinformatics resources. Nature protocols 4: 44–57.
37. de Graeff P, Crijns A, ten Hoor K, Klip H, Hollema H, et al. (2008) The erbb signalling pathway: protein expression and prognostic value in epithelial ovarian cancer. British Journal of Cancer 99: 341–349.
38. Park J, Chen X, Trop C, Davidson B, Shih IM, et al. Notch3 over expression is related to the recurrence of ovarian cancer and confers resistance to carboplatin .
39. Yamamura S, Matsumura N, Mandai M, Huang Z, Oura T, et al. (2012) The activated transforming growth factor-beta signaling pathway in peritoneal metastases is a potential therapeutic target in ovarian cancer. International Journal of Cancer 130: 20–28.
40. Satoh F, Mimata H, Nomura T, Fujita Y, Shin T, et al. (2001) Autocrine expression of neurotrophins and their receptors in prostate cancer. International Journal of Urology 8: s28–s34.
41. Kinkade C, Castillo-Martin M, Puzio-Kuter A, Yan J, Foster T, et al. (2008) Targeting akt/mtor and erk mapk signaling inhibits hormone-refractory prostate cancer in a preclinical mouse model. The Journal of Clinical Investigation 118: 3051–3064.
42. Gioeli D, Mandell J, Petroni G, Frierson HJ, Weber M (1999) Activation of mitogen-activated protein kinase associated with prostate cancer progression. Cancer Research 59: 279–284.
43. Abreu-Martin M, Chari A, Palladino A, Craft N, Sawyers C (1999) Mitogen-activated protein kinase kinase kinase 1 activates androgen receptor-dependent transcription and apoptosis in prostate cancer. Molecular and Cellular Biology 19: 5143–5154.
44. da Silva H, Amaral E, Nolasco E, de Victo N, Atique R, et al. (2013) Dissecting major signaling pathways throughout the development of prostate cancer. Prostate Cancer 2013: 23 pages.
45. Gupta S, Iljin K, Sara H, Mpindi J, Mirtti T, et al. (2007) Fzd4 as a mediator of erg oncogene- induced wnt signaling and epithelial-to-mesenchymal transition in human prostate cancer cells. Cancer Research 70: 6735–6745.
46. Wikstrm P, Stattin P, Franck-Lissbrant I, Damber JE, Bergh A (1998) Transforming growth factor beta1 is associated with angiogenesis, metastasis, and poor clinical outcome in prostate cancer. The Prostate 37: 19–29.
47. Adler H, McCurdy M, Kattan M, Timme T, et al. (1999) Elevated levels of circulating interleukin-6 and transforming growth factor-$\beta 1$ in patients with metastatic prostatic carcinoma. The Journal of Urology 161: 182–187.
48. Shariat S, Shalev M, Menesses-Diaz A, Kim I, Kattan M, et al. (2001) Preoperative plasma levels of transforming growth factor beta1 (tgf-$\beta 1$) strongly predict progression in patients undergoing radical prostatectomy. Journal of Clinical Oncology 19: 2856–2864.
49. Wu YM, Robinson D, Kung HJ (2004) Signal pathways in up-regulation of chemokines by tyrosine kinase mer/nyk in prostate cancer cells. Cancer Research 64: 7311–7320.

9

Inferring Tree Causal Models of Cancer Progression with Probability Raising

Loes Olde Loohuis[1]*◑, Giulio Caravagna[2]◑, Alex Graudenzi[2]◑, Daniele Ramazzotti[2]◑, Giancarlo Mauri[2], Marco Antoniotti[2], Bud Mishra[3]

1 Center for Neurobehavioral Genetics, University of California Los Angeles, Los Angeles, United States of America, **2** Dipartimento di Informatica Sistemistica e Comunicazione, Università degli Studi, Milano-Bicocca, Milano, Italy, **3** Courant Institute of Mathematical Sciences, New York University, New York, United States of America

Abstract

Existing techniques to reconstruct tree models of progression for accumulative processes, such as cancer, seek to estimate causation by combining correlation and a frequentist notion of temporal priority. In this paper, we define a novel theoretical framework called CAPRESE (CAncer PRogression Extraction with Single Edges) to reconstruct such models based on the notion of probabilistic causation defined by Suppes. We consider a general reconstruction setting complicated by the presence of noise in the data due to biological variation, as well as experimental or measurement errors. To improve tolerance to noise we define and use a shrinkage-like estimator. We prove the correctness of our algorithm by showing asymptotic convergence to the correct tree under mild constraints on the level of noise. Moreover, on synthetic data, we show that our approach outperforms the state-of-the-art, that it is efficient even with a relatively small number of samples and that its performance quickly converges to its asymptote as the number of samples increases. For real cancer datasets obtained with different technologies, we highlight biologically significant differences in the progressions inferred with respect to other competing techniques and we also show how to validate conjectured biological relations with progression models.

Editor: Lars Kaderali, Technische Universität Dresden, Medical Faculty, Germany

Funding: This work was supported by the National Science Foundation grants CCF-0836649 and CCF-0926166 and by Regione Lombardia (Italy) under the research projects RetroNet through the ASTIL [12-4-5148000-40]; U.A 053 and NEDD Project [ID14546A Rif SAL-7] Fondo Accordi Istituzionali 2009. The funders had no role in study design, data collection and analysis, decision to publish, or preparation of the manuscript.

Competing Interests: The authors have declared that no competing interests exist.

* Email: l.oldeloohuis@gmail.com

◑ These authors contributed equally to this work.

Introduction

Cancer is a disease of evolution. Its initiation and progression are caused by dynamic somatic alterations to the genome manifested as point mutations, structural alterations, DNA methylation and histone modification changes [1].

These genomic alterations are generated by random processes, and since individual tumor cells compete for space and resources, the fittest variants are naturally selected for. For example, if through some mutations a cell acquires the ability to ignore anti-growth signals from the body, this cell may thrive and divide, and its progeny may eventually dominate some part(s) of the tumor. This *clonal expansion* can be seen as a *discrete state* of the cancer's progression, marked by the acquisition of a set of genetic events. Cancer progression can then be thought of as a sequence of these discrete steps, where the tumor acquires certain distinct properties at each state. Different progression sequences are possible, but some are more common than others, and not every order is viable [2].

In the last two decades, many specific genes and genetic mechanisms that are involved in different types of cancer have been identified (see e.g. [3,4] for an overview of common cancer genes and [5,6] for specific genetic analyses of ovarian carcinoma and lung adenocarcinoma, respectively), and *therapies* targeting the activity of these genes are now being developed at a fast pace [2]. However, unfortunately, the *causal and temporal relations* among the genetic events driving cancer progression remain largely elusive.

The main reason for this state of affairs is that information revealed in the data is usually obtained only at one (or a few) points in time, rather than over the course of the disease. Extracting this dynamic information from the available *cross-sectional* data is challenging, and a combination of mathematical, statistical and computational techniques is needed. In recent years, several methods to extract progression models from cross-sectional data have been developed, starting from the seminal work on single-path-models by Fearon and Vogelstein [7]. In particular, different models of oncogenetic trees were developed over the years. At the core of some of these methods, e.g. [8,9], is the use of *correlation* to identify relations among genetic events. These techniques reconstruct *tree* models of progression as independent acyclic paths with branches and no confluences. Distinct models of oncogenetic trees are instead based on *maximum likelihood estimation*, e.g., [10,11,12]. More general *Markov chain* models, e.g., [13], describe more flexible probabilistic networks, despite the computationally expensive parameter estimation. Other recent models are Conjunctive Bayesian Networks, CBNs [14,15], that extract *directed acyclic graphs*, yet imposing specific constraints on the joint occurrence of events. Finally, in a slightly different context, temporal models were reconstructed from time-course gene expression data [16,17].

In this paper we present a novel theoretical framework called CAPRESE (CAncer PRogression Extraction with Single Edges) to reconstruct cumulative progressive phenomena, such as cancer progression. We assume the original problem setting of [8], and propose a new a technique to infer *probabilistic progression trees* from cross-sectional data. Unlike maximum likelihood estimation-based techniques, our goal is the extraction of the *minimal* progression model explaining the order in which mutations occur and accumulate. The method is technology agnostic, i.e., it can be applied to dataset derived from all types of (epi-)genetic data such as deep exome sequencing, bisulfite sequencing, SNP arrays, etc., (see Results), and takes as input a set of pre-selected genetic events of which the presence or the absence of each event is recorded for each sample.

CAPRESE is based on two main ingredients: 1) rather than using *correlation* to infer progression structures, we base our technique on a notion of *probabilistic causation*, and 2), to increase robustness against noise, we adopt a *shrinkage-like estimator* to measure causation among any pair of events. More specifically, with respect to our first ingredient, we adopt the notion of (prima facie) causation proposed by Suppes in [18]. Its basic intuition is simple: event a causes event b if (*i*) a occurs *before* b and (*ii*) the occurrence of a *raises the probability* of observing b. This is a very basic notion of probabilistic causation that in itself does not address many of the problems associated with it (such as asymmetry, common causes, and screening off [19]), and includes *spurious* as well as *genuine* causes. However, as it turns out, this basic notion combined with a filter for independent progressions starting from the same root, is an excellent tool to guide progression extraction from cross-sectional data – one that outperforms the commonly used correlation-based methods.

Probabilistic causation was used in biomedical applications before (e.g., to find driver genes from CNV data in [20], and to extract causes from biological time series data in [21]), but, to the best of our knowledge, never to infer *progression models* in the *absence* of direct temporal information.

The extraction problem is complicated by the presence of both false positive and false negative observations (see [22] for a discussion on this issue based on the reconstruction by [8]), such as the one provided by the intrinsic variability of biological processes (e.g., *genetic heterogeneity*) and *experimental errors*. This poses a problem, because while probability raising is a very precise tool, it, by itself, is not robust enough against noise. Conditional on the amount of noise, we will rely both on probabilistic causation and on a more robust (but less precise) correlation-based metric in an optimal way. To do this we introduce our second ingredient, a *shrinkage-like estimator* to measure causation among any pair of events. The intuition behind this estimator, which is closely related to a shrinkage estimator from [23], is to find the optimal balance between probability raising on the one hand and correlation on the other, depending on the amount of noise.

We prove correctness of our algorithm by showing that with increasing sample sizes, the reconstructed tree asymptotically converges to the correct one (Theorem 3). Under mild constraints on the noise rates, this result holds for the reconstruction problem in the presence of uniform noise as well.

We also study the performance of CAPRESE in more realistic settings with limited sample sizes. Using synthetic data, we show that under these conditions, our algorithm outperforms the state-of-the-art tree reconstruction algorithm of [8] (see Results). In particular, our shrinkage-like estimator provides, on average, an increased robustness to noise which ensures it to outperform oncotrees [8]. Performance is defined in terms of *structural similarity* between the reconstructed tree and the actual tree, rather than on their induced distribution as is done, e.g., in [11]. This metric is especially appropriate for the goal of reconstructing a progression model where data-likelihood fit is secondary to "calling" the possibly minimal set of causal relations.

Also, we show that CAPRESE works well already with a relatively low number of samples and that its performance quickly converges to its asymptote as the number of samples increases. This outcome hints at the applicability of the algorithm with relatively small datasets without compromising its efficiency.

We remark that further analyses on synthetic data suggests that CAPRESE outperforms a well known bayesian probabilistic graphical model as well (i.e., *Conjunctive Bayesian Networks* [14,15]), which was originally conceived for the reconstruction of more complex topologies, e.g. DAGs, but was proven effective in reconstructing tree topologies as well [24] (see Results).

Finally, we apply our technique to alterations assessed with both Comparative Genomic Hybridization and Next Generation Sequencing techniques (see Results). In the former case, we show that the algorithm of [8] and CAPRESE highlight biologically important differences in ovarian, gastrointestinal and oral cancer, but our inferences are statistically more significant. In the latter, we validate a recently discovered relation among two key genes involved in leukemia.

Methods

Problem setting

The set-up of the reconstruction problem is as follows. Assuming that we have a set G of n mutations (*events*, in probabilistic terminology) and s samples, we represent a cross-sectional dataset as an $s \times n$ binary matrix in which an entry $(k,l)=1$ if the mutation l was observed in sample k, and 0 otherwise. The problem we solve in this paper is to extract a set of edges E yielding a progression *tree* $\mathcal{T}=(G\cup\{\blacklozenge\},E,\blacklozenge)$ from this matrix which, we remark, only implicitly provides information of progression timing. The root of $\mathcal{T}$ is modeled using a (special) event $\blacklozenge \notin G$ such that *heterogenous progression paths* or *forests* can be reconstructed. More precisely, we aim at reconstructing a *rooted tree* that satisfies: (*i*) each node has at most one incoming edge, (*ii*) the root has no incoming edges (*iii*) there are no *cycles*.

Each progression tree subsumes a distribution of observing a subset of the mutations in a cancer sample that can be formalized as follows:

Definition 1. (Tree-induced distribution) *Let $\mathcal{T}$ be a tree and $\alpha : E \to [0,1]$ a labeling function denoting the independent probability of each edge, $\mathcal{T}$ generates a distribution where the probability of observing a sample with the set of alterations $G^* \subseteq G$ is*

$$\mathcal{P}(G^*) = \prod_{e \in E'} \alpha(e) \cdot \prod_{\substack{(u,v)\in E \\ u\in G^*, v\notin G}} [1-\alpha(u,v)] \tag{1}$$

where all events in G^* are assumed to be reachable from the root $\blacklozenge$, and $E' \subseteq E$ is the set of edges connecting the root to the events in G^*.

We would like to emphasize two properties related to the tree-induced distribution. First, the distribution subsumes that, given any oriented edge ($a \to b$), an observed sample contains alteration b with probability $\mathcal{P}(a)\mathcal{P}(b)$, that is the probability of observing b after a. For this reason, if a causes b, the probability of observing a will be greater than the probability of observing b accordingly to the temporal priority principle which states that all causes must precede, in time, their effects [25].

Second, the input dataset is a set of samples generated, ideally, from an unknown distribution induced by an unknown tree or forest that we aim at reconstructing. However, in some cases, it could be that no tree exists whose induced distribution generates *exactly* those input data. When this happens, the set of observed samples slightly diverges from any tree-induced distribution. To model these situations a notion of *noise* can be introduced, which depends on the context in which data are gathered. Adding noise to the model complicates the reconstruction problem (see Results).

The *oncotree* approach. In [8] Desper *et al.* developed a method to extract progression trees, named *"oncotrees"*, from static CNV data. In [22] Szabo *et al.* extended the setting of Desper's reconstruction problem to account for both *false positives* and *negatives* in the input data. In these oncotrees, nodes represent CNV events and edges correspond to possible progressions from one event to the next.

The reconstruction problem is exactly as described above, and each tree is rooted in the special event ♦. The choice of which edge to include in a tree is based on the estimator

$$w_{a \to b} = \log\left[\frac{\mathcal{P}(a)}{\mathcal{P}(a)+\mathcal{P}(b)} \cdot \frac{\mathcal{P}(a,b)}{\mathcal{P}(a)\mathcal{P}(b)}\right], \tag{2}$$

which assigns to each edge $a \to b$ a weight accounting for both the relative and joint frequencies of the events – thus measuring *correlation*. The estimator is evaluated after including ♦ to each sample of the dataset. In this definition the rightmost term is the (symmetric) *likelihood ratio* for a and b occurring together, while the leftmost is the asymmetric *temporal priority* measured by rate of occurrence. This implicit form of timing assumes that, if a occurs *more often* than b, then it likely occurs *earlier*, thus satisfying

$$\frac{\mathcal{P}(a)}{\mathcal{P}(a)+\mathcal{P}(b)} > \frac{\mathcal{P}(b)}{\mathcal{P}(a)+\mathcal{P}(b)}.$$

An oncotree is the rooted tree whose total weight (i.e., sum of all the weights of the edges) is maximized, and can be reconstructed in $O(|G|^2)$ steps using Edmond's algorithm [26]. By construction, the resulting graph is a proper tree rooted in ♦: each event occurs only once, *confluences* are absent, i.e., any event is caused by at most one other event. This method has been used to derive progressions for various cancer datasets e.g., [27,28,29]), and even though several methods that extend this framework exists (e.g. [9,11,15]), to the best of our knowledge, it is currently the only method that aims to solve exactly the same problem as the one investigated in this paper and thus provide a benchmark to compare against.

A probabilistic approach to causation

We briefly review the approach to probabilistic causation, on which our method is based. For an extensive discussion on this topic we refer to [19].

In his seminal work [18], Suppes proposed the following notion.

Definition 2. (Probabilistic causation, [18]). *For any two events c and e, occurring respectively at times t_c and t_e, under the mild assumptions that $0 < \mathcal{P}(c), \mathcal{P}(e) < 1$, the event c is a prima facie cause of the event e if it occurs before the effect and the cause raises the probability of the effect, i.e.,*

$$t_c < t_e \quad \text{and} \quad \mathcal{P}(e|c) > \mathcal{P}(e|\bar{c}). \tag{3}$$

As discussed in [19] the above conditions are not, in general, sufficient to claim that event c is a cause of event e. In fact a prima facie cause is either *genuine* or *spurious*. In the latter case, the fact that the conditions hold in the observations is due either to coincidence or to the presence of a certain third *confounding factor*, related both to c and to e [18]. Genuine causes, instead, satisfy Definition 2 and are not screened-off by any confounding factor. However, they need not be direct causes. See Figure 1.

Note that we consider cross-sectional data where no information about t_c and t_e is available, so in our reconstruction setting we are restricted to consider solely the *probability raising* (PR) property, i.e., $\mathcal{P}(e|c) > \mathcal{P}(e|\bar{c})$, which makes it harder to discriminate among genuine and spurious causes. Now we review some of its properties.

Proposition 1. (Dependency). *Whenever the* PR *holds between two events a and b, then the events are* statistically dependent *in a positive sense, i.e.,*

$$\mathcal{P}(b|a) > \mathcal{P}(b|\bar{a}) \Leftrightarrow \mathcal{P}(a,b) > \mathcal{P}(a)\mathcal{P}(b). \tag{4}$$

This and the next proposition are well-known facts of the PR; their derivation as well as the proofs of all the results we present is in the File S1. Notice that the opposite implication holds as well: when the events a and b are still dependent but in a negative sense, i.e., $\mathcal{P}(a,b) < \mathcal{P}(a)\mathcal{P}(b)$, the PR does not hold, i.e., $\mathcal{P}(b|a) < \mathcal{P}(b|\bar{a})$.

We would like to use the asymmetry of the PR to determine whether a pair of events a and b satisfy a causation relation so to place a before b in the progression tree but, unfortunately, the PR satisfies the following property.

Proposition 2. (Mutual PR). $\mathcal{P}(b|a) > \mathcal{P}(b|\bar{a}) \Leftrightarrow \mathcal{P}(a|b) > \mathcal{P}(a|\bar{b})$.

That is, if a raises the probability of observing b, then b raises the probability of observing a too.

Nevertheless, in order to determine causes and effects among the genetic events, we can use our *degree of confidence* in our estimate of probability raising to decide the direction of the causation relationship between pairs of events. In other words, if a raises the probability of b *more* than the other way around, then a is a more likely cause of b than b of a. Notice that this is sound as long as each event has *at most* one cause; otherwise, *frequent late events* with more than one cause, which are rather common in biological progressive phenomena, should be treated differently. As mentioned, the PR is not symmetric, and the *direction* of probability raising depends on the relative frequencies of the events. We make this asymmetry precise in the following proposition.

Proposition 3. (Probability raising and temporal priority). *For any two events a and b such that the probability raising $\mathcal{P}(a|b) > \mathcal{P}(a|\bar{b})$ holds, we have*

$$\mathcal{P}(a) > \mathcal{P}(b) \Leftrightarrow \frac{\mathcal{P}(b|a)}{\mathcal{P}(b|\bar{a})} > \frac{\mathcal{P}(a|b)}{\mathcal{P}(a|\bar{b})}. \tag{5}$$

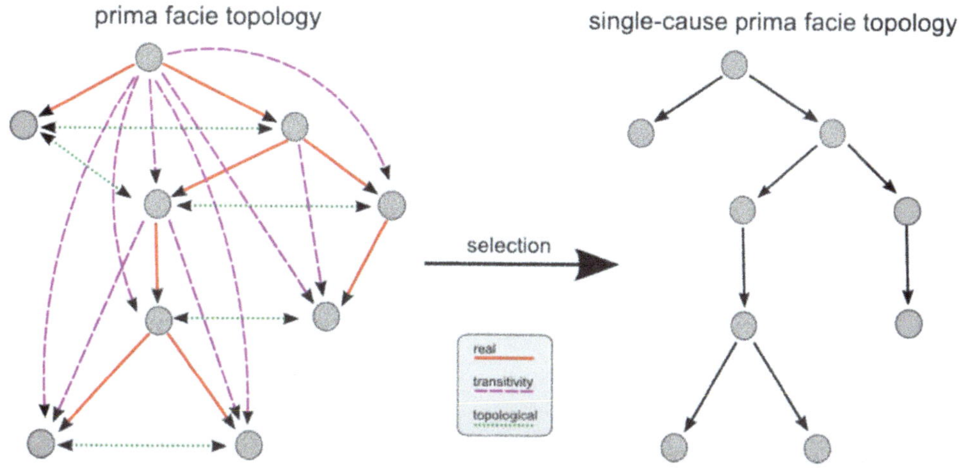

Figure 1. Prima facie topology. Example prima facie topology where all edges (a,b) represent prima facie causes, according to Definition 3: a is a probability raiser of b and it occurs more frequently. In left, we filter out spurious causes and select only the real ones among the genuine, yielding a single-cause prima facie topology.

That is, given that the PR holds between two events, a raises the probability of b *more* than b raises the probability of a, if and only if a is observed more frequently than b. Notice that we use the ratio to assess the PR inequality. The proof of this proposition is technical and can be found in the File S1. From this result it follows that if we measure the timing of an event by the rate of its occurrence (that is, $\mathcal{P}(a) > \mathcal{P}(b)$ implies that a happens before b), this notion of PR subsumes the same notion of temporal priority induced by a tree. We also remark that this is also the temporal priority made explicit in the coefficients of Desper's method. Given these results, we define the following notion of causation.

Definition 3. *We state that a is a prima facie cause of b if a is a probability raiser of b, and it occurs more frequently:*

$$\mathcal{P}(b|a) > \mathcal{P}(b|\bar{a}) and \mathcal{P}(a) > \mathcal{P}(b).$$

We term *prima facie topology* a directed acyclic graph (over some events) where each edge represents a prima facie cause. When at most a single incoming edge is assigned to each event (i.e., an event has at most a *unique cause*, in the real world), we term this structure *single-cause prima facie topology*. Intuitively, this last class of topologies correspond to the trees or, more generally forests when they have disconnected components, that we aim at reconstructing.

Before moving on to introducing our algorithm let us discuss our definition of *causation*, its role in the definition of the reconstruction problem and some of its limitations. As already mentioned, it may be that for some prima facie cause c of an event e, there is a third event a prior to both, such that a causes c and ultimately c causes e. Alternatively, a may cause both c and e independently, and the causation relationship observed from c to e is merely *spurious*. In the context of the tree-reconstruction problem, namely when it is assumed that each event has at most a unique cause, the aim is to filter out the spurious edges from a general prima facie topology, so to extract a single-cause prima facie structure (see Figure 1).

Definition 3 summarizes Suppes basic notion of prima facie cause, while it is ignoring deeper discussions of causation that aim at distinguishing between actual genuine and spurious causes, e.g. screening-off, background context, d-separation [30,31,19]. For our purposes however, the above definition is sufficient when (*i*) all the significant events are considered, i.e., all the genuine causes are observed as in a closed-world assumption, and (*ii*) we aim at extracting the *order* of progression among them (or determine that there is no apparent relation), rather than extracting causalities *per se*. Note that these assumptions are strong and might be weakened in the future (see Discussions), but are shared by us and [8].

Finally, we recall a few algebraic requirements necessary for our framework to be well-defined. First of all, the PR must be computable: every mutation a should be observed with probability strictly $0 < \mathcal{P}(a) < 1$. Moreover, we need each pair of mutations (a,b) to be *distinguishable* in terms of PR, that is, for each pair of mutations a and b, $\mathcal{P}(a|b) < 1$ or $\mathcal{P}(b|a) < 1$ similarly to the above condition. Any non-distinguishable pair of events can be merged as a single composite event. From now on, we will assume these conditions to be verified.

Performance measure and synthetic datasets

We made use of *synthetic data* to evaluate the performance of CAPRESE as a function of dataset size and the false positive and negative rates. Many distinct synthetic datasets were created for this purpose, as explained below. The algorithm's performance was measured in terms of *Tree Edit Distance* (TED, [32]), i.e., the minimum-cost sequence of node edit operations (relabeling, deletion and insertion) that transforms the reconstructed trees into the ones generating the data. The choice of this measure of evaluation is motivated by the fact that we are interested in the *structure* behind the progressive phenomenon of cancer evolution and, in particular, we are interested in a measure of the genuine causes that we miss and of the spurious causes that we fail to recognize (and eliminate). Also, since topologies with similar distributions can be structurally different we choose to measure performance using structural distance rather than a distance in terms of distributions. Within the realm of 'structural metrics' however, we have also evaluated the performance with the *Hamming Distance* [33], another commonly used structural metric, and we obtained analogous results (not shown here).

Synthetic data generation and experimental setting. Synthetic datasets were generated by sampling from various random trees constrained to have depth $\log(|G|)$, since

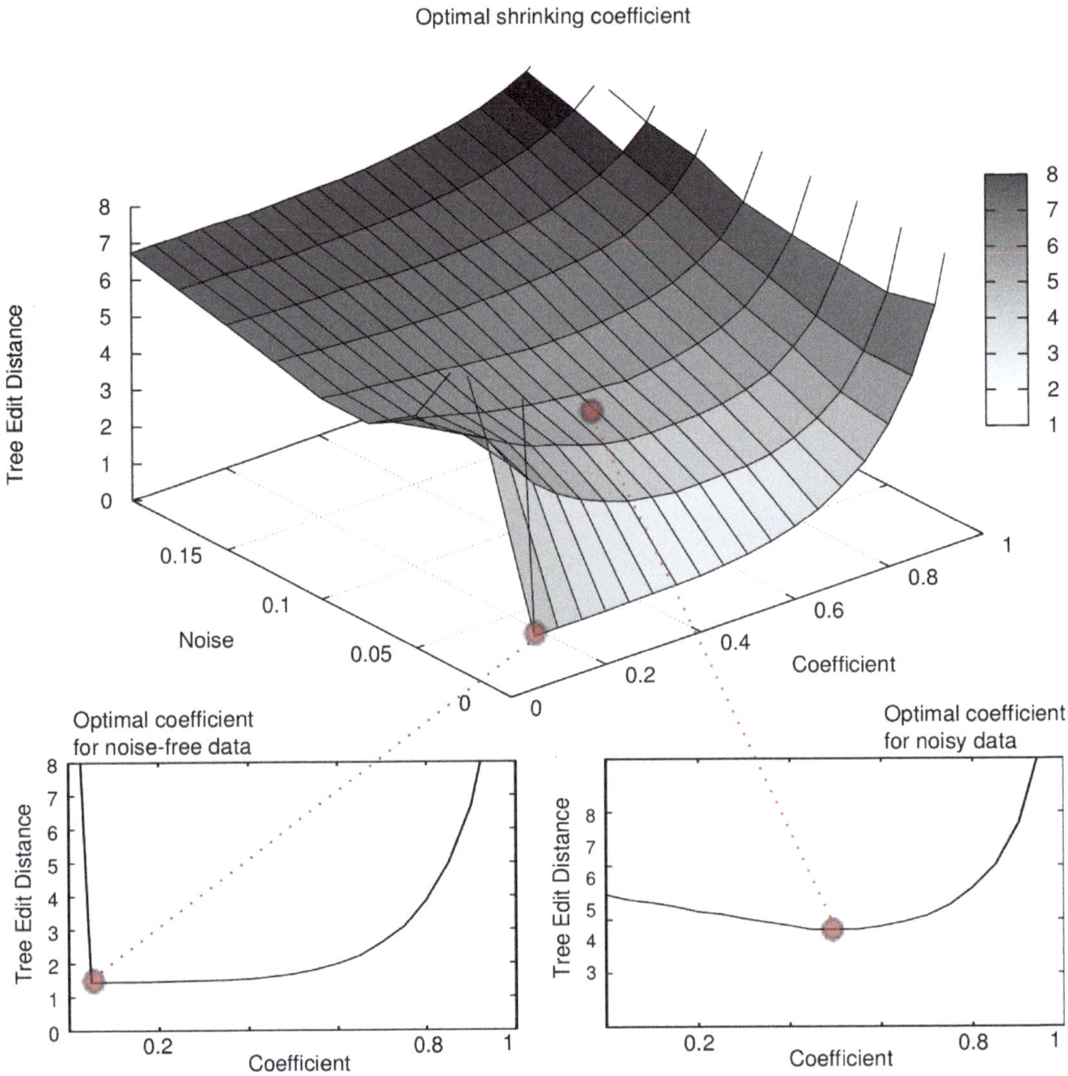

Figure 2. Optimal shrinkage-like coefficient for reconstruction performance. We show here the performance in the reconstruction of trees (TED surface) with $n = 150$ samples as a function of the shrinkage-like coefficient λ. Notice the global optimal performance for $\lambda \to 0$ when $\nu \to 0$ and for $\lambda \approx 1/2$ when $\nu > 0$.

wide branches are harder to reconstruct than straight paths, and by sampling event probabilities in [0.05,0.95] (see File S1).

Unless explicitly specified, in all the experiments we used 100 distinct random trees (or forests, accordingly to the test to perform) of 20 events each. This seems a fairly reasonable number of events and is in line with the usual size of reconstructed trees, e.g. [34,35,36,37]. The *scalability* of the techniques was tested against the number of samples by ranging $|G|$ from 50 to 250, with a step of 50, and by replicating 10 independent datasets for each parameters setting (see the caption of the figures for details).

We included a form of *noise* in generating the datasets, in order to account for (*i*) the realistic presence of *biological noise* (such as the one provided by bystander mutations, genetic heterogeneity, etc.) and (*ii*) *experimental errors*. A noise parameter $0 \leq \nu < 1$ denotes the probability that any event assumes a random value (with uniform probability), after sampling from the tree-induced distribution. Algorithmically this process generates, on average, $|G|\nu/2$ random entries in each sample (e.g. with $\nu = 0.1$ we have, on average, one error per sample). We wish to assess whether these noisy samples can mislead the reconstruction process, even for low values of ν. Notice that assuming a uniformly distributed noise may appear simplistic since some events may be more robust, or easy to measure, than others. However, introducing in the data both *false positives* (at rate $\epsilon_+ = \nu/2$) and *negatives* (at rate $\epsilon_- = \nu/2$) makes the inference problem substantially harder, and was first investigated in [22].

In the Results section, we refer to datasets generated with rate $\nu > 0$ as noisy synthetic dataset. In the numerical experiments, ν is usually discretized by 0.025, (i.e., 2.5% noise).

Results

Extracting progression trees with probability raising and a shrinkage-like estimator

The CAPRESE reconstruction method is described in Algorithm 1. The algorithm is similar to Desper's and Szabo's algorithm, the main difference being an alternative weight function based on a shrinkage-like estimator.

Algorithm 1. CAPRESE: a tree-like reconstruction with a shrinkage-like estimator.

1: consider a set of n genetic events G plus a special event ◆, added to each sample of the dataset;

2: define a $m \times n$ matrix M where each entry contains the shrinkage-like estimator $m_{i \to j} = (1-\lambda)\cdot \frac{\mathcal{P}(j|i) - \mathcal{P}(j|\bar{i})}{\mathcal{P}(j|i) + \mathcal{P}(j|\bar{i})} + \lambda \cdot \frac{\mathcal{P}(i,j) - \mathcal{P}(i)\mathcal{P}(j)}{\mathcal{P}(i,j) + \mathcal{P}(i)\mathcal{P}(j)}$ according to the observed probability of the events i and j;

3: [PR causation] define a tree $\mathcal{T} = (G \cup \{◆\}, E, ◆)$ where $(i \to j) \in E$ for $i,j \in G$ if and only if: $m_{i \to j} > 0$ and $m_{i \to j} > m_{j \to i}$ and $\forall i' \in G, m_{i,j} > m_{i',j}$.

4: [Independent progressions filter] define $G_j = \{x \in G | \mathcal{P}(x) > \mathcal{P}(j)\}$, replace edge $(i \to j) \in E$ with edge $(◆ \to j)$ if, for all $x \in G_j$, it holds $\frac{1}{1+\mathcal{P}(j)} > \frac{\mathcal{P}(x)}{\mathcal{P}(x)+\mathcal{P}(j)} \frac{\mathcal{P}(x,j)}{\mathcal{P}(x)\mathcal{P}(j)}$.

Definition 4. (Shrinkage-like estimator). *We define the shrinkage-like estimator $m_{a \to b}$ of the confidence in the causation relationship from a to b as*

$$m_{a \to b} = (1-\lambda)\alpha_{a \to b} + \lambda \beta_{a \to b}, \tag{6}$$

where $0 \leq \lambda \leq 1$ *and*

$$\alpha_{a \to b} = \frac{\mathcal{P}(b|a) - \mathcal{P}(b|\bar{a})}{\mathcal{P}(b|a) + \mathcal{P}(b|\bar{a})} \qquad \beta_{a \to b} = \frac{\mathcal{P}(a,b) - \mathcal{P}(a)\mathcal{P}(b)}{\mathcal{P}(a,b) + \mathcal{P}(a)\mathcal{P}(b)}. \tag{7}$$

This estimator is similar in spirit to a shrinkage estimator (see [23]) and combines a normalized version of PR, the *raw estimate* α, with a *correction factor* β (in our case a correlation-based measure of temporal distance among events), to define a proper order in the confidence of each causation relationship. Our λ is the analogous of the *shrinkage coefficient* and can have a Bayesian interpretation based on the strength of our belief that a and b are causally relevant to one another and the evidence that a raises the probability of b. In the absence of a closed form solution for the optimal value of λ, one may rely on cross-validation of simulated data. The power of shrinkage (and our shrinkage-like estimator) lies in the possibility of determining an optimal value for λ to balance the effect of the correction factor on the raw model estimate to ensure optimal performances on ill posed instances of the inference problem. A crucial difference, however, between our estimator and classical shrinkage, is that our estimator aims at improving the performance of the *overall* reconstruction process, not limited to the performance of the estimator itself as is the case in shrinkage. That is, the metric m induces an ordering to the events reflecting our confidence for their causation. Furthermore, since we make no assumption about the underlying distribution, we learn it empirically by cross-validation. In the next sections we show that the shrinkage-like estimator is an effective way to get such an ordering especially when data are noisy. In CAPRESE we use a pairwise matrix version of the estimator.

The raw estimator and the correction factor. By considering only the raw estimator α, we would include an edge $(a \to b)$ in the tree consistently in terms of (*i*) Definition 3 (Methods) and (*ii*) if a is the best probability raiser for b. When $\mathcal{P}(a) = \mathcal{P}(b)$ the events a and b are indistinguishable in terms of temporal priority, thus α is not sufficient to decide their causal relation, if any. This intrinsic ambiguity is unlikely in practice even if, in principle, it is possible. Notice that this formulation of α is a monotonic normalized version of the PR ratio.

Proposition 4. (Monotonic normalization). *For any two events a and b we have*

$$\mathcal{P}(a) > \mathcal{P}(b) \Leftrightarrow \frac{\mathcal{P}(b|a)}{\mathcal{P}(b|\bar{a})} > \frac{\mathcal{P}(a|b)}{\mathcal{P}(a|\bar{b})} \Leftrightarrow \alpha_{a \to b} > \alpha_{b \to a}. \tag{8}$$

This raw model estimator satisfies $-1 \leq \alpha_{a \to b}, \alpha_{b \to a} \leq 1$: when it tends to -1 the pair of events appear disjointly (i.e., they show an anti- causation pattern), when it tends to 0 no causation or anti-causation can be inferred and the two events are statistically independent and, when it tends to 1, the causation relationship between the two events is genuine. Therefore, α provides a quantification of the degree of confidence for a PR causation relationship. In fact, for any given possible causation edge (a,b), the term $\mathcal{P}(b|\bar{a})$ gives an estimate of the *error rate* of b, therefore the numerator of the raw model α provides an estimate of how often b is actually caused by a. The α estimator is then normalized to range between -1 and $+1$.

However, α does not provide a general criterion to disambiguate among genuine causes of a given event. We show a specific case in which α is not a sufficient estimator. Let us consider, for instance, a causal linear path: $a \to b \to c$. In this case, when evaluating the candidate parents a and b for c we have: $\alpha_{a \to c} = \alpha_{b \to c} = 1$, so a and b are genuine causes of c, though we would like to select b, instead of a. Accordingly, we can only infer that $t_a < t_c$ and $t_b < t_c$, i.e., a partial ordering, which does not help to disentangle the relation among a and b with respect to c.

In this case, the β coefficient can be used to determine which of the two genuine causes occurs closer, in time, to c (b, in the example above). In general, such a correction factor provides information on the *temporal distance* between events, in terms of statistical dependency. In other words, the higher the β coefficient, the closer two events are. Therefore, when dealing with noisy data and limited sample sizes, there are situations where, by using the α estimator alone, we could infer a wrong transitive edge to be the most likely cause even in the presence of the real cause. For this reason, we reduce the α estimator to the correction factor β, which, for each given edge (a,b), is normalized within -1 and $(1-\max[\mathcal{P}(a),\mathcal{P}(b)])/(1+\max[\mathcal{P}(a),\mathcal{P}(b)]) < +1$.

The shrinkage-like estimator m then results in the combination of the raw PR estimator α and of the β correction factor, which respects the temporal priority induced by α.

Proposition 5. (Coherence in dependency and temporal priority). *The β correction factor is symmetrical and subsumes the same notion of dependency of the raw estimator α, that is*

$$\mathcal{P}(a,b) > \mathcal{P}(a)\mathcal{P}(b) \Leftrightarrow \alpha_{a \to b} > 0 \Leftrightarrow \beta_{a \to b} > 0 \quad and \ \beta_{a \to b} = \beta_{b \to a}. \tag{9}$$

The independent progressions filter. As in Desper's approach, we also add a *root* ◆ with $\mathcal{P}(◆) = 1$ in order to separate different progression paths, i.e., the different sub-trees rooted in ◆. CAPRESE initially builds a unique tree by using the estimator; typically, the most likely event will be at the top of the progression even if there may be rare cases where more than one event has no valid parent, in these cases we would already be reconstructing a forest. In the reconstructed tree, all the edges represent the most confident prima facie cause, although some of those could still be spurious causes. Then the correlation-like weight between any node j and ◆ is computed as

$$\frac{\mathcal{P}(\blacklozenge)}{\mathcal{P}(\blacklozenge)+\mathcal{P}(j)}\frac{\mathcal{P}(\blacklozenge,j)}{\mathcal{P}(\blacklozenge)\mathcal{P}(j)}=\frac{1}{1+\mathcal{P}(j)}.$$

If this quantity is greater than the weight of j with each upstream connected element i, we consider the best prima facie cause of j to be a spurious cause and we substitute the edge $(i \to j)$ with the edge $(\blacklozenge \to j)$. Note that in this work we are ignoring deeper discussions of probabilistic causation that aim at distinguishing between actual genuine causes and spurious causes. Instead, we remove spurious causes by using a filter based on correlation because the probability raising of the omnipresent event $\blacklozenge$ is not well defined (see Methods). In addition, we remark that the evaluation for an edge to be a genuine or a spurious cause takes into account all the given events. Because of this, if events are added or removed from the dataset, the same edge can be defined to be genuine or spurious as the set of events included in the model is varied arbitrarily. However, since we do not consider the problem of selecting the set of progression events, we assume that all and only the relevant events for the problem at hand are already known a priori and included in the model.

Finally, note that this filter is indeed implying a non-negative threshold for the shrinkage-like estimator, when an edge is valid.

Theorem 1. (Independent progressions). *Let* $G^* = \{a_1, \ldots, a_k\} \subset G$ *a set of* k prima facie causes *for some* $b \notin G^*$*, and let* $a^* = \max_{a_i \in G^*}\{m_{a_i \to b}\}$*. The reconstructed tree by CAPRESE contains edge* $\blacklozenge \to b$ *instead of* $a^* \to b$ *if, for all* $a_i \in G^*$

$$\mathcal{P}(a_i,b) < \mathcal{P}(a_i)\mathcal{P}(b)\frac{1}{1+\mathcal{P}(b)} + \frac{\mathcal{P}(b)^2}{1+\mathcal{P}(b)}. \tag{10}$$

The proof of this theorem can be found in the File S1. What this theorem suggests is that, in principle, by examining the level of statistical dependency of each pair of events, it would be possible to determine how many trees compose the reconstructed forest. Furthermore, it suggests that CAPRESE could be defined by first processing the independent progressions filter, and then using m to build the independent progression trees in the forest.

To conclude, the algorithm reconstructs a well defined tree (or, more in general, forest).

Theorem 2. (Algorithm correctness). *CAPRESE reconstructs a well defined tree* T *without disconnected components, transitive connections and cycles.*

Additionally, asymptotically with the number of samples, the reconstructed tree is the correct one.

Theorem 3. (Asymptotic convergence). *Let* $T = (G \cup \{\blacklozenge\}, E, \blacklozenge)$ *be the forest to reconstruct from a set of* s *input samples, given as the input matrix* D*. If* D *is strictly sampled from the distribution induced by* T *and infinite samples are available, i.e.,* $s \to \infty$*, CAPRESE with* $\lambda \to 0$ *correctly reconstructs* T*.*

The proof of these Theorems are also in the File S1. These theorems considered datasets where the observed and theoretical probabilities match, because of $s \to \infty$. However, data often contains false positives and negatives (i.e., data are noisy) and resistance to their effects is desirable in any inferential technique. With this in mind, we prove a corollary of the theorem analoguos to a result appearing in [22].

Corollary 1. (Uniform noise). *Let the input matrix* D *be strictly sampled from the distribution induced by* T *with sample size* $s \to \infty$*, but let it be corrupted by noise levels of false positives* ϵ_+ *and false negatives* ϵ_-*. Let* $p_{\min} = \min_{x \in G}\{\mathcal{P}(x)\}$*, CAPRESE correctly reconstructs* T *for* $\lambda \to 0$ *whenever*

$$\epsilon_+ < \sqrt{p_{\min}}(1-\epsilon_+-\epsilon_-)$$

and $\epsilon_+ + \epsilon_- < 1$.

Essentially, this corollary states that CAPRESE (and so the estimator m) is robust against a noise affecting all samples equally. Also, the fact that it holds for $\lambda \to 0$ is sound with the theory of shrinkage estimators for which, asymptotically, the corrector factor is not needed to regularize the ill posed problem.

Optimal shrinkage-like coefficient

Theorem 3 and Corollary 1 state that with infinite samples and mild constraints on the false positive/negative rates we get optimal results with $\lambda \to 0$. Precisely, for the uniform noise model that we applied to synthetic data (see Methods) we have $\epsilon_+ = \epsilon_- = v/2$, thus the hypothesis required by Corollary 1 is

$$v < \frac{\sqrt{p_{\min}}}{1/2 + \sqrt{p_{\min}}}.$$

For $p_{\min} = 0.05$, which we set in data generation (see File S1), this inequality implies correct reconstruction for $v < 0.3$ (a 15% error rate), with infinite samples. However, we are interested in performance and the optimal value of λ in situations in which we have finite sample sizes as well. Here, we empirically estimate the optimal λ value, both in the case of trees and forests, as a function of noise and sample size. In the next section, we assess performance of our algorithm empirically.

In Figure 2, we show the variation of the performance of CAPRESE as a function of λ, for datasets with 150 samples generated from tree topologies. The optimal value, i.e., lowest Tree Edit Distance (TED, see Methods), for noise-free datasets (i.e., $v=0$) is obtained for $\lambda \to 0$, whereas for the noisy datasets a series of U-shaped curves suggests a unique optimum value for $\lambda \to 1/2$, immediately observable for $v < 0.15$. Identical results are obtained when dealing with forests (not shown here). In addition, further experiments with n varying around the typical sample size ($n = 150$) show that the optimal λ is largely insensitive to the dataset size (see Figure 3). Thus we have limited our analysis to datasets with the typical sample size that is characteristic of data currently available.

Summarizing, Figures 2 and 3 suggest that for sample size below 250 without false positives and negatives the PR raw estimate α suffices to drive reconstruction to good results (TED is 0 with 250 samples), i.e.,

$$m_{a \to b} \overset{\lambda \to 0}{\approx} \alpha_{a \to b} \tag{11}$$

which is obtained by setting λ to a very small value, e.g. 10^{-2}, in order to consider at least a small contribution of the correction factor too. Conversely, when $v > 0$, the best performance is obtained by averaging the shrinkage-like effect, i.e.,

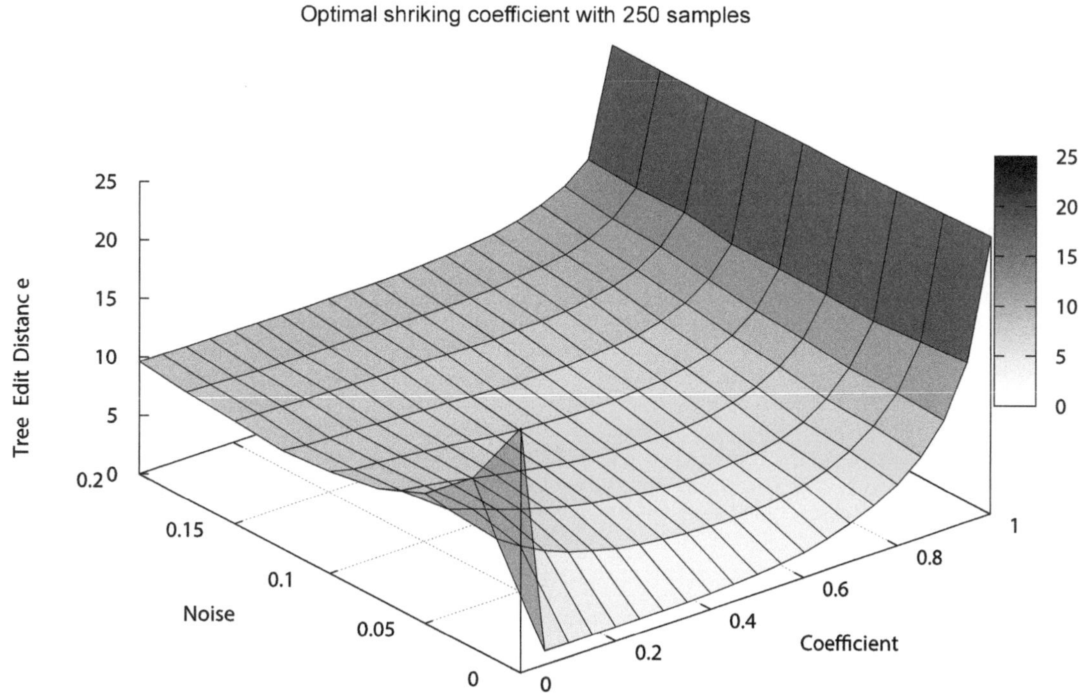

Figure 3. Optimal λ with datasets of different size. We show the analogous of Figure 2 with 50 and 250 samples. The estimation of the optimal shrinkage-like coefficient λ appears to be irrespective of the sample size.

$$m_{a\to b} \overset{\lambda=1/2}{=} \frac{\alpha_{a\to b}}{2} + \frac{\beta_{a\to b}}{2}. \quad (12)$$

These results suggest that, in general, a unique optimal value for the shrinkage-like coefficient can be determined, even in situations not captured by Theorem 3 and Corollary 1.

Performance of CAPRESE compared to *oncotrees*

An analogue of Theorem 3 holds for Despers's oncotrees (Theorem 3.3, [8]), and an analogue of Corollary 1 holds for Szabo's extension with uniform noise (Reconstruction Theorem 1, [22]). Thus, with infinite samples both approaches reconstruct the correct trees/forests. With finite samples and noise, however, their performance may show different patterns, as speed of convergence may vary. We investigate this issue in the current section.

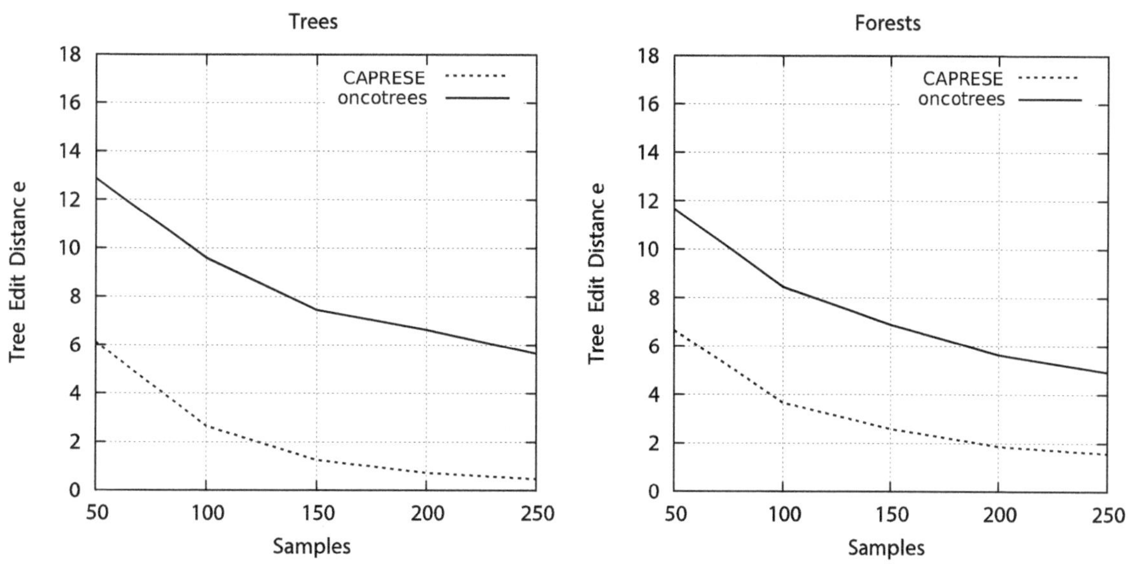

Figure 4. Comparison on noise-free synthetic data. Performance of CAPRESE (dashed line) and oncotrees (full line) in average TED when data are generated by random trees (left) and forests (right). In this case $v=0$ (no false positives/negatives) and $\lambda \to 0$ in the estimator m.

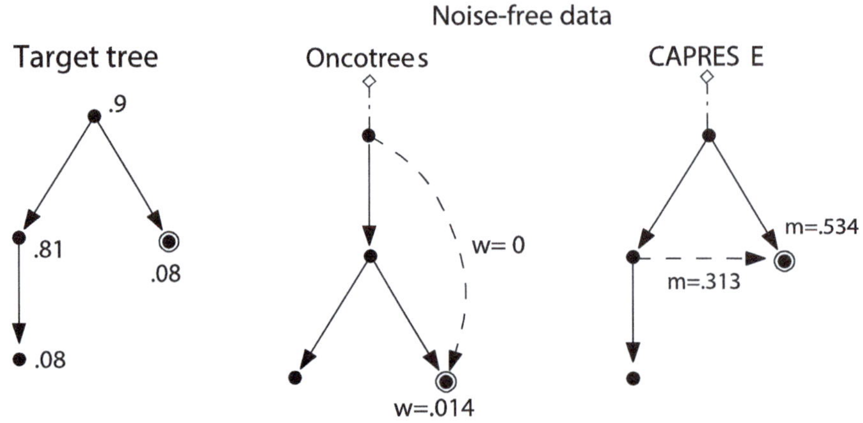

Figure 5. Example of reconstructed trees. Example of reconstruction from a dataset with 100 samples generated by the left tree (the theoretical probabilities are shown, i.e., the doubly-circled event appears in a sample with probability.08), with $\nu=0$. In the sampled dataset oncotrees mislead the cause of the doubly-circled mutation ($w=0$ for the true edge and $w=0.014$ for the wrong one). CAPRESE infers the correct cause (the values of the estimator m with $\lambda=1/2$ are shown, similar results are obtained for $\lambda \to 1$).

In Figure 4 we compare the performance of CAPRESE with oncotrees, for the case of noise-free synthetic data with the optimal shrinkage-like coefficient: $\lambda \to 0$, equation (11). Since Szabo's algorithm is equivalent to Desper's without false negatives and positives, we rely solely on Szabo's implementation [22]. In Figure 5 we show an example of reconstructed tree where CAPRESE infers the correct tree while oncotrees mislead a causation relation.

In general, one can observe that the TED of CAPRESE is, on average, always bounded above by the TED of oncotrees, both in the case of trees and forests. For trees, with 50 samples the average TED of CAPRESE is around 6, whereas for Desper's technique it is around 13. The performance of both algorithms improves as long as the number of samples is increased: CAPRESE has the best performance (i.e., TED ≈ 0) with 250 samples, while oncotrees have TED around 6. When forests are considered, the difference between the performance of the algorithms reduces slightly, but also in this case CAPRESE clearly outperforms oncotrees.

Notice that the improvement due to the increase in the sample size seems to reach a *plateau*, and the initial TED for our estimator seems rather close to the plateau value. This empirical analysis suggests that CAPRESE has already good performances with few samples, a favorable adjoint to Theorem 3. This result has some important practical implications, particularly considering the scarcity of available biological data.

In Figure 6 we extend the comparison to *noisy* datasets. In this case, we used the optimal shrinkage-like coefficient: $\lambda \to 1/2$, equation (12). The results confirm what observed without false positives and negatives, as CAPRESE outperforms oncotrees up to $\nu=0.15$, for all the sizes of the sample sets. In the File S1 we show similar plots for the noise-free case.

We can thus draw the conclusion that our algorithm performs better with finite samples and noise, since less samples are required

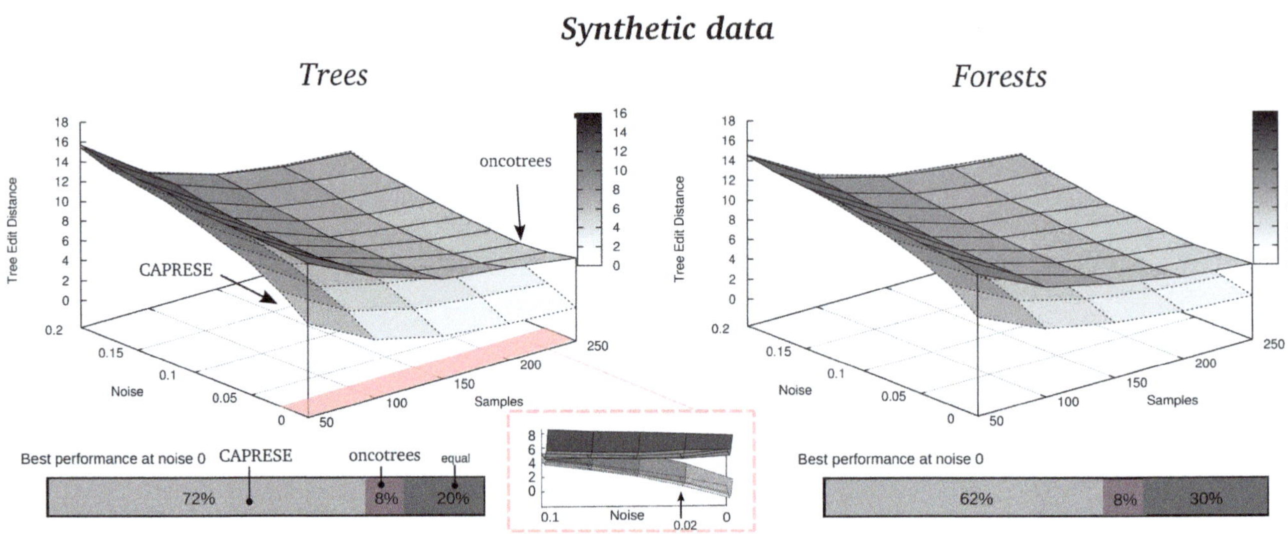

Figure 6. Reconstruction with noisy synthetic data and $\lambda=1/2$. Performance of CAPRESE and oncotrees as a function of the number of samples and noise ν. According to Figure 2 the shrinkage-like coefficient is set to $\lambda=1/2$. The magnified image shows the convergence to Desper's performance for $\nu \approx 0.1$. The barplot represents the percentage of times the best performance is achieved at $\nu=0$.

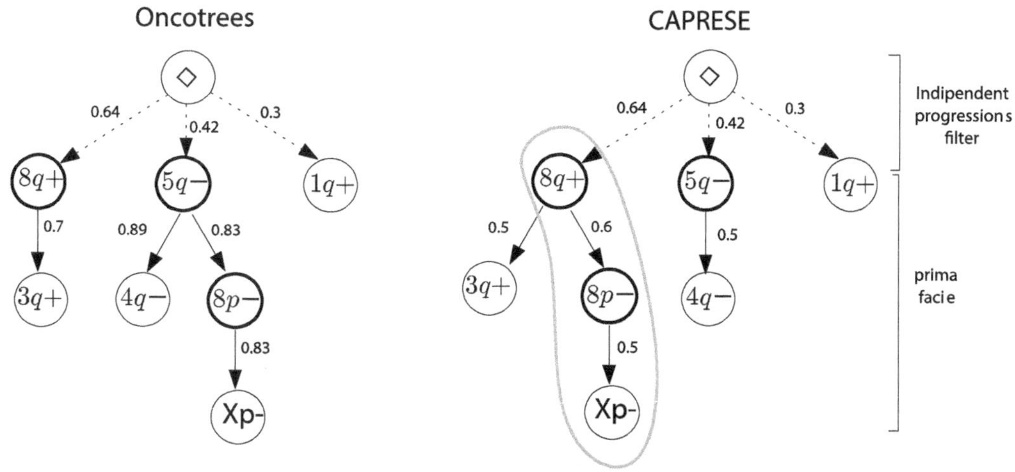

Figure 7. Reconstruction of ovarian cancer progression. Trees reconstructed by oncotrees and CAPRESE (with $\lambda \to 0$, with $\lambda = 1/2$ the same tree is reconstructed). The set of CGH events considered are gains on $8q$, $3q$ and $1q$ and losses on $5q$, $4q$, $8p$ and Xp. Events on chromosomes arms containing the key genes for ovarian cancer are in bolded circles. In the left tree all edge weights are the observed probabilities of events. In the right the full edges are the causation inferred with the PR and the weights represent the scores used by CAPRESE. Weights on dashed lines are as in the left tree.

to get good performances and a higher resistance to false positives and negatives is shown.

Performance of CAPRESE compared to *Conjunctive Bayesian Networks*

Inspired by Desper's seminal work, Beerenwinkel and others developed methods to estimate the constraints on the order in which mutations accumulate during cancer progression, using a probabilistic graphical model called *Conjuntive Bayesian Networks* (CBN) [14,15]. While the goal of this research was to reconstruct *direct acyclic graphs* and not trees per se, evidence presented in [24] suggests that, in the absence of noise, these models perform better than oncotrees even at reconstructing *trees*. For this reason, we performed experiments similar to the ones suggested above, comparing CAPRESE to the extension of CBN called *hidden-CBN* (h-CBN) that accounts for noisy genotype observations [15]. This method combines CBNs with a simulated annealing algorithm for structure search and a denoising of the genotypes via the maximum a posteriori estimates to compute the most likely progression. One aspect that complicates a comparison between CAPRESE and (h-)CBN is that the methods assume different models. For example, at the heart of CBN is a monotonicity assumption (i.e., an event can only occur if all its predecessors have occurred) not assumed by CAPRESE. Despite the differences between the model assumptions, we present a preliminary comparison between the methods in Appendix S3, indicating that we not only outperform oncotrees, but h-CBNs as well. In particular, this suggests that CAPRESE converges much faster than h-CBNs with respect to the sample size, also in the presence of noise.

We also analyze the rate of *false positives/negatives* reconstructed by CAPRESE when (synthetic) data are sampled from DAGs (Appendix S3). The rate of *false positives* goes to 0 as the sample size increases, implying that CAPRESE is capable of reconstructing a tree subsumed by the underlying causal DAG topology. In addition, the number of *false negatives* approaches a value proportional to the connectivity of the model from which the data was generated. This is expected, since CAPRESE will assign at most one cause to each considered event. However, it should be noted that further experiments with samples selected from a wider array of topologies should be performed to confirm these results and compare both methods in full. While not within the scope of the current paper, these issues will be addressed in future work.

Case studies

In the next subsections we apply CAPRESE to real cancer data obtained by *Comparative Genomic Hybridization* (CGH) and *Next Generation Sequencing* (NGS). This shows the potential application of reconstruction techniques to various types of mutational profiles and various cancers.

Performance on cancer CGH datasets

Encouraged by the results in previous sections, we test our reconstruction approach on a real *ovarian cancer* dataset made available within the oncotree package [8]. The data was collected through the public platform SKY/M-FISH [38], used to allow investigators to share molecular cytogenetic data. The data was obtained by using the CGH technique on samples from *papillary serous cystadenocarcinoma* of the ovary. This technique uses fluorescent staining to detect CNV data at the resolution of chromosome arms. While the recent emergence of NGS approaches make the dataset itself rather outdated, the underlying principles remain the same and the dataset provides a valid test-case for our approach. The seven most commonly occurring events are selected from the 87 samples, and the set of events are the following gains and losses on chromosomes arms $G = \{8q+, 3q+, 1q+, 5q-, 4q-, 8p-, Xp-\}$ (e.g., $4q-$ denotes a deletion of the q arm of the 4th chromosome).

In Figure 7 we compare the trees reconstructed by the two approaches. Our technique differs from Desper's by predicting the causal sequence of alterations

$$8q+ \rightarrow 8p- \rightarrow Xp-,$$

when used either $\lambda \to 0$ or $\lambda = 1/2$. Notice that among the samples in the dataset some are not generated by the distribution induced by the recovered tree, thus comparing the reconstruction for both λs is necessary.

Table 1. Estimated confidence for ovarian progression.

Oncotrees (overall confidence 8.3%)

→	$8q+$	$3q+$	$5q-$	$4q-$	$8p-$	$1q+$	$Xp-$
◆	**.99**	.06	**.51**	.22	.004	**.8**	.06
$8q+$	0	**.92**	.08	0.16	.04	.02	.007
$3q+$	.002	0	.04	0	0	.09	.04
$5q-$	.001	.002	0	**.52**	**.39**	.009	.16
$4q-$	0	0	.27	0	.14	.05	.11
$8p-$	0	0	.07	.08	0	.004	**.59**
$1q+$	0	0	0	.004	0	0	0
$Xp-$	0	0	.003	.003	.04	.01	0

CAPRESE (overall confidence 8.6%)

→	$8q+$	$3q+$	$5q-$	$4q-$	$8p-$	$1q+$	$Xp-$
◆	**.99**	.06	**.51**	.22	.004	**.8**	.06
$8q+$	0	**.92**	.06	.16	**.62**	.01	.008
$3q+$	.002	0	.03	.002	0	.09	.04
$5q-$	.001	.002	0	**.5**	.26	.009	.17
$4q-$	0	0	.29	0	.09	.05	.12
$8p-$	0	0	.07	.08	0	.004	**.59**
$1q+$	0	0	0	.004	0	0	0
$Xp-$	0	.001	.003	.004	.01	.01	0

Frequency of edge occurrences in the non-parametric bootstrap test, for the trees shown in Figure 7. Bold entries are the edges recovered by the algorithms.

At this point, we do not have a biological interpretation for this result. However, we do know that common cancer genes reside in these regions, e.g. the tumor suppressor gene PDGFR on $5q$ and the oncogene MYC on $8q$), and loss of heterozygosity on the short arm of chromosome 8 is quite common (see, e.g., http://www.genome.jp/kegg/). Recently, evidence has been reported that $8p$ contains many cooperating cancer genes [39].

In order to assign a confidence level to these inferences we applied both parametric and non-parametric *bootstrapping methods* to our results. Essentially, these tests consist of using the reconstructed trees (in the parametric case), or the probability observed in the dataset (in the non-parametric case) to generate new synthetic datasets, and then reconstructs again the progressions (see, e.g., [40] for an overview of these methods and [41] for the use of bootstrap for evalutating the confidence of oncogenetic

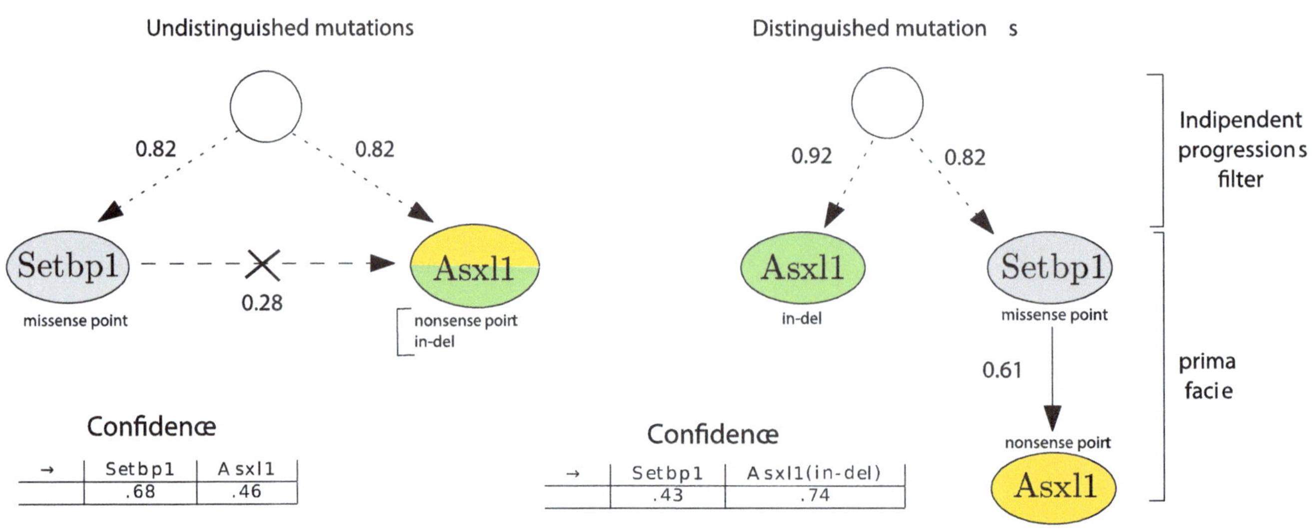

Figure 8. Validating the Setbp1 - ASXL1 relation in atypical Chronic Myeloid Leukemia. Progression models where ASXL1 indel and non-sense point are merged (left) and separate (right) suggest that a missense point mutation hitting SETBP1 can cause a non-sense point mutation in ASXL1, that the observed ASXL1 mutations might be independent and that indel ASXL1 is an early event with high confidence.

trees.). The confidence is given by the number of times the trees in Figure 7 are reconstructed from the generated data. A similar approach can be used to estimate the confidence of every edge separately. For oncotrees the *exact tree* is obtained 83 times out of 1000 non-parametric resamples, so its estimated confidence is 8.3%. For CAPRESE the confidence is 8.6%. In the parametric case with false positive and false negative error rates of 0.21 and 0.027, following [22], the confidence of oncotrees is 17% while the confidence of our method is much higher: 32%. When error rates are forced to 0 the confidence of oncotrees raises to 86.6% and 90.9% respectively.

For the non-parametric case, edges confidence is shown in Table 1. Most notably, our algorithm reconstructs the inference $8q+ \rightarrow 8p-$ with high confidence (confidence 62%, and 26% for $5q- \rightarrow 8p-$), while the confidence of the edge $8q+ \rightarrow 5q-$ is only 39%, almost the same as $8p- \rightarrow 8q+$ (confidence 40%). The confidences are similar with either $\lambda \rightarrow 0$ or $\lambda = 1/2$.

Analysis of other CGH datasets. We report the differences between the reconstructed trees also based on datasets of gastrointestinal and oral cancer ([35,37] respectively). In the case of gastrointestinal stromal cancer, among the 13 CGH events considered in [35] (gains on $5p$, $5q$ and $8q$, losses on $14q$, $1p$, $15q$, $13q$, $21q$, $22q$, $9p$, $9q$, $10q$ and $6q$), oncotrees identify the path progression

$$1p- \rightarrow 15q- \rightarrow 13q- \rightarrow 21q-$$

while CAPRESE reconstructs the branch

$$1p- \rightarrow 15q- 1p- \rightarrow 13q- \rightarrow 21q-.$$

In the case of oral cancer, among the 12 CGH events considered in [37] (gains on $8q$, $9q$, $11q$, $20q$, $17p$, $7p$, $5p$, $20p$ and $18p$, losses on $3p$, $8p$ and $18q$), the reconstructed trees differ since oncotrees identifies the path

$$8q+ \rightarrow 20q+ \rightarrow 20p+$$

while our algorithm reconstructs the path

$$3p- \rightarrow 7p+ \rightarrow 20q+ \rightarrow 20p+ .$$

These examples show that CAPRESE provides important differences in the reconstruction compared to oncotrees.

Performance on cancer NGS datasets

In this section we show the application of reconstruction techniques to the validation of a specific relation among recurrent mutations involved in *atypical Chronic Myeloid Leukemia* (ACML).

In [42] Piazza *et al.* used high-throughput *exome sequencing technology* to identity somatically acquired mutations in 64 ACML patients, and found a previously unidentified recurring *missense point mutation* hitting SETBP1. By re-sequencing SETBP1 in samples with ACML and other common human cancers, they found that around 25% of the ACML patients tested positive for SETBP1, while most of the other types of tumors were negative. Assessing the possible relationship between SETBP1 variants and the mutations in many driver ACML oncogenes such as (e.g., ASXL1, TET2, KRAS, etc.) no significant association or mutual exclusion with SETBP1 was found but for ASXL1, which was frequently mutated together with SETBP1, hinting at a potential relation among the events. In particular, ASXL1 was presenting either a *non-sense point* or a *indel* type of somatic mutation.

Hence, we reconstructed ACML progression models from the datasets provided in [42], with the goal of assessing a *potential causal dependency* between mutated SETBP1 and ASXL1. A more extensive analysis is postponed, as we only seek to clearly illustrate the functionalities of the algorithm here.

As a first case (Figure 8, left), we treated the ASXL1 missense point and indel mutations as indistinguishable, and we merged the two events in the dataset. Afterwards, we separated the two types of mutations for ASXL1 (Figure 8, right).

In particular, it is interesting to notice that, when the ASXL1 mutations are considered equivalent, the inference suggests that the mutations belong to two independent progression paths (i.e., the independent progression filters "breaks" every potential causal relation among the events). Conversely, when the mutations are kept separate, the progression model suggests that: (*i*) the missense point mutation hitting SETBP1 can cause a non-sense point mutation in ASXL1 and (*ii*) the observed ASXL1 mutations seems to be independent. Concerning edges confidence, as before assessed via non-parametric bootstrap, it is worth noting that the confidence in the indel ASXL1 mutation being an early event raises consistently in the latter case.

All in all, it seems that a progression model allows to test the significance of the association firstly observed in [42] and also refines the knowledge by suggesting a specific causal and temporal relations among events. With this this in mind, ad-hoc sequencing experiments might be set up to assess these predictions, eventually providing a strong evidence that could be used to, e.g., synthesize a progression-specific ACML-effective drug.

Discussion

In this work we have introduced a novel framework for the reconstruction of the causal topologies underlying cumulative progressive phenomena, based on the *probability raising* notion of causation. Besides such a probabilistic notion, we also introduced the use of a *shrinkage-like estimator* to efficiently unravel ambiguous causal relations, often present when data are noisy. As a first step towards the definition of our new framework, we have here presented an effective novel technique called CAPRESE (CAncer PRogression Extraction with Single Edges) for the reconstruction of tree or, more generally, forest models of progression which combines probabilistic causation and a shrinkage-like estimation.

We prove correctness of CAPRESE by showing asymptotic convergence to the correct tree. Under mild constraints on the noise rates, this result holds for the reconstruction problem in the presence of uniform noise as well. Moreover, we also compare our technique to the standard tree reconstruction algorithm based on correlation (i.e., Oncontrees) and to a more general bayesian probabilistic graphical model (i.e., Conjunctive Bayesian Networks), and show that CAPRESE outperforms the state-of-the-art on synthetic data, also exhibiting a noteworthy efficiency with relatively small datasets. Furthermore, we tested our technique on ovarian, gastrointestinal and oral cancer CGH data and NGS leukemia data. The CGH analysis suggested that our approach can infer, with high confidence, novel causal relationships which would remain unpredictable in a correlation-based attack. The NGS analysis allowed validating a causal and temporal relation among key mutations in atypical chronic myeloid leukemia.

One of the strong points of CAPRESE is that it can be applied to genomic data of any kind, even heterogeneous, and at any resolution, as shown. In fact, it simply requires a set of samples in which the presence or the absence of some alterations supposed to be involved in a causal cumulative process have been assessed. Notice also that the results of our technique can be used not only to describe the *progression* of the process, but also to *classify* different progression types. In the case of cancer, for instance, this genome-level classifier could be used to group patients according to the position of the detected individual genomic alterations in the progression model (e.g., at a specific point of the tree) and, consequently, to set up a genome-specific *therapy design* aimed, for instance, at blocking or slowing certain progression paths instead of others, as was studied in [43].

Several future research directions are possible. First, more complex models of progression, e.g. directed acyclic graphs, could be inferred with probability raising and compared to the standard approaches of [14,15,44], as we explained in the introduction. These models, rather than trees, could explain the common phenomenon of *preferential progression paths* in the target process via, e.g., *confluence* among events. In the case of cancer, for instance, these models would be certainly more suitable than trees to describe the accumulation of mutations.

Second, the shrinkage-like estimator itself could be improved by introducing, for instance, different correction factors. In addition, an analytical formulation of the optimal shrinkage-like coefficient could be investigated by starting from the hypotheses which apply to our problem setting, along the lines of [45].

Third, advanced statistical techniques such as *bootstrapping* [40] could be used to account for more sophisticated models of noise within data, so as to decipher complex causal dependencies.

Finally, a further development of the framework could involve the introduction of *timed data*, in order to extend our techniques to settings where a temporal information on the samples is available.

Software availability

The implementation of CAPRESE is part of the TRanslational ONCOlogy (TRONCO) R package and is available for download at standard R repositories.

Acknowledgments

We are grateful for the many excellent comments we received from anonymous reviewers.

Author Contributions

Conceived and designed the experiments: LO GC AG DR GM MA BM. Performed the experiments: LO GC AG DR. Analyzed the data: LO GC AG DR. Wrote the paper: LO GC AG DR MA BM GM. Software implementation: DR.

References

1. Hanahan D, Weinberg RA (2011) Hallmarks of cancer: The next generation. Cell 144: 646–674.
2. Luo J, Solimini NL, Elledge SJ (2009) Principles of cancer therapy: Oncogene and non-oncogene addiction. Cell 136: 823–837.
3. Vogelstein B, Kinzler K (2004) Cancer genes and the pathways they control. Nature medicine 10: 789–799.
4. Frank SA (2007) Dynamics of Cancer. Princeton University Press.
5. Bell D, Berchuck A, Birrer M, Chien J, Cramer D, et al. (2011) Integrated genomic analyses of ovarian carcinoma. Nature.
6. Imielinski M, et al. (2012) Mapping the hallmarks of lung adenocarcinoma with massively parallel sequencing. Cell 150: 1107–1120.
7. Vogelstein B, Fearon ER, Hamilton SR, Kern SE, Preisinger AC, et al. (1988) Genetic alterations during colorectal-tumor development. New England Journal of Medicine 319: 525–532.
8. Desper R, Jiang F, Kallioniemi O, Moch H, Papadimitriou C, et al. (1999) Inferring tree models for oncogenesis from comparative genome hybridization data. Journal of Computational Biology 6: 37–51.
9. Desper R, Jiang F, Kallioniemi O, Moch H, Papadimitriou C, et al. (2000) Distance-based reconstruction of tree models for oncogenesis. Journal of Computational Biology 7: 789–803.
10. von Heydebreck A, Gunawan B, Füzesi L (2004) Maximum likelihood estimation of oncogenetic tree models. Biostatistics 5: 545–56.
11. Beerenwinkel N, Rahnenführer J, Däumer M, Hoffmann D, Kaiser R, et al. (2005) Learning multiple evolutionary pathways from cross-sectional data. Journal of Computational Biology 12: 584–598.
12. Beerenwinkel N, Rahnenführer J, Kaiser R, Hoffmann D, Selbig J, et al. (2005) Mtreemix: a software package for learning and using mixture models of mutagenetic trees. Bioinformatics 21: 2106–2107.
13. Hjelm M, Höglund M, Lagergren J (2006) New probabilistic network models and algorithms for oncogenesis. Journal of Computational Biology 13: 853–865.
14. Beerenwinkel N, Eriksson N, Sturmfels B (2007) Conjunctive bayesian networks. Bernoulli: 893–909.
15. Gerstung M, Baudis M, Moch H, Beerenwinkel N (2009) Quantifying cancer progression with conjunctive bayesian networks. Bioinformatics 25: 2809–2815.
16. Gupta A, Bar-Joseph Z (2008) Extracting dynamics from static cancer expression data. IEEE/ACM Transactions on Computational Biology and Bioinformatics 5: 172–182.
17. Ramakrishnan N, Tadepalli S, Watson LT, Helm RF, Antoniotti M, et al. (2010) Reverse engineering dynamic temporal models of biological processes and their relationships. PNAS 107: 12511–12516.
18. Suppes P (1970) A probabilistic theory of causality. North Holland Publishing Company.
19. Hitchcock C (2012) Probabilistic causation. In: Zalta E, editor, The Stanford Encyclopedia of Philosophy. Winter 2012 edition.
20. Ionita I, Daruwala R, Mishra B (2006) Mapping Tumor-Suppressor genes with multipoint statistics from Copy-Number–Variation data. American Journal of Human Genetics 79: 13–22.
21. Kleinberg S (2012) Causality, Probability, and Time. Cambridge University Press.
22. Szabo A, Boucher K (2002) Estimating an oncogenetic tree when false negatives and positives are present. Mathematical biosciences 176: 219–236.
23. Efron B (2013) Large-Scale Inference: Empirical Bayes Methods for Estimation, Testing, and Prediction. Cambridge University Press.
24. Hainke K, Rahnenführer J, Fried R (2012) Cumulative disease progression models for cross-sectional data: A review and comparison. Biometrical Journal 54: 617–640.
25. Reichenbach H (1956) The Direction of Time. University of California Press.
26. Edmonds J (1967) Optimum branchings. Journal of Research of the National Bureau of Standards B 71: 233–240.
27. Kainu T, et al. (2000) Somatic deletions in hereditary breast cancers implicate 13q21 as a putative novel breast cancer susceptibility locus. Proceedings of the National Academy of Sciences 97: 9603–9608.
28. Huang Q, Yu G, McCormick S, Mo J, Datta B, et al. (2002) Genetic differences detected by comparative genomic hybridization in head and neck squamous cell carcinomas from different tumor sites: construction of oncogenetic trees for tumor progression. Genes, Chromosomes and Cancer 34: 224–233.
29. Radmacher M, Simon R, Desper R, Taetle R, Schäffer A, et al. (2001) Graph models of oncogenesis with an application to melanoma. Journal of theoretical biology 212: 535–548.
30. Cartwright N (1979) Causal laws and effective strategies. Noûs 13: 419–437.
31. Pearl J (2000) Causality: Models, Reasoning, and Inference. Cambridge University Press.
32. Zhang K, Shasha D (1989) Simple fast algorithms for the editing distance between trees and related problems. SIAM journal on computing 18: 1245–1262.
33. Hamming RW (1950) Error-detecting and error-correcting codes. Bell System Technical Journal 29: 147–160.
34. Samuelson E, Karlsson S, Partheen K, Nilsson S, Szpirer C, et al. (2012) Bac cgh-array identified specific small-scale genomic imbalances in diploid dmba-induced rat mammary tumors. BMC cancer 12: 352.
35. Gunawan B, et al. (2007) An oncogenetic tree model in gastrointestinal stromal tumours (gists) identifies different pathways of cytogenetic evolution with prognostic implications. The Journal of pathology 211: 463–470.
36. Longerich T, Mueller M, Breuhahn K, Schirmacher P, Benner A, et al. (2012) Oncogenetic tree modeling of human hepatocarcinogenesis. International Journal of Cancer 130: 575–583.
37. Pathare S, Schäffer A, Beerenwinkel N, Mahimkar M (2009) Construction of oncogenetic tree models reveals multiple pathways of oral cancer progression. International journal of cancer 124: 2864–2871.

38. Knutsen T, Gobu V, Knaus R, Padilla-Nash H, Augustus M, et al. (2005) The interactive online sky/m-fish & cgh database and the entrez cancer chromosomes search database: Linkage of chromosomal aberrations with the genome sequence. Genes, Chromosomes and Cancer 44: 52–64.
39. Xue W, et al. (2012) A cluster of cooperating tumor-suppressor gene candidates in chromosomal deletions. Proceedings of the National Academy of Sciences 109: 8212–8217.
40. Efron B (1982) The jackknife, the bootstrap and other resampling plans, volume 38. SIAM.
41. Szabo A, Boucher KM (2008) Oncogenetic trees. Handbook of Cancer Models with Applications to Cancer Screening, Cancer Treatment and Risk Assessment World Scientific.
42. Piazza R, Valletta S, Winkelmann N, Redaelli S, Spinelli R, et al. (2013) Recurrent setbp1 mutations in atypical chronic myeloid leukemia. Nature Genetics 45: 18–24.
43. Olde Loohuis L, Witzel A, Mishra B (2014) Cancer hybrid automata: Model, beliefs & therapy. Information and Computation 236: 68–86.
44. Gerstung M, Eriksson N, Lin J, Vogelstein B, Beerenwinkel N (2011) The temporal order of genetic and pathway alterations in tumorigenesis. PloS one 6: e27136.
45. Efron B, Morris C (1973) Stein's estimation rule and its competitors–an empirical bayes approach. Journal of the American Statistical Association 68: 117–130.

Withaferin A Alone and in Combination with Cisplatin Suppresses Growth and Metastasis of Ovarian Cancer by Targeting Putative Cancer Stem Cells

Sham S. Kakar[1,2*], Mariusz Z. Ratajczak[2,3], Karen S. Powell[4], Mana Moghadamfalahi[5], Donald M. Miller[2,3], Surinder K. Batra[6], Sanjay K. Singh[1,2]

1 Department of Physiology and Biophysics, University of Louisville, Louisville, Kentucky, United States of America, 2 James Graham Brown Cancer Center, University of Louisville, Louisville, Kentucky, United States of America, 3 Department of Medicine, University of Louisville, Louisville, Kentucky, United States of America, 4 Research Resources Center, University of Louisville, Louisville, Kentucky, United States of America, 5 Department of Pathology, University of Louisville, Louisville, Kentucky, United States of America, 6 Department of Biochemistry and Molecular Biology, Eppley Institute for Research in Cancer and Allied Diseases, University of Nebraska Medical Center, Omaha, Nebraska, United States of America

Abstract

Currently, the treatment for ovarian cancer entails cytoreductive surgery followed by chemotherapy, mainly, carboplatin combined with paclitaxel. Although this regimen is initially effective in a high percentage of cases, unfortunately within few months of initial treatment, tumor relapse occurs because of platinum-resistance. This is attributed to chemo-resistance of cancer stem cells (CSCs). Herein we show for the first time that withaferin A (WFA), a bioactive compound isolated from the plant Withania somnifera, when used alone or in combination with cisplatin (CIS) targets putative CSCs. Treatment of nude mice bearing orthotopic ovarian tumors generated by injecting human ovarian epithelial cancer cell line (A2780) with WFA and cisplatin (WFA) alone or in combination resulted in a 70 to 80% reduction in tumor growth and complete inhibition of metastasis to other organs compared to untreated controls. Histochemical and Western blot analysis of the tumors revealed that inclusion of WFA (2 mg/kg) resulted in a highly significant elimination of cells expressing CSC markers - CD44, CD24, CD34, CD117 and Oct4 and downregulation of Notch1, Hes1 and Hey1 genes. In contrast treatment of mice with CIS alone (6 mg/kg) had opposite effect on those cells. Increase in cells expressing CSC markers and Notch1 signaling pathway in tumors exposed to CIS may explain recurrence of cancer in patients treated with carboplatin and paclitaxel. Since, WFA alone or in combination with CIS eliminates putative CSCs, we conclude that WFA in combination with CIS may present more efficacious therapy for ovarian cancer.

Editor: Deodutta Roy, Florida International University, United States of America

Funding: NIH/NCI CA124630, James Graham Brown Cancer Center Research Funds, School of Medicine Basic Research program Research Grant. The funders had no role in study design, data collection and analysis, decision to publish, or preparation of the manuscript.

Competing Interests: Co-author Surinder Batra is a PLOS ONE Editorial Board member. This does not alter the authors' adherence to all the PLOS ONE policies on sharing data and materials.

* Email: sskaka01@louisville.edu

Introduction

Epithelial ovarian cancer (EOC) remains the leading cause of death in women among gynecologic cancers and is the 5th highest cause of cancer-related deaths in women in the United States [1,2]. The majority of ovarian cancers are diagnosed at advanced stage due to the mainly non-specific symptoms. Currently, the treatment for ovarian cancer entails cytoreductive surgery followed by chemotherapy, employing mainly platinum/taxane combination [3]. Although this regimen is initially effective in a high percentage of cases (70 to 80%), unfortunately 70% of women develop recurrent cancer within few months of initial treatment as a result of platinum-resistance [4,5]. In addition, cisplatin (CIS) is associated with multiple severe side effects such as nausea, vomiting, myelosuppression, hepatotoxicity, neurotoxicity, nephrotoxicity and ototoxicity [4,6–9]. Therefore, need for new treatment options that target cancer cells and in particular putative cancer stem cells is mandatory either at first-line setting or even more at the first- and second-line management of recurrent ovarian cancer.

In our previous studies [10], we showed for a first time that withaferin A (WFA), a bioactive compound isolated from the plant Withania somnifera, when used alone or in combination with CIS had a time- and dose-dependent synergistic effect on inhibition of cell proliferation and induction of cell death, thus reducing required dosage of cisplatin. We also showed that while WFA achieves its antitumor effect through generation of ROS leading to DNA damage, CIS achieves its effects though direct binding to DNA causing the formation of DNA adducts. Combination treatment also resulted in a significant enhancement of reactive oxygen species (ROS) production and DNA damage.

WFA has been a part of Indian traditional medicine for centuries. It is available in US over-the-counter as a dietary supplement and is known to treat various disorders due to its anti-inflammatory [11,12], anti-bacterial [13], and cardio protective properties [14]. In recent years, WFA has been suggested as a potential anti-cancer compound shown to prevent tumor growth, angiogenesis, and metastasis [15,16] in various types of cancer [17–26]. Mechanisms by which WFA attains its anticancer activity include inactivation of Akt and NF-κB [27] to achieve apoptosis, decrease in pro-survival protein Bcl-2 [28], G2/M cell cycle arrest [29,30], generation of reactive oxygen species (ROS) [31,32], induction of Par-4 [17], activation of caspase 3 and 9 activities, DNA damage [10], inhibition of HSP90 [20], regulation of FOXO3a and Bim [15] inhibition of Notch-1 [33] and down regulation of expression of HPV E6 and E7 oncoproteins [19].

Development of drug resistance and recurrence of ovarian cancer has been a major clinical problem. A number of mechanisms that induce drug resistance have been proposed. Over the last several years, there has been increasing evidence that "cancer stem cells (CSCs)", are the most important trigger of tumor progression, chemo-resistance and relapse after initial treatment [34,35]. First evidence for the existence of cancer stem cells came in the year 1997, with the identification of leukemia stem cells [36,37]. In the year 2003, Al-Hajj et al. [38] experimentally demonstrated the hierarchical stem cell origin in breast cancer. However, until recently the existence of putative cancer stem cells within solid tumors had remained controversial [39]. In recent studies using murine models for brain, skin and intestinal tumors, three independent groups have provided convincing evidence for the existence of CSCs in tumors and their role in tumor expansion [40–42]. Accordingly, CSCs within tumor mass undergo self-renewal and give rise to heterogeneous cancer lineages that comprise tumor tissue. CSCs purified accordingly to some surface markers are able to form tumors when injected into nude mice [36,43,44]. Since, ovarian cancer is very heterogeneous; different cell surface markers have been reported for putative ovarian CSCs. Most commonly reported include CD24, CD34, CD44, CD133, CD117, ALDH1, Oct4, MyD88 and EpCAM [45–53]. Since, CSCs are considered to be major players responsible for developing drug resistance and hence leading to cancer recurrence [52,53], targeting CSCs and inhibiting their self-renewal will lead to reduction of cancer growth [33].

In our current study, we show for the first time that WFA alone or in combination with CIS if employed to treat mice bearing human orthotopic ovarian tumors not only suppresses tumor growth but targets cells expressing CSC markers as well as inhibits Notch1 and its downstream signaling genes (Hes1 and Hey1) that have been reported to play a crucial role in self-renewal and maintenance of CSCs (33).

Material and Methods

Cell line and cell culture

Ovarian epithelial cancer cell line A2780 was initially obtained from Denise Connolly (Fox Chase Cancer Center) and was maintained in RPMI 1640 medium containing insulin and supplemented with penicillin/streptomycin (100 IU/ml and 100 μg/ml) and 10% fetal bovine serum (FCS) (Hyclone, Atlanta, GA) as described previously [10].

Cell migration Boyden chamber assays

Cell migration in vitro was assayed by determining the ability of cells to migrate through a synthetic basement membrane. The procedure used was as described previously [54]. Briefly, polycarbonate filters (8 μM) were placed in modified Boyden chamber. A2780 cells in log phase were trypsinized and plated in 6 wells plates. After 24 h of plating, cells were treated with WFA and CIS both alone and in combination as described previously [10]. After 24 h of treatment, cells were trypsinized and suspended in serum free medium. A total of 2×10^5 cells were transferred to the top chamber. The medium containing 5% FBS was added to the lower chamber. The cells were incubated at 37°C for 24 h and allowed to migrate through the membrane. Non-migrated cells were removed with a clean cotton swab. Migrated cells on other side of the membrane were stained with crystal violet and counted in three different fields under Olympus microscope. The experiments were repeated for three times. The values represented are the mean ± SEM of three independent experiments.

Generation of orthotopic ovarian tumors in nude mice and treatment with WFA and CIS both alone and in combination

Orthotopic ovarian tumors were generated by injecting ovarian cancer cell line A2780 directly into ovary as described by Nunez Cruz et al. [55]. Briefly, A2780 (1×10^6) cells were directly injected into left ovary of 5 to 6 weeks old nu/nu female mice (Jackson Laboratory) under aseptic conditions and under light anesthesia. After 10 days of post-cell injection, mice were treated with 1) vehicle control (10% DMSO and 90% glyceryl trioctanoate), 2) WFA 2 mg/kg, 3), CIS 6 mg/kg, and 4) WFA 2 mg/kg plus CIS 6 mg/kg. Five animals randomly were included in each group. CIS in saline was injected i.p. once a week, whereas WFA was injected i.p. every other day. After 4 weeks of treatment, animals were sacrificed; tumor and other tissues such as un-injected ovary, lung, kidney, liver, adrenal and heart were collected from each mouse. Tumors were weighted at the time of collection. The tumors and other tissues were divided into two parts, one part was snap frozen, and second part was fixed in 10% buffered formalin. The animals' experiments were approved by the University of Louisville, Institutional Animal Care and Use Committee (IACUC) (protocol # 12063).

Formalin fixed tumor and tissues were processed and embedded in paraffin using standard protocols as described previously [56]. Five μM thick sections of the embedded tumors and tissues were prepared and stained with Hematoxylin and Eosin (H&E). Sections in triplicates were examined under microscope and photographed. Histopatholoigcal analysis of sections was performed by a trained pathologist Dr. Mana Moghadamfalahi.

Immunohistochemistry

Formalin fixed paraffin embedded tissues were deparaffinized in xylene and rehydrated in a decreasing graded series of ethanol as described previously [56]. Sections were heated at 95°C in 10 mM sodium citrate (pH 6.0) for 20 min, cooled to room temperature and then rinsed in PBS. Sections were incubated with 0.3% hydrogen peroxide in methanol for 10 min at room temperature to quench endogenous peroxidase followed by two rinses in PBS (5 min each), and were blocked with normal goat serum using reagents from ABC kit from Vector Laboratories for 60 min at room temperature following the instructions from the supplier. The blocking solution was removed by draining and sections were incubated with specific antibody with appropriate dilution according to instructions from the suppliers at 4°C for overnight in a humidified chamber. The antibodies for CD24 (cat # SAB14202713), CD44 (cat # SAB1405590), CD117 (cat # SAB4300489) and Oct4 (cat # P0873) were obtained from Sigma-Aldrich, and antibody for CD34 (cat # sc-19587) was obtained from Santa Cruz Biotechnology. After rinsing the sections three times (5 min each) with PBS, sections were incubated with biotinylated anti-rabbit (for polyclonal antibodies) or anti-mouse (for monoclonal antibodies) from the ABC kits (Vector Laboratories) at room temperature for 45 min followed by incubation with streptavidin. After three rinses (5 min each) with PBS, sections were incubated with 3,3′-diaminobenzidine (DAB, Sigma) to develop color. The sections were examined under Nikon Elipse E400 microscope and photographed.

Protein isolation and western blot analysis

A2780 cells were plated into 6 well plates. After 24 h of plating, cells were treated with WFA and CIS both alone and in combination as described previously (10). After 48 h of treatment, cells were lysed in chilled lysis buffer [50 mM Tris-HCl (pH 7.5), 150 mM NaCl, 0.1% NP-40, 1 mM Na_3VO_4, and 1 mM NaF) supplemented with Complete Mini Protease Inhibitor tablet (Roche Molecular Biochemicals, Indianapolis, IN). To prepare extract from normal and tumor tissues, tissues were suspended in lysis buffer and homogenized on ice using Polytron homogenizer followed by centrifugation at 10,000 rpm for 5 min. The supernatants were collected and protein concentration in each sample was determined using Bradford method (BioRad Laboratories) according to supplier's instructions. Forty μg of protein from each sample was fractionated on SDS-polyacrylamide gels and transferred to nitrocellulose membranes as described previously [56]. Blocking of nonspecific proteins was performed by incubation of the membranes with 5% nonfat dry milk in Tris buffered saline Tween-20 (TBST) for 1 h at room temperature. The membranes were incubated with specific antibody with appropriate dilution as suggested by the suppliers. Antibody for Notch 1 (cat # N6786), Hey1 (cat # SAB1404975) and β-actin (cat # A3854) were obtained from Sigma-Aldrich, and antibody for Hes1 (cat # sc-165996) was obtained from Santa Cruz Biotechnology. The membranes were washed three times (5 min each) with TBST, followed by incubation with horseradish peroxidase conjugated secondary antibody (1:5,000 dilution) in TBST. The membranes were rinsed three times (5 min each) with TBST and the immuno-reactive bands were visualized by enhanced chemiluminescence. Membranes were stripped off for 10 min with methanol containing 3% H_2O_2 and probed with β-actin antibody in order to serve as an internal control.

Statistical analysis

Statistical comparison of data was carried out by the student's t test (for single comparison). Probability of $p<0.05$ determined from the two-sided test was considered significant. The statistical analysis was carried out by using SPSS 10.0 software.

Results

WFA/CIS combination inhibits cell migration in vitro

Various steps are involved in tumor progression and metastasis including detachment of tumor cells from the primary tumor site, transmigration into lymph- or blood vessels, attachment to endothelium at distant sites of metastasis followed by seeding into new location and subsequent expansion. To examine the effect of WFA and CIS on A2780 cell migration, we treated the A2780 cells with WFA and CIS both alone and in combination for 48 h. As shown in Fig. 1, by employing Boyden chambers we noticed that the treatment of cells with WFA or CIS alone inhibited cell migration in a dose-dependent manner as compared to untreated control cells. While treatment of cells with 20 μM CIS inhibited cell migration, addition of WFA (0.5 μM or 1.5 μM) to CIS resulted in enhanced inhibition of cell migration, suggesting that

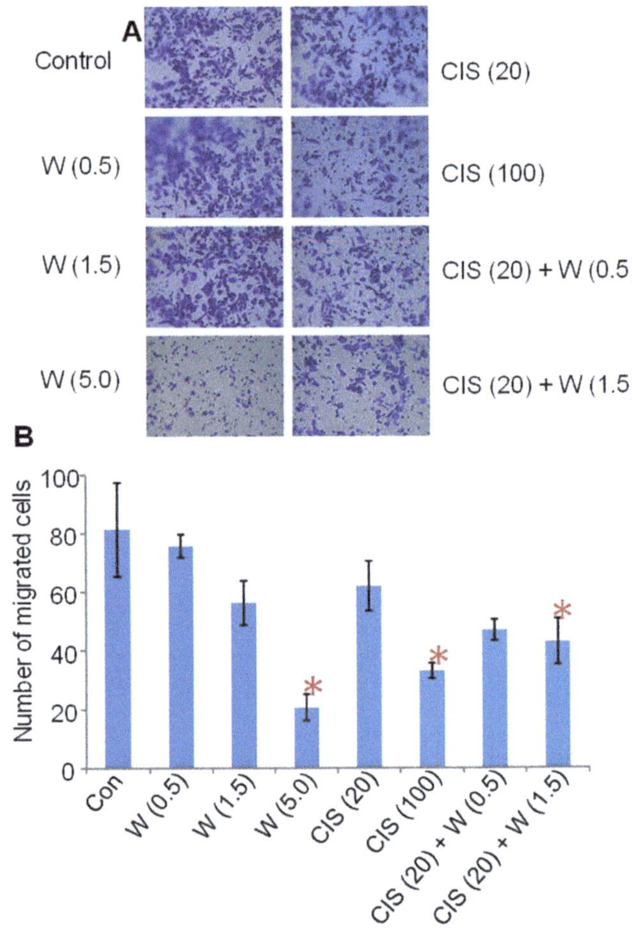

Figure 1. Effect of WFA and CIS both alone and in combination on cell migration. A2780 cells were treated with different concentration of WFA and CIS both alone and in combination for 48 h. The cells were trypsinized and subjected for cell migration using Boyden chamber. Cells were stained with crystal violet and photographed (A). The stained cells were counted under microscope using three different areas; values shown are mean ± SD of three independent experiments. * Represents significant compared to control at $p \leq 0.05$ (B). Con = control, W = WFA. Values shown in parenthesis are μM.

WFA combined with CIS is more effective than each agent employed.

WFA/CIS combination suppresses tumor growth and metastasis in nude mice

In our *in vitro* studies, we showed that treatment of CIS-sensitive cell lines (A2780 and CaOV3) as well as CIS-resistance cell line (A2780/CP70) with WFA and CIS both alone and in combination inhibited cell proliferation in a time- and dose-dependent manner and induced cell apoptosis and DNA damage. Moreover, the combined effect of WFA and CIS was synergistic [10]. To assess the efficacy of WFA/CIS combination on tumor growth and metastasis in vivo, we tested the effect of WFA and CIS both alone and in combination on tumor growth and metastasis in nude mice bearing inoculated orthotopic human ovarian tumors. Murine orthotopic tumors were established by injecting A2780 cells directly into left ovary of 5 to 6 week old nu/nu female mice. Beginning from day 10 after inoculation of tumor cells, animals were treated with WFA and CIS both alone and in combination as detailed in Materials and Methods section. After 4 weeks of treatment, animals were sacrificed. We noticed that the control mock-treated animals developed highly vascularized and large tumors (Fig. 2). At the same time 4 out of 5 WFA (2 mg/kg) alone-treated animals developed tumors that were significantly smaller in size. Similarly, 3 out of 5 animals treated with CIS (6 mg/kg) developed tumors that were significantly smaller in size as compared to mock-treated controls. Moreover, treatment of animals with WFA (2 mg/kg) in combination with CIS (6 mg/kg) resulted in 70 to 80% reduction in tumor weight compared to untreated control animals (Fig. 2) and out of 5 mice, only three mice developed tumors. No significant differences in tumor weight were observed in mice treated with WFA and CIS alone or in combination (Fig 2).

H&E histo-pathological analysis of un-injected opposite ovaries, livers, and lungs showed metastasis to livers and ovaries in mock-treated animals only. Metastatic cells comprised ~10% of cells in those organs (Fig. 3). In contrast no metastases were observed in WFA and CIS treated groups. These results suggest that combination of low dose of WFA (2 mg/kg) with suboptimal dose of CIS (6 mg/kg) is highly effective in suppressing tumor growth and metastasis of orthotopic ovarian tumors in nude mice. This indicates that it would be possible to reduce therapeutic dose of CIS when combined with WFA in humans to ameliorate side effects associated with high dosage of CIS.

WFA alone or in combination with CIS eliminates putative cancer stem cells in orthotopic ovarian tumors

Chemo-resistance and recurrence of ovarian cancer is a major problem and cause of death. In recent years, a concept of CSCs in solid cancers including ovarian cancers has been proposed [57,58]. CSCs have been reported to be responsible for chemo-resistance, tumor growth and recurrence of cancer after treatment. Putative CSCs have been reported as cancer initiating cells capable to develop tumors when injected into nude mice [57]. To test if WFA when used alone or in combination with CIS targets CSCs, we performed immunohistochemical analysis of the tumors collected from the mock-treated animals and animals treated with WFA and CIS both alone and in combination using the antibodies for markers expressed by putative CSCs including CD44, CD24, CD34, CD117 and Oct4 [56]. As shown in Figs. 4–6, we observed ~10–20% of cells positive for CD44, CD24, CD34, CD117 and Oct4 in tumors collected from untreated animals. However, treatment of animals with WFA (2 mg/kg) resulted in a highly significant reduction in number of those cells. In contrast, treatment of animals with CIS alone at a dose of 6 mg/kg resulted in significant increase in CD44, CD24, CD34, CD117 and Oct 4 positive cells (60%) (Figs. 4–6). More importantly, treatment of animals with WFA in combination with CIS (6 mg/kg) significantly reduced number of cells expressing CSC markers.

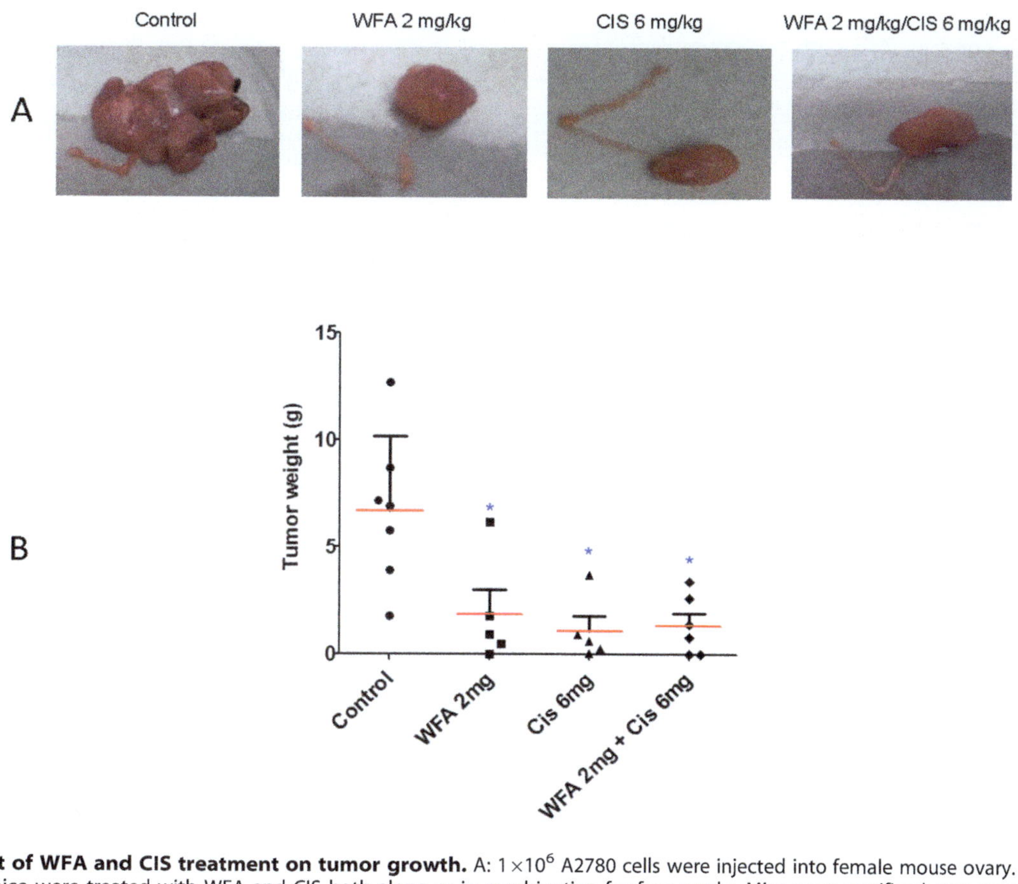

Figure 2. Effect of WFA and CIS treatment on tumor growth. A: 1×10^{6} A2780 cells were injected into female mouse ovary. After 10 days of post-injection, mice were treated with WFA and CIS both alone or in combination for four weeks. Mice were sacrificed; tumors were excised out, photographed and weighted. Tumors shown are representative from each group. B: Tumors weight was plotted from each group. Horizontal line represents median weight of each group. Treated group showed significantly lower weight than untreated mice. Results are mean (red line) and $\pm$ SD (vertical bar). * Represents significant compared to control at $p\leq0.05$.

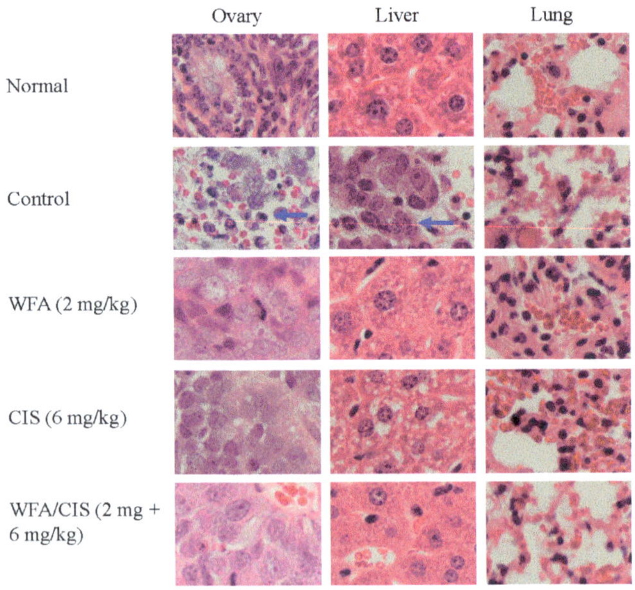

Figure 3. Effect of WFA and CIS both alone and in combination on tumor metastasis. Mice were treated with WFA and CIS as indicated in Figure 2. Tumors and other tissues sections were stained with H&E and examined by a trained pathologist. Metastasis (shown by arrows) was observed in un-injected ovaries and livers and represent approximate 10% of the cells.

WFA alone or in combination with CIS down regulates the expression of CSC-related markers

To confirm our immuno-histochemical analysis of CD44, CD24, CD34, CD117 and Oct4 positive cells in orthotopic tumors, we performed Western blot analysis of the tumor extracts using specific antibody for markers detected by immuno-histochemical staining. As shown in Fig. 7, expression of CD24, CD34, CD44, and Oct4 antigens was significantly down-regulated in tumors collected from animals treated with WFA alone as compared to tumors from mock-treated animals. In contrast a significant increase in expression of CD24, CD34, CD44 and Oct4 was observed in tumor extracts from animals treated with CIS (6 mg/kg) as compared to mock-treated mice or mice treated with WFA (2 mg/kg) alone. Interestingly, treatment of animals with WFA (2 mg/kg) in combination with CIS (6 mg/kg) resulted in a significant elimination of cells expressing CD44, CD24, CD34 and Oct4 antigens.

Increase in number of cells expressing markers of putative CSCs in tumors collected from animals treated with CIS as analyzed by immuno-staining as well as Western blot analysis suggests that treatment by CIS may increase number of cells expressing these markers and may explain development of chemo-resistance and reoccurrence of ovarian cancer in patients treated with CIS or its derivative such as carboplatin in combination with paclitaxel that are commonly used in chemotherapy. In contrast elimination of cells expressing CSC markers in tumors on treatment with WFA alone or in combination with CIS (6 mg/kg) demonstrates that WFA is highly effective in eliminating cells expressing CSC markers.

WFA alone or in combination with CIS inhibits Notch 1 and its downstream signaling genes (Hes1 and Hey1)

Self-renewal, drug resistance and differentiation are key characteristics of CSCs. Sonic Hedgehog (Shh), Notch1, Twist1, Snail and Wnt1 signaling transduction pathways play major roles in the self-renewal of these cells [33,59–68]. WFA has been reported to inhibit Notch-1 and downstream signaling genes (Hes1 and Hey1) [33,68]. Notch 1 signaling pathway is associated with regulation of cell fate at several distinct developmental stages and has been implicated in cancer initiation and progression [63,69,70]. In our present study as shown in Fig. 8, we noticed highly significant inhibition of expression of Notch 1 and its downstream signaling genes Hes1 and Hey1 in tumors collected from mice treated with WFA (2 mg/kg) as compared to tumors from control mock-treated animals. In contrast, animals treated with CIS (6 mg/kg) showed a highly significant increase in levels of Notch1, Hes1 and Hey1 genes. What is important, tumors collected from mice treated with WFA (2 mg/kg) in combination with CIS (6 mg/kg) showed significant decreased levels of Notch1 as well as Hes1 and Hey1 proteins (Fig. 8), suggesting downregulation of Notch1 signaling by WFA alone or in combination with CIS leading to elimination of putative CSCs.

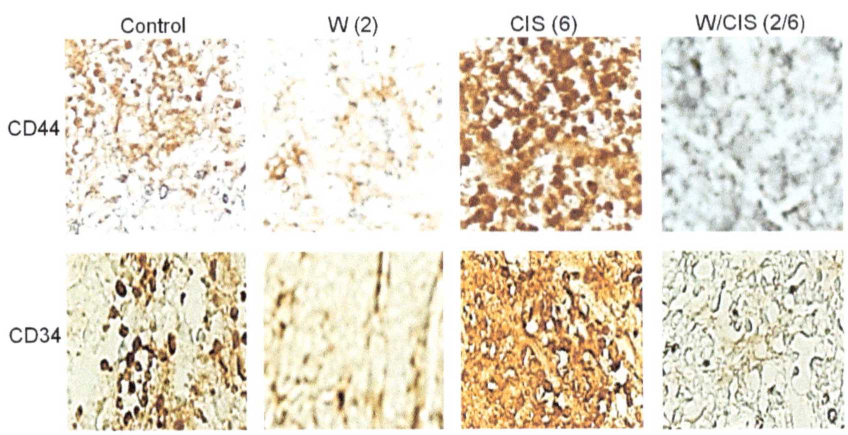

Figure 4. Immunohistochemical analysis of CD44 and CD34 positive cells in tumors collected from mock treated mice (control) and mice treated with WFA and CIS both alone and in combination. The data shown is representative of two independent experiments. W = WFA. Values shown in parenthesis are mg/kg.

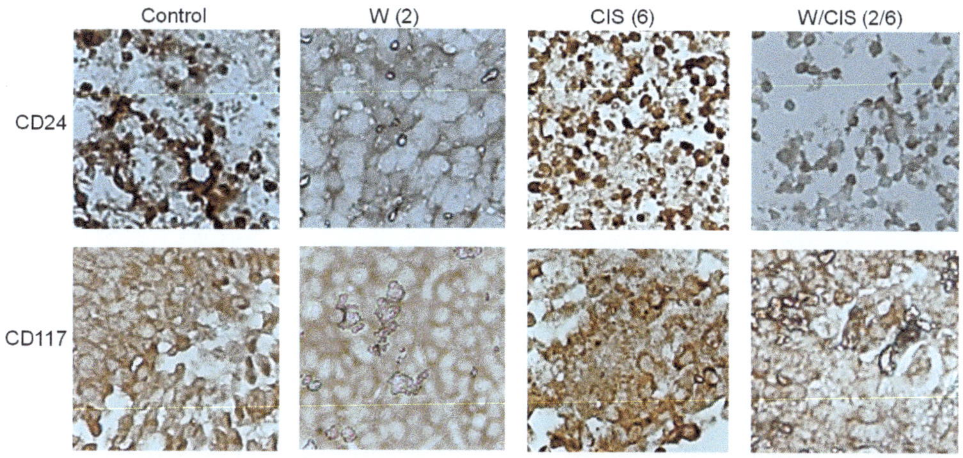

Figure 5. Immunohistochemical analysis of CD24 and CD117 positive cells in tumors collected from mock treated mice (control) and mice treated with WFA and CIS both alone and in combination. The data shown is representative of two independent experiments. W = WFA. Values shown in parenthesis are mg/kg.

Discussion

The most common first line chemotherapy used for ovarian cancer after cytoreductive surgery is carboplatin in combination with paclitaxel. Initial response rate to this combination is very high (70 to 80%), however within 6 to 20 months after initial treatment tumor relapse and patients become resistance to CIS [71]. Resistance to CIS has been associated with number of mechanisms such as increase in glutathione and metallothionein levels, decrease in drug uptake, increase in DNA repair mechanisms (due to enhanced expression of excision repair genes) and tolerance of the formation of platinum-DNA adducts [72]. Change in status of p53 has also been reported to play important role in sensitivity of CIS [73,74].

In recent years, several investigators have reported a presence of small population of CSCs in tumor tissues to be responsible for induction of chemo-resistance and recurrence of cancer [75–77]. The convincing evidence for the role of CSCs in ovarian cancer was provided by Bapat et al. [45] who showed the presence of CSCs at single cell level in the ascites of an ovarian cancer patient, that could sequentially propagate tumor over several generations. Consistent with this, many other investigators reported the presence of CSCs in ovarian cancer cell lines, patients' ovarian tumors and tumor associated-ascites [57,76,77]. As a follow up of these observations CSCs have been isolated based on the presence of some extracellular markers. Most common makers used for ovarian CSCs include CD44, CD24, CD34, CD117 and CD133. CSCs also express ALDH1, Oct4, Myd88 and EpCAM [47,51,57,60,78,79]. An increase in number of CSCs in ovarian tumors correlates with a poor prognosis, including shorter overall and disease free survival [80–82]. Development of chemo-resistance of ovarian cancer could be explained by enrichment for CSCs [77,83–85]. In a recent study, Abubaker et al. [53] demonstrated using two ovarian cancer cell lines (epithelial OVCA433 and mesenchymal HEY) enrichment for a population of cells with high expression of CSC markers at the protein as well as mRNA levels after treatment with CIS, paclitaxel and the combination of both. In addition, these investigators showed

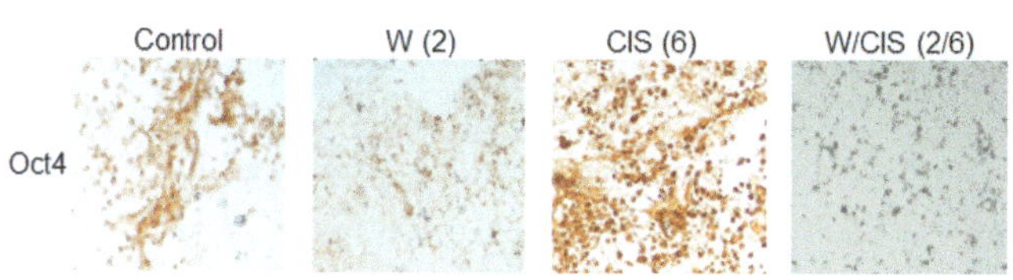

Figure 6. Immunohistochemical analysis of Oct4 positive cells in tumors collected from mock treated mice (control) and mice treated with WFA and CIS both alone and in combination. The data shown is representative of two independent experiments. W = WFA. Values shown in parenthesis are mg/kg.

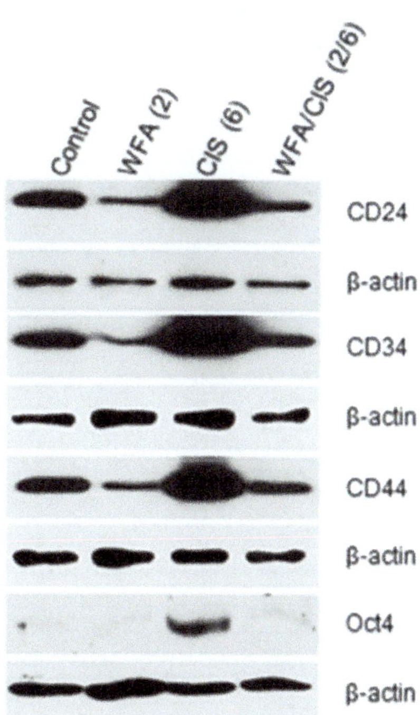

Figure 7. Western lot analysis of CD24, CD34, CD44, and Oct4 proteins from tumors collected from mock treated mice and mice treated with WFA and CIS both alone and in combination. Beta-actin was used as an internal control. The data shown is representative of two independent experiments. Con = control, W = WFA. Values shown in parenthesis are mg/kg.

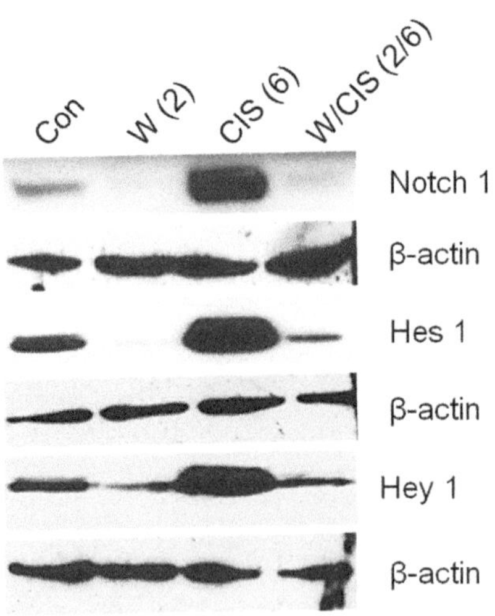

Figure 8. Western blot analysis of Notch1, Hes1 and Hey 1 proteins from tumors collected from mock treated mice and mice treated with WFA and CIS both alone and in combination. Beta-actin was used as an internal control. The data shown is representative of two independent experiments. Con = control, W = WFA. Values shown in parenthesis are mg/kg.

increase in tumorigenic properties of ovarian cancer cells in response to chemotherapy drugs. In the present study, we show somehow in agreement with those studies [53] that the number of CSCs increases in animals bearing orthotopic ovarian tumors treated with CIS at 6 mg/kg. This increase in CSCs population in ovarian tumors of mice with CIS may explain the development of chemo-resistance and reoccurrence of ovarian cancer in patients treated with CIS or its derivative carboplatin employed in combination with paclitaxel.

Increase in number of CSCs in tumors inoculated in nude mice followed by CIS treatment is result of amplification of CSCs present in human cancer cell line A2780. On other hand growing tumor will attract host-derived normal stem cells that will provide stroma and vasculature for expanding tumor tissue. These cells could provide trophic signals for CSCs, and this is currently investigated in our laboratories.

In the past years a great deal of efforts has been devoted to develop drugs that can kill cancer cells as well as CSCs in order to reduce chemo-resistance and recurrence of cancer after treatment. WFA as reported exhibits an inhibitory effect against several different types of cancer cells. However, its effect on CSCs has not been explored so far. In our previous study [10], we demonstrated that WFA when used alone or in combination with CIS inhibits cell proliferation and induce cell death of both CIS-sensitive (A2780 and CaOV3) as well as CIS-resistant (A2780/CP70) cell lines. In our present follow-up study we show that WFA (2 mg/kg) when used alone or in combination with CIS to treat mice bearing orthotopic ovarian tumor reduced tumor growth by 70 to 80% and prevented metastasis to other organs. In addition, treatment of mice bearing orthotopic ovarian tumors with WFA alone or WFA + CIS eliminated cells that express CSC markers. (CD44, CD24, CD34, CD117 and Oct4). In contrast the number of these cells as mentioned above increased in our hands after treatment by CIS alone. Thus, our results clearly demonstrate that combination of low dose of WFA (2 mg/kg) with suboptimal dose of CIS (6 mg/kg) is highly effective in suppressing the tumor growth and elimination of putative CSCs "expanded" by CIS treatment. Since, therapeutic dose of CIS is 8 mg/kg [19], WFA in combination with CIS has potential to be highly effective and efficacious therapy for ovarian cancer and may ameliorate CIS-therapy related side effects.

Self-renewal, drug resistance and differentiation are key characteristics of CSCs and several developmental pathways such as Sonic Hedgehog (Shh), Notch, Wnt and TGFβ, Twist, and Snail which have been shown to be crucial in these processes [33,59–67,86]. WFA has been reported to inhibit Notch1 and downstream signaling genes (Hes1 and Hey1) [43,77] that have been implicated in cancer initiation and progression [63,69,70].

In our present study, we show for a first time highly significant inhibition of Notch1 and its downstream signaling proteins Hes1 and Hey1 in tumors collected from animals treated with WFA (2 mg/kg) as compared to tumors from mock-treated animals. In contrast, animals treated with CIS (6 mg/kg) alone showed a significant increase in levels of Notch1, Hes1 and Hey1 genes which is consistent with the increase in number of CSCs, suggesting an important role of Notch1 transduction pathway in amplification of those cells. More importantly, treatment of animals with WFA (2 mg/kg) + CIS (6 mg/kg) prevented increase of Notch1, Hes1 and Hey1 expression, suggests that such combined therapy ameliorates unwanted effect of CIS treatment alone and unwanted expansion of CSCs. Thus, treatment of patients that have become resistance to CIS and have developed recurrence cancer could be benefited by WFA treatment alone or in combination with CIS.

Conclusions

The silent observation from this study is that treatment of mice bearing human ovarian tumors with CIS results in an unwanted expansion of cells that express CSC markers, what may lead to CIS resistance and recurrence of ovarian tumor. In contrast, WFA if employed alone or in combination with CIS ameliorates this unwanted effect. The data obtained from our study suggest that WFA alone or in combination with CIS may serve as a safer and more efficacious therapy for both first line and second line options for ovarian cancer.

Acknowledgments

We thank Renu Kakar for expert technical assistance.

Author Contributions

Conceived and designed the experiments: SSK. Performed the experiments: SSK SKS KSP. Analyzed the data: SKS. Wrote the paper: SSK. Contributed reagents/material/planning of experiments: SKB. Edited the manuscript: MZR. Provided input in planning the experiments: DMM. Histopathological analysis of tumors and normal tissues MM.

References

1. Siegel R, Naishadham D, Jemal A (2013) Cancer statistics. CA Cancer J Clin 63: 11–30.
2. Hunn J, Rodriguez GC (2012) Ovarian cancer: etiology, risk factors, and epidemiology. Clin Obstet Gynecol 55: 3–24.
3. National Comprehensive Cancer Network. NCCN Clinical Practice Guidelines in Oncology. Ovarian Cancer. Version 1.2013. Available: HTTP://www.nccn.org/professionals/physician_gls/pdf/ovarian.pdf
4. Piccart MJ, Bertelsen K, Stuart G, Cassidy J, Mangioni C, et al. (2003) Long-term follow-up confirms a survival advantage of the paclitaxel-cisplatin regimen over the cyclophosphamide-cisplatin combination in advanced ovarian cancer. Int J Gynecol Cancer 13 Suppl 2: 144–148.
5. Matsuo K, Lin YG, Roman LD, Sood AK (2010) Overcoming platinum resistance in ovarian carcinoma. Expert Opin Investig Drugs 19: 1339–1354.

6. Galluzzi L, Senovilla L, Vitale I, Michels J, Martins I, et al. (2012) Molecular mechanisms of cisplatin resistance. Oncogene 31: 1869–1883.
7. El-Awady SE, Moustafa YM, Abo-Elmatty DM, Radwan A (2011) Cisplatin-induced cardiotoxicity: Mechanisms and cardioprotective strategies. Eur J Pharmacol 650: 335–41.
8. Kintzel PE (2001) Anticancer drug-induced kidney disorders. Drug Saf 24(1): 19–38.
9. Lieberthal W, Triaca V, Levine J (1996) Mechanisms of death induced by cisplatin in proximal tubular epithelial cells: apoptosis vs. necrosis. Am J Physiol 270: F700–708.
10. Kakar SS, Jala VR, Fong MY (2012) Synergistic cytotoxic action of cisplatin and withaferin A on ovarian cancer cell lines. Biochem Biophys Res Commun 423: 819–825.
11. Fugner A (1973) Inhibition of immunologically induced inflammation by the plant steroid withaferin A. Arzneimittelforschung 23: 932–935.
12. Rasool M, Varalakshmi P (2006) Immunomodulatory role of Withania somnifera root powder on experimental induced inflammation: An in vivo and in vitro study. Vascul Pharmacol 44: 406–410.
13. Scartezzini P, Speroni E (2000) Review on some plants of Indian traditional medicine with antioxidant activity. J Ethnopharmacol 71: 23–43.
14. Gupta SK, Mohanty I, Talwar KK, Dinda A, Joshi S, et al. (2004) Cardioprotection from ischemia and reperfusion injury by Withania somnifera: a hemodynamic, biochemical and histopathological assessment. Mol Cell Biochem 260: 39–47.
15. Stan SD, Hahm ER, Warin R, Singh SV (2008) Withaferin A causes FOXO3a- and Bim-dependent apoptosis and inhibits growth of human breast cancer cells in vivo. Cancer Res 68: 7661–7669.
16. Mohan R, Hammers HJ, Bargagna-Mohan P, Zhan XH, Herbstritt CJ, et al. (2004) Withaferin A is a potent inhibitor of angiogenesis. Angiogenesis 7: 115–122.
17. Srinivasan S, Ranga RS, Burikhanov R, Han SS, Chendil D (2007) Par-4-dependent apoptosis by the dietary compound withaferin A in prostate cancer cells. Cancer Res 67: 246–253.
18. Stan SD, Zeng Y, Singh SV (2008) Ayurvedic medicine constituent withaferin a causes G2 and M phase cell cycle arrest in human breast cancer cells. Nutr Cancer 60 Suppl 1: 51–60.
19. Munagala R, Kausar H, Munjal C, Gupta RC (2011) Withaferin A induces p53-dependent apoptosis by repression of HPV oncogenes and upregulation of tumor suppressor proteins in human cervical cancer cells. Carcinogenesis 32: 1697–16705.
20. Yu Y, Hamza A, Zhang T, Gu M, Zou P, et al. (2010) Withaferin A targets heat shock protein 90 in pancreatic cancer cells. Biochem Pharmacol 79: 542–551.
21. Mayola E, Gallerne C, Esposti DD, Martel C, Pervaiz S, et al. (2011) Withaferin A induces apoptosis in human melanoma cells through generation of reactive oxygen species and down-regulation of Bcl-2. Apoptosis 16: 1014–1027.
22. Choi MJ, Park EJ, Min KJ, Park JW, Kwon TK (2011) Endoplasmic reticulum stress mediates withaferin A induced apoptosis in human renal carcinoma cells. Toxicol In Vitro 25: 692–698.
23. Samadi AK, Mukerji R, Shah A, Timmermann BN, Cohen MS (2010) A novel RET inhibitor with potent efficacy against medullary thyroid cancer in vivo. Surgery 148: 1228–1236.
24. Samadi AK, Tong X, Mukerji R, Zhang H, Timmermann BN, et al. (2010) Withaferin A, a cytotoxic steroid from Vassobia breviflora, induces apoptosis in human head and neck squamous cell carcinoma. J Nat Prod 73: 1476–1481.
25. Shah N, Kataria H, Kaul SC, Ishii T, Kaur G, et al. (2009) Effect of the alcoholic extract of Ashwagandha leaves and its components on proliferation, migration, and differentiation of glioblastoma cells: combinational approach for enhanced differentiation. Cancer Sci 100: 1740–1747.
26. Oh JH, Lee TJ, Kim SH, Choi YH, Lee SH, et al. (2008) Induction of apoptosis by withaferin A in human leukemia U937 cells through down-regulation of Akt phosphorylation. Apoptosis 13: 1494–1504.
27. Oh JH, Kwon TK (2009) Withaferin A inhibits tumor necrosis factor-alpha-induced expression of cell adhesion molecules by inactivation of Akt and NF-kappaB in human pulmonary epithelial cells. Int Immunopharmacol 9: 614–619.
28. Mayola E, Gallerne C, Esposti DD, Martel C, Pervaiz S, et al. (2011) Withaferin A induces apoptosis in human melanoma cells through generation of reactive oxygen species and down-regulation of Bcl-2. Apoptosis 16: 1014–27.
29. Roy RV, Suman S, Das TP, Luevano JE, Damodaran C (2013) Withaferin A, a steroidal lactone from Withania somnifera, induces mitotic catastrophe and growth arrest in prostate cancer cells. J Nat Prod 76: 1909–1915.
30. Malik F, Kumar A, Bhushan S, Khan S, Bhatia A, et al. (2007) Reactive oxygen species generation and mitochondrial dysfunction in the apoptotic cell death of human myeloid leukemia HL-60 cells by a dietary compound withaferin A with concomitant protection by N-acetyl cysteine. Apoptosis 12: 2115–2133.
31. Lee TJ, Um HJ, Min do S, Park JW, Choi KS, et al. (2009) Withaferin A sensitizes TRAIL-induced apoptosis through reactive oxygen species-mediated up-regulation of death receptor 5 and downregulation of c-FLIP. Free Radic Biol Med 46: 1639–1649.
32. Hahm ER, Moura MB, Kelley EE, Van Houten B, Shiva S, et al. (2011) Withaferin a-induced apoptosis in human breast cancer cells is mediated by reactive oxygen species. PLoS One 6: e23354.
33. Koduru S, Kumar R, Srinivasan S, Evers MB, Damodaran C (2010) Notch-1 inhibition by Withaferin-A: a therapeutic target against colon carcinogenesis. Mol Cancer Ther 9: 202–210.
34. Hermann PC, Huber SL, Heeschen C (2008) Metastatic cancer stem cells: a new target for anti-cancer therapy? Cell Cycle 7: 188–193.
35. Dean M, Fojo T, Bates S (2005) Tumour stem cells and drug resistance. Nat Rev Cancer 5: 275–284.
36. Bonnet D, Dick JE (1997) Human acute myeloid leukemia is organized as a hierarchy that originates from a primitive hematopoietic cell. Nat Med 3: 730–737.
37. Lapidot T, Sirard C, Vormoor J, Murdoch B, Hoang T, et al. (1994) A cell initiating human acute myeloid leukemia after transplantation into SCID mice. Nature 367: 645–648.
38. Al-Hajj M, Wicha MS, Benito-Hernandez A, Morrison SJ, Clarke MF (2003) Prospective identification of tumorigenic breast cancer cells. Proc Natl Acad Sci U S A 100: 3983–3988.
39. Medema JP (2013) Cancer stem cells: the challenges ahead. Nat Cell Biol 15: 338–344.
40. Chen L, Kasai T, Li Y, Sugii Y, Jin G, et al. (2012) A model of cancer stem cells derived from mouse induced pluripotent stem cells. PLoS One 7: e33544.
41. Driessens G, Beck B, Caauwe A, Simons BD, Blanpain C (2012) Defining the mode of tumour growth by clonal analysis. Nature 488: 527–530.
42. Schepers AG, Snippert HJ, Stange DE, van den Born M, van Es JH, et al. (2012) Lineage tracing reveals Lgr5+ stem cell activity in mouse intestinal adenomas. Science 337(6095): 730–735.
43. Quintana E, Shackleton M, Sabel MS, Fullen DR, Johnson TM, et al. (2008) Efficient tumour formation by single human melanoma cells. Nature 456: 593–598.
44. Dalerba P, Cho RW, Clarke MF (2007) Cancer stem cells: models and concepts. Annu Rev Med 58: 267–284.
45. Bapat SA, Mali AM, Koppikar CB, Kurrey NK (2005) Stem and progenitor-like cells contribute to the aggressive behavior of human epithelial ovarian cancer. Cancer Res 65: 3025–3029.
46. Kurrey NK, Amit K, Bapat SA (2005) Snail and Slug are major determinants of ovarian cancer invasiveness at the transcription level. Gyne Oncol 97: 155–165.
47. Zhang S, Balch C, Chan MW, Lai HC, Matei D, et al. (2008) Identification and characterization of ovarian cancer-initiating cells from primary human tumors, Cancer Res 68: 4311–4320.
48. Deng S, Yang X, Lassus H, Liang S, Kaur S, et al. (2010) Distinct expression levels and patterns of stem cell marker, aldehyde dehydrogenase isoform 1 (ALDH1), in human epithelial cancers. PLoS ONE 5: e10277.
49. Silva IA, Bai S, McLean K, Yang K, Griffith K, et al. (2011) Aldehyde dehydrogenase and CD133 define angiogenic ovarian cancer stem cells that portend poor patient survival, Cancer Res 71: 3991–4001.
50. Dyall S, Gayther SA, Dafou D (2010) Cancer stem cells and epithelial ovarian cancer. J Oncol 2010: 105269.
51. Alvero AB, Chen R, Fu HH, Montagna M, Schwartz PE, et al. (2009) Molecular phenotyping of human ovarian cancer stem cells unravels the mechanisms for repair and chemoresistance. Cell Cycle 8: 158–166.
52. Clarke MF, Dick JE, Dirks PB, Eaves CJ, Jamieson CH, et al. (2006) Cancer stem cells–perspectives on current status and future directions: AACR Workshop on cancer stem cells. Cancer Res 66: 9339–9344.
53. Abubaker K, Latifi A, Luwor R, Nazaretian S, Zhu H, et al. (2013) Short-term single treatment of chemotherapy results in the enrichment of ovarian cancer stem cell like cells leading to an increased tumor burden. Mol Cancer 12: 24.
54. Malik MT, Kakar SS (2006) Regulation of angiogenesis and invasion by human Pituitary tumor transforming gene (PTTG) through increased expression and secretion of matrix metalloproteinase-2 (MMP-2). Mol Cancer 5: 61.
55. Nunez-Cruz S, Connolly DC, Scholler N (2010) An orthotopic model of serous ovarian cancer in immunocompetent mice for in vivo tumor imaging and monitoring of tumor immune responses. J Vis Exp 28.pii: 2146.
56. Fong MY, Jin S, Rane M, Singh RK, Gupta R, et al. (2012) Withaferin A synergizes the therapeutic effect of doxorubicin through ROS-mediated autophagy in ovarian cancer. PLoS One 7: e42265.
57. Tomao F, Papa A, Strudel M, Rossi L, Lo Russo G, et al. (2014) Investigating Molecular Profiles of Ovarian Cancer: An Update on Cancer Stem Cells. J Cancer 5: 301–310.
58. Ramdass B, Duggal R, Minev B, Chowdhary A, Koka P (2013) Functional role of solid tumor stem cells in disease etiology and susceptibility to therapeutic interventions. J Stem Cells 8: 189–231.
59. Ponnusamy MP, Batra SK (2008) Ovarian cancer: emerging concept on cancer stem cells. J Ovarian Res, 1: 4.
60. Alvero AB, Fu HH, Holmberg J, Visintin I, Mor L, et al. (2009) Stem like ovarian cancer cells can serve as tumor vascular progenitors. Stem Cells 7: 2405–2413.
61. Reya T, Clevers H (2005) Wnt signaling in stem cells and cancer. Nature 434: 843
62. Liu S, Dontu G, Mantle ID, Patel S, Ahn NS, et al. (2006) Hedgehogsignaling and Bmi-1 regulate self-renewal of normal and malignant human mammary stem cells. Cancer Res 66: 6063–6071.
63. Dontu G, Jackson KW, McNicholas E, Kawamura MJ, Abdallah WM, et al. (2004) Role of Notch signaling in cell-fate determination of human mammary stem/progenitor cells, Breast Cancer Res 6: 605–615.

64. Giles RH, van Es JH, Clevers H (2003) Caught up in a Wnt storm: wnt signaling in cancer, Biochim Biophys Acta 1653: 1–24.
65. Mimeault M, Batra SK (2012) Novel biomarkers and therapeutic targets for optimizing the therapeutic management of melanomas. World J Clin Oncol 3: 32–42.
66. Wu KJ, Yang MH (2011) Epithelial-mesenchymal transition and cancer stemness: the Twist1-Bmi1connection. Biosci Rep 31: 449–455.
67. Jain P, Alahari SK (2011) Breast cancer stem cells: a new challenge for breast cancer treatment. Front Biosci 16: 1824–1832.
68. Suman S, Das TP, Damodaran C (2013) Silencing NOTCH signaling causes growth arrest in both breast cancer stem cells and breast cancer cells. Br J Cancer, 109: 2587–2596.
69. Shi W, Harris AL (2006) Notch signaling in breast cancer and tumor angiogenesis: cross-talk and therapeutic potentials. J Mammary Gland Biol Neoplasia 11: 41–52.
70. Gangopadhyay S, Nandy A, Hor P, Mukhopadhyay A (2013) Breast cancer stem cells: a novel therapeutic target. Clin Breast Cancer 13: 7–15.
71. Lengyel E (2010) Ovarian cancer development and metastasis. Am J Pathol 177: 1053–1064.
72. Christen RD, Isonishi S, Jones JA, Jekunen AP, Hom DK, et al. (1994) Signaling and drug sensitivity. Cancer Metastasis Rev 13: 175–189.
73. Brown R, Clugston C, Burns P, Edlin A, Vasey P, et al. (1993) Increased accumulation of p53 protein in cisplatin-resistant ovarian cell lines. Int J Cancer 55: 678–684.
74. Perego P, Giarola M, Righetti SC, Supino R, Caserini C, et al. (1996) Association between cisplatin resistance and mutation of p53 gene and reduced bax expression in ovarian carcinoma cell systems. Cancer Res 56: 556–62.
75. Hollier BG, Evans K, Mani SA (2009) The epithelial-to-mesenchymal transition and cancer stem cells: a coalition against cancer therapies. J Mammary Gland Biol Neoplasia 14: 29–43.
76. Ahmed N, Abubaker K, Findlay J, Quinn M (2010) Epithelial mesenchymal transition and cancer stem cell-like phenotypes facilitate chemoresistance in recurrent ovarian cancer. Curr Cancer Drug Targets 10: 268–278.
77. Latifi A, Luwor RB, Bilandzic M, Nazaretian S, Stenvers K, et al. (2012) Isolation and characterization of tumor cells from the ascites of ovarian cancer patients: molecular phenotype of chemoresistant ovarian tumors. PLoS One 7: e46858.
78. Gao MQ, Choi YP, Kang S, Youn JH, Cho NH (2010) CD24+ cells from hierarchically organized ovarian cancer are enriched in cancer stem cells. Oncogene 29: 2672–2680.
79. Landen CN Jr, Goodman B, Katre AA, Steg AD, Nick AM, et al. (2010) Targeting aldehyde dehydrogenase cancer stem cells in ovarian cancer. Mol Cancer Ther 9: 3186–3199.
80. Guo X, Xiong L, Sun T, Peng R, Zou L, et al. (2012) Expression features of SOX9 associate with tumor progression and poor prognosis of hepatocellular carcinoma. Diagn Pathol 7: 44.
81. Surowiak P, Materna V, Maciejczyk A, Kaplenko I, Spaczynski M, et al. (2006) CD46 expression is indicative of shorter revival-free survival for ovarian cancer patients. Anticancer Res 26: 4943–4948.
82. Oh DH, Kim SH, Jung S, Sung YK, Bang SY, et al. (2011) Precuneus hypoperfusion plays an important role in memory impairment of patients with systemic lupus erythematosus. Lupus 20: 855–860.
83. Steg AD, Bevis KS, Katre AA, Ziebarth A, Dobbin ZC, et al. (2012) Stem cell pathways contribute to clinical chemoresistance in ovarian cancer. Clin Cancer Res 18: 869–881.
84. Szotek PP, Pieretti-Vanmarcke R, Masiakos PT, Dinulescu DM, Connolly D, et al. (2006) Ovarian cancer side population defines cells with stem cell-like characteristics and Mullerian Inhibiting Substance responsiveness. Proc Natl Acad Sci U S A 103: 11154–11159.
85. Vathipadiekal V, Saxena D, Mok SC, Hauschka PV, Ozbun L, et al. (2012) Identification of a potential ovarian cancer stem cell gene expression profile from advanced stage papillary serous ovarian cancer. PLoS One 7: e29079.
86. Kwon MJ, Shin YK (2013) Regulation of ovarian cancer stem cells or tumor-initiating cells. Int J Mol Sci 14: 6624–6648.

The Use of Laser Microdissection in the Identification of Suitable Reference Genes for Normalization of Quantitative Real-Time PCR in Human FFPE Epithelial Ovarian Tissue Samples

Jing Cai[1], Tao Li[1], Bangxing Huang[1,2], Henghui Cheng[3], Hui Ding[1], Weihong Dong[1], Man Xiao[1], Ling Liu[1], Zehua Wang[1]*

1 Department of Obstetrics and Gynecology, Union Hospital, Tongji Medical College, Huazhong University of Science and Technology, Wuhan, China, **2** Department of Pathology, Union Hospital, Tongji Medical College, Huazhong University of Science and Technology, Wuhan, China, **3** Department of Pathology, Tongji Hospital, Tongji Medical College, Huazhong University of Science and Technology, Wuhan, China

Abstract

Quantitative real-time PCR (qPCR) is a powerful and reproducible method of gene expression analysis in which expression levels are quantified by normalization against reference genes. Therefore, to investigate the potential biomarkers and therapeutic targets for epithelial ovarian cancer by qPCR, it is critical to identify stable reference genes. In this study, twelve housekeeping genes (ACTB, GAPDH, 18S rRNA, GUSB, PPIA, PBGD, PUM1, TBP, HRPT1, RPLP0, RPL13A, and B2M) were analyzed in 50 ovarian samples from normal, benign, borderline, and malignant tissues. For reliable results, laser microdissection (LMD), an effective technique used to prepare homogeneous starting material, was utilized to precisely excise target tissues or cells. One-way analysis of variance (ANOVA) and nonparametric (Kruskal-Wallis) tests were used to compare the expression differences. NormFinder and geNorm software were employed to further validate the suitability and stability of the candidate genes. Results showed that epithelial cells occupied a small percentage of the normal ovary indeed. The expression of ACTB, PPIA, RPL13A, RPLP0, and TBP were stable independent of the disease progression. In addition, NormFinder and geNorm identified the most stable combination (ACTB, PPIA, RPLP0, and TBP) and the relatively unstable reference gene GAPDH from the twelve commonly used housekeeping genes. Our results highlight the use of homogeneous ovarian tissues and multiple-reference normalization strategy, e.g. the combination of ACTB, PPIA, RPLP0, and TBP, for qPCR in epithelial ovarian tissues, whereas GAPDH, the most commonly used reference gene, is not recommended, especially as a single reference gene.

Editor: Michael R. Emmert-Buck, National Cancer Institute, National Institutes of Health, United Statesof America

Funding: This work was supported by China Postdoctoral Science Foundation (Grant No. 2012T50650) and the Natural Science Foundation of Hubei Province of China (Grant No. 2013CFB128). The funders had no role in study design, data collection and analysis, decision to publish, or preparation of the manuscript.

Competing Interests: The authors have declared that no competing interests exist.

* E-mail: zehuawang@163.net

These authors contributed equally to this work.

Introduction

Despite advances in the understanding of potential biomarkers and therapeutic targets, effective screening techniques and therapies of ovarian cancer remain a challenging task, partly due to tissue heterogeneity. Numerous studies have analyzed genetic alterations or gene expression profiles in ovarian cancer by making the comparison between cancerous tissue and normal ovarian tissue. In a normal ovary, epithelial cells, from which the carcinomas primarily originate, only account for a very small percentage of the ovarian cell population, while stromal cells occupy the overwhelming majority [1]. Thus, it is unreliable to analyze gene expression based on RNA or DNA preparations from whole ovarian tissue [2]. To ensure the accuracy and reliability of results, the procurement of homogeneous cells is immensely important.

Laser microdissection (LMD) is a tool that facilitates the microscopic isolation of objective regions without contamination or unwanted tissue components [3,4]. The dissected tissues, as homogeneous starting materials, can be used for a variety of analyses, such as transcriptomic and proteomic studies [5]. During this process, the use of Rnase-free reagents and cresyl violet staining are recommended to minimize RNA degradation and maintain tissue morphology, respectively [6,7]. Although fresh cryosections are preferred for nucleic acids extraction using LMD, fresh sections are usually scarce in basic and clinical research. Formalin-fixed, paraffin-embedded tissues (FFPE), which represent an alternative for nucleic acids extraction and downstream experiments, such as quantitative real-time PCR (qPCR), are more widely available in clinical laboratories.

To date, innumerable papers have embraced qPCR as an indispensable method to quantify gene expression at the transcription level because of its high sensitivity, reproducibility,

Table 1. Candidate reference genes evaluated in this study.

Gene symbol	Gene name	Accession number	Function
GAPDH	Glyceraldehyde-3-phosphate dehydrogenase	NM-001256799.1	gluconeogenesis and Glycolysis
ACTB	Actin, beta	NM-001101.3	Cytoskeletal structural protein
18S	18S ribosomal RNA	NR-003286	Ribosomal RNA
B2M	Beta-2-microglobulin	NM-004048.2	Cytoskeletal protein in cell locomotion
GUSB	Glucuronidase, beta	NM-000181.3	Lysosomal exoglycosidase
PBGD	Porphobilinogen deaminase	NM-001258209.1	Heme biosynthetic pathway
PUM1	Pumilio homolog 1 (Drosophila)	NM-014676.2	RNA binding
PPIA	Peptidylprolyl isomerase A	NM-021130.3	Cyclosporin binding protein
TBP	TATA box binding protein	NM-001172085.1	Transcription by RNA polymerases
HRPT1	Hypoxanthine phosphoribosyltransferase 1	NM-000194.2	Metabolic salvage of purines
RPLPO	Ribosomal protein, large, P0	NM-001002.3	Ribosomal protein
RPL13A	Ribosomal protein L13a	NM-001270491.1	Ribosomal protein

and throughput [8–10]. In this approach, when comparing gene expression profiles, accurate normalization is a prerequisite for reliable results. Therefore, the identification of suitable reference genes is crucial in qPCR assays. An ideal reference gene or housekeeping gene (HKG) should be stably expressed in all specimens regardless of tissue type, pathological stage and/or experimental treatment [11,12]. Regrettably, the commonly used reference genes have shown variability in expression in different tissues and cells [13–16].

Thus far, two reports have been published that explored the identification of reference genes for the normalization of qPCR results in ovarian tissues. After examining 20 normal ovarian tissue specimens and 20 serous ovarian cancer specimens, Li *et al.* recommended a combination of PPIA and GUSB genes as a reliable normalization strategy [17]. Fu *et al.* recommended a combination of RPLP0 and RPL4 afer investigating 52 normal, benign, and malignant ovarian tissues samples [18]. However, both studies did not account for tissue heterogeneity and their results were inconsistent.

To understand the current use of reference genes, we performed a PubMed search using the MeSH terms "real-time PCR" and "ovarian cancer" and obtained 128 available articles published from January 1st, 2010 to March 10th, 2013; among the articles, 25 various reference genes were used without any preliminary evaluation of suitability. Although studies have recommended the combination use of reference genes, only 17 of the 128 (13.3%) studies used two or more reference genes for data normalization. In addition, within the other 111 (86.7%) studies that applied a single reference gene, GAPDH was the most frequently used (52, 40.6%), followed by ACTB (33, 25.8%), 18S rRNA (5, 3.9%), and B2M (3, 2.3%). Other genes, such as TBP, PBGD, RPLP0, PUM1 and GUSB, were only used twice (1.6%) or once (0.78%) among the studies that applied a single reference gene.

In summary, the use of reference genes for qPCR is inconsistent, and standardization is urgent, especially for the evaluation of gene expression in tissues with high heterogeneity, such as ovarian tumors. In this study, we collected epithelial components from FFPE ovarian tissues with varying degrees of neoplasia via LMD to identify universal reference genes for qPCR in ovarian epithelial tumor studies.

Materials and Methods

Ethics Statement Results

The present study was approved by the ethical committee of Union Hospital, Tongji Medical College, Huazhong University of Science and Technology, China. All patients or their next of kin have provided written informed consent for the collection of samples and subsequent researches.

Patients and samples

Between January 2011 and July 2013, we collected a total of 50 tissue samples comprising eight normal ovarian tissues (mean age 41.5 years, age range 28 to 63 years), ten benign neoplasms (three serous neoplasms and seven mucinous neoplasms; mean age 35.3 years, age range 14 to 57 years), seven borderline neoplasms (four serous neoplasms and three mucinous neoplasms; mean age 35.57 years, age range 24 to 60 years), 25 malignant epithelial tumors (12 serous adenocarcinomas, three mucinous adenocarcinomas, six endometrioid carcinomas, and four clear cell tumors; mean age 50.2 years, age range 22 to 64 years). The normal tissue samples were excised from patients receiving an adnexectomy due to adenomyosis or myoma or excised from patients receiving a wedge biopsy of the ovaries. The tumor tissues were obtained during surgery, and cases with preoperative treatment were excluded. All specimens used in this study were pathologically verified.

LMD

Serial sections (n = 3–20, 8 μm) were cut from each FFPE sample and stored at 4°C until use. A 4-μm thick section was also cut for H&E staining. Immediately before LMD, the sections were deparaffinized, stained with 1% cresyl violet (Sigma-Aldrich, St. Louis, Missouri, USA) for 1 minute, dehydrated through 75%, 95%, and 100% alcohol grades for 30 seconds each, and finally immersed in xylene for 3 minutes and air-dried for 1 minute. The microdissection was performed using the Arcturus^{XT} LCM instrument (Applied Biosystems-Life Technologies, Carlsbad, CA, USA) following the manufacturer's protocol. An AutoScan^{TM} analysis software module was implemented when using the ArcturusXT LCM instrument, which allowed the user to visually inspect the regions of interest. Approximately 5000 cells were captured per specimen and subsequently used for the following studies.

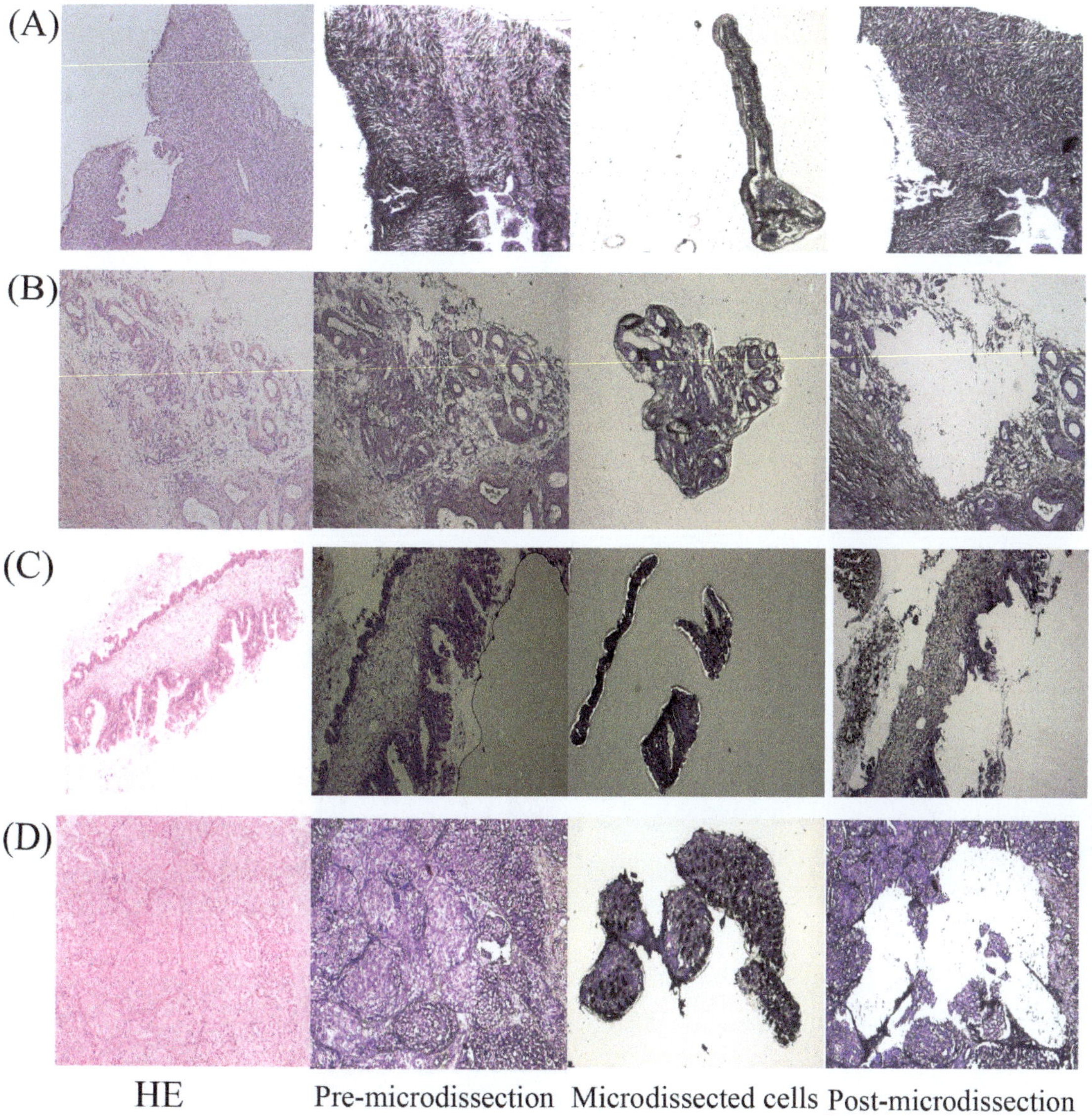

Figure 1. LMD mediated isolation of epithelial cells. (A–D) Ovarian tissue specimens, ordered by normal, benign, borderline, and malignant pathological categories, were used for target cells isolation. Panels from left to right are as follows: sections stained with H&E prior to LMD; sections stained with cresyl violet before LMD; cells captured on the collecting caps; sections after LMD (×100).

RNA isolation and cDNA synthesis

Total RNA from homogenized tissues was isolated using the RNeasy FFPE kit (Qiagen, Hilden, Germany) according to the manufacturer's protocol. The quality and integrity of the total RNA were measured using the Nanodrop 2000 (Thermo Scientific, Wilmington, DE, USA) and by electrophoresis on a 1% agarose gel. The total RNA (100 ng) was reverse-transcribed into cDNA using a PrimeScript RT reagent kit (TaKaRa Biotechnology, Shiga, Japan) with random hexamer primers and oligo(dT). All reactions were carried out at 37°C for 15 min followed by 85°C for 5 s to inactivate the enzymes.The cDNA was stored at −20°C until use.

Quantitative real-time PCR

Reference genes (n = 12) frequently used in the last three years in ovarian cancer research were selected to identify the most stable gene for qPCR normalization. Information regarding the 12 candidate genes is provided in Table 1. Primers were generated from published papers or designed using Primer 5 software, and the specificity of each primer was confirmed by primer-BLAST searches. qPCR was performed on an Applied Biosystems StepOnePlus Real-time PCR system (Applied Biosystems, Foster City, CA, USA) using SYBR Green Real-time PCR Master Mix (Toyobo, Osaka, Japan) according to the manufacturer's recommendations. Negative controls (no template in PCR) were performed for each gene, and a melting curve was constructed for each primer to confirm product specificity.

Standard curves of a five-fold dilution series were performed for all candidate genes, and the amplification efficiency and correlation coefficient (R^2) were generated based on the slope of each standard curve. The equation used to calculate the efficiency was as follows: E% = $[10^{(-1/\text{slope})}-1]$%. The delta-$C_t$ method was used

Table 2. Primer related information.

Gene symbol	Primer sequences (forward/reverse)	Annealing temperature(°C)	PCR efficiency (%)	R^2	Amplicon length(bp)
GAPDH	F:TGAACGGGAAGCTCACTGG R:TCCACCACCCTGTTGCTGTA	60	95.1	0.999	307
ACTB	F:GCCAACACAGTGCTGTCTGG R:GCTCAGGAGGAGCAATGATCTTG	60	98.7	1	121
18S	F:CGGCTACCACATCCAAGGAA R:GCTGGAATTACCGCGGCT	64	99.5	1	186
B2M	F:CGCTACTCTCTCTTTCTGGC R:AGACACATAGCAATTCAGGAAT	56	105	0.997	113
GUSB	F:AGCCAGTTCCTCATCAATGG R:GGTAGTGGCTGGTACGGAAA	56	105	0.999	160
PBGD	F:AGTGTGGTGGGAACCAGC R:CAGGATGATGGCACTGAACTC	56	103	0.999	144
PUM1	F:CAGGCTGCCTACCAACTCAT R:GTTCCCGAACCATCTCATTC	60	96.8	0.999	211
PPIA	F:GTGGTGTTTGGCAAAGTGAA R:TCGAGTTGTCCACAGTCAGC	60	103	0.999	116
TBP	F:TGCACAGGAGCCAAGAGTGAA R:CACATCACAGCTCCCCACCA	60	95.9	0.999	132
HRPT1	F:TGACACTGGCAAAACAATGCA R:GGTCCTTTTCACCAGCAAGCT	60	102	0.999	94
RPLP0	F:TTAAACCCTGCGTGGCAATCC R:CCACATTCCCCCGGATATGA	60	99.2	0.999	296
RPL13A	F:CCTGGAGGAGAAGAGGAAAGAGA R:TTGAGGACCTCTGTGTATTTGTCAA	60	100.8	0.999	126

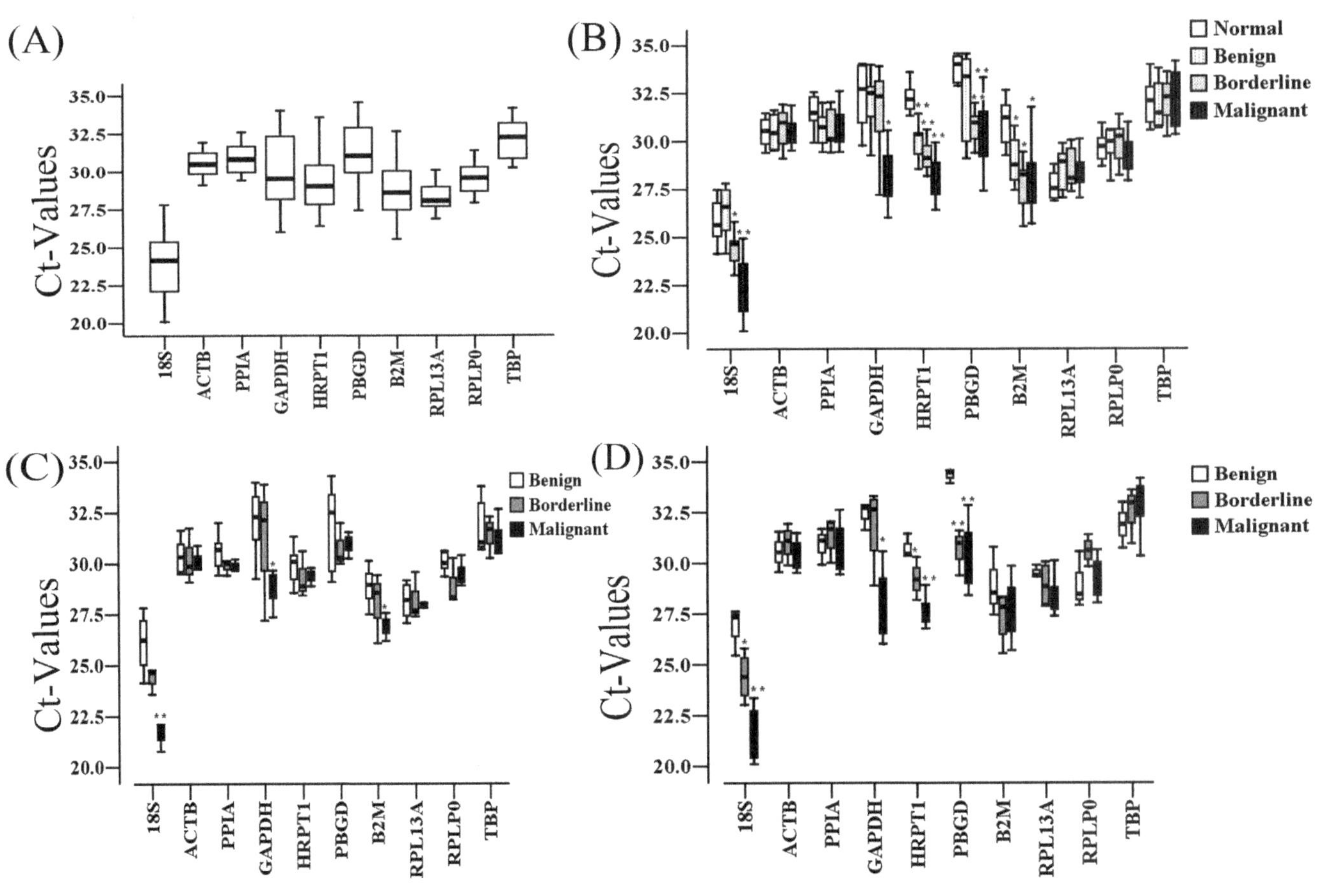

Figure 2. Expression levels of candidate reference genes in ovarian tissues. (A) C_t values of the 10 reference genes in fifty ovarian tissues. Boxes reveal the lower and upper quartiles with medians; bars represent the range of the data. (B) Expression changes of the 10 genes in ovarian tissues with four different groups were investigated by one-way ANOVA and the Kruskal-Wallis test. *$P<0.05$ vs. normal tissues, **$P<0.01$ vs. normal tissues. (C–D) Expression differences of the 10 genes in mucinous (C) and serous (D) ovarian tissues in three groups were analyzed. *$P<0.05$ vs. benign tissues, **$P<0.01$ vs. benign tissues.

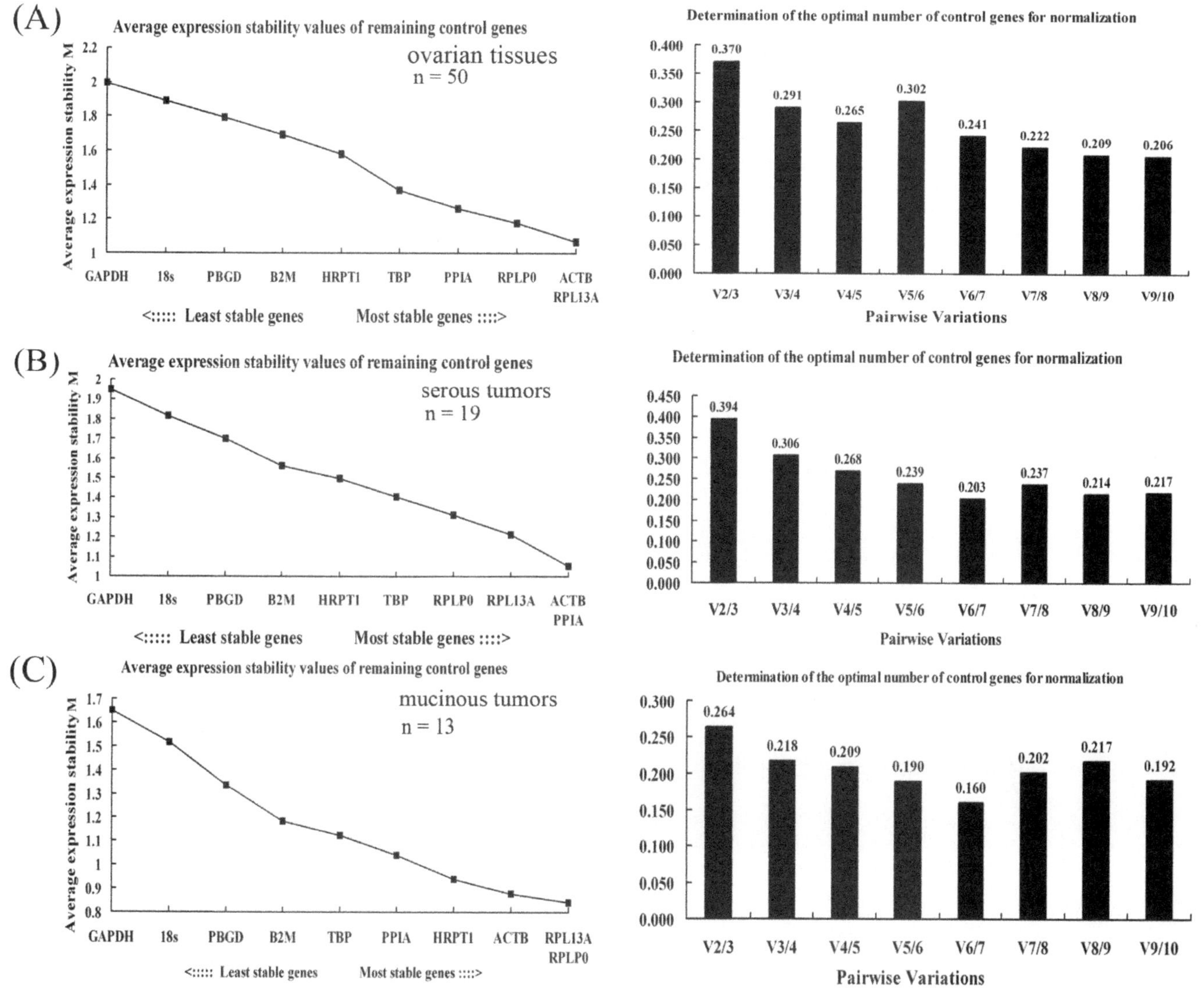

Figure 3. Determination of the expression stability (*M*) of the 10 candidate genes using the geNorm applet. (A) Left, the least stable gene was excluded stepwise by calculating *M* values across 50 ovarian tissues. The average expression stability values and the associated order from least to most stable expression are presented on the y-axis and x-axis, respectively. Right, the determination of the optimal number of internal control genes for normalization depending on the pairwise variation (V) analyses. (B–C) Selection of the most suitable reference genes for normalization in serous (B) and mucinous (C) ovarian tissues using the geNorm program.

to calculate the relative quantification (Q) of the amplification of the candidate genes according to the following formula: $Q = E^{-(sampleCt-minCt)}$, where $minC_t$ = the lowest C_t value observed in a group analyzed for a given primer.

Stability analysis

Statistical analysis was carried out with SPSS 13.0 statistic software (SPSS, Chicago, IL, USA). Differences were appropriately analyzed by one-way analysis of variance (ANOVA) or a nonparametric (Kruskal-Wallis) test. $P<0.05$ was considered statistically significant. For the stability analysis of the candidate reference genes, two freely available software programs were applied: NormFinder (http://www.mdl.dk/publicationsnormfinder.htm) and geNorm version 3.5 (http://medgen.ugent.be/~jvdesomp/genorm/). NormFinder, a Microsoft Excel add-in, focuses on calculating a stability value based on intra- and inter-group expression variations for candidate reference genes. A low value represents a low combined variation and, thereby, reveals high expression stability [19]. GeNorm, another Microsoft Excel application, provides a gene stability measure (*M*) and ranks the tested genes by stepwise exclusion of the gene with the highest *M* value. In addition, geNorm calculates the pairwise variations, V_n/V_{n+1}, between each combination of sequential normalization factors (NF), which allows for the identification of the optimal number of reference genes for accurate normalization [16].

Results

LMD, quality control, and amplification efficiency

Using LMD, approximately 5000 epithelial cells were isolated from each of the normal, benign, borderline, and malignant ovarian tissues (Fig. 1). Results showed that epithelial cells only occupied a small percentage of the whole ovarian tissues, especially the normal ovary. To guarantee the reliability of the results, only

Table 3. Candidate reference genes were ranked according to their expression stability values calculated by geNorm and NormFinder programs.

geNorm		NormFinder	
Gene	**Stability value**	**Gene**	**Stability value**
RPL13A	1.066	PPIA	0.592
ACTB	1.066	RPLPO	0.592
RPLPO	1.176	ACTB	0.660
PPIA	1.259	HRPT1	0.706
TBP	1.367	B2M	0.748
HRPT1	1.580	TBP	0.751
B2M	1.693	PBGD	0.758
PBGD	1.794	RPL13A	0.772
18S	1.889	18S	0.821
GAPDH	1.994	GAPDH	0.993

high quality RNA samples were included in the subsequent qPCR reactions. The purity and integrity of the RNA samples were characterized by the A260/280 ratio, which ranged from 1.8 to 2.06 (1.92±0.074) and the 28S/18S ratio (>1.7) on a 1% agarose gel. The amplification efficiencies and correlation coefficients (R^2) of the12 HKGs ranged from 95.1 to 105% and from 0.997 to 1, respectively (Table 2).

Expression levels of candidate HKGs in epithelial ovarian tissues

The PUM1 and GUSB genes demonstrated C_t values above 35 cycles in most of the 50 samples and were expressed at low levels; therefore, PUM1 and GUSB were excluded from further analyses. The remaining 10 HKGs displayed a wide range of expression. The 18S rRNA gene demonstrated the lowest mean C_t value (C_t = 24), while the TATA-binding protein gene (TBP) exhibited the highest mean C_t value (C_t = 32.1) (Fig. 2A). One-way ANOVA and the Kruskal-Wallis test were used to compare expression differences that were caused by disease progression. Five genes (ACTB [p = 0.93], PPIA [p = 0.21], RPL13A [p = 0.14], RPLPO [p = 0.26], and TBP [p = 0.89]) were expressed equivalently in all the 50 specimens from normal, benign, borderline, and malignant tissues; whereas, the expression of the other five HKGs (GAPDH, 18S rRNA, PBGD, HRPT1, and B2M) varied (P<0.05, Fig. 2B). Additionally, the expression levels of B2M, ACTB, PPIA, RPL13A, RPLPO, and TBP were not correlated with patient age (correlation coefficient = -0.195–0.133; P = 0.174–0.809).

Furthermore, the expression of the 10 HKGs was slightly different between the mucinous and serous neoplasms. Apart from ACTB, PPIA, RPL13A, RPLPO, and TBP, HRPT1 (P = 0.57) and PBGD (P = 0.70) demonstrated relatively equivalent expression in the 13 mucinous ovarian tumors (benign tissues, n = 7; borderline tissues, n = 3; malignant tissues, n = 3, Fig. 2C); whereas, the expression of B2M (P = 0.29) was not significantly different in the 19 serous neoplasms (benign, n = 3; borderline, n = 4; malignant, n = 12, Fig. 2D).

Determination of HKG expression stability

The C_t values of all 10 candidate reference genes were transformed to relative quantities using the delta-C_t method and subjected to two application tools, geNorm and NormFinder. GeNorm calculates the stability of genes (*M*) by pairwise

Table 4. Stability values of candidate genes in serous tissue samples.

geNorm		NormFinder	
Gene	**Stability value**	**Gene**	**Stability value**
PPIA	1.055	RPL13A	0.504
ACTB	1.055	HRPT1	0.602
RPL13A	1.214	ACTB	0.703
RPLPO	1.313	PPIA	0.784
TBP	1.405	B2M	0.860
HRPT1	1.498	RPLPO	0.983
B2M	1.560	TBP	1.051
PBGD	1.701	PBGD	1.052
18S	1.815	18S	1.158
GAPDH	1.948	GAPDH	1.222

Table 5. Stability values of candidate genes in mucinous tissue samples.

geNorm		NormFinder	
Gene	**Stability value**	**Gene**	**Stability value**
RPL13A	0.842	HRPT1	0.366
RPLPO	0.842	RPL13A	0.427
ACTB	0.878	ACTB	0.443
HRPT1	0.940	TBP	0.467
PPIA	1.040	PBGD	0.476
TBP	1.122	RPLPO	0.478
B2M	1.184	B2M	0.482
PBGD	1.335	PPIA	0.576
18S	1.516	18S	0.952
GAPDH	1.649	GAPDH	0.956

comparisons and then ranks these genes according to their M values. With M values below the geNorm default threshold of 1.5, TBP, PPIA, RPLP0, ACTB, and RPL13A exhibited high expression stability (Fig. 3A and Table 3). ACTB and RPL13A were identified as the two most stable genes; whereas, GAPDH was the least stable one. Additionally, the geNorm software recommended the combination of four genes (PPIA, RPLP0, ACTB, and RPL13A), which yielded a V4/5 value of 0.265 (Fig. 3A), as a much more reliable normalization strategy.

The NormFinder program analysis revealed varied M values ranging from 0.592 to 0.993 (Table 3). GAPDH was still determined to be the least stable gene in our analysis. Whereas PPIA and RPLP0 were identified as the most stable genes, followed by ACTB, HRPT1, and B2M, which were different from the geNorm results. However, HRPT1 ($M=0.706$) and B2M ($M=0.748$) should be excluded because each gene was expressed with statistically significant differences in the 50 ovarian tissues. As an alternative to HRPT1 and B2M, the NormFinder results determined that TBP ($M=0.751$) should be used as a reference gene.

Additionally, the stability of the 10 candidate genes in mucinous and serous neoplasms was also evaluated by these two programs. ACTB, PPIA, RPL13A, RPLP0, TBP, and B2M achieved high expression stability (Fig. 3B, Table 4), which suggested that they were adequate for normalizing gene expression data among ovarian serous tumors. With M values less than 1.5, HRPT1, RPL13A, ACTB, TBP, PBGD, and RPLP0 were recommended as a dependable normalizing combination for ovarian mucinous tumors (Fig. 3C, Table 5).

Discussion

Although the combination of LMD and qPCR analysis has been used in ovarian cancers for biomarker and therapeutic target identification [20,21], for the first time this combination has been employed to HKG selection for ovarian sample research. We confirmed that epithelial cells only occupied a small percentage of the normal ovary, which demonstrated the importance of LMD. From the 12 candidate reference genes we studied, the combination use of ACTB, PPIA, RPLP0, and TBP was identified as a relatively superior normalization strategy, while GAPDH was insufficient for accurate normalization when considering its overexpression in ovarian cancer. These results contribute to reliable normalized qPCR gene expression data in epithelial ovarian cancer.

In this study, we collected approximately 5000 cells from each specimen using an LMD system for RNA extraction and subsequent qPCR. To minimize RNA degradation, the LMD operation must be performed as quickly as possible [6]. Additionally, the use of staining methods that might influence tissue morphology and RNA quality was determined carefully. Cresyl violet, a hydrophilic stain that binds to negatively charged nucleic acids, is recommended as an adequate stain for the identification of target cells and RNA preservation using LMD for qPCR [6,7]. Furthermore, the RNeasy FFPE kit, which optimizes RNA isolation from microdissected FFPE tissue sections, was also used in this study. Briefly, the comprehensive use of these reagents allowed us to preserve tissue morphology, maximize RNA yield, and protect RNA integrity.

To evaluate candidate gene stability, we employed two statistical models, geNorm and NormFinder [16,19]. GeNorm identified ACTB, RPL13A, RPLP0, and PPIA as the most stably expressed reference combination in the 50 ovarian samples, while NormFinder highlighted PPIA, RPLP0, ACTB, and HRPT1, followed by B2M and TBP. Given that HRPT1 and B2M were expressed differently in the 50 specimens, which suggested that these two genes were not eligible reference genes, the combination of ACTB, RPLP0, PPIA, and TBP was recommended for use in epithelial ovarian cancer studies. Additionally, to determine the optimal number of reference genes required for normalization, geNorm defines a pairwise variation of 0.15 as the cutoff value, under which the inclusion of an additional gene is unnecessary. However, as Vandesompele *et al.* reported, the proposed 0.15 value must not be considered in a strict sense but rather as a theory guidance [16]. In the present study, the V4/5 value was 0.265, which increased when a gene was included or excluded (V3/4 = 0.29, V5/6 = 0.30). Therefore, the combination of four genes was a preferred choice for normalizing qPCR data in epithelial ovarian cancer. The selection of reference genes for mucinous and serous ovarian cancer also encountered this situation, and the same comprehensive choice was made.

Stability orders of the 10 candidate reference genes determined by NormFinder and geNorm were not completely consistent, which could be explained by the various principles used by each of them. The principle of geNorm is that the expression ratio of two ideal candidate reference genes is identical in all specimens, in spite of disease degree or experimental condition. The geNorm software is suitable for the identification of a combination of at least two genes rather than a single gene. The variation in the expression ratio of two internal control genes reveals that one or both genes is (are) not equivalently expressed, which results in increased variation in the ratio corresponding to decreased expression stability [16]. NormFinder orders the set of HKGs according to their expression stability in a given experimental design and given sample set. It estimates the expression variation of both the intra- and inter-group and provides a stability value for each candidate gene. Compared to geNorm, this applet is less affected by HKG co-regulation. Therefore, in studies with identified inconsistent results, the NormFinder program is preferred to the other programs [19]. Accordingly, in this study, TBP should be superior to RPL13A and, therefore, added into the stable combination for normalization in epithelial ovarian cancer studies.

Additionally, some similar results were attained based on the two applets we used. PPIA, ACTB, and RPLP0 were identified as the most stable genes, and GAPDH and 18S rRNA were considered to be the least stable ones in epithelial ovarian tissues. However, in previous studies [17,18], ACTB was considered as an unstable normalizer, and 18S rRNA was highlighted as a stable gene which were contrary to our results. This inconsistency is likely due to the differences in the starting materials (whole tissues vs. LMD materials) and in the composition of the samples. In addition, PPIA and the ribosomal protein gene RPLP0 were identified as the most stable reference genes in ovarian tissues by Li *et al.* and Fu *et al.*, respectively. Furthermore, in accordance with our results, Li *et al.* reported that GAPDH was significantly increased in malignant ovarian tissues. The altered expression of GAPDH was also found in other types of neoplasia, such as human glioma, atopic bronchial epithelial cells, and squamous cervical cancer [22–24].

In conclusion, for an accurate gene expression assay in ovarian tumor tissues, homogeneous tissues as starting materials and normalization based on multiple validated reference genes, such as PPIA, RPLP0, ACTB, and TBP, are recommended.

Acknowledgments

We would like to thank the Department of Obstetrics and Gynecology, Union Hospital, Wuhan, China.

Author Contributions

Conceived and designed the experiments: ZW JC. Performed the experiments: TL HC HD. Analyzed the data: JC TL BH HC WD MX. Contributed reagents/materials/analysis tools: WD LL. Wrote the paper: TL JC. Final approval of manuscript: ZW JC.

References

1. Ono K, Tanaka T, Tsunoda T, Kitahara O, Kihara C, et al. (2000) Identification by cDNA microarray of genes involved in ovarian carcinogenesis. Cancer research 60: 5007–5011.
2. Szaniszlo P, Wang N, Sinha M, Reece LM, Van Hook JW, et al. (2004) Getting the right cells to the array: Gene expression microarray analysis of cell mixtures and sorted cells. Cytometry Part A 59: 191–202.
3. Bonner RF, Emmert-Buck M, Cole K, Pohida T, Chuaqui R, et al. (1997) Laser capture microdissection: molecular analysis of tissue. Science (New York, NY) 278: 1481, 1483.
4. Suarez-Quian C, Goldstein S, Pohida T, Smith P, Peterson J, et al. (1999) Laser capture microdissection of single cells from complex tissues. Biotechniques 26: 328–335.
5. Espina V, Wulfkuhle JD, Calvert VS, VanMeter A, Zhou W, et al. (2006) Laser-capture microdissection. Nature Protocols 1: 586–603.
6. Clément-Ziza M, Munnich A, Lyonnet S, Jaubert F, Besmond C (2008) Stabilization of RNA during laser capture microdissection by performing experiments under argon atmosphere or using ethanol as a solvent in staining solutions. Rna 14: 2698–2704.
7. Golubeva Y, Salcedo R, Mueller C, Liotta LA, Espina V (2013) Laser Capture Microdissection for Protein and NanoString RNA Analysis. Cell Imaging Techniques. Springer. pp. 213–257.
8. Huggett J, Dheda K, Bustin S, Zumla A (2005) Real-time RT-PCR normalisation; strategies and considerations. Genes and immunity 6: 279–284.
9. Nolan T, Hands RE, Bustin SA (2006) Quantification of mRNA using real-time RT-PCR. Nature Protocols 1: 1559–1582.
10. Peters I, Helps C, Hall E, Day M (2004) Real-time RT-PCR: considerations for efficient and sensitive assay design. Journal of immunological methods 286: 203–217.
11. Bonefeld BE, Elfving B, Wegener G (2008) Reference genes for normalization: a study of rat brain tissue. Synapse 62: 302–309.
12. Dheda K, Huggett J, Chang J, Kim L, Bustin S, et al. (2005) The implications of using an inappropriate reference gene for real-time reverse transcription PCR data normalization. Analytical biochemistry 344: 141–143.
13. Lee JH, Fitzgerald JB, DiMicco MA, Grodzinsky AJ (2005) Mechanical injury of cartilage explants causes specific time dependent changes in chondrocyte gene expression. Arthritis & Rheumatism 52: 2386–2395.
14. Schmittgen TD, Zakrajsek BA (2000) Effect of experimental treatment on housekeeping gene expression: validation by real-time, quantitative RT-PCR. Journal of biochemical and biophysical methods 46: 69–81.
15. Selvey S, Thompson E, Matthaei K, Lea RA, Irving MG, et al. (2001) β-Actin—an unsuitable internal control for RT-PCR. Molecular and cellular probes 15: 307–311.
16. Vandesompele J, De Preter K, Pattyn F, Poppe B, Van Roy N, et al. (2002) Accurate normalization of real-time quantitative RT-PCR data by geometric averaging of multiple internal control genes. Genome biology 3: research0034.
17. Li Y-L, Ye F, Hu Y, Lu W-G, Xie X (2009) Identification of suitable reference genes for gene expression studies of human serous ovarian cancer by real-time polymerase chain reaction. Analytical biochemistry 394: 110–116.
18. Fu J, Bian L, Zhao L, Dong Z, Gao X, et al. (2010) Identification of genes for normalization of quantitative real-time PCR data in ovarian tissues. Acta biochimica et biophysica Sinica 42: 568–574.
19. Andersen CL, Jensen JL, Ørntoft TF (2004) Normalization of real-time quantitative reverse transcription-PCR data: a model-based variance estimation approach to identify genes suited for normalization, applied to bladder and colon cancer data sets. Cancer research 64: 5245–5250.
20. Flesken-Nikitin A, Choi K-C, Eng JP, Shmidt EN, Nikitin AY (2003) Induction of carcinogenesis by concurrent inactivation of p53 and Rb1 in the mouse ovarian surface epithelium. Cancer research 63: 3459–3463.
21. Kelly MG, Alvero AB, Chen R, Silasi D-A, Abrahams VM, et al. (2006) TLR-4 signaling promotes tumor growth and paclitaxel chemoresistance in ovarian cancer. Cancer research 66: 3859–3868.
22. He J-Q, Sandford AJ, Wang I-M, Stepaniants S, Knight DA, et al. (2008) Selection of housekeeping genes for real-time PCR in atopic human bronchial epithelial cells. European Respiratory Journal 32: 755–762.
23. Kreth S, Heyn J, Grau S, Kretzschmar HA, Egensperger R, et al. (2010) Identification of valid endogenous control genes for determining gene expression in human glioma. Neuro-oncology 12: 570–579.
24. Zhou J, Cai J, Huang Z, Ding H, Wang J, et al. (1899) Proteomic identification of target proteins following Drosha knockdown in cervical cancer. Oncology Reports 2013 doi: 10.3892/or. 2013. 2672

12

Somatic Mutations Favorable to Patient Survival Are Predominant in Ovarian Carcinomas

Wensheng Zhang[1], Andrea Edwards[1], Erik Flemington[2]*, Kun Zhang[1]*

1 Department of Computer Science, Xavier University of Louisiana, New Orleans, Louisiana, United States of America, 2 Tulane Cancer Center, Tulane School of Medicine, New Orleans, Louisiana, United States of America

Abstract

Somatic mutation accumulation is a major cause of abnormal cell growth. However, some mutations in cancer cells may be deleterious to the survival and proliferation of the cancer cells, thus offering a protective effect to the patients. We investigated this hypothesis via a unique analysis of the clinical and somatic mutation datasets of ovarian carcinomas published by the Cancer Genome Atlas. We defined and screened 562 macro mutation signatures (MMSs) for their associations with the overall survival of 320 ovarian cancer patients. Each MMS measures the number of mutations present on the member genes (except for TP53) covered by a specific Gene Ontology (GO) term in each tumor. We found that somatic mutations favorable to the patient survival are predominant in ovarian carcinomas compared to those indicating poor clinical outcomes. Specially, we identified 19 (3) predictive MMSs that are, usually by a nonlinear dose-dependent effect, associated with good (poor) patient survival. The false discovery rate for the 19 "positive" predictors is at the level of 0.15. The GO terms corresponding to these MMSs include "lysosomal membrane" and "response to hypoxia", each of which is relevant to the progression and therapy of cancer. Using these MMSs as features, we established a classification tree model which can effectively partition the training samples into three prognosis groups regarding the survival time. We validated this model on an independent dataset of the same disease (Log-rank p-value $<2.3\times10^{-4}$) and a dataset of breast cancer (Log-rank p-value $<9.3\times10^{-3}$). We compared the GO terms corresponding to these MMSs and those enriched with expression-based predictive genes. The analysis showed that the GO term pairs with large similarity are mainly pertinent to the proteins located on the cell organelles responsible for material transport and waste disposal, suggesting the crucial role of these proteins in cancer mortality.

Editor: Shannon M. Hawkins, Baylor College of Medicine, United States of America

Funding: Research reported in this publication was supported by a National Institutes of Health grant (NIGMS-2G12MD007595), an US Department of Army grant (W911NF-12-1-0066) and a seed grant from the Louisiana Cancer Research Consortium. The funders had no role in study design, data collection and analysis, decision to publish, or preparation of the manuscript.

Competing Interests: The authors have declared that no competing interests exist.

* Email: eflemin@tulane.edu (EF); kzhang@xula.edu (KZ)

Introduction

Ovarian cancer is the fifth-leading cause of cancer death among women in the United States [1]. The disease is often called a "silent killer" since its occurrence is usually not detected until an advanced stage. About 70% of the deaths occur in patients with advanced-stage, high-grade serous ovarian carcinomas [2]. The mortality has not been significantly improved in the past three decades [3]. Except for the detection delay and inaccessible location of the ovaries, other factors accounting for the persistent mortality include the poor understanding of the underlying biology and a lack of reliable biomarkers [4].

The formation of tumors largely results from cell growth that gets out of control [5]. In the human genome, there are many different types of genes that control cell growth in a very systematic, precise way. When these genes have an error in their DNA codes, the RNA or proteins that they encode may not function properly. Typically, a series of several mutations to certain classes of genes is usually required before a normal cell will transform into a cancer cell [6]. Nevertheless, some observed mutations may be neutral or even beneficial to patient survival. This perception can be considered from at least two perspectives. First, some mutations may be deleterious to the growth and proliferation of cancer cells, thus offering a protective mechanism to the patients. Second, some mutations may include the actual causal factors for relatively less-malignant subtypes of the same disease. For example, previous studies showed that cases with BRCA1/2 mutations have better overall survival than those with wild type BRCA1/2 in patients with ovarian carcinoma [7,8].

To date, the Cancer Genome Atlas (TCGA) [9] has generated and released comprehensive genomic, epigenomic and proteomic data of clinically annotated high-grade serous ovarian carcinomas (Ov-HGSCs). These rich data provide an unprecedented opportunity to investigate the genetic mechanisms underlying the variance in the survival of cancer patients and to advance the clinical prognosis and therapy of the disease. Besides the BRCA1/2 genotypes, the TCGA ovarian cancer paper [7] showed that gene expression-based sample clusters are also associated with the survival outcomes. Moreover, recent years have witnessed numerous studies that focus on the re-analysis of the TCGA data.

In these works, miscellaneous predictive signatures for survival outcomes have been identified. These signatures include the expression measures of coding and miRNA genes [10], genotypes of germline single-nucleotide polymorphisms (SNPs) [11], methylation patterns of genes in key cancer pathways [12], DNA copy number variations (CNV) [13] and the occurrences of chromosome aberrations [14].

As shown in [7], most of the Ov-HGSCs had 8 to 209 somatic mutations. These mutations, detected by exome sequencing, were present in 8945 genes, and 92% of them were validated by experiments using alternative technologies. However, most of the observed variants may be passenger mutations not involved in the formation and progression of ovarian cancer. Hidden among observed mutations are the individual-specific tumor drivers and the genetic alterations positively or adversely impacting the growth and survival of cancer cells. The identification of the clinically important mutations (genes) is far from completed. A major challenge impeding the effective statistical analysis of the somatic mutation spectrum (SMS) is the data sparseness issue. This is particularly implied by the fact that, among the 510 consensus cancer genes collected in the Catalogue Of Somatic Mutations In Cancer database [15], only six are significant in terms of their mutation frequencies over the 326 tumors. Nevertheless, two recent studies have demonstrated the potential to train a predictive model for survival outcomes of ovarian cancer patients using SMS [16,17]. In this study, we conducted a unique analysis of the recently updated TCGA's clinical and SMS datasets of ovarian cancer. Our study provides significant insights into the treatment of ovarian cancer and may open novel avenues for molecular prognosis and prediction.

Results

Predictive macro mutation signatures for patient survival

We developed a novel method to unravel the relationships between the somatic mutations and the survival time of cancer patients. First, by assuming that the DNA alterations on the genes of a similar function may have equivalent or complementary impacts on the growth and proliferation of cancer cells, we defined 562 macro mutation signatures (MMS), each of which corresponds to a highly-specific Gene Ontology (GO) term with 50 to 500 member genes. For each patient (i.e. a carcinoma sample), the MMS quantities were calculated as the number of the mutations on the genes (except for TP53) covered by the cognate GO term. When a gene involves in multiple GO terms, the mutation(s) present on each gene were counted with respect to each cognate MMS. In this way, we circumvented the sparsity issue inherent to the raw somatic mutation data (see Introduction section). After that, the MMSs were screened for their associations with the overall survival (OS) months of the cancer patients. More specifically, the associations were evaluated by performing the Log-rank test and Cox Proportional Hazards (Cox-PH) regression analysis on the mutation and clinical datasets of 320 training samples. In the implementation, quantities of the MMSs were capped by a ceiling value of 2, which represented that a tumor had at least two mutations present on the member genes covered by the corresponding GO term. Capping the MMS values was performed to alleviate the influence of leverage data points, which were related to un-ordinarily high MMS values and usually occurred in highly-specific GO terms. In the Cox-PH analysis, along with a focused MMS, the ages of the patients at the initial diagnosis and a binary measurement variable indicating the presence of somatic mutation on TP53 gene, which had a modestly significant ($p<0.05$) effect on the patient survival as shown in our preliminary analysis of the same data, were included as covariates. In the Log-rank test, the three possible values (0, 1, 2) of a specific MMS were factorized as the indicators of three groups.

The analysis of the training set ($N = 320$) demonstrated strong evidence for the existence of an association between the MMSs and survival outcomes. As shown in Figure 1-A and 1-B, the distributional profiles of the p-values (from both the Log-rank test and Cox-PH regression) for the MMSs are deviated from a uniform distribution U (0, 1). Interestingly, most of the regression coefficients (i.e., beta values), especially those corresponding to small p-values, are negative (Figure 1-C). In the Cox-PH model, a negative regression coefficient indicates that the hazard function decreases (or equivalently, survival time increases) as the quantity of the corresponding predictive variable increases [18]. In this regard, we concluded that somatic mutations favorable to the survival of cancer patients are predominant in ovarian carcinoma compared to those indicating poor clinical outcomes. As shown in Figure 1-D and 1-E, this statement is also valid in terms of the number of the involved GO terms and the sizes of the relevant gene sets (Table S1).

Neither Log-rank test nor Cox-PH regression analysis are perfect for evaluating the associations between a MMS and the clinical outcome. The former ignores the patients' ages at the initial diagnosis, which intuitively influence survival time. The latter assumes that the quantity of the hazard functions is linearly dependent on the preprocessed MMS values, which is not true in many cases. Therefore, we determined the top significant MMSs (GO terms) by an alternative method. That is, we selected 20 MMSs if (1) their p-values from both the Log-rank test and Cox-PH analysis are less than 0.05 and (2) the resulting composite p-value (see Method section) is less than 0.025. Among those MMSs, 19 are "positive" predictors for survival time. Considering that the selection criteria may be too stringent for the potential MMSs adversely affecting overall survival outcomes, we chose another two MMSs. These two "negative" predictors, with Log-rank p-values less than 0.01, are relevant to two small patient sets of poor survival and correspond to GO:0045666 and GO:0042393, respectively. In this way, we established a predictor set consisting of 22 MMSs (Table 1).

We addressed the multiple-testing problem in the identification of predictive MMSs for patient survival by calculating false discovery rate (FDR) with a permutation-based algorithm (see Material and Methods section). In the implementation, we considered not only the skewness of the distribution of the effect parameters estimated from the original datasets (Figure 1C), but also the asymmetry of their null distribution established from the randomly permutated datasets (Figure S1). Because only one negative predictor (MMS) was rigorously selected, the analysis was focused on the 19 MMSs associated with good clinical outcomes. The result showed that, when those MMSs are stated to be significant, the FDR could be controlled at the level of 0.15.

Based on the definitions, we partition the cognate GO terms of the 19 positive predictors (MMSs) into six groups: (1) the gene products (proteins) locate in the cell organelles (membrane) responsible for waste disposal (lysosome) and material transport (recycling endosome); (2) the gene products locate in the sub-cellular structures playing roles in mitosis (nucleosome, spindle pole, centrosome); (3) the gene products perform function in cell division (mitosis and cytokinesis); (4) the gene products are involved in cellular responses to nutrient and hypoxia; (5) the gene products play roles in cancer pathways (integrin-mediated signaling pathway and positive regulation of ERK1 and ERK2 cascade); and (6) others. Numerous records regarding those GO

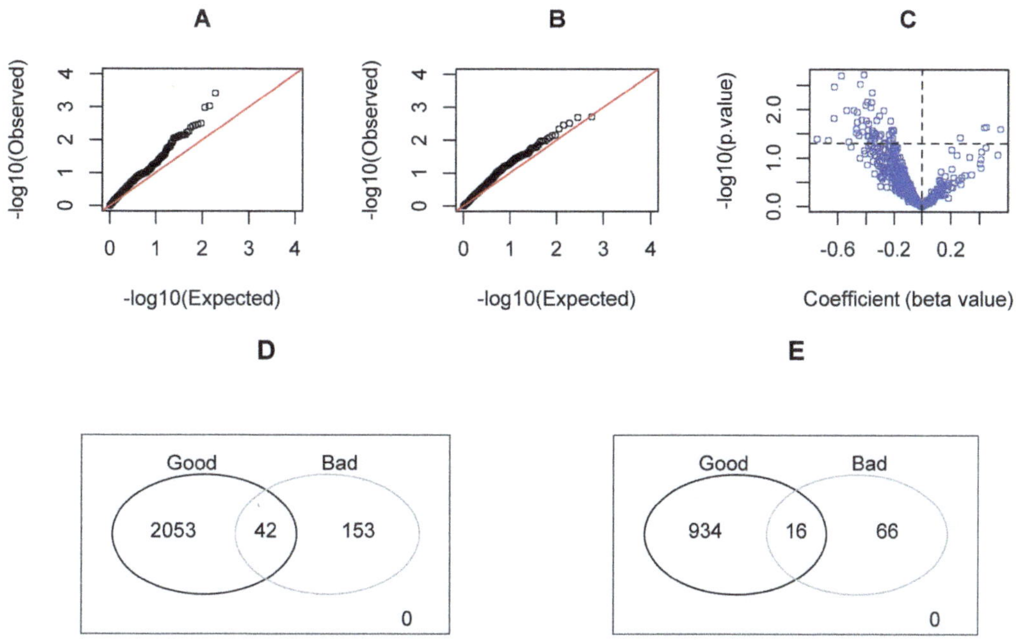

Figure 1. The profile for the associations between the somatic mutations and survival time of patients with ovarian cancer. A (B): The Q-Q plot of the p-values from Log-rank test (Cox-PH regression) for the 562 considered MMSs. C: The volcano plot of the Cox-PH p-values and regression coefficients for the 562 considered MMSs. The horizontal dot line marks p = 0.05. D: The Venn diagram for the entire set of genes covered by the 22 selected MMSs. Specifically, the good (bad) genes are the genes involved in the GO terms corresponding to the 19 (3) positive (negative) MMSs which predict good (poor) clinical outcomes. A gene can belong to both the positive and negative MMSs, therefore may be double counted. E: The Venn diagram for the subset of the genes which are covered by the 22 selected MMSs. Each of the genes has the mutation burden in at least one training sample.

terms' relevance to the formation, progression and therapy of tumors can be located in the literature (see Discussion section).

By looking into the Kaplan-Meier survival curves, we found a "dose-effect" relationship between the somatic mutations and survival outcomes. That is, for a specific GO term, a single mutation on the member genes usually does not make much difference to the patient survival time but two or multiple mutations do (Figure 2).

Robustness analysis of the selected predictors

In order to test the robustness of our main result, we randomly split the 320 training samples into two equal-size subsets, and estimated the effects of the 22 predictive signatures on each subset separately. The result showed that the sign (positive or negative) of the estimated regression coefficients of hazard functions on the MMSs were consistent with those estimated using the entire training set (upper left plot of Figure S2).

We further tested if each of the 22 selected MMSs can individually predict the survival of cancer patients in the validation set. The results showed that, just the predictors ranked at the second, third and fifth places had a marginally significant p-value (upper right and bottom plots of Figure S2). While this analysis only provided a minor support to our findings in the last subsection, the result is aligned to our expectation. This is because the insufficiencies of the training set, i.e. the small sample size (N = 140) and un-validated mutations, could lead to a lower statistical power.

A classification tree model for patient survival prediction

The findings presented above inspired us to build a classification tree to predict the patient survival using the 22 identified MMSs. More specifically, based on the measures of all three negative predictors, we can separate a poor-prognosis group from the entire set of training samples whose members meet $\max^{j} (N_j^i) \geq 2$, where N_j^i indicates the value of the jth negative MMS on the ith sample. Then, based on the values of the top k positive predictors and the same criterion, i.e. $\max^{k} (P_k^i) \geq 2$ with P_k^i indicating the value of the jth positive MMS on the ith sample, a good-prognosis group can be split from the remaining samples that constitute an intermediate-prognosis group. See Figure S3 for an illustration. The threshold for the combined MMS values in the partition was heuristically chosen according to the pattern of dose-dependent effect of several MMSs of high interest to patient survival, as showed in Figure 2 and described in the ending paragraph of the first result subsection.

As shown in Figure 3, the patient groups generated by the tree model are significantly differentiated with respect to the times of overall survival (OS) and progression-free survival (PFS). Regardless of the k value (5 or 10), the Log-rank test p-value is less than 1.2×10^{-10} for OS and is less than 1.6×10^{-7} for PFS. From the Kaplan-Meier survival curves, we found that, for the poor-prognosis group, the upper limits of OS and PFS are 50 and 20 months, respectively. They are also the time points when the differences in the survival probabilities between the good-prognosis group and intermediate prognosis group become sharper. It is worth noting that, the choice of k value is somewhat arbitrary. The value determines the size of the predicted good-prognosis group that has a better survival curve compared to the intermediate-prognosis group. Therefore, a prior knowledge about the proportion of good-prognosis samples would help with the specification of k value.

Table 1. The summary of significant MMSs for the overall survival of patients with Ov-HGSCs.

GO (MMS) ID	β	Cox-PH p-value	Log-rank p-value	CP	N1	N2	GO Name
Positive predictors							
GO:0000786	−0.67	4.4E-02	4.3E-05	1.4E-03	65	25	nucleosome
GO:0005765	−0.28	1.1E-02	3.7E-04	2.0E-03	232	135	lysosomal membrane
GO:0050900	−0.42	1.9E-03	3.8E-03	2.7E-03	110	92	leukocyte migration
GO:0007229	−0.44	3.0E-03	8.0E-03	4.9E-03	77	80	integrin-mediated signaling pathway
GO:0010923	−0.54	1.1E-02	3.1E-03	5.7E-03	51	49	negative regulation of phosphatase activity
GO:0007584	−0.63	3.4E-03	1.1E-02	6.1E-03	67	54	response to nutrient
GO:0007067	−0.36	4.5E-03	8.5E-03	6.2E-03	245	126	mitosis
GO:0007160	−0.41	8.2E-03	7.0E-03	7.6E-03	79	75	cell-matrix adhesion
GO:0000910	−0.58	2.0E-03	3.0E-02	7.8E-03	64	54	cytokinesis
GO:0006928	−0.49	1.0E-02	5.9E-03	7.8E-03	97	60	cellular component movement
GO:0001666	−0.31	1.4E-02	7.4E-03	1.0E-02	153	115	response to hypoxia
GO:0000922	−0.39	7.0E-03	1.6E-02	1.1E-02	86	77	spindle pole
GO:0031965	−0.33	1.7E-02	8.6E-03	1.2E-02	162	108	nuclear membrane
GO:0005813	−0.21	2.6E-02	7.4E-03	1.4E-02	353	165	centrosome
GO:0004674	−0.23	1.7E-02	1.3E-02	1.5E-02	374	217	protein serine/threonine kinase activity
GO:0070374	−0.36	3.1E-02	9.1E-03	1.7E-02	97	57	positive regulation of ERK1 and ERK2 cascade
GO:0044325	−0.37	9.1E-03	3.5E-02	1.8E-02	71	87	ion channel binding
GO:0055037	−0.63	1.5E-02	2.7E-02	2.0E-02	60	37	recycling endosome
GO:0004843	−0.46	1.8E-02	2.9E-02	2.3E-02	55	39	ubiquitin-specific protease activity
Negative predictors							
GO:0051436	0.55	2.5E-02	1.0E-03	5.1E-03	65	27	negative regulation of ubiquitin-protein ligase activity involved in mitotic cell cycle
GO:0045666	0.15	4.0E-01	3.6E-03	3.8E-02	68	50	positive regulation of neuron differentiation
GO:0042393	0.17	3.6E-01	7.1E-03	5.0E-02	62	47	histone binding

β: the regression coefficients estimated by the Cox-PH model. **CP**: the composite p-value, which is the square root of the product of the Log-rank test p-value and the corresponding Cox-PH p-value. **N1**: the number of member genes covered by the corresponding MMS or GO term. **N2**: the number of mutated member genes present in at least one training sample. Note that a single gene can be covered by more than one GO term.

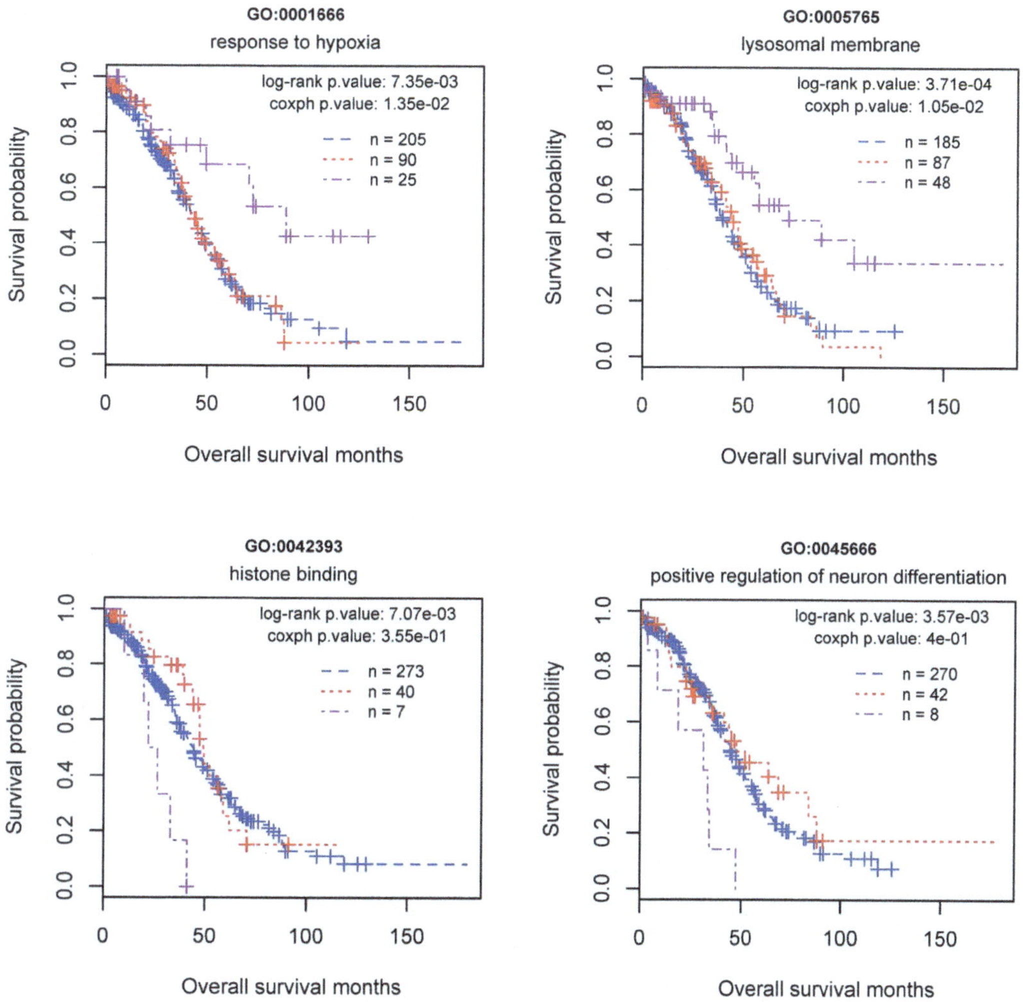

Figure 2. The illustration of the dose-dependent effect of somatic mutations on survival outcomes. Each plot demonstrates the relationship between the overall survival months and a specific macro mutation signature (MMS) that corresponds to a GO term. The purple curve represents the patients each of whom has at least two somatic mutations on the member genes of the indicated MMS (i.e., GO term). The red curve represents the patients each of whom has one somatic mutation on the member genes of the indicated MMS. The blue curve represents the patients without any somatic mutation on the member genes of the indicated MMS.

Model validation using independent datasets

We validated the tree model by applying it to an independent dataset of Ov-HGSCs. As shown in Figure 4, the survival curves of the patients in the three (good-, poor- and intermediate-prognosis) groups resemble those observed for the training set. The group effect on overall survival time is significant (Log-rank test p-value <0.001). When k is 5, the good prognosis group in this validation set has the same OS survival probability (~30%) as that in the training samples. Moreover, interestingly, although the underlying negative predictors are not defined on a stringent statistical criterion, both the survival profile of the poor-prognosis group and the patient percentage ($5/140 = 3.8\%$) of in this group are similar to those ($14/320 = 4.5\%$) of the training set. It is worthy of note that, in the TCGA database, the observed somatic mutations of the samples in the validation set have not been confirmed by other methods yet. The average number of mutations in this set is approximately 80, much higher than those (~50 observed and ~46 validated) of the training set. Hereby, the classification results are more sensitive to the number of used predictors.

Recent studies showed that the formation of ovarian tumors shares common cancer drivers with breast tumors. We assume that these two diseases may be similar regarding the biological mechanisms underlying the variance in the patient survival time. We look into this issue by applying the identified predictors for Ov-HGSCs to the TCGA data of invasive breast carcinomas. As shown in Figure 5, we can identify a good-prognosis group using the top positive predictors but cannot separate a poor-prognosis group via the negative predictors. The difference in the survival probability between the good-prognosis patents and other patients becomes evident at the point of 75 months, 25 months more than the time for ovarian carcinomas.

Comparison between mutation signatures and expression signatures

By analyzing the TCGA clinical and mRNA expression data of Ov-HGSCs, we identified 333 expression predictors (genes) for the overall survival time of patients with the p-values less than 0.01. 28 functionally specific non-redundant GO terms, either at level-4 or level-5 as categorized by DAVID [19], were over-represented

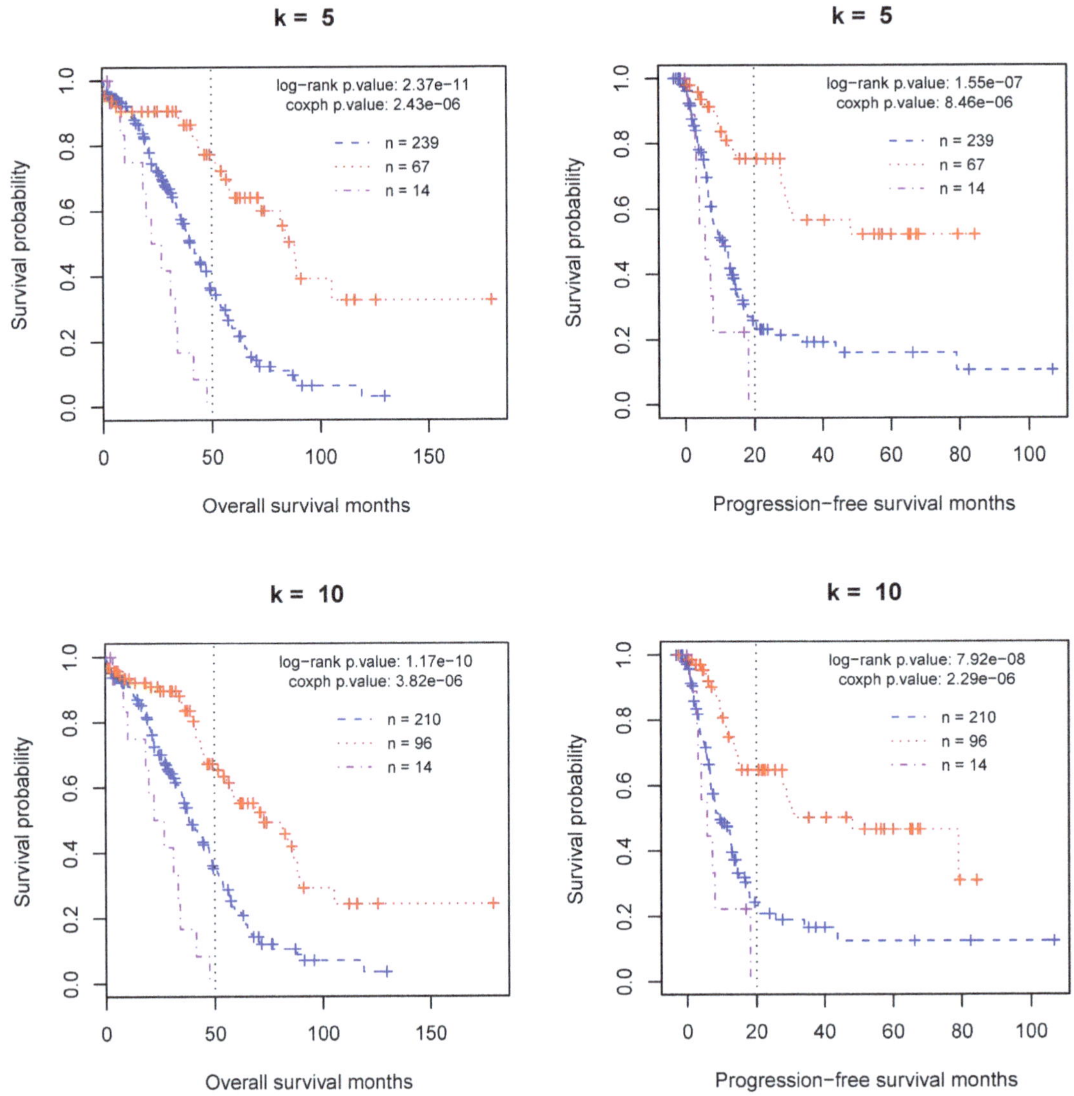

Figure 3. The classification of the training set of ovarian cancer patients by the proposed tree model. In each plot, the considered predictors include all three negative MMSs and the most significant (or top) *k* (5 or 10) positive MMSs as summarized in Table 1. The purple, red and blue curves represent the predicted poor, good, and intermediate-prognosis groups, respectively.

(FDR <0.1) by these genes. Hereafter, we named those 28 GO terms macro expression signatures (MESs). The matrix of the semantic similarity between the MESs and macro mutation signatures (MMSs), i.e. the GO terms corresponding to the 22 significant MMSs, was evaluated using the algorithm documented in [20]. As shown in Figure 6, the similarity coefficients are low in general. Four MES::MMS pairs have the coefficients over 0.5. They are: GO:0005788 (endoplasmic reticulum lumen) versus GO:0055037 (recycling endosome); GO:0005788 versus GO:0005665 (lysosomal membrane); GO:0051427 (human receptor binding) versus GO:00044325 (ion channel binding), GO:0051427 versus GO:0042393 (histone binding). Moreover, five MESs, relevant to the regulation of cellular process and cell death, show modest levels of similarity to seven MMSs, which correspond to some specific molecular functions and biological processes including integrin-mediated signaling pathway (GO:0007229) and positive regulation of ERK1 and ERK2 cascade (GO:0070374). These results suggest that: (1) only several survival-relevant somatic mutations impact the clinical outcomes via the modification of the expression level of the host genes; and (2) the proteins located on the cell organelles responsible for material transport and waste disposal may be crucial for the survival of cancer patients in that both the modification of properties (due to a non-synonymous mutation) and the change of expression level in cancer cells can significantly influence the clinical outcomes.

Discussion

Over the last few decades, cancer researchers have pinpointed hundreds of cancer genes [21,22], including oncogenes and cancer suppressor genes, and established a number of DNA-alteration based theories for carcinogenesis [5,23]. Nevertheless, the genetic determination of survival outcomes for patients with malignant tumors has been less investigated yet. By analyzing 320 ovarian tumor samples, we found that somatic mutations favorable to the patient survival are predominant in ovarian carcinoma compared to those indicating poor clinical outcomes. This observation

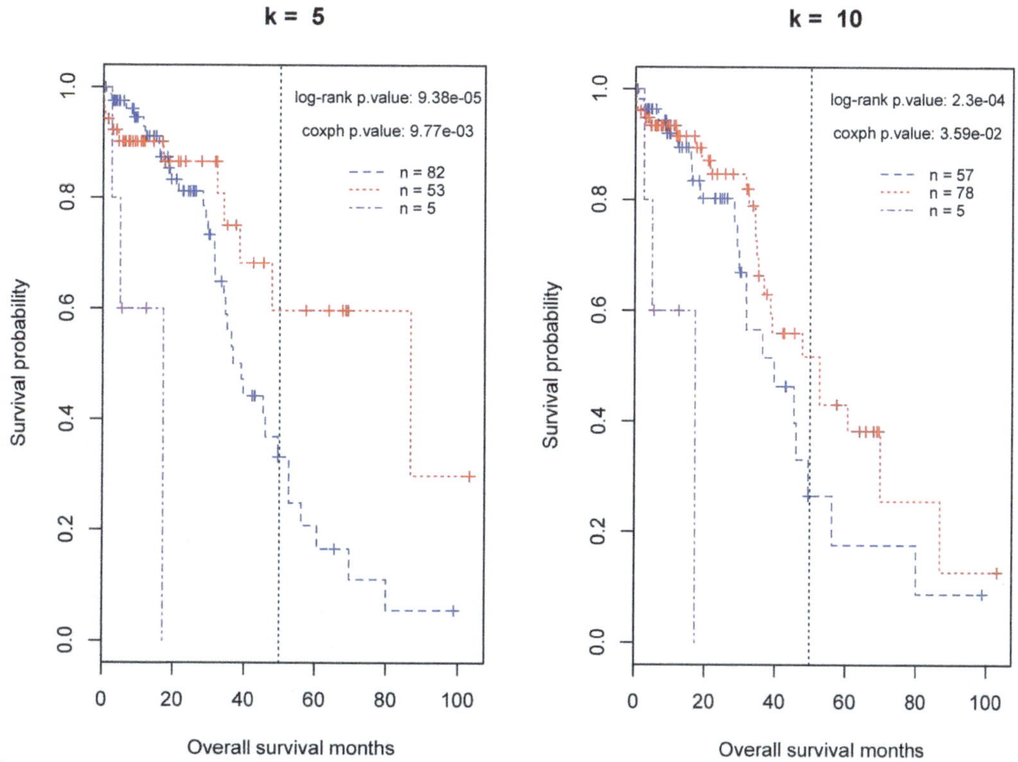

Figure 4. The classification of the validation set of ovarian cancer patients by the proposed tree model. In each plot, the considered predictors include all three negative MMSs and the most significant (or top) *k* (5 or 10) positive MMSs as summarized in Table 1. The purple, red and blue curves represent the predicted poor, good, and intermediate-prognosis groups, respectively.

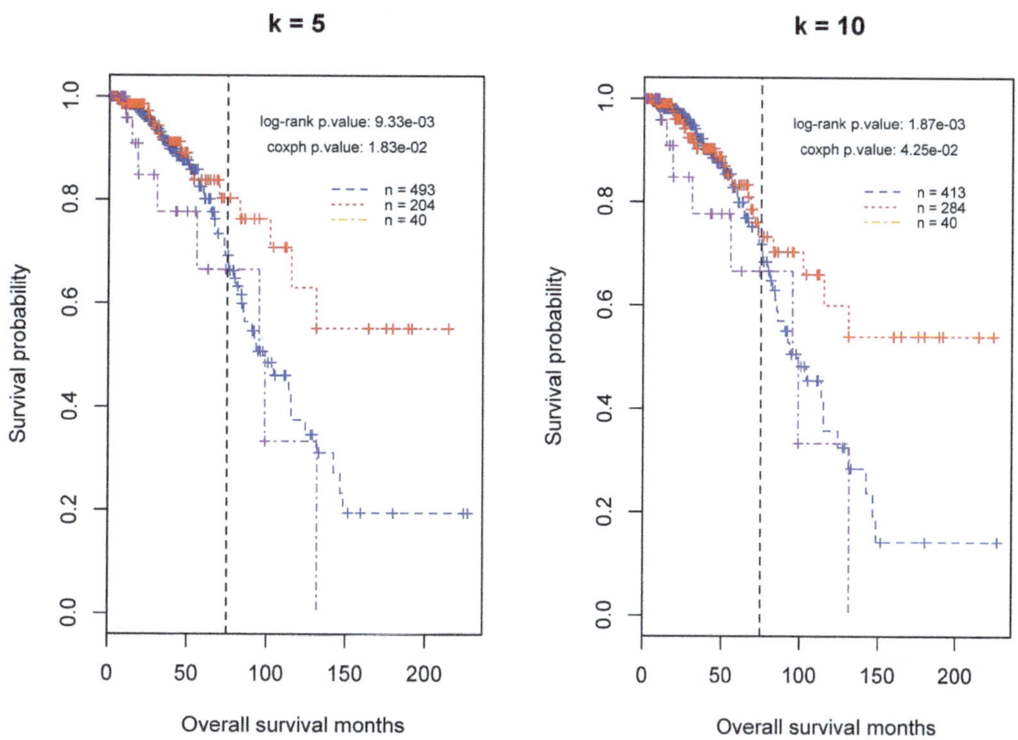

Figure 5. The classification of breast cancer patients by the proposed tree model. In each plot, the considered predictors include all three negative MMSs and the most significant (or top) *k* (5 or 10) positive MMSs as summarized in Table 1. The purple, red and blue curves represent the predicted poor, good, and intermediate-prognosis groups, respectively.

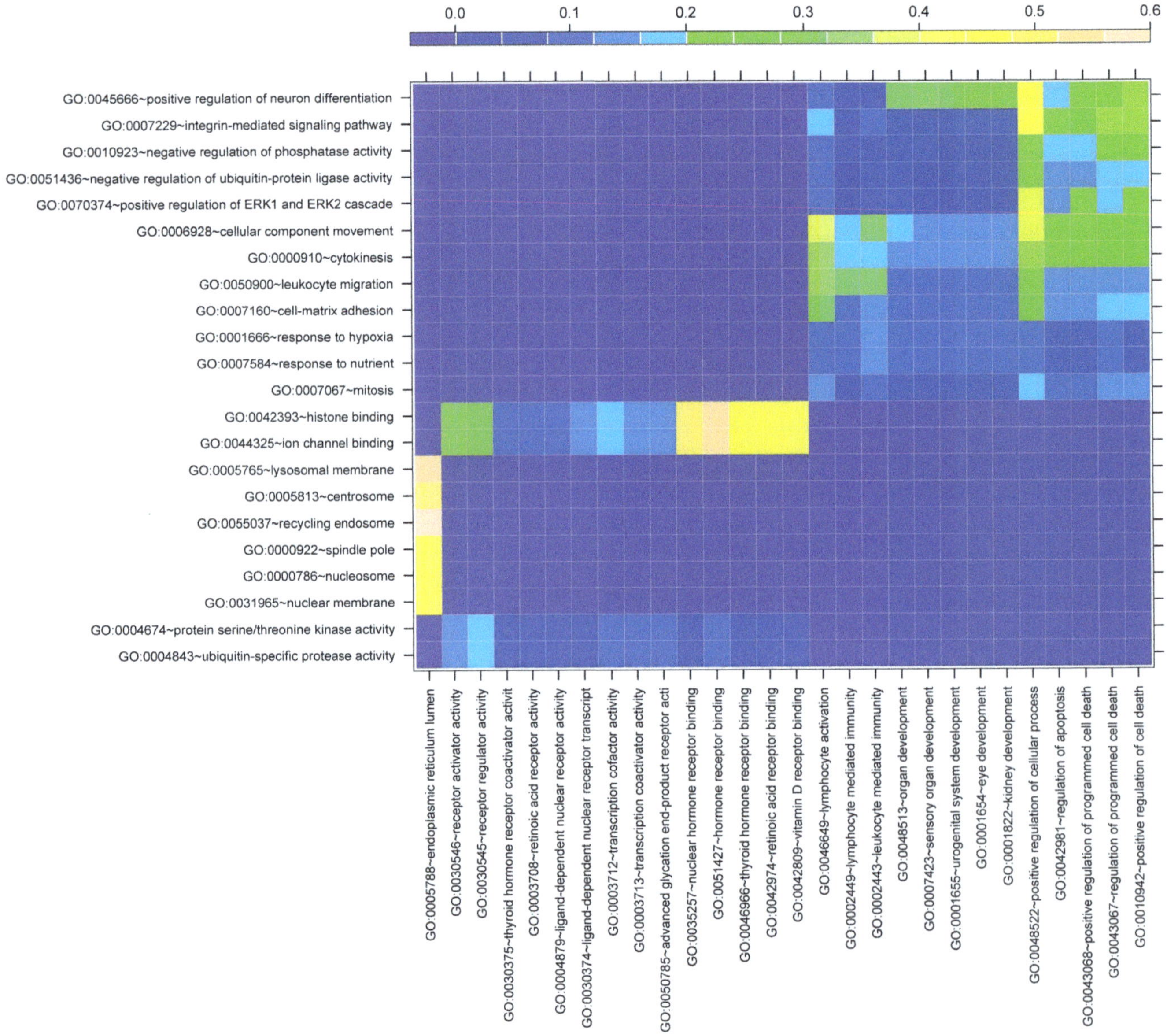

Figure 6. The visualization of the semantic similarity between the MESs and MMSs. The similarity is measured by a coefficient in the range of 0 to 1. 1 is the theoretical maximum of the similarity coefficient. For the GO term pairs considered here, the values are consistently less than 0.6.

highlights the vulnerability of cancer cells to "extra" mutations. That is, while the cancer-driver mutations prompt cancer cells to divide in an uncontrolled way or offer them selection advantage over the adjacent normal cells, the extra mutations may restrict the continuous proliferation in certain microenvironments. When the restriction occurs in some important organs such as liver and spleen, where ovarian metastases usually lead to mortality, the extra mutations may benefit the patient survival. Such a mechanism can be elucidated by a further scrutiny of our results. For example, among the predictive MMSs identified for good prognosis, there is one that measures the mutation events occurring on the genes involved in the biological process of "response to hypoxia" [24]. It is well known that the activation of anaerobic glycolysis (the Warburg effect) provides most of the building blocks required to duplicate the cellular components of a dividing cell; therefore, it is also essential for carcinogenesis [25,26]. If the properties of one or multiple protein(s) involved in anaerobic glycolysis are altered, the tumors may lose the ability to produce enough energy for maintaining their growth. As a result, the carcinogenesis can be retarded.

On the other hand, in many cases, cancer cells acquire mutations to constitutively activate their survival pathway and to develop chemo-resistance. This mechanism seems to cast a shadow on our explanation to the main conclusion of this study. However, the dilemma could be resolved to some extent if we assume that only a few new driver mutations occur as the responses to the treatments. This assumption is supported by our preliminary analysis which showed that the average numbers of somatic mutations in Ov-HGSCs don't substantially increase across the development stages (from II to IV).

Our analysis suggests that the proteins located on the cell organelles responsible for material transport and waste disposal bear a special importance for cancer mortality since both the modification of properties (due to a non-synonymous mutation) and the change of expression level in cancer cells can significantly impact the clinical outcomes. In particular, the identified predictors for good clinical outcomes include the MMS corresponding to the cell component GO term "lysosomal membrane". This result provides the genetic insight into and clinical support for a promising cancer therapy strategy, in which the lysomoses of cancer cells can be treated as the drug targets. The strategy arose from the perception that the altered lysosomal trafficking and increased expression of the lysosomal proteases termed cathepsins may form an "Achilles heel" for cancer cells by sensitizing them to death pathways involving lysosomal membrane permeabilization and the release of cathepsins into the cytosol [27,28,29,30]. A recent study on the screening of a small molecule drug library provided strong evidence for this mechanism. The authors found that over half of the 11 compounds that induced significant cell death in p53-null colon cancer cells triggered lysosomal membrane permeabilization and cathepsin-mediated killing of tumor cells [31]. We speculate that these compounds may functionally resemble the mutations present on the genes related to lysosomal membrane. We further surmise that, for an ovarian cancer patient with a single mutation on the lysosomal membrane related genes, an additional functional disruption of these genes caused by the anti-cancer compounds (or by other treatments) may offer the patient a better chance for survival, which is similar to those patients denoted by the purple curve in the upper right plot of Figure 2.

Resistance to apoptosis and chemotherapy is a critical factor in cancer recurrence and patient relapse. Several studies over the last decade have demonstrated that ECM/integrin signaling provides a survival advantage to various cancer cell types against numerous chemotherapeutic drugs and against antibody/radiotherapy therapy [32,33,34]. Our result implies that such an advantage for cancer cells can be interrupted by the mutations occurred on the cognate genes. As shown in Table 1, the MMS corresponding to the biological process of "integrin-mediated signaling pathway" is a positive predictor for the survival time of Ov-HGSC patients. Furthermore, we find that the mutations on the genes that positively regulate ERK1/2 cascade [35] can be deleterious to the continuous proliferation of cancer cells in the sense that the patients with such mutations had a longer survival time. These observations suggest that even the mutations whose host genes play a role in a cancer pathway may benefit the survival of cancer patients.

Another novel finding from this study is the dose-dependent effect of somatic mutations on survival outcomes. In light of this observation, we established a classification tree model to predict the survival profiles of the Ov-HGSC patients. The model is robust and performs comparably to the classifiers created using gene expression and other -omic data [10,11,12,13,36]. The phenomenon that a single mutation does not make much difference to a biological process but two (or multiple) mutations do may be explained by genome evolution. That is, evolution often created "backup" genes (or gene fragments) that perform the normal functions of a specific gene (or gene fragment) and a biological aberration occurs only when both the gene (or fragment) and its backups are altered [37,38]. In fact, this mechanism may explain why the formation and malignancy of cancer require multiple mutations. To clarify this point, it is worth noting that a lethal biological aberration for tumor cells can imply a favorable change for the cancer patients and vice versa.

The proposed classification method can be implemented in a flexible way. For example, using the MMS corresponding to the GO term "histone binding" as the only predictor, a group of seven patients whose overall survival time is consistently less than 50 months can be identified from the Ov-HGSC training samples (Figure 2: bottom left plot). Each of these poor-survival patients has a short list of "lethal" mutations. Specifically, for the first sample of this group, there are three lethal mutations present on the genes NOC2L, CHD8 and CHAF1B. For the other six samples, the host genes of the lethal mutations are (L3MBTL2, L3MBTL2, L3MBTL2), (UIMC1, RNF20), (UIMC1, RNF20), (HJURP, NCAPD2), (NASP, PKN1), (MCM2, NCAPD2), respectively. Among the eleven member genes, three have been identified as prognostic indicators of breast or gastric cancers in previous studies. The evidences include: overexpression of MCM2 in gastric tumors predicted poor prognosis in the patients [39]; knock down of HJURP reduced the sensitivity of breast cancer patients to radiation treatment [40]; the loss of CHD8 may be an indicator for biological aggressiveness in gastric cancer [41]. Another two, i.e. UIMC1and CHAF1B, are cancer-relevant. The former codes BRCA1-A subunit RAP80 [42], a protein important for genomic stability [43]. The latter codes the chromatin assembly factor-1/p60, a proliferation marker in various malignant tumors with prognostic value in renal, endometrial and cervical carcinomas [44]. Therefore, further investigation on the functions and interaction of the proteins coded by these genes may facilitate the inference of the personalized mechanisms for the mortality of ovarian carcinomas.

Recent studies found cancer-driving changes shared across tumor types [45]. A well-known hallmark is the genetic similarity between breast cancer and ovarian cancer. For example, the major driver genes BRCA1/2 for breast cancer are frequently (10~20%) mutated in the cancer cells of the patients with ovarian tumors [7]. Moreover, somatic mutations on TP53 (a major cancer driver gene in Ov-HGSCs) have been observed in the breast cancer samples of all subtypes, including luminal A, B, basal-like, and Her2-enriched [46]. Interestingly, we found that the top predictive MMSs identified using the clinical data and SMS of Ov-HGSC can predict the survival time of breast cancer patients. However, the three predictors for poor-prognostic outcomes of ovarian cancer are invalid when applied to breast cancer. Intuitively, more significant predictive macro signatures for breast cancer could be identified using the information of the patients of the same disease but this work is out of our scope.

To date, survival prediction using the gene expression signatures for breast or ovarian cancer patients has been the subject of much research [47,48,49,50,51,52,53]. However, most of the reported predictive expression signatures cannot be consistently validated by the analysis on the independent datasets (cohorts) [54]. Our comparative analysis suggests that only a few survival-related somatic mutations impact the clinical outcomes by modifying the expression level of the host genes. A potential reason for the robustness deficiency in the expression-based prognostic signatures is the temporal and/or spatial gap between the sampling of the disease tissue and the occurrence of the lethal metastasis of cancer cells. We speculate that mutation prognostic signatures, such as those we identified, have an advantage over an expression-based signature in the sense that they are less likely subject to progression history and location transition of cancer cells.

At last, we note that there are some uncertainties in our results. First, a few genes (N = 16), such as FN1, are involved in both positive and negative predictors for patient survival. Those genes account for 1.6% (16/1016) of all the genes which have at least one mutation in the training set and are covered by the 22 significant MMSs. Second, the false discovery rate of the predictive MMSs is slightly high (at the level of 0.15 for the 19 MMSs associated with good clinical incomes). In other words, a small portion of those MMSs might be falsely identified.

Nevertheless, these issues are relatively minor to affect our conclusions regarding the predominance of somatic mutations favorable to patient survival and the prognostic usefulness of the identified predictive MMSs as a whole.

Material and Methods

Somatic mutation dataset for Ov-HGSC training samples (Data-1)

The dataset of 321 tumor samples was generated from three *mat*-format files (version 2.4)in the TCGA database [9]. The archives containing these files are *"broad.mit.edu_OV.IlluminaGA_DNASeq.Level_2.100.1.0"*, *"hgsc.bcm.edu_OV.SOLiD_DNASeq.Level_2.1.6.0"*, and *"genome.wustl.edu_OV.IlluminaGA_DNASeq.Level_2.1.3.0"*, respectively. Among the total 16306 mutations identified by exome-sequencing, 14960 have been validated using other methods and were used in our study. Most validated mutations belong to four single nucleotide mutation categories, namely missense_mutation (68.09%), silence (21.39%), nonsense_mutation (4.26%) and splice_site (2.20%). Among them, 257 validated mutations occurred on the gene TP53 of 225 samples. The cancer samples contained in this dataset were also used in [7]. There is a trivial difference between the SMS analyzed in our study and that used in [8].

Somatic mutation dataset for Ov-HGSC validation samples (Data-2)

This mat-format dataset (version 2.4) was obtained from the archive *"genome.wustl.edu_OV.IlluminaGA_DNASeq.Level_2.2.1.0"* at TCGA [9]. In total, there are 142 tumor samples and 11342 mutations, of which 111 are present on the gene TP53. None of these mutations has been validated yet. The mutation distribution over variant types is similar to that of the training set (Data -1). The entire mutation profiling was used in the study.

Somatic mutation dataset for breast invasive carcinoma samples (Data-3)

The dataset containing 776 tumor samples [55] was downloaded from TCGA [9]. The corresponding *mat*-format file is located in the archive *"genome.wustl.edu_BRCA.IlluminaGA_DNASeq.Level_2.5.3.0"*. In total, there are 47243 mutations. The mutation distribution over variant types is similar to that of *Data-1*. Among these somatic mutations identified by exome-sequencing, only 6397 have been validated using other methods. The entire mutation profiling was used in the study.

Clinical dataset for Ov-HGSC training samples (Data-4)

This dataset is contained in the supplement, *"Copy of TCGA-OV-Clinical-Table_S1.2.xlsx"*, of the TCGA paper [7]. We downloaded it from the Nature website. The dataset consists of the clinical information of 488 Ov-HGSC patients (samples), of which 320 had the somatic mutations collected in *Data-1*. This dataset was used because it contains the progression-free survival time (PFS) which are not present in the matrix data archive of [9]. While the tumor-stage and tumor-grade attributes are also available in the dataset, neither [7] nor our preliminary analysis showed that their effects on the survival time were statistically significant. Hereby, these two attributes were not considered as predictive variables in the study.

Clinical dataset for Ov-HGSC validation samples

This dataset was downloaded from [9]. Out of 573 patients in this set, 140 had the somatic mutations collected in *Data-2*.

Clinical dataset for breast invasive carcinoma samples

The dataset was downloaded from TCGA database. Out of 971 patients in this set, 737 had the somatic mutations collected in *Data-3*.

GO dataset

The gene function annotation data for human was downloaded (on Oct 8, 2013) from The Gene Ontology (GO) website [56]. In the dataset, 18920 genes (symbols) were annotated to 13863 GO terms. We used a heuristic method to select the GO terms considered in this study. That is, a GO term was selected if the number of genes annotated to this term was between 50 and 500. The reason for doing so is twofold. First, if a GO term has only a few genes, the values of its corresponding MMS may be too sparse to perform an efficient statistical inference. Second, if there are too many genes annotated to a GO term, the functional category can be rather broad to infer meaningful biological insight from the results. While this setting was somewhat arbitrary, it won't introduce the selection bias that might substantially impact the conclusion.

Gene expression dataset for Ov-HGSC training samples

The mRNA expression levels of the tumor sample contained in *Data-1* were measured on three different platforms, i.e. Affymetrix Human Exon1.0 ST Array, Agilent 244K Whole Genome Expression Array and Affymetrix HT-HG-U133A Array. In the study, the combined gene expression dataset of 11684 genes present on all three platforms was used. The dataset is a supplement of [7] and was downloaded from the Nature website.

Methods for survival analysis

Survival analysis was performed using the statistical functions included in R package "survival" [57,58]. For univariate survival analysis with a factorized MMS as the predictor, the function "*survdiff*" was implemented to generate the Log-rank test p-value. It worth noting that, when "*survdiff*" was applied to the breast cancer dataset in which the cases of death at an early stage are rare due to right censoring, we let the *rho* parameter equal to negative 2, *i.e.* assigned each death a weight of $S(t)^{-2}$, where S(t) is the Kaplan-Meier estimate of survival. The Kaplan-Meier survival curves (in Figures 2, 3, 4, 5 and S1), with the censored observations being marked by a vertical tick, were obtained via the function "*survfit*". Multivariate survival analysis was conducted using the function "*coxph*" which implements Cox PH regression.

Identification of MMSs for survival prediction

We identified the predictive MMSs for overall survival time using the procedure presented in the Result section, and ranked them according to the composite p-value *CP*. The *CP* value for a MMS was calculated as the square root of the product of the p-values obtained from the Log-rank test and the corresponding Cox-PH analysis.

Identification of expression predictors for survival time

The association between the patient survival time and the gene expression levels was evaluated by the Cox PH regression. Similar to the analysis for the association between a MMS and the survival time, the patient age at the initial diagnosis was included in the model as a covariate.

Comparison between macro mutation signatures and expression signatures

The similarity matrix for the macro mutation signatures (MMSs) and macro expression signatures (MESs) was calculated by the function "*goSim*" in the R package "GOSemSim" [59]. In the employed method [20], the semantics of GO terms are encoded into a numeric format and the different semantic contributions of the distinct relations are considered.

Estimation of FDR

By adapting the methods used in [60,61], we developed a permutation-based algorithm to estimate the false discovery rate (FDR) for the 19 predictive MMSs associated with good clinical outcomes. First, we generated 500 shuffled datasets via randomly permutating the clinical records of the 320 training samples while keeping their mutation profile untouched. Then, we repeated the survival analysis by the same method used in the identification of predictive MMSs, and recorded the Log-rank p-values (p_{rank}), Cox-PH p-values (p_{cox}), the complex p-values (p_{cp}) as well as the regression coefficients (i.e. the beta values c) for all the 562 addressed MMSs. By doing so, we established the null distributions for p_{rank}, p_{cox}, p_{cp} and c, respectively. Finally, we compared the true distributions of p-values and regression coefficients to the corresponding null distributions to estimate false discovery rate by the following equation.

$$FDR = \frac{P(p_{rank}^{(0)} < z_{rank}, p_{cox}^{(0)} < z_{cox}, p_{cp}^{(0)} < z_{cp}, c < 0)}{P(p_{rank}^{(1)} < z_{rank}, p_{cox}^{(1)} < z_{cox}, p_{cp}^{(1)} < z_{cp}, c < 0)} \quad (1)$$

In (1), $p_*^{(0)}$ is a p-value from the null distribution and the subscript index * represents "rank", "cox" or "cp"; $p_*^{(1)}$ is a p-value from the true distribution; z_* is the threshold specified for the identification of predictive MMSs, and it is set to be 0.05, 0.05 or 0.025 for p_{rank}, p_{cox} or p_{cp}, respectively. The numerator is the fraction of p-values from the null distributions that fall below the thresholds (z_*) with the cognate regression coefficients less than 0. The denominator is the corresponding fraction for the estimates of p-values and regression coefficients based on the original dataset.

Availability

R codes for the statistical analysis are available upon request.

Supporting Information

Figure S1 The asymmetry of the null distributions of the effect parameters. The volcano plot of the Cox-PH p-values and regression coefficients for the 562 considered MMSs is based on the results of five randomly shuffled datasets.

Figure S2 Robustness analysis of the predictive MMSs. Top-left: The scatter plot shows the regression coefficients estimated from the two equal-size subsets of 320 training samples using the same Cox-PH model in the identification of the predictors. The solid squares (triangle) represent the 19 (1) MMSs which were rigorously selected and associated with good (poor) clinical outcomes. The solid circles represent the two MMSs which were selected in a less-rigorous way and were associated with poor clinical outcomes. The MMSs focused in the top right and bottom plots of this figure are marked with red. **Top-right (bottom-left, bottom-right)**: The results were obtained by analyzing 140 training samples. Each plot demonstrates the relationship between overall survival months and a specific macro mutation signature (MMS) that corresponds to a GO term. The purple curve represents the patients each of whom has at least two somatic mutations on the member genes of the indicated MMS (i.e., GO term). The red curve represents the patients each of whom has one somatic mutation on the member genes of the indicated MMS. The blue curve represents the patients without any somatic mutation on the member genes of the indicated MMS.
(TIF)

Figure S3 An illustration of the proposed classification tree model for patient survival prediction. This sample tree is generated using the three negative predictors (N_j, $1 \le j \le 3$) and five positive predictors (P_k, $1 \le k \le 5$) as the features. *S* represents the entire sample (or patient) set. *B* represents the predicted poor-prognosis set of patients. $\bar{B}$represents the remaining patient set after *B* is excluded. *G* represents the predicted patient set with good-prognosis. M represents the intermediate-prognosis set of patients, which is the remaining section of *S* after *B* and *G* are excluded. Note that in this sample tree, the feature tested at each internal node is a feature set instead of a single feature, which is different from the traditional classification/decision tree model.
(TIF)

Table S1 The genes involved in the GO terms corresponding to the predictive MMSs.
(XLSX)

Acknowledgments

The results presented here are based upon data published by The Cancer Genome Atlas managed by the NCI and NHGRI. Information regarding TCGA can be found at http://cancergenome.nih.gov. The authors are grateful to the four reviewers for their insightful comments which greatly improved this paper.

Author Contributions

Conceived and designed the experiments: WZ KZ. Performed the experiments: WZ. Analyzed the data: WZ KZ. Wrote the paper: WZ AE EF KZ. Helped with experiment design: EF AE.

References

1. Siegel R, Ma J, Zou Z, Jemal A (2014) Cancer statistics, 2014. CA Cancer J Clin 64: 9–29.
2. Goff BA, Mandel L, Muntz HG, Melancon CH (2000) Ovarian carcinoma diagnosis. Cancer 89: 2068–2075.
3. Bast RC Jr, Hennessy B, Mills GB (2009) The biology of ovarian cancer: new opportunities for translation. Nat Rev Cancer 9: 415–428.
4. Li J, Fadare O, Xiang L, Kong B, Zheng W (2012) Ovarian serous carcinoma: recent concepts on its origin and carcinogenesis. J Hematol Oncol 5: 8.
5. Bunz F (2008) Principles of cancer genetics. Dordrecht?: Springer. xi, 325 p. p.
6. Fearon ER, Vogelstein B (1990) A genetic model for colorectal tumorigenesis. Cell 61: 759–767.
7. TCGA (2011) Integrated genomic analyses of ovarian carcinoma. Nature 474: 609–615.
8. Birkbak NJ, Kochupurakkal B, Izarzugaza JM, Eklund AC, Li Y, et al. (2013) Tumor mutation burden forecasts outcome in ovarian cancer with BRCA1 or BRCA2 mutations. PLoS One 8: e80023.
9. TCGA website. Available: http://cancergenome.nih.gov/. Accessed 2013 Oct 22.
10. Delfino KR, Rodriguez-Zas SL (2013) Transcription factor-microRNA-target gene networks associated with ovarian cancer survival and recurrence. PLoS One 8: e58608.
11. Braun R, Finney R, Yan C, Chen QR, Hu Y, et al. (2013) Discovery analysis of TCGA data reveals association between germline genotype and survival in ovarian cancer patients. PLoS One 8: e55037.

12. Dai W, Zeller C, Masrour N, Siddiqui N, Paul J, et al. (2013) Promoter CpG island methylation of genes in key cancer pathways associates with clinical outcome in high-grade serous ovarian cancer. Clin Cancer Res 19: 5788–5797.
13. Engler DA, Gupta S, Growdon WB, Drapkin RI, Nitta M, et al. (2012) Genome wide DNA copy number analysis of serous type ovarian carcinomas identifies genetic markers predictive of clinical outcome. PLoS One 7: e30996.
14. Cope L, Wu RC, Shih Ie M, Wang TL (2013) High level of chromosomal aberration in ovarian cancer genome correlates with poor clinical outcome. Gynecol Oncol 128: 500–505.
15. COSMIC website. Available: http://cancer.sanger.ac.uk/cancergenome/projects/cosmic/. Accessed 2013 Oct 20.
16. Sohn I, Jung WY, Sung CO (2012) Somatic hypermutation and outcomes of platinum based chemotherapy in patients with high grade serous ovarian cancer. Gynecol Oncol 126: 103–108.
17. Sohn I, Sung CO (2013) Predictive modeling using a somatic mutational profile in ovarian high grade serous carcinoma. PLoS One 8: e54089.
18. Korosteleva O (2009) Clinical statistics: introducing clinical trials, survival analysis, and longitudinal data analysis. Sudbury, Mass.: Jones and Bartlett Publishers. vii, 120 p. p.
19. Huang da W, Sherman BT, Tan Q, Collins JR, Alvord WG, et al. (2007) The DAVID Gene Functional Classification Tool: a novel biological module-centric algorithm to functionally analyze large gene lists. Genome Biol 8: R183.
20. Wang JZ, Du Z, Payattakool R, Yu PS, Chen CF (2007) A new method to measure the semantic similarity of GO terms. Bioinformatics 23: 1274–1281.
21. Santarius T, Shipley J, Brewer D, Stratton MR, Cooper CS (2010) A census of amplified and overexpressed human cancer genes. Nat Rev Cancer 10: 59–64.
22. Futreal PA, Coin L, Marshall M, Down T, Hubbard T, et al. (2004) A census of human cancer genes. Nat Rev Cancer 4: 177–183.
23. Weinberg RA (2007) The biology of cancer. New York, NY: Garland Science.
24. Kunz M, Ibrahim SM (2003) Molecular responses to hypoxia in tumor cells. Mol Cancer 2: 23.
25. Lopez-Lazaro M (2010) A new view of carcinogenesis and an alternative approach to cancer therapy. Mol Med 16: 144–153.
26. Vander Heiden MG, Cantley LC, Thompson CB (2009) Understanding the Warburg effect: the metabolic requirements of cell proliferation. Science 324: 1029–1033.
27. Repnik U, Stoka V, Turk V, Turk B (2012) Lysosomes and lysosomal cathepsins in cell death. Biochim Biophys Acta 1824: 22–33.
28. Tardy C, Codogno P, Autefage H, Levade T, Andrieu-Abadie N (2006) Lysosomes and lysosomal proteins in cancer cell death (new players of an old struggle). Biochim Biophys Acta 1765: 101–125.
29. Guicciardi ME, Leist M, Gores GJ (2004) Lysosomes in cell death. Oncogene 23: 2881–2890.
30. Fehrenbacher N, Jaattela M (2005) Lysosomes as targets for cancer therapy. Cancer Res 65: 2993–2995.
31. Erdal H, Berndtsson M, Castro J, Brunk U, Shoshan MC, et al. (2005) Induction of lysosomal membrane permeabilization by compounds that activate p53-independent apoptosis. Proc Natl Acad Sci U S A 102: 192–197.
32. Aoudjit F, Vuori K (2001) Integrin signaling inhibits paclitaxel-induced apoptosis in breast cancer cells. Oncogene 20: 4995–5004.
33. Park CC, Zhang HJ, Yao ES, Park CJ, Bissell MJ (2008) Beta1 integrin inhibition dramatically enhances radiotherapy efficacy in human breast cancer xenografts. Cancer Res 68: 4398–4405.
34. Aoudjit F, Vuori K (2012) Integrin signaling in cancer cell survival and chemoresistance. Chemother Res Pract 2012: 283181.
35. Wortzel I, Seger R (2011) The ERK Cascade: Distinct Functions within Various Subcellular Organelles. Genes Cancer 2: 195–209.
36. Liu Y, Sun Y, Broaddus R, Liu J, Sood AK, et al. (2012) Integrated analysis of gene expression and tumor nuclear image profiles associated with chemotherapy response in serous ovarian carcinoma. PLoS One 7: e36383.
37. Kafri R, Bar-Even A, Pilpel Y (2005) Transcription control reprogramming in genetic backup circuits. Nat Genet 37: 295–299.
38. Ihmels J, Collins SR, Schuldiner M, Krogan NJ, Weissman JS (2007) Backup without redundancy: genetic interactions reveal the cost of duplicate gene loss. Mol Syst Biol 3: 86.
39. Liu M, Li JS, Tian DP, Huang B, Rosqvist S, et al. (2013) MCM2 expression levels predict diagnosis and prognosis in gastric cardiac cancer. Histol Histopathol 28: 481–492.
40. Hu Z, Huang G, Sadanandam A, Gu S, Lenburg ME, et al. (2010) The expression level of HJURP has an independent prognostic impact and predicts the sensitivity to radiotherapy in breast cancer. Breast Cancer Res 12: R18.
41. Sawada G, Ueo H, Matsumura T, Uchi R, Ishibashi M, et al. (2013) CHD8 is an independent prognostic indicator that regulates Wnt/beta-catenin signaling and the cell cycle in gastric cancer. Oncol Rep 30: 1137–1142.
42. Yan Z, Kim YS, Jetten AM (2002) RAP80, a novel nuclear protein that interacts with the retinoid-related testis-associated receptor. J Biol Chem 277: 32379–32388.
43. Wu J, Liu C, Chen J, Yu X (2012) RAP80 protein is important for genomic stability and is required for stabilizing BRCA1-A complex at DNA damage sites in vivo. J Biol Chem 287: 22919–22926.
44. Mascolo M, Vecchione ML, Ilardi G, Scalvenzi M, Molea G, et al. (2010) Overexpression of Chromatin Assembly Factor-1/p60 helps to predict the prognosis of melanoma patients. BMC Cancer 10: 63.
45. Weinstein JN, Collisson EA, Mills GB, Shaw KR, Ozenberger BA, et al. (2013) The Cancer Genome Atlas Pan-Cancer analysis project. Nat Genet 45: 1113–1120.
46. Silwal-Pandit L, Vollan HK, Chin SF, Rueda OM, McKinney S, et al. (2014) TP53 Mutation Spectrum in Breast Cancer Is Subtype Specific and Has Distinct Prognostic Relevance. Clin Cancer Res 20: 3569–3580.
47. van de Vijver MJ, He YD, van't Veer LJ, Dai H, Hart AA, et al. (2002) A gene-expression signature as a predictor of survival in breast cancer. N Engl J Med 347: 1999–2009.
48. Finak G, Bertos N, Pepin F, Sadekova S, Souleimanova M, et al. (2008) Stromal gene expression predicts clinical outcome in breast cancer. Nat Med 14: 518–527.
49. Li J, Lenferink AE, Deng Y, Collins C, Cui Q, et al. (2010) Identification of high-quality cancer prognostic markers and metastasis network modules. Nat Commun 1: 34.
50. Berchuck A, Iversen ES, Lancaster JM, Pittman J, Luo J, et al. (2005) Patterns of gene expression that characterize long-term survival in advanced stage serous ovarian cancers. Clin Cancer Res 11: 3686–3696.
51. Partheen K, Levan K, Osterberg L, Horvath G (2006) Expression analysis of stage III serous ovarian adenocarcinoma distinguishes a sub-group of survivors. Eur J Cancer 42: 2846–2854.
52. Bonome T, Levine DA, Shih J, Randonovich M, Pise-Masison CA, et al. (2008) A gene signature predicting for survival in suboptimally debulked patients with ovarian cancer. Cancer Res 68: 5478–5486.
53. Tothill RW, Tinker AV, George J, Brown R, Fox SB, et al. (2008) Novel molecular subtypes of serous and endometrioid ovarian cancer linked to clinical outcome. Clin Cancer Res 14: 5198–5208.
54. Venet D, Dumont JE, Detours V (2011) Most random gene expression signatures are significantly associated with breast cancer outcome. PLoS Comput Biol 7: e1002240.
55. TCGA (2012) Comprehensive molecular portraits of human breast tumours. Nature 490: 61–70.
56. GO website. Available: http://www.geneontology.org/. Accessed 2013 Oct 8.
57. Therneau T (2013) A Package for Survival Analysis in S. R package version 2.37–4. http://CRANR-projectorg/package=survival
58. Therneau TM, Grambsch PM (2000) Modeling survival data: extending the Cox model. New York: Springer. xiii, 350 p. p.
59. Yu G, Li F, Qin Y, Bo X, Wu Y, et al. (2010) GOSemSim: an R package for measuring semantic similarity among GO terms and gene products. Bioinformatics 26: 976–978.
60. Zhang W, Edwards A, Flemington EK, Zhang K (2013) Inferring polymorphism-induced regulatory gene networks active in human lymphocyte cell lines by weighted linear mixed model analysis of multiple RNA-Seq datasets. PLoS One 8: e78868.
61. Pickrell JK, Marioni JC, Pai AA, Degner JF, Engelhardt BE, et al. (2010) Understanding mechanisms underlying human gene expression variation with RNA sequencing. Nature 464: 768–772.

CD117 Expression in Fibroblasts-Like Stromal Cells Indicates Unfavorable Clinical Outcomes in Ovarian Carcinoma Patients

Ruixia Huang[1,2], Dan Wu[3], Yuan Yuan[4], Xiaoran Li[1,2], Ruth Holm[1], Claes G. Trope[5,6], Jahn M. Nesland[1,2], Zhenhe Suo[1,2]*

1 Departments of Pathology, The Norwegian Radium Hospital, Oslo University Hospital, Oslo, Norway, **2** Department of Pathology, Institute of Clinical Medicine, Faculty of Medicine, University of Oslo, Oslo, Norway, **3** Department of Gynecology, International Peace Maternity and Child Health Hospital, Medical College of Shanghai, Jiaotong University, Shanghai, China, **4** Department of Pathology, Capital Medical University, Beijing, China, **5** Department of Gynecology, Institute of Clinical Medicine, Faculty of Medicine, University of Oslo, Oslo, Norway, **6** Department of Gynecology, The Norwegian Radium Hospital, Oslo University Hospital, Oslo, Norway

Abstract

The stem cell factor (SCF) receptor CD117 (c-kit), is widely used for identification of hematopoietic stem cells and cancer stem cells. Moreover, CD117 expression in carcinoma cells indicates a poor prognosis in a variety of cancers. However the potential expression in tumor microenvironment and the biological and clinical impact are currently not reported. The expression of CD117 was immunohistochemically evaluated in a serial of 242 epithelial ovarian cancer (EOC) cases. Thirty-eight out of 242 cases were CD117 positive in fibroblast-like stromal cells and 22 cases were positive in EOC cells. Four cases were both positive in fibroblast-like stromal cells and EOC cells for CD117. CD117 expression in fibroblast-like stromal cells in ovarian carcinoma was closely linked to advanced FIGO stage, poor differentiation grade and histological subtype ($p<0.05$), and it was significantly associated with poor overall survival (OS) and progression free survival (PFS) (Kaplan-Meier analysis; $p<0.05$, log-rank test). CD117 expression in ovarian carcinoma cells was not associated with these clinicopathological variables. The CD117 positive fibroblast-like stromal cells were all positive for mesenchymal stem/stromal cell (MSC) marker CD73 but negative for fibroblast markers fibroblast activation protein (FAP) and α smooth muscle actin (α-SMA), indicating that the CD117+/CD73+ fibroblast-like stromal cells are a subtype of mesenchymal stem cells in tumor stroma, although further characterization of these cells are needed. It is concluded herewith that the presence of CD117+/CD73+ fibroblast-like stromal cells in ovarian carcinoma is an unfavorable clinical outcome indication.

Editor: Jung Weon Lee, Seoul National University, Republic Of Korea

Funding: This study was financially supported by grants from Inger and John Fredriksen Foundation, Norwegian Radium Hospital Research Foundation and The Norwegian Cancer Society. The funders had no role in study design, data collection and analysis, decision to publish, or preparation of the manuscript.

Competing Interests: The authors have declared that no competing interests exist.

* Email: zhenhes@medisin.uio.no

Introduction

Epithelial ovarian cancer (EOC) is the most lethal gynecologic malignancy worldwide [1,2]. Most women with EOC are diagnosed at an advanced stage. The 5-year survival is less than 30% for the women diagnosed at advanced stage [2]. Cancer stem cells (CSCs) represent a subpopulation of tumor cells responsible for tumor initiation, progression, invasion, metastasis and relapse, and are capable of cell renewal. Thus, therapies targeting CSCs are being considered a promising way to control cancer.

Tumor microenvironment is the cellular environment in which tumor cells exist, including blood vessels, immune cells, fibroblasts, macrophages, extracellular matrix (ECM) and other molecules, etc. The stromal cells interact with each other in a complex net by secreting distinct, abnormal molecules into ECM and contribute to tumor growth and invasiveness [3,4,5,6,7]. Tumor stromal cells from different tissue have different gene expression profiles and hence contribute to tumor heterogeneity [8]. According to Albini, et. al, the microenvironment of a cancer is an integral part of its anatomy and physiology, and functionally, one cannot totally dissociate this microenvironment from what have traditionally been called "cancer cells" [9]. Therefore, it is now necessary to develop new tumorpreventive methods to target tumor microenvironment and hence to interfere carcinogenesis [9].

CD117, also known as proto-oncogene c-Kit or tyrosine-protein kinase Kit, is a transmembrane cytokine receptor expressed on the surface of hematopoietic stem cells and other cell types. It is normally phosphorylated and activated by binding to its ligand stem cell factor (SCF). It is a widely used stemness marker for recognition of cancer stem cells in various tumors, including ovarian carcinoma, endometrial cancer, osteosarcoma [10,11,12] and others. The unfavorable outcome for cancer patients with CD117 expression in cancer cells is well established [10,11], whereas, the role of CD117 expression in stromal cells is rarely reported.

To better understand CD117 expression in ovarian carcinoma cells and stromal cells and the clinicopathological associations, we investigated CD117 expression in 242 formalin-fixed paraffin-

Table 1. The primary antibodies used for IHC.

Name	Company	Catalog number	Resource	Dilution	Retrieval solution	Positive control
CD117	Dako	A4502	Rabbit	1:400	HPH	Human seminoma tissue
FAP	Abcam	Ab53066	Rabbit	1:300	HPH	Human colon tissue
α-SMA	BioGenex	MU128-UC	Mouse	1:750	HPH	Human appendix tissue
CD73	LSBio	LS-C138754	Rabbit	1:1600	LPH	Human tonsil tissue

embedded (FFPE) tumor tissue samples, which were obtained routinely from surgical dissection of patients diagnosed with EOC in The Norwegian Radium Hospital, Oslo University Hospital. Furthermore, we analyzed the associations between CD117 expression and clinicopathological characters, including age, histological subtype, differentiation grade, FIGO stage, overall survival (OS) and progression free survival (PFS). CD117 expressions in stromal cells and tumor cells and the clinicopathological analyses were investigated respectively.

Materials and Methods

Ethics Statement

The Regional Committee for Medical Research Ethics South of Norway (S-06277a), The Social- and Health Directorate (06/3280) and The Data Inspectorate (06/5345) approved the study. All the patients involved provided their written consent to participate in this study, and all the written consents were filed in The Norwegian Radium Hospital, Oslo University Hospital.

Clinical samples

Two-hundred and forty-two surgically dissected ovarian carcinoma samples were randomly enrolled in this study. All patients were operated at The Norwegian Radium Hospital, Oslo University Hospital from March 1983 to May 2001. FFPE ovarian carcinoma tissues were obtained from the files of the Department of Pathology, and 3μm sections were cut and used for morphological examination and immunohistochemistry (IHC). The ages of the patients range from 19 to 89 years, and the median age is at 58 years old. The patients were followed up until January 1st 2012. All patients were clinically staged following the recommendations of International Federation of Gynecology and Obstetrics (FIGO) [13]. The primary tumors were histologically graded as well, moderately and poorly differentiated according to WHO recommendations [13]. Disease progression was determined based on the definitions outlined by the Gynecologic Cancer Intergroup [14].

Immunohistochemistry (IHC)

The Dako Envision FLEX+ system (K8012; Dako, Glostrup, Denmark) and the Dako Autostainer were used for IHC. Paraffin sections were deparaffinized and epitopes unmasked in PT link with high pH/low pH target retrieval solution (Dako), and then blocked with peroxidase blocking (Dako) for 5 minutes. The slides were incubated with primary antibody 30 minutes at room temperature, following up with rabbit/mouse linker (Dako) according to the resource of primary antibody for 15 minutes and HRP for 30 minutes at room temperature. Slides were then stained with 3, 3′-diaminobenzidine tetrahydrochloride (DAB) for 10 minutes and counter-stained with hematoxylin, dehydrated, and mounted in Richard-Allan Scientific Cyto seal XYL (Thermo Scientific, Waltham, MA, USA). Already known each antibody positive tissue was used as positive control in the same procedure. The same positive control slide was used as a negative control incubated with the same concentration of non-immune rabbit/mouse IgG replacing the primary antibody. The information for each primary antibody is shown in Table 1.

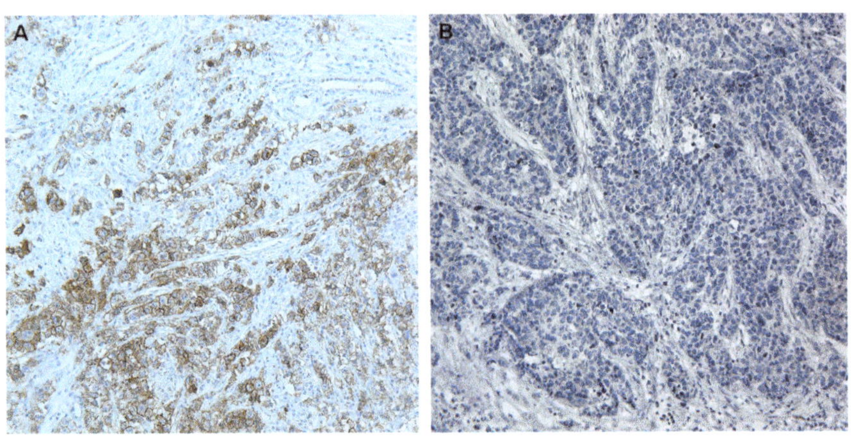

Figure 1. (A) Known CD117-positive seminoma tissue is always positive for CD117 and used as positive control in this study. (B) Section from the same seminoma tissue is negative by incubating with the corresponding non-immune rabbit IgG in the same concentration, instead of rabbit anti-CD117 antibody. Both pictures were taken at 200×.

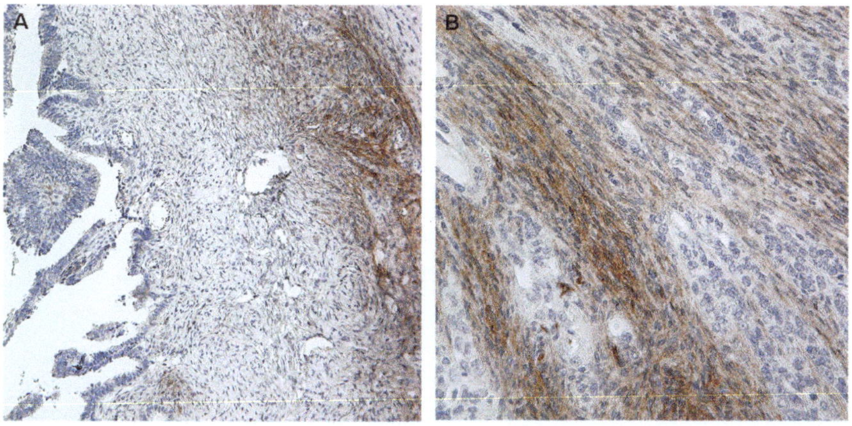

Figure 2. CD117 positive fibroblast-like stromal cells surrounding ovarian carcinoma cells were shown (A:200×, and B: 400×).

IHC scoring system

CD117 immunodetection was evaluated and grouped as positive and negative in carcinoma cells and stromal cells for each slide. Slides were grouped as positive for tumor cells if over 10 percent of tumor cells were stained. Likewise, slides were grouped as positive for stromal cells if over 10 percent of stromal cells were stained. The morphology and immunostaining judgment were confirmed by two pathologists.

Statistical analyses

SPSS software (version 18.0) was used for data analyses. Associations between categorical variables were assessed by Chi-square tests (Pearson and linear-by-linear as appropriate). Survival analysis was estimated using the Kaplan-Meier method, and groups were compared with log-rank tests. For all the analyses, associations were considered to be significant if the p value was $<$ 0.05.

Results

Immunodetection of CD117 in ovarian carcinoma tissues

Generally, CD117 immunoreactivity was observed in some EOC cells and stromal cells, including endothelial cells, fibroblast-like stromal cells and blood cells. It was found out that out of 242 cases 38 were positive in fibroblast-like stromal cells and 22 cases were positive for CD117 in EOC cells. Four cases were positive in both fibroblast-like stromal cells and EOC cells. Positive control and negative control were shown in Figure 1. CD117 immnoreactivity was limited to cytoplasm and membrane in both fibroblast-like stromal cells (Figure 2) and tumor cells (Figure 3). Nuclear staining was not observed. It was commonly observed if possible, tumor cells in the same case were variably stained (Figure 3B), and some cases were scattered immunostaining. CD117 positive fibroblast-like stromal cells were further identified by mesenchymal stem/stromal cell (MSC) marker CD73 (NT5E) and cancer associated fibroblast (CAF) markers fibroblast activation protein (FAP) and α-smooth muscle actin (α-SMA). All CD117 positive stromal cells were negative for both FAP and α-SMA, but positive for CD73 (Figure 4).

CD117 expression in fibroblast-like stromal cells and clinical impact

The associations between CD117 expression in fibroblast-like stromal cells and the clinicopathological variables are demonstrated in Table 2. CD117 expression in fibroblast-like stromal cells was significantly associated with late FIGO stage, poor differentiation stage, and histological subtypes ($p<0.05$). No significant difference was observed for age (patients diagnosed at $\geq$ 60 years and $\leq$59 years ($p=0.411$)). CD117 expression in fibroblast-like

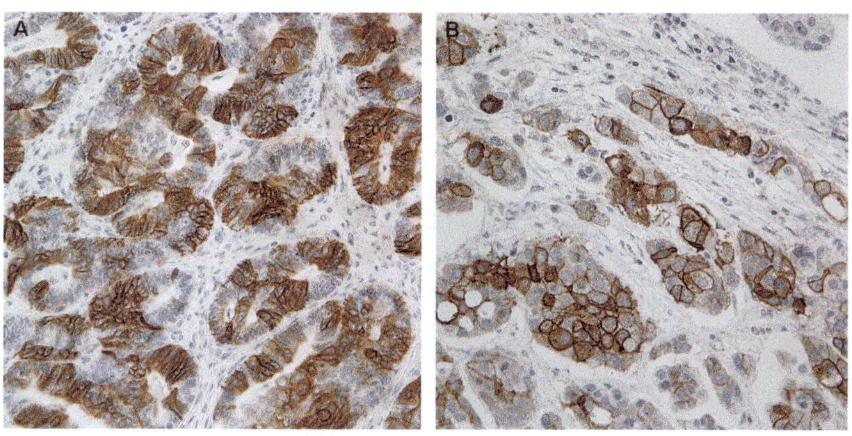

Figure 3. Variable expression of CD117 in ovarian carcinoma cells is demonstrated. The magnitude was 200× for (A) and 400× for (B).

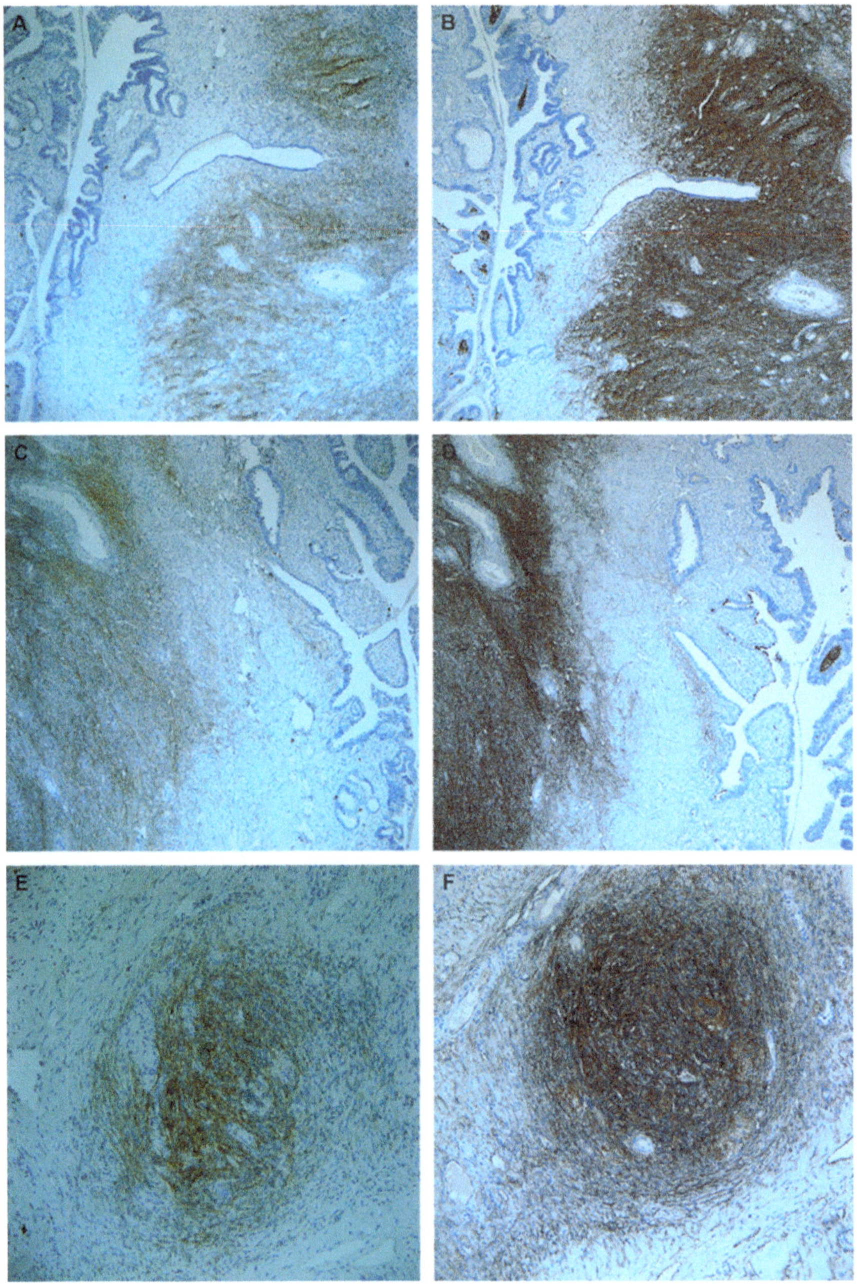

Figure 4. Three pairs of slides stained with CD117 and CD73 for each pair were randomly picked and demonstrated. Each pair of the slides was from the same tumor tissue in our database. CD117+ fibroblast-like stromal cells (A,C,E) were all positive for CD73 (B,D,F). (A,B,C,D) were taken at 100× and (E, F) were taken at 200×.

stromal cells was observed in 4.3% (2/46) of EOC patients in FIGO stage I/II compared to 18.4% (36/196) of patients in FIGO stage III/IV, and the difference is significant ($p = 0.019$). For histological grade, 0% (0/19) of well differentiated EOC samples was CD117 positive in fibroblast-like stromal cells, compared to 11.3% (7/62) in moderately differentiated EOC samples and 21.1% (28/133) in poorly differentiated EOC samples. Thus, CD117 immunoreactivity was closely associated with differentiation grade ($p = 0.010$). Ovarian serous carcinomas and the group of undifferentiated EOC, mixed EOC and others showed more CD117-positive fibroblast-like stromal cells than the group of mucinous EOC, endometrial EOC and clear cell carcinoma ($p = 0.012$).

CD117 expression in EOC cells and clinical impact

For CD117 expression in EOC cells, we did not observe any statistical difference in different age groups ($p = 0.632$), FIGO stage groups ($p = 0.267$), differentiation grade groups ($p = 0.306$) or histological subtype groups ($p = 0.439$) (Table 3).

Table 2. Associations between CD117 expression in fibroblast-like stromal cells and clinicopathological features (N = 242).

	Total N	CD117 expression, n (%) negative	positive	*p* value
Age group				0.411
≤59	121	104 (86.0)	17 (14.0)	
≥60	111	91 (82.0)	20 (18.0)	
missing	10			
FIGO stage				0.019
I+II	46	44 (95.7)	2 (4.3)	
III+IV	196	160 (81.6)	36 (18.4)	
Differentiation grade				0.010
well	19	19 (100)	0 (0)	
moderately	62	55 (88.7)	7 (11.3)	
poorly	133	105 (78.9)	28 (21.1)	
missing	28			
Histological subtype				0.012
serous	163	131 (80.4)	32 (19.6)	
MUC+END+CLE	48	47 (97.9)	1 (2.1)	
UND+MIX+others	27	23 (85.2)	4 (14.8)	
missing	4			

MUC, Mucinous carcinoma; END, Endometrioid carcinoma; CLE, Clear cell carcinoma; UND, Undifferentiated carcinoma; MIX, Mixed carcinoma.

Survival analyses

Progression free survival (PFS) and overall survival (OS) were used to analyze survival time in our study (Table 4). The patient group with CD117 expression in fibroblast-like stromal cells had a significantly shorter OS (Figure 5A) and PFS (Figure 5B) than the patient group not expressing CD117 in fibroblast-like stromal cells.

When comparing the two patient groups with positive and negative CD117 expression in tumor cells, we did find a trend for

Table 3. Associations between CD117 expression in EOC cells and clinicopathological features (N = 242).

	Total N	CD117 expression, n (%) negative	positive	*p* value
Age group				0.632
≤59	121	109 (90.1)	12 (9.9)	
≥60	111	102 (91.9)	9 (8.1)	
missing	10			
FIGO stage				0.267
I+II	46	44 (95.7)	2 (4.3)	
III+IV	196	176 (89.8)	20 (10.2)	
Differentiation grade				0.306
well	19	17 (89.5)	2 (10.5)	
moderately	62	59 (95.2)	3 (4.8)	
poorly	133	116 (87.2)	22 (12.8)	
missing	28			
Histological subtype				0.439
serous	163	149 (91.4)	14 (8.6)	
MUC+END+CLE	48	42 (87.5)	6 (12.5)	
UND+MIX+others	27	26 (96.3)	1 (3.7)	
missing	4			

MUC, Mucinous tumor; END, Endometrioid carcinoma; CLE, Clear cell carcinoma; UND, Undifferenciated tumor; MIX, Mixed epithelial tumor.

Table 4. CD117 expression and survival (years).

	Mean		Median		*p* value
	Extimate	95% CI	Extimate	95% CI	
OS:CD117 in tumor cells					
Negative (n = 211)	5.649	4.494 to 6.805	1.719	1.267 to 2.172	0.113
Positive (n = 21)	2.995	0.948 to 5.041	0.715	0.000 to 1.652	
OS:CD117 in fibroblast-like stromal cells					
Negative (n = 195)	5.922	4.686 to 7.159	1.719	1.165 to 2.274	0.031
Positive (n = 37)	2.978	1.269 to 4.688	1.098	0.605 to 1.591	
PFS:CD117 in tumor cells					
Negative (n = 211)	4.592	3.405 to 5.774	0.665	0.516 to 0.814	0.204
Positive (n = 21)	2.274	0.332 to 4.217	0.216	0.000 to 0.560	
PFS:CD117 in fibroblast-like stromal cells					
Negative (n = 195)	4.484	3.574 to 6.105	0.706	0.483 to 0.929	0.016
Positive (n = 37)	2.180	0.415 to 3.946	0.397	0.221 to 0.573	

the CD117-positive group to have a worse OS (Figure 5C) and PFS (Figure 5D) probability, but no statistical significance was achieved.

Discussion

In our study 9% of EOC cases expressed CD117 in carcinoma cells, with a relatively lower positive frequency compared to 15% positivity in ovarian serous carcinoma in a previous study [15]. Garrity and coworkers [16] have pointed out the variable positivity using different antibodies, showing 6% positivity using rabbit anti-human CD117 antibody from one company compared to 33% positivity with stronger staining background using rabbit anti-human CD117 from another antibody. In our current study, we firstly tested 4 commercial anti-human CD117 antibodies and chose the optimized one with high specificity and low background staining as revealed by the previous study [17]. Further IHC procedure optimization was performed in order to ensure high sensitivity for this antibody as well.

CD117 is mostly reported in mast cells/myeloid cells (mastocytoma/acute myeloid leukemia) [18], germ cells (seminoma) [19], Cajal cell (gastrointestinal stromal tumors) [20,21] and some epithelial cells [22,23,24,25]. CD117 expression in tumor stromal cells is neglected and rarely reported. In our series, we disclosed for the first time that CD117 expression in fibroblast-like stromal cells had a statistical association with poor clinical outcomes.

The importance of microenvironment for tumor growth is well established [26,27,28,29]. Fibroblast cells, as predominant component in the microenvironment, act synergistically with carcinoma cells to prepare the microenvironment according to the "seed and soil" theory [29,30]. Fibroblasts in mammals comprise a highly heterogeneous group of cells, and reflect a substantial genetic diversity [31]. Similar to organ fibrosis, the fibroblasts at the site of a carcinoma remain perpetually activated, and this subpopulation of fibroblasts are designated cancer-associated fibroblasts (CAFs) [32]. FAP and α-SMA are widely used among other markers to mark CAFs in tumors. FAP is selectively expressed on fibroblasts within the tumor stroma or on CAFs [33,34]. α-SMA is positive in most of smooth muscle cells and fibroblasts in the stroma of the epithelial cancer [35,36]. In our study, the CD117+ fibroblast-like stromal cells were neither positive for FAP nor positive for α-SMA, which shadows forth that these morphologically fibroblast-like stromal cells were not supposed to be fibroblasts actually.

To further identify these cells, mesenchymal stem/stromal cell (MSC) marker CD73 (NT5E) were immune-evaluated. More intriguingly, All CD117+ fibroblast-like stromal cells were positive for CD73. Mesenchymal stem cells (MSCs) were initially isolated from the bone marrow and demonstrated the multipotency to differentiate into a variety of cell types [37,38]. MSCs recruited into the tumors as the progenitors of stromal cells may play a significant role in the regulation of both solid and haematological malignancies [39]. It is still an open discussion about how to define MSCs, because no single marker is specific to identify MSCs to date [40]. Cultured MSCs are uniformly and strongly positive for CD105, CD90, and CD73, regardless of their passage or time in culture [41], and it has been one of the minimal criteria to identify MSC [40,42]. Moreover, the morphology of MSCs was reported to be fibroblast-like [43,44]. Bone marrow-derived MSCs selectively express FAP but not other resources [45], and slightly express α-SMA [46]. But MSCs in tumor stroma are currently not reported to express these two markers. As a result, to our point of view, there is a possibility for these CD117+/CD73+ fibroblast-like stromal cells to be MSC-derived, although currently we are not able to confirm this suppose.

The effect of MSCs on tumor growth is still controversial, but Ljujic, et. al believes MSCs are capable to home to tumor cites and promote tumor growth in mice [47]. CD73, also known as ecto-5′-nucleotidase, is an enzyme that in humans is encoded by the NT5E gene and commonly serves to convert adenosine monophosphate (AMP) to adenosine. Through the increasing adenosine, CD73 contribute to immunosuppressive effects of anti-tumor T cells [48] and regulate adaptive responses upon hypoxia[49]. Furthermore, CD73 expression in tumor cells and tumor environment are required for tumor angiogenesis [50].The percentage of CD73+ Natural killer (NK) NK cells increases significantly on coculture with MSCs and thus acquires the ability to convert AMP into adenosine [51]. Epithelial mesenchymal transition (EMT) is a fundamental biologic process during which epithelial cells lose their polarity and change to a mesenchymal phenotype [52,53,54]. The mesenchymal state facilitates cells with the capacity of migrating to distant organs and maintain stemness,

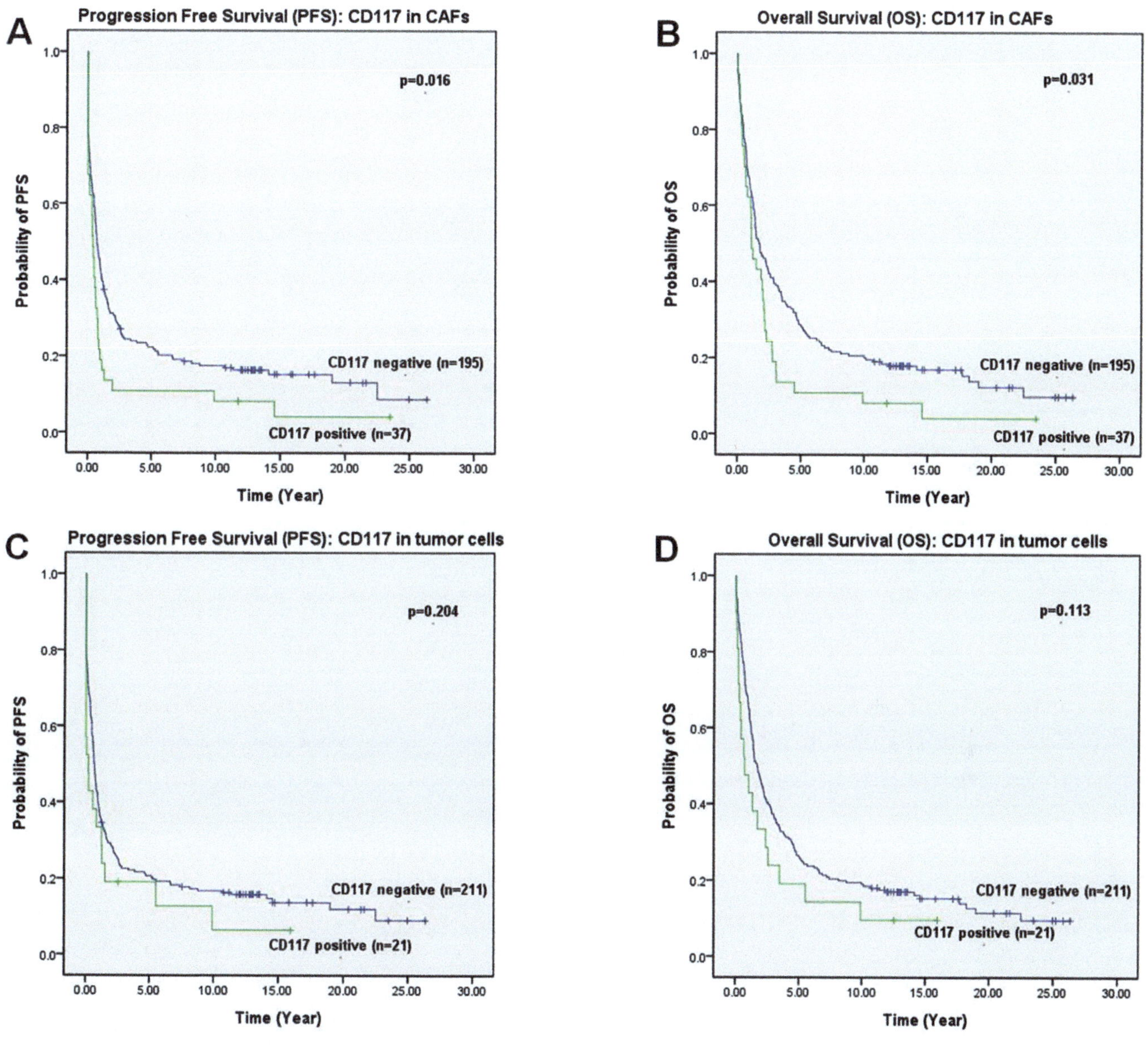

Figure 5. The survival probabilities of CD117 expression in ovarian carcinoma cells and fibroblast-like stromal cells were demonstrated. PFS (A) and OS (B) probabilities are shown for the group of CD117 positive and negative in fibroblast-like stromal cells. CD117 negativity in stromal cells shows a significantly better survival probabilities ($p<0.05$). PFS (C) and OS (D) probabilities are revealed for CD117 expression in ovarian carcinoma cells. No significant difference was observed for survival probabilities between CD117+ tumor cell group and CD117- tumor cell group ($p>0.05$).

allowing the initiation of metastasis [53]. CD73 may contribute to induce EMT by the regulation of EMT-related key factors including cadherin-1 (CDH1) and vimentin (VIM) [55].

The traditional defined MSCs, including bone marrow-derived MSCs (BM-MSCs) and human embryonic stem cell-derived mesenchymal stroma cells (hES-MSCs), express CD73 but rarely express CD117 [56,57]. On the other hand, CD117 was also regarded as one of MSC markers [11,58]. In our study, we found that CD117 expressed in fibroblast-like stromal cells in ovarian carcinomas was significantly linked to poor clinical characters and survival time. Although these CD117 positive stromal cells were negative for both fibroblast markers FAP and α-SMA, it was confirmed in our study that these cells were positive for mesenchymal stem cell marker CD73, which strongly indicates their mesenchymal stem cells in nature. To the best of our knowledge, this is the first report of CD117+/CD73+ tumor stromal cells with negative clinical consequences.

To conclude, it is verified in our study that CD117+/CD73+ fibroblast-like stromal cells are significantly associated with poor clinical manifestations and poor survival probability in ovarian carcinomas, but CD117 expression in tumor cells does not show any clinical significance. Thus, it is worthy of further study for CD117 positive and CD73 positive stromal cells in EOCs in order to explore their potential application in prognostic prediction and targeting therapy.

Acknowledgments

We are grateful to Ellen Hellesylt, Mette Synnøve Førsund, Mai Nguyen and Don Trinh for immunohistochemistry technical support.

Author Contributions

Conceived and designed the experiments: R. Huang DW YY JMN ZS. Performed the experiments: R. Huang. Analyzed the data: R. Huang DW YY XL R. Holm JMN ZS. Contributed reagents/materials/analysis tools: CGT ZS. Wrote the paper: R. Huang DW YY XL R. Holm CGT JMN ZS.

References

1. Downs LS Jr, Judson PL, Argenta PA, Ghebre R, Geller MA, et al. (2008) A prospective randomized trial of thalidomide with topotecan compared with topotecan alone in women with recurrent epithelial ovarian carcinoma. Cancer 112: 331–339.
2. Guppy AE, Nathan PD, Rustin GJ (2005) Epithelial ovarian cancer: a review of current management. Clin Oncol (R Coll Radiol) 17: 399–411.
3. Ghesquiere B, Wong BW, Kuchnio A, Carmeliet P (2014) Metabolism of stromal and immune cells in health and disease. Nature 511: 167–176.
4. Liu ET (2007) Stromal effects in breast cancer. N Engl J Med 357: 2537–2538.
5. McMillin DW, Negri JM, Mitsiades CS (2013) The role of tumour-stromal interactions in modifying drug response: challenges and opportunities. Nature Reviews Drug Discovery 12: 217–228.
6. Kang Y (2013) Imaging signaling pathways and tumor-stromal interactions in cancer metastasis. Journal of Nuclear Medicine 54: 32–32.
7. Tod J, Jenei V, Thomas G, Fine D (2013) Tumor-stromal interactions in pancreatic cancer. Pancreatology 13: 1–7.
8. Pollack IF (2013) Tumor-Stromal Interactions in Medulloblastoma. New England Journal of Medicine 368: 1942–1943.
9. Albini A, Sporn MB (2007) The tumour microenvironment as a target for chemoprevention. Nat Rev Cancer 7: 139–147.
10. Zhang X, Kyo S, Nakamura M, Mizumoto Y, Maida Y, et al. (2014) Imatinib sensitizes endometrial cancer cells to cisplatin by targeting CD117-positive growth-competent cells. Cancer Lett 345: 106–114.
11. Adhikari AS, Agarwal N, Wood BM, Porretta C, Ruiz B, et al. (2010) CD117 and Stro-1 identify osteosarcoma tumor-initiating cells associated with metastasis and drug resistance. Cancer Res 70: 4602–4612.
12. Chen D, Zhang Y, Wang J, Chen J, Yang C, et al. (2013) MicroRNA-200c overexpression inhibits tumorigenicity and metastasis of CD117+CD44+ ovarian cancer stem cells by regulating epithelial-mesenchymal transition. J Ovarian Res 6: 50.
13. Cho KR, Shih Ie M (2009) Ovarian cancer. Annu Rev Pathol 4: 287–313.
14. Zivanovic O, Sima CS, Iasonos A, Hoskins WJ, Pingle PR, et al. (2010) The effect of primary cytoreduction on outcomes of patients with FIGO stage IIIC ovarian cancer stratified by the initial tumor burden in the upper abdomen cephalad to the greater omentum. Gynecol Oncol 116: 351–357.
15. Schmandt RE, Broaddus R, Lu KH, Shvartsman H, Thornton A, et al. (2003) Expression of c-ABL, c-KIT, and platelet-derived growth factor receptor-beta in ovarian serous carcinoma and normal ovarian surface epithelium. Cancer 98: 758–764.
16. Garrity MM, Gibbons SJ, Smyrk TC, Vanderwinden JM, Gomez-Pinilla PJ, et al. (2009) Diagnostic challenges of motility disorders: optimal detection of CD117+ interstitial cells of Cajal. Histopathology 54: 286–294.
17. Went PT, Dirnhofer S, Bundi M, Mirlacher M, Schraml P, et al. (2004) Prevalence of KIT expression in human tumors. J Clin Oncol 22: 4514–4522.
18. Ma D, Stence AA, Bossler AB, Hackman JR, Bellizzi AM (2013) Identification of KIT activating mutations in paediatric solitary mastocytoma. Histopathology 64: 218–225.
19. Gallegos I, Valdevenito JP, Miranda R, Fernandez C (2010) Immunohistochemistry expression of P53, Ki67, CD30, and CD117 and presence of clinical metastasis at diagnosis of testicular seminoma. Appl Immunohistochem Mol Morphol 19: 147–152.
20. de Silva CM, Reid R (2003) Gastrointestinal stromal tumors (GIST): C-kit mutations, CD117 expression, differential diagnosis and targeted cancer therapy with Imatinib. Pathol Oncol Res 9: 13–19.
21. Doyle LA, Hornick JL (2014) Gastrointestinal stromal tumours: from KIT to succinate dehydrogenase. Histopathology 64: 53–67.
22. Ismail RS, Cada M, Vanderhyden BC (1999) Transforming growth factor-beta regulates Kit ligand expression in rat ovarian surface epithelial cells. Oncogene 18: 4734–4741.
23. Kim DJ, Lee MH, Park TI, Bae HI (2006) Expression and mutational analysis of c-kit in ovarian surface epithelial tumors. J Korean Med Sci 21: 81–85.
24. Song N, Chen G, Zhang P, Liu M, He WX, et al. (2012) Diagnostic and clinical significance of KIT(CD117) expression in thymic epithelial tumors in China. Asian Pac J Cancer Prev 13: 2745–2748.
25. Petrini I, Zucali PA, Lee HS, Pineda MA, Meltzer PS, et al. (2010) Expression and mutational status of c-kit in thymic epithelial tumors. J Thorac Oncol 5: 1447–1453.
26. Kalluri R (2003) Basement membranes: structure, assembly and role in tumour angiogenesis. Nat Rev Cancer 3: 422–433.
27. Hanahan D, Weinberg RA (2000) The hallmarks of cancer. Cell 100: 57–70.
28. Tlsty TD, Coussens LM (2006) Tumor stroma and regulation of cancer development. Annu Rev Pathol 1: 119–150.
29. Cheng JD, Weiner LM (2003) Tumors and their microenvironments: tilling the soil. Commentary re: A. M. . Scott et al., A Phase I dose-escalation study of sibrotuzumab in patients with advanced or metastatic fibroblast activation protein-positive cancer. Clin. Cancer Res., 9: 1639–1647, 2003. Clin Cancer Res 9: 1590–1595.
30. Langley RR, Fidler IJ (2011) The seed and soil hypothesis revisited–the role of tumor-stroma interactions in metastasis to different organs. Int J Cancer 128: 2527–2535.
31. Chang HY, Chi JT, Dudoit S, Bondre C, van de Rijn M, et al. (2002) Diversity, topographic differentiation, and positional memory in human fibroblasts. Proc Natl Acad Sci U S A 99: 12877–12882.
32. Kalluri R, Zeisberg M (2006) Fibroblasts in cancer. Nat Rev Cancer 6: 392–401.
33. Brennen WN, Isaacs JT, Denmeade SR (2012) Rationale behind targeting fibroblast activation protein-expressing carcinoma-associated fibroblasts as a novel chemotherapeutic strategy. Mol Cancer Ther 11: 257–266.
34. Fearon DT (2014) The carcinoma-associated fibroblast expressing fibroblast activation protein and escape from immune surveillance. Cancer Immunol Res 2: 187–193.
35. Wang S, Ma N, Kawanishi S, Hiraku Y, Oikawa S, et al. (2014) Relationships of alpha-SMA-positive fibroblasts and SDF-1-positive tumor cells with neoangiogenesis in nasopharyngeal carcinoma. Biomed Res Int 2014: 507353.
36. Wu MH, Hong HC, Hong TM, Chiang WF, Jin YT, et al. (2011) Targeting galectin-1 in carcinoma-associated fibroblasts inhibits oral squamous cell carcinoma metastasis by downregulating MCP-1/CCL2 expression. Clin Cancer Res 17: 1306–1316.
37. in 't Anker PS, Noort WA, Scherjon SA, Kleijburg-van der Keur C, Kruisselbrink AB, et al. (2003) Mesenchymal stem cells in human second-trimester bone marrow, liver, lung, and spleen exhibit a similar immunophenotype but a heterogeneous multilineage differentiation potential. Haematologica 88: 845–852.
38. Pittenger MF, Mackay AM, Beck SC, Jaiswal RK, Douglas R, et al. (1999) Multilineage potential of adult human mesenchymal stem cells. Science 284: 143–147.
39. Stagg J (2008) Mesenchymal stem cells in cancer. Stem Cell Rev 4: 119–124.
40. Lv FJ, Tuan RS, Cheung KM, Leung VY (2014) Concise review: the surface markers and identity of human mesenchymal stem cells. Stem Cells 32: 1408–1419.
41. Boxall SA, Jones E (2012) Markers for characterization of bone marrow multipotential stromal cells. Stem Cells Int 2012: 975871.
42. Dominici M, Le Blanc K, Mueller I, Slaper-Cortenbach I, Marini F, et al. (2006) Minimal criteria for defining multipotent mesenchymal stromal cells. The International Society for Cellular Therapy position statement. Cytotherapy 8: 315–317.
43. Potdar P, Sutar J (2010) Establishment and molecular characterization of mesenchymal stem cell lines derived from human visceral & subcutaneous adipose tissues. J Stem Cells Regen Med 6: 26–35.
44. Haniffa MA, Collin MP, Buckley CD, Dazzi F (2009) Mesenchymal stem cells: the fibroblasts' new clothes? Haematologica 94: 258–263.
45. Bae S, Park CW, Son HK, Ju HK, Paik D, et al. (2008) Fibroblast activation protein alpha identifies mesenchymal stromal cells from human bone marrow. Br J Haematol 142: 827–830.
46. Hung SC, Kuo PY, Chang CF, Chen TH, Ho LL (2006) Alpha-smooth muscle actin expression and structure integrity in chondrogenesis of human mesenchymal stem cells. Cell Tissue Res 324: 457–466.
47. Ljujic B, Milovanovic M, Volarevic V, Murray B, Bugarski D, et al. (2013) Human mesenchymal stem cells creating an immunosuppressive environment and promote breast cancer in mice. Scientific Reports 3.
48. Allard B, Turcotte M, Stagg J (2012) CD73-generated adenosine: orchestrating the tumor-stroma interplay to promote cancer growth. J Biomed Biotechnol 2012: 485156.
49. Synnestvedt K, Furuta GT, Comerford KM, Louis N, Karhausen J, et al. (2002) Ecto-5′-nucleotidase (CD73) regulation by hypoxia-inducible factor-1 mediates permeability changes in intestinal epithelia. J Clin Invest 110: 993–1002.
50. Allard B, Turcotte M, Spring K, Pommey S, Royal I, et al. (2013) Anti-CD73 therapy impairs tumor angiogenesis. Int J Cancer 134: 1466–1473.
51. Chatterjee D, Tufa DM, Baehre H, Hass R, Schmidt RE, et al. (2014) Natural killer cells acquire CD73 expression upon exposure to mesenchymal stem cells. Blood 123: 594–595.
52. Sleeman JP, Thiery JP (2011) SnapShot: The epithelial-mesenchymal transition. Cell 145: 162 e161.
53. Thiery JP, Acloque H, Huang RY, Nieto MA (2009) Epithelial-mesenchymal transitions in development and disease. Cell 139: 871–890.

54. Thiery JP (2002) Epithelial-mesenchymal transitions in tumour progression. Nat Rev Cancer 2: 442–454.
55. Xiong L, Wen Y, Miao X, Yang Z (2013) NT5E and FcGBP as key regulators of TGF-1-induced epithelial-mesenchymal transition (EMT) are associated with tumor progression and survival of patients with gallbladder cancer. Cell Tissue Res 355: 365–374.
56. Li O, Tormin A, Sundberg B, Hyllner J, Le Blanc K, et al. (2013) Human embryonic stem cell-derived mesenchymal stroma cells (hES-MSCs) engraft in vivo and support hematopoiesis without suppressing immune function: implications for off-the shelf ES-MSC therapies. PLoS One 8: e55319.
57. Park JS, Chang DY, Kim JH, Jung JH, Park J, et al. (2013) Retrovirus-mediated transduction of a cytosine deaminase gene preserves the stemness of mesenchymal stem cells. Exp Mol Med 45: e10.
58. Hermida-Gomez T, Fuentes-Boquete I, Gimeno-Longas MJ, Muinos-Lopez E, Diaz-Prado S, et al. (2010) Quantification of cells expressing mesenchymal stem cell markers in healthy and osteoarthritic synovial membranes. J Rheumatol 38: 339–349.

14

Primary Ovarian Carcinomas and Abdominal Metastasis Contain 4,6-Disulfated Chondroitin Sulfate Rich Regions, Which Provide Adhesive Properties to Tumour Cells

Myrtille J. E. Vallen[1,2]*, Samuel Schmidt[3], Arie Oosterhof[1], Johan Bulten[4], Leon F. A. G. Massuger[2], Toin H. van Kuppevelt[1]

1 Department of Biochemistry, Radboud Institute for Molecular Life Sciences, Radboud University Medical Center, Nijmegen, The Netherlands, **2** Department of Obstetrics and Gynaecology, Radboud University Medical Center, Nijmegen, The Netherlands, **3** Department of Cell Biology, Nijmegen Center for Molecular Life Sciences, Radboud University Medical Center, Nijmegen, The Netherlands, **4** Department of Pathology, Radboud University Medical Center, Nijmegen, The Netherlands

Abstract

High mortality in ovarian cancer patients is primarily caused through rapid metastasis of the tumour, but the underlying mechanisms are poorly understood. Glycosaminoglycans, are abundantly present in tumours and chondroitin sulfate-E (CSE), a highly 4,6-sulfated glycosaminoglycan, has been indicated to play a role in carcinogenesis. In this study we investigated the presence of CSE in ovarian cancer metastasis and studied its role in tumour cell adhesiveness and migration. CSE was studied immunohistochemically in primary ovarian carcinomas and abdominal metastases using the single chain antibody GD3G7. The role of CSE was studied in 2D (scratch assays) and 3D (collagen matrices, spheroids) systems using SKOV3 cells applying 1: overexpression of CSE by stable transfection with DNA encoding GalNAc4S-6 sulfotransferase, 2: enzymatic removal of CS, and 3: addition of CSE. In ovarian cancer tissue, CSE expression was predominantly seen in the stromal compartment of both primary ovarian carcinomas and metastases, with a comparable degree of intensity and extent. Overexpression of CSE disaccharide units by tumour cells increased their adhesive properties which was especially seen in tumour spheroid formation. Increased expression of CSE reduced cell migration. Addition of free CSE had similar effects. The data presented here indicate that CSE is associated with metastatic lesions and that it provides tumours with adhesive properties. CSE rich motifs are put forward as a potential target for ovarian cancer therapy.

Editor: Nikos K. Karamanos, University of Patras, Greece

Funding: This work was supported by the Dutch Cancer Society (2008-4058). The funders had no role in study design, data collection and analysis, decision to publish, or preparation of the manuscript.

Competing Interests: The authors have declared that no competing interests exist.

* Email: m.vallen@obgyn.umcn.nl

Introduction

Ovarian cancer is the fifth leading cause of cancer death in women worldwide. Each year this disease accounts for approximately 225,000 new patients and 140,000 deaths [1]. Despite advances in cytoreductive surgery and modern chemotherapy, five-year survival rates are not improving. This high lethality is primarily due to the fact that patients are diagnosed with advanced stage disease (FIGO III–IV), when the tumour is already widely spread [2,3]. Unlike other tumours, haematogenous dissemination of ovarian cancer cells is rare. Instead, ovarian carcinomas mainly disseminate via the transcoelomic route. Tumour cells and cell aggregates (spheroids) are shed from the primary tumour into the peritoneal space, where they preferably seed and attach to the peritoneum and omentum [4,5].

In order for ovarian cancer cells to establish metastatic depositions, they need to aggregate and attach to the mesothelial lining. These initial steps in ovarian cancer progression are still poorly understood [6] and only little is known about the molecules involved in ovarian cancer cell adhesion [7]. There is increasing evidence that molecules in the extracellular matrix (ECM) play a crucial role in adhesiveness, and that the tumour stroma is a key player in this respect. It has been indicated that tumour cells may even bring their own soil, thereby providing a specific tumour niche and facilitating metastasis [8].

The ECM is a highly organized three-dimensional structure which maintains tissue integrity and is actively involved in many important physiological and pathological processes e.g. the binding of growth factors and adapting mechanical properties [9]. Tumour cells are known to interfere with the normal biosynthesis of the ECM and as a consequence modify its biochemical composition [10]. Proteoglycans and glycosaminoglycans are major constituents of the ECM and the cell membrane, mediating cell-cell and cell-matrix interactions. Proteoglycans are a complex group of glycoproteins, which contain a core protein with one or more covalently bound sulfated glycosaminoglycan chains. Based on the chemical backbone of glycosaminoglycans a number of classes can be discerned including dermatan sulfate (DS)/chondroitin sulfate (CS), heparan sulfate (HS)/heparin and keratan sulfate (KS). Hyaluronan (HA) is a special class of glycosaminoglycans not bound to a protein core. Normal ovary contains large amounts of DS [11,12], however, during ovarian carcinogenesis the predominant glycosaminoglycan reverts to CS [13], a phenomenon seen in various types of cancer [14,15]. Within the class of CS a large heterogeneity exists due to the presence of differently sulfated disaccharide units including CSA (4-sulfated), CSC (6-sulfated), CSD (2,6-disulfated) and CSE (4,6-disulfated). In cancerous tissue alterations in the sulfation level and type of the disaccharide units have been observed [16–21].

Using an antibody recognizing a motif that is rich in CSE units (GD3G7), we recently showed strong upregulation of CSE in primary ovarian carcinomas which correlated with poor prognostic parameters such as high grade, and advanced FIGO stage [19]. Interference with CSE, either by blockage using GD3G7 or by enzymatic degradation of CS chains, strongly inhibited metastatic growth in a mouse Lewis lung carcinoma model [22]. In addition, murine osteosarcoma cells containing high levels of CSE formed more metastatic liver tumour nodules compared to cells with lower levels, an effect that could be inhibited by preincubation of cells with the GD3G7 antibody or by preadministration with CS rich in CSE units [23].

The final step in the biosynthesis of the CSE subunit depends on the enzyme *N*-acetyl galactosamine 4-sulfate 6-*O*-sulfotransferase (GalNAc4S-6ST), which forms CSE by transferring an additional sulfate group to CSA [24]. An increase of GalNAc4S-6ST mRNA has been observed in patients with colorectal and astrocytic tumours [25,26]. In astrocytic tumours elevated levels of GalNAc4S-6ST mRNA correlated with poor patient outcome. Down regulation of the expression of GalNAc4S-6ST in a Lewis lung carcinoma cell line resulted in reduced adhesiveness of cells to ECM molecules and suppression of metastatic lung carcinoma [27].

In this study, we first examined CSE expression in primary ovarian carcinomas and ovarian metastasis in the peritoneal cavity. We then addressed the mechanistic role of CSE, a.o. by establishing SKOV3 cell lines stably transfected with DNA encoding GalNAc4S-6ST and studying adhesiveness and cell migration using 2D and 3D model systems.

Materials and Methods

Human tumour tissue and cell lines

Paraffin embedded tumour material from 25 ovarian cancer patients (serous subtype) was obtained from the archives of the Department of Pathology at Radboud University Medical Centre. From all patients we collected representative tumour slides including primary carcinoma and abdominal metastases (omental and peritoneal tumour depositions). All slides were reviewed by an experienced gyneco-pathologist (JB) using H&E sections. The age at diagnosis, CA125 level at diagnosis, menopausal status, FIGO stage [28], tumour grade [29] and primary debulking result (defined as complete or incomplete) were recorded (Table 1).

The human ovarian cancer SKOV3 cell line was generously provided by Dr. L.G. Poels (Radboud University Medical Center). Originally this SKOV3 cell line was obtained from the American Type Culture Collection (ATCC, Manassas, VA). Cells were cultured and maintained in Dulbecco's modified Eagle's medium (DMEM) supplemented with 10% fetal calf serum (FCS) (Life Technologies Paisley, UK) and penicillin/streptomycin (100 U/ml). Cells were incubated in a humidified atmosphere containing 5% CO_2 at 37°C.

Immunohistochemistry

Five µm paraffin sections were immunohistochemically analysed according to the ABC-method as described previously [19]. In brief, sections were de-paraffinised in xylene, hydrated with graded ethanol and blocked for endogenous peroxidase activity. After rinsing in phosphate-buffered saline (PBS) containing 0.1% Tween-20 (PBS-T), sections were incubated in 0.1 M citrate buffer (pH 5.8) and blocked with 2% bovine serum albumin (BSA, fraction V, Sigma-Aldrich) in PBS-T. Next, sections were incubated successively with primary anti-CS antibodies, secondary mouse anti-VSV antibody P5D4, and tertiary biotinylated horse-anti-mouse IgG (Vector Laboratories Inc.). After incubation with ABC-reagents (Vectastain ABC anti-mouse-IgG kit, Vector Laboratories Inc.), bound antibodies were detected using 3-amino-9-ethylcarbazole (AEC). Sections were counterstained with haematoxylin and mounted with Kaiser's glycerol gelatin (Merck, Darmstadt, Germany). Different single chain CS-antibodies were applied, including IO3H10 (overall staining for CS) [30], GD3A12 (staining for dermatan sulfate) [11], and GD3G7 (staining for 4,6-disulfated CS (CSE)) [31].

For immunofluorescence of SKOV3 cell lines, cells were plated on 10-wells glass slides (Nutacon, Portsmouth, NH) and grown to confluency. Cells were washed with PBS and fixed with 100% ice cold methanol. After blocking with PBS-T and 1% BSA, sections were incubated with primary antibody for 60 min. Bound antibodies were detected by secondary anti-VSV tag mouse antibody P5D4 and visualized by a tertiary antibody step including goat antimouse IgG Alexa Fluor 488 (Invitrogen, Paisley, Scotland), Finally, cryosections were fixed in 100% ethanol, air-dried and mounted in mowiol-488 (Calbiochem, La Jolla, CA).

Generation of stably transfected SKOV-3 cell lines with DNA encoding for GalNAc4S-6ST

pFLAG-CMV2-hGalNAc4S-6ST, generously provided by Prof. Osami Habuchi, (Kariya, Japan), pBluescript SK II (Stratagene, La Jolla, USA) and pIRES-EGFP (Invitrogen, Paisley, Scotland) were used to construct the pIRES2-EGFP-GalNAc4S-6ST plasmid. An intermediate step was incorporated in the cloning procedure to generate compatible restriction sites (S. 1). Restriction enzymes *EcoRI, HindIII and XhoI* were purchased from New England Biolabs, Beverly, MA. Transfection of the SKOV3 was performed using Lipofectamine$^{TM\ 2000}$ (Invitrogen, San Diego, CA) according to the manufacturer's protocol. Geneticine G418 (Invitrogen, San Diego, CA) resistant cell clones were isolated and expanded for further characterization. For comparative purposes we selected two clones (C5 and C6) containing an empty vector (pIRES2-EGFP(-)) and three clones (F5, F7 and F9) with full vector (pIRES2-EGFP-GalNAc4S-6ST).

To establish the incorporation of the pIRES2-EGFP-GalNAc4S-6ST into genomic DNA, total genomic DNA was isolated from SKOV3 cells using a Qiagen AllPrep DNA/RNA micro kit (Qiagen GmbH, Hilden, Germany) according to manufacturer's specifications. The concentration of DNA was determined using a Nanodrop 2000c spectrophotometer (NanoDrop products, Wilmington, DE, USA). Primer sets covering exon-exon boundaries were designed using Primer 3 [32] based on the reference sequence obtained from the UCSC human genome browser (http://genome.ucsc.edu/), assembly February 2009 (GRCh37/hg19). Two primer sets for human GalNAc4S-6ST and 1 for the housekeeping gene human acidic ribosomal phosphoprotein P0 (RPLP0) were used (Biolegio (Nijmegen, The Netherlands). The primer sequences were as follow: hGalNAc4S-6ST, 5′-GACGCAGGACTTCATCCAC-'3 (forward), 5′-AGCAACAGTTTCTCATTCTTCG-'3 (forward), 5'GCGGATTTATTCGAACTTGC-'3 (reverse) and 5′-ATCAAAGCCTCCTGCTTCTC-'3 (reverse), and for RPLP0, 5′-CACCATTGAAATCCTGAGTGATGT-'3 (forward) and 5′-TGACCAGCCCAAAGGAGAAG-′3 (reverse). Real-Time quantitative polymerase chain reaction

Table 1. General patient characteristics.

	Panel (n = 25)
Age (median, range)	57 (23–84)
CA125 at diagnosis (median, range)	433.9 (53.9–8203.0)
Menopausal status	
Pre-	9
Post-	16
FIGO	
I	-
II	2
III	20
IV	2
Unknown	1
Grade	
I	-
II	2
III	23
Primary cytoreductive surgery	
Complete	9
Incomplete	14
Not reported	2

(QPCR) was carried out with 5 ng DNA, using CFX Real Time PCR detection system and Bio-Rad CFX manager software version 1.6 for quantification with Sybr Green and melting curve analysis (Bio-Rad Laboratories, Inc., Hercules, CA). Amplifications were performed starting with a 10 min template denaturation step at 95°C, followed by 40 cycles of denaturation at 95°C for 15 s and combined primer annealing/extension at 60°C for 60 s.

Reverse phase-high performance liquid chromatography (RP-HPLC) disaccharide analysis

Cells were plated in T175 flasks, grown to 80–90% confluency and detached using ethylenediaminetetraacetic acid (EDTA) and a police man scraper to harvest extracellular matrix components. The preparation was incubated with chondroitinase-ABC (Sigma Aldrich, St. Louis, USA) in digestion buffer (250 mM Tris, 20 mM $MgAc_2$, pH 8.0) at a final concentration of 1 IU/ml (37°C, 24 h). Samples were vacuum dried and reconstituted with 0.1 M aminoacridone (AMAC) solution in glacial acetic acid/DMSO (3:17, v/v). 1 M $NaCNBH_3$ was added and the samples were incubated for 6 h at 45°C. Finally, 50% (v/v) dimethyl sulfoxide was added and the samples were stored at −80°C. The final disaccharide composition of CS was evaluated by quantitative analysis of the AMAC labeled digests using RP-HPLC. A gradient elution was performed using a binary solvent system as described by Ambrosius *et al* [33]. Equilibration of the Waters X-Bridge Shield column (100×4.6 mm ID) took place with 98% 60 mM ammonium acetate (NH_4Ac), pH 5.6 and 2% acetonitril for 7 min. After injection of the samples the following program was used: 1 min at equilibration condition, a linear gradient step to 4% acetonitril in two min, a separation gradient step to 15% acetonitril in 23 min, a washing step in 1 min to 60% acetonitril followed by another 5 min at 60% and returning to equilibration conditions in 1 min. Flow rate was 1.5 ml/min and monitoring was performed with a fluorescence detector (λ_{ex} 442 nm, λ_{em} 520 nm).

2D scratch assay

For 2D-migration analysis a scratch assay was applied. Transfected and not-transfected SKOV3 cells were detached by EDTA, resuspended in DMEM medium containing 10% FCS and plated onto 12-well plates (5×10^4 per well). Cells were grown to confluency and subsequently starved in a serum free DMEM medium for 24 hrs. After starvation, one artificial gap (scratch) was made using a sterile plastic 10 µl micropipette tip. Next, tissue culture medium was removed and cells were washed in sterile PBS to eliminate detached cells and debris. Experiments were performed by incubating the cells with normal medium or normal medium supplemented with CSE (Seikagaku, Tokyo, Japan) (50 and 100 µg/ml). Cell migration was monitored taking digital photographs at different time-points with a phase contrast microscope. All experiments were performed three or more times.

Spheroid formation, the 'hanging'- drop method

In accordance with the predominant metastatic pattern of ovarian carcinomas in the abdomen, we studied SKOV3 cell behavior not only as single cells but also as tumour cell aggregates (spheroids). Multicellular spheroids are thought to represent an important way for tumour dissemination in ovarian cancer. In addition, compact spheroid formation provides a protective shield for tumour cells. For that purpose, cells from subconfluent cultures were detached with 2 mM EDTA and multicellular spheroids were generated using the hanging-drop method [34]. In brief, cells were resuspended in DMEM growth medium supplemented with 10% methylcellulose to a final cell concentration of $\pm4\times10^4$ cells/ml and incubated in hanging droplets (25 µl) overnight. After cell aggregation, spheroids were washed in phosphate buffered saline (PBS) and used for migration assays. To further study the adhesive properties of CS wildtype SKOV3 cells in hanging drops were digested with specific glycosaminoglycan degrading enzymes including chondroitinase ABC (Sigma Aldrich, St. Louis, USA), chondroitinase B and chondroitinase AC (IBEX Technologies, Montreal, Canada).

Spheroid cell migration in 3-D collagen matrices

Spheroids ($\pm1\times10^3$ cells) prepared from different SKOV3 clones were incorporated into 3D collagen matrices as described before [35,36]. In brief, SKOV3 spheroids were suspended in a solution containing 1.6 mg/ml bovine collagen type I (Inamed Biomaterials, Fremond, CA), 7% minimal essential medium and 3% bicarbonate in DMEM. The mix was gently transferred into a 6 well plate and allowed to polymerize for 20–30 minutes in an incubator at 37°C with 5% CO_2. After polymerization the freshly prepared gels were covered with DMEM medium.

To study the influence of CSE on tumour cell migration, a protocol for CS decoration of the fibrillar type I collagen was developed. For this, an intermediate step was incorporated in which CSE (final concentration either 50 or 100 ug/ml) was added to the MEM bicarbonate suspension prior to collagen addition ((S2A). Inclusion of this step resulted in collagen fibrils associated with (FITC-labeled) CSE (AMS biotechnology, Abington UK), as demonstrated with confocal microscopy (S2B). To our knowledge, this is the first time a complex re-assembled meshwork of collagen fibrils homogeneously decorated with a negatively charged glycosaminoglycans is visualized. SKOV3 cell migration was microscopically recorded with an inverted microscope (Leitz Fluovert, Cologne, Germany) at 37°C and photographs were taken at time points 0, 12 and 24 hrs. All experiments were performed three or more times.

Cell viability was checked for single cells contained in DMEM supplemented with 50 or 100 μg/ml CSE using WST-1 analysis and cell counting based on nigrosin staining. Both CSE concentrations did not significantly affect cell viability (data not shown).

Results

Chondroitin sulfate expression in primary and secondary ovarian tumours

The clinical characteristics of the patient panel are summarized in table 1. Median age at the time of diagnosis was 57 (range 23–84) and the majority of women was postmenopausal. Our study panel consisted solely of patients suffering from high grade (II–III), serous ovarian carcinomas.

CS and DS are present throughout both the tumoural and non-tumoural stroma. This was demonstrated using antibodies IO3H10 (overall CS staining) and GD3A12 (overall DS staining) (fig. 1B and C) [11,30]. We also applied antibody GD3G7 which defines a specific epitope harboring contiguous 4,6 disulfated (CSE) disaccharide units, a rare CS modification. In accordance with our previous studies [19,31], GD3G7 expression in ovarian carcinomas was predominantly seen in the intratumoural stroma, the basement membrane zone underlying tumour cells, and the region surrounding (pathological) blood vessels. A CSE gradient was seen at places where tumour tissue is adjacent to non-tumourous tissue (fig. 1D and E).

In general, primary ovarian tumours and abdominal secondary tumours showed a similar staining pattern. Both intensity and extent of CSE staining were comparable. In figure 2 GD3G7 epitope expression is shown for a primary tumour (fig. 2A), and three secondary metastatic tumour depositions, one on the contralateral ovary (fig. 2B), one in the omentum (fig. 2C) and one in the Douglas pouch' (fig. 2D). All metastatic localizations were strongly positive for the GD3G7 epitope. Again, GD3G7 expression was predominantly present in the intratumoural stroma, the stroma directly surrounding tumour depositions, and small (tumour) blood vessels. When the mesothelial lining and its underlying basement membrane were associated with tumour cells, an evident strong staining with GD3G7 was seen (arrow fig. 2B).

Expression of chondroitin sulfate-E by SKOV3 cells transfected with DNA encoding GalNAc4S-6STGalNAc4S-6ST

To study the effect of CSE on tumour cell behavior we transfected cells with DNA encoding GalNAc4S-6ST, the enzyme involved in the biosynthesis of 4,6-disulfated disaccharides. We selected three stably transfected clones with the vector containing GalNAc4S-6ST and two clones containing an empty vector. These cell lines and wild-type SKOV3 cells were analysed for the presence of CSE using antibody GD3G7 and by disaccharide analysis of CS.

Using confluent cells, the wildtype SKOV3 cells as well the cells containing the empty vector showed weak to moderate (peri)cellular staining with antibody GD3G7 (fig. 3A–C), whereas cells transfected with the DNA encoding GalNAc4S-6ST showed more abundant staining, including areas of very strong staining intensity (fig 3D–F).

To analyse the disaccharide composition of CS we applied RP-HPLC with AMAC labelling. This technique allows separation and quantification of 8 different CS disaccharides based on their degree of sulfation. Overall, SKOV3 wildtype and empty vector clones were comparable for their CS disaccharide composition, including the CSE (4,6-di sulfated disaccharide) unit. When the CS disaccharide composition of full vector cell lines was compared with the control cell lines, CSE content was significantly elevated (p-value $= 0.026$) (fig. 4), which was in line with the increased staining by GD3G7 (fig. 3). In addition, there was a tendency ($p = 0.081$), for a decrease in CSA disaccharide units (4S), which is the substrate of GalNAc4S-6ST.

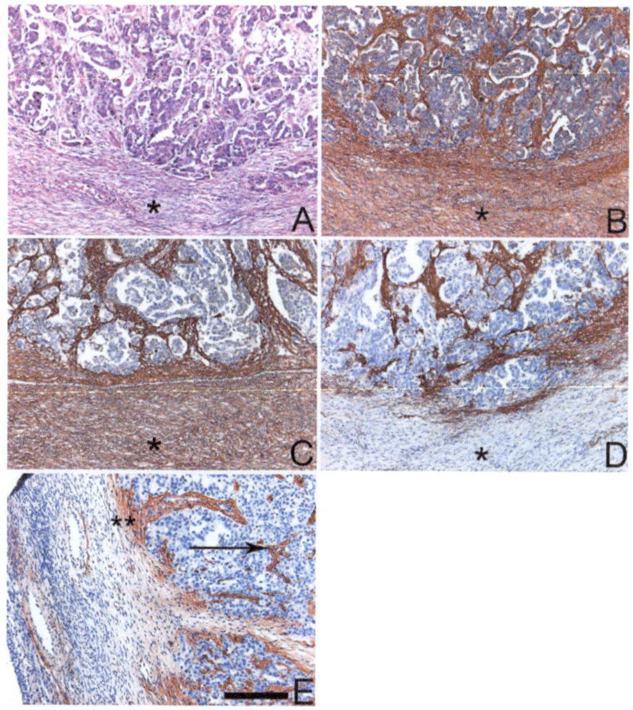

Figure 1. Strong staining for CSE in tumours. Sections of paraffin embedded primary serous ovarian carcinoma were stained for CS, DS and CSE using antibodies IO3H10, GD3A12 and GD3G7, respectively. A) Haematoxylin-Eosin staining showing tumourous versus non-tumourous regions. Non-tumourous regions are indicated with an asterisk (*). B–E) Overall staining for CS (B: antibody IO3H10), DS (C:antibody GD3A12) and CSE (D, E antibody GD3G7). Note overall staining for CS and DS, but strong CSE staining in intratumoural stroma, including small tumour capillaries (E, arrows). Also note mild staining of large blood vessels in non-tumourous areas (E) Staining for CSE indicated a gradient of CSE at the boundary of tumour and non-tumourous tissue (**). Bar: 100 μm.

Chondroitin sulfate (E) provides adhesive properties

Strong adhesive properties are an important survival tool of tumours. To investigate the role of CS in this respect, we prepared spheroids, cell aggregates often associated with tumour metastasis. Wildtype SKOV3 cells in hanging drops were digested with specific glycosaminoglycan degrading enzymes including chondroitinase ABC (cleaves both CS and DS), chondroitinase B (cleaves DS) and chondroitinase AC (cleaves CS). When either of chondroitinase ABC or AC was added, spheroid formation was inhibited for approximately 48 hours (fig. 5A). After 48 hours this effect disappeared, likely because of reduced enzyme activity. By contrast, chondroitinase B did not influence cell aggregation. Indicating that spheroid formation is CS but not DS dependent. To study the specific effect of CSE on spheroid formation, spheroids prepared from cells overexpressing CSE were evaluated.

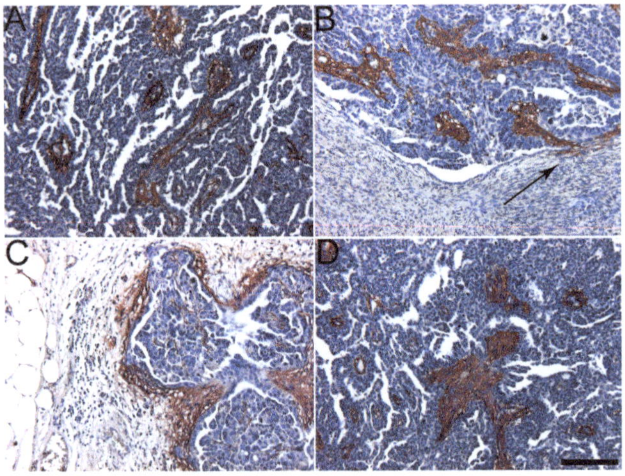

Figure 2. Strong staining for CSE in transcoelomic, ovarian metastasis (antibody GD3G7). A) Primary tumour, B) contralateral ovary, C) omentum, D) Douglas' pouch all displayed strong staining for CSE. Note the staining at sites where the mesothelial lining and its underlying basal membrane were associated with intruding tumour cells (B, arrow). Bar: 100 μm.

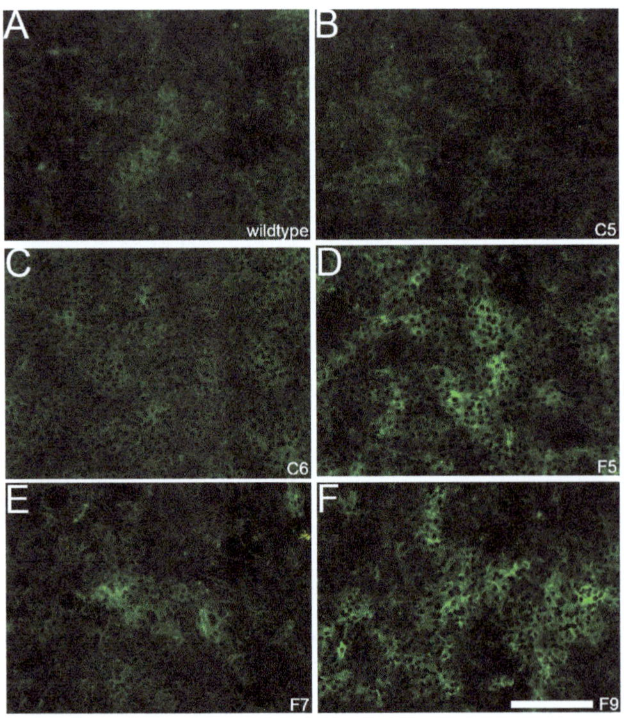

Figure 3. Increase of staining for CSE in SKOV3 cells transfected with GalNAc4S-6ST (antibody GD3G7). SKOV3 wildtype (A) and transfection control (empty vector) SKOV3(-) cells (C5 (B) and C6 (C)) showed weak (peri)cellular expression of CSE, whereas SKOV3 cells transfected with DNA encoding GalNAc4S-6ST (F5(D), F7(E), F9(F)) showed strong expression for CSE expression, especially in more dense regions. Bar: 100 μm.

In comparison with to spheroids prepared from wild type cells or empty vector cells, CSE overexpressing spheroids displayed a more roundish appearance and showed a more smooth surface (fig. 5B), suggesting a more firm attraction of cells.

Chondroitin sulfate E reduces cell migration

Since cell migration is an intermediate step in the metastatic process of ovarian cancer, the role of CSE was examined in 2D and 3D migration assays. We studied the migrative properties of wildtype and transfected SKOV3 cells in a 2D system using a scratch assay (fig. 6). Both wildtype SKOV3 cells and SKOV3 cells containing the empty vector closed the artificial wound within 24 hours. SKOV3 cells overexpressing CSE did not (fig. 6A). These cells closed the gap approximately 12 to 24 hours later. An inhibitory effect on migration was also seen when CSE was supplemented to the culture medium of wildtype SKOV3 cells (fig. 6B).

To study the effect of CSE on cell migration in 3D systems, spheroids were prepared from wildtype and transfected SKOV3 cells and embedded in a collagenous matrix. Wildtype SKOV3 cells migrated out of the spheroid primarily as single cells and sometimes following collective strand formation. The same was seen for spheroids prepared from SKOV3 cells harboring an empty vector. However, SKOV3 cells overexpressing CSE were hardly able to migrate out of the spheroid, nor as single cells, nor as collective strands (fig. 7A). In an alternative approach, we prepared collagenous matrices in the presence of CSE, resulting in collagen fibrils associated with CSE. In such matrices wildtype SKOV3 cells showed very restricted cell migration (fig. 7B), further indicating the cell migrative inhibiting effect of CSE.

Discussion

High lethality in ovarian cancer is primarily due to rapid metastasis of the tumour. In this study we observed manifest presence of CSE, a CS harbouring 4,6-disulfated disaccharides, in both primary and metastatic ovarian tumours, and we propose a functional role for CSE in tumour cell adhesion in ovarian cancer spheroids.

CS likely possesses a number of roles in the micro-environment of (tumour) cells and upregulation of highly sulfated CS (such as CSE) has been described for various tumours. Through the binding of glycosaminoglycans with effector molecules such as cytokines, chemokines, and growth factors [37], chondroitin sulfates (especially CSE) are able to regulate many cellular mechanisms in both physiological and pathological conditions, including proliferation and angiogenesis. The metastatic cascade involves detachment, adhesion and migration/invasion, and encompasses various interactions between tumour cells and components of the ECM [38].

Ovarian cancer dissemination predominantly occurs via intra-abdominal spread of the tumour. Exfoliated tumour cells are carried via peritoneal fluid or ascites to secondary sites in the abdominal cavity [39]. Spheroid formation may represent an important intermediate survival mechanism facilitating ovarian cancer dissemination. Compact formation of spheroids by ovarian cancer cells has been associated with more aggressive and invasive characteristics [40,41]. In addition, decreased penetrance of immune cells and therapeutics provides spheroids with an important advantage for survival [42]. In this study, we found that CS has a role in spheroid formation, and overexpression of CSE disaccharide units improves the adhesive properties of tumour cells. Our results are in line with the finding that down-regulating of GalNAc4S-6ST in Lewis lung carcinoma cells

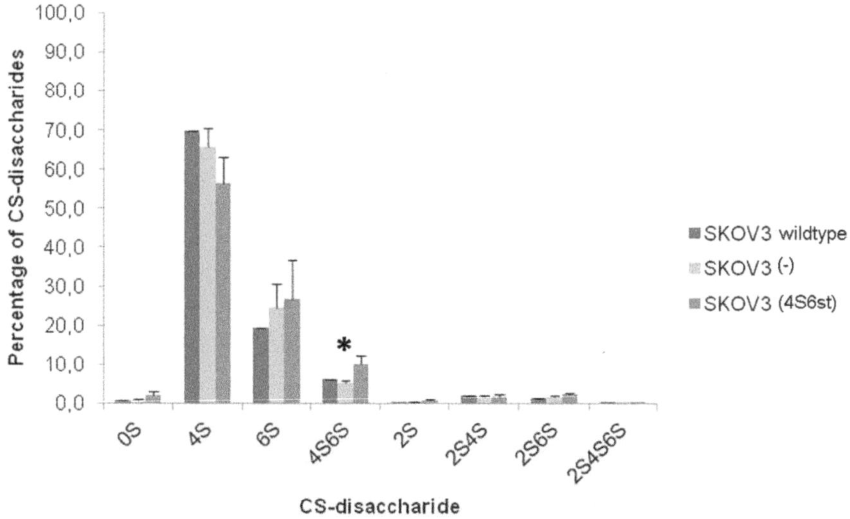

Total amount of CS-disaccharides in different cell cultures (ρmol per 1 million cells)

Cell culture	0S	4S	6S	4S6S	2S	2S4S	2S6S	2S4S6S	Total amount
Wildtype SKOV3	0.0514 (0.7%)	4.8172 (69.9%)	1.3321 (19.3%)	0,4219 (6.1%)	0,0166 (0.2%)	0,1388 (2.0%)	0,1048 (1.5%)	0,0074 (0.11%)	6.89 (100%)
SKOV3(-) C5	0.0688 (0.6%)	6.9073 (62.1%)	3.2150 (28.9%)	0,5080 (4.6%)	0,0264 (0.2%)	0,2070 (1.9%)	0,1750 (1.6%)	0,0076 (0.07%)	11.12 (100%)
SKOV3(-) C6	0.0478 (1.0%)	3.4506 (69.2%)	1.0089 (20.2%)	0,2884 (5.8%)	0,0170 (0.3%)	0,0753 (1.5%)	0,0953 (1.9%)	0,0065 (0.13%)	4.99 (100%)
SKOV3(4S6ST) F5	0.0933 (0.9%)	5.0700 (50.4%)	3.7684 (37.5%)	0,8061 (8.0%)	0,0410 (0.4%)	0,0910 (0.9%)	0,1771 (1.8%)	0,0092 (0.09%)	10.06 (100%)
SKOV3(4S6ST) F7	0.1669 (2.4%)	3.8022 (54.8%)	1.7555 (25.3%)	0,8562 (12.3%)	0,0398 (0.6%)	0,1463 (2.1%)	0,1598 (2.3%)	0,0094 (0.14%)	6.94 (100%)
SKOV3(4S6ST) F9	0.1157 (2.7%)	2.7138 (63.7%)	0.7707 (18.1%)	0,4216 (9.9%)	0,0451 (1.1%)	0,0774 (1.8%)	0,1110 (2.6%)	0,0033 (0.08%)	4.26 (100%)

Figure 4. Reversed phase high performance liquid chromatography (RP-HPLC) for CS disaccharides. Chondroitin sulfate disaccharide composition of wild type, cells transfected with an empty vector (C5, C6), and cells transfected with a vector containing GalNAc4S-6ST (F5, F7, F9). Significantly higher CSE disaccharide content (*) was found in cells transfected with GalNAc4S-6ST (one-way ANOVA; level of significance $p<0.05$).

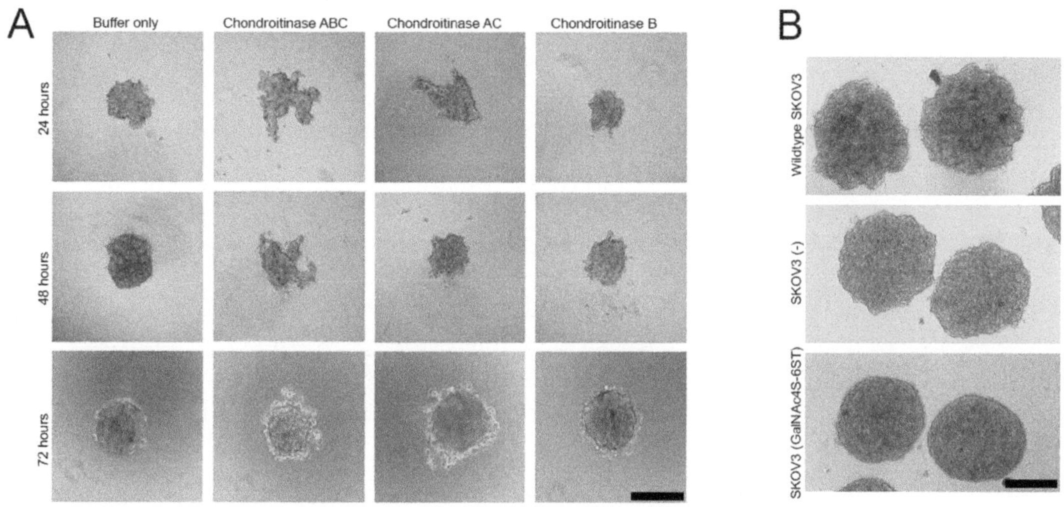

Figure 5. Spheroid formation by SKOV3 cells depends on chondroitin sulfate. A) Spheroid formation (tumour cell aggregation) was inhibited by enzymatic digestion using either of chondroitinase-ABC or –AC but not by chondroitinase B. Bar: 200 μm B) Spheroids formed by wild type SKOV3 cells and cells transfected with GalNAc4S-6ST and empty vector. Note the smooth and roundish appearance of GalNAc4S-6ST transfected cells. Bar: 100 μm.

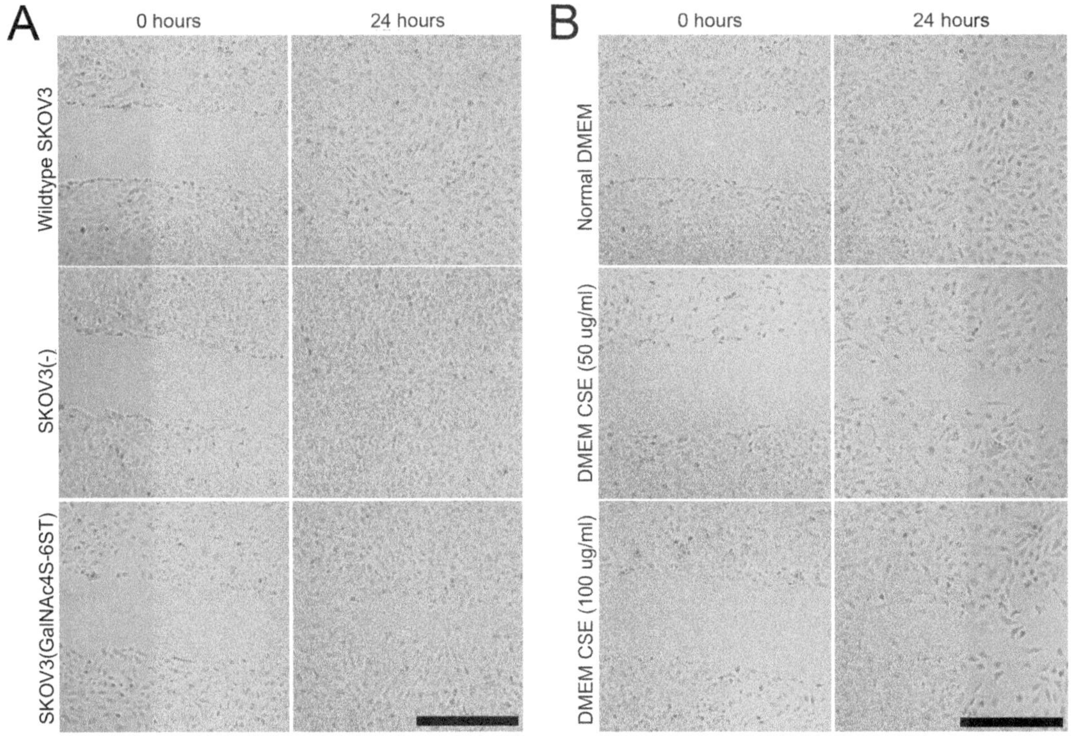

Figure 6. CSE inhibits artificial wound closure in 2D scratch assays. A) Wildtype SKOV3 cells and cell transfected with empty vector closed the artificial wound within 24 hours, whereas cells transfected with GalNAc4S-6ST cells did not. B) Addition of CSE to wildtype SKOV3 cells inhibited cell migration, showing limited gap-closure after 24 hours. Bar: 200 μm.

reduced adhesion and restricted the formation of novel tumor noduli [27]. Like lung cancer, the majority of malignant tumours spread through hematogenous or lymphogenous pathways, and upregulation of CSE may play a role. Blood born metastatic tumour cells with adhesive properties are more likely to develop tumour noduli at secondary sites. In addition, the formation of a physical barrier (pericellular matrix containing CSE) may provide a protective environment against the immune system and chemotherapy.

In vivo, CSE expression is predominantly seen in the stromal compartment of both primary ovarian carcinomas and metastasis. The stromal compartment is actively involved in tumour progression and metastasis. The presence of large intratumoural stroma areas has been correlated with poor prognosis in ovarian cancer patients [43]. Tumour cells create a tumour-facilitating micro-environment by altering the pre-existent stroma. In addition, tumour cells create ECM during spheroid formation [44]. CS, as part of the tumour micro-environment, accumulates in the stromal compartment of many solid tumours, including ovarian carcinoma [13,45]. The "seed and soil" hypothesis proposes that an appropriate host micro-environment (the soil) is needed for the optimal growth and spread of tumour cells (the seed) [46]. Recently, it was suggested that tumour cells might bring their own soil [8]. For this matter, spheroids may provide the ideal vehicle to bring soil (metastatic niche) to a secondary tumour site. This metastatic niche includes ECM components, growth factors and activated fibroblasts (CAFs), all active facilitators for tumour growth and metastasis formation [8]. Identifying adhesion molecules that are responsible for adherence (such as CSE) between cancer cells, stroma and CAFs may provide new targets for anti-metastasis therapy.

Strong CSE expression was observed at the "invasion front" of metastatic lesions (fig. 2). The upregulation of CSE at the secondary site may be a tumour cell induced modification of host cell ECM in such a way that it presents the appropriate soil for tumour growth and angiogenesis. The binding properties of CSE for a large variety of tumour associated growth factors such as FGF2 and VEGF, but also important adhesion molecules including N-cadherin and E-cadherin may be instrumental in this regard. [47,48] In addition, CSE may be one of the adhesion molecules involved in the adherence between cancer cells and stroma. It was shown that pretreatment of ovarian cancer cells with the chondroitin sulfate cleaving enzyme chondroitinase ABC decreased cell adhesion to the ECM proteins fibronectin, type IV collagen and laminin, and mesothelial cells [49,50].

Although tumour cells are the prime targets of cytostatic therapy, the tumour stroma has been suggested as an attractive target for cancer treatment as well. CSE, which is accumulated in tumour stroma, could be a specific target in this respect. Blockage, inhibition or enzymatic degradation of CSE could interfere with tumour cell aggregation, growth factor binding, and metastasis. Enzymatic degradation of CS by chondroitinase AC has been shown to inhibit melanoma proliferation and invasion [51]. However, conflicting data are available to the effect of enzymatic degradation of all chondroitin and dermatan sulfate by intra-tumoral injections of chondroitinase ABC. For instance, enzymatic degradation of *all* CS/DS by intra-tumoural injections of chondroitinase ABC results in the development of secondary tumours and increased lung metastases [52]; in solid Ehrlich ascites tumors, however, growth was restricted after chondroitinase ABC injection [53]. This suggests that targeting specific

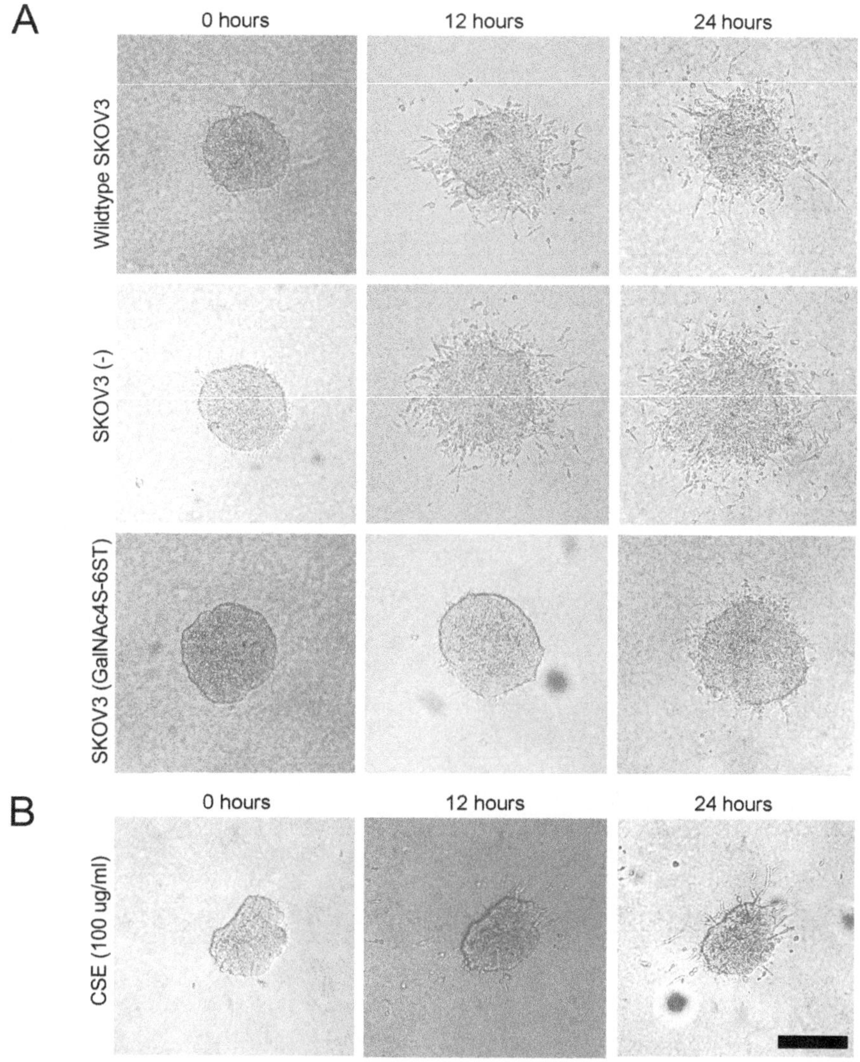

Figure 7. CSE inhibits SKOV3 cell migration out of spheroids in 3D collagen matrices. A) Wildtype and cells transfected with an empty vector (-) showed cell migration out of spheroids, whereas migration of cells transfected with GalNAc4S-6STwas almost absent. B) Strong restriction of migration of wildtype SKOV3 cells out of spheroids in CSE decorated collagen matrices. Bar: 200 μm.

chondroitin sulfates, rather than all of them, is key to a potential anti-tumour strategy.

The data presented here indicate that a specific 4,6-disulfated CS motif (CSE) is associated with metastatic lesions and that this structural motif provides tumours with adhesive properties. If specifically addressed, the CS motif may be a potential target for ovarian cancer therapy.

Supporting Information

Information S1 Cloning strategy to obtain GalNAc4S-6ST containing pIRES2-EGFP plasmid. A) pFLAG-CMV2-hGalNAc4S-6ST plasmid was double digested with restriction enzymes *EcoRI* and *HindIII* to obtain the GalNAc4S-6ST insert. The pBluescript SK II (-) vector was double digested with restriction enzymes *EcoRI* and *HindIII*, and the GalNAc4S-6ST insert was ligated vector, generating an intermediate vector. B) The intermediate vector and the pIRES2-EGFP plasmid were double digested with restriction enzymes *EcoRI* and *IXhoI, and* GalNAc4S-STt ligated into the pIRES2-EGFP plasmid.

Information S2 Generation of 3D collagen matrices with homogeneously coated chondroitin sulfate E chains, and culturing of SKOV3 spheroids for cell migration studies. A) The spheroids were embedded into a matrix of type I collagen as described previously [54], but with an additional step for administration of the chondroitin sulfate E (CSE, 1 mg/ml) into the minimum essential medium (MEM)/bicarbonate (BIC) solution before adding the bovine type I collagen. SKOV3 spheroids in DMEM medium were transfered into the collagen I/ chondroitin sulfate E solution reaching a final concentration of collagen-spheroid suspension of 1.67 mg/mI. The suspension was quickly pre-polymerized for 5 minutes at 37°C, 5% CO_2 and eventually allowed to polymerize at 37°C for 20–30 min (5% $C0_2$) in a self-constructed cell migration chamber [54]. The type I collagen–chondroitin sulfate matrices were analyzed by using an

Olympus FV1000 confocal laser scanning microscope excitation at 488 nm and emission detection of 520/50 nm (for FITC-labeled chondroitin sulfate) and confocal reflection contrast was used for detection of collagen fibers. For that, laser light (633 nm) at a low intensity was introduced into the sample. B) Confocal microscopy showing matrix decoration with chondroitin sulfate E (CSE). Upper row; non-decorated type I bovine collagen matrix. Left: Collagen reflection (white), middle: Background (green (FITC) channel), right: Overlay of reflection and background signal. Lower row; CSE-decorated bovine collagen I matrix. Left: Collagen reflection, middle: CSE-FITC (green (FITC) channel), right: Overlay of reflection and CSE signal.

Acknowledgments

We want to give our special thanks to Prof. Dr. Osami Habuchi (Aichi University of Education, Kariya, Japan) for kindly providing the pFLAG-CMV2-hGalNAc4S-6ST plasmid.

Author Contributions

Conceived and designed the experiments: MJEV SS LFAGM THvK. Performed the experiments: MJEV SS AO JB. Analyzed the data: MJEV AO SS THvK LFAGM. Contributed reagents/materials/analysis tools: AO THvK. Wrote the paper: MJEV SS LFAGM THvK JB.

References

1. Jemal A, Bray F, Center M, Ferlay J, Ward E, et al. (2011) Global cancer statistics. CA Cancer J Clin 61: 69–90.
2. Cho KR, Shih I (2009) Ovarian cancer. AnnuRevPathol 4: 287–313.
3. (2011) Ovarian cancer, five-year stage-specific relative survival rates (2004-2008). J Natl Cancer Inst 103: 1287.
4. Tan DS, Agarwal R, Kaye SB (2006) Mechanisms of transcoelomic metastasis in ovarian cancer. Lancet Oncol 7: 925–934.
5. Lengyel E (2010) Ovarian cancer development and metastasis. Am J Pathol 177: 1053–1064.
6. Naora H, Montell DJ (2005) Ovarian cancer metastasis: integrating insights from disparate model organisms. Nat Rev Cancer 5: 355–366.
7. Gardner MJ, Jones LM, Catterall JB, Turner GA (1995) Expression of cell adhesion molecules on ovarian tumour cell lines and mesothelial cells, in relation to ovarian cancer metastasis. Cancer Lett 91: 229–234.
8. Duda DG, Duyverman AM, Kohno M, Snuderl M, Steller EJ, et al. (2010) Malignant cells facilitate lung metastasis by bringing their own soil. Proc Natl Acad Sci U S A 107: 21677–21682. doi: 21610.21073/pnas.1016234107. Epub 1016232010 Nov 1016234122.
9. Tlsty TD, Coussens LM (2006) Tumor stroma and regulation of cancer development. Annu Rev Pathol 1: 119–150.
10. Freedman RS, Deavers M, Liu J, Wang E (2004) Peritoneal inflammation - A microenvironment for Epithelial Ovarian Cancer (EOC). J Transl Med 2: 23.
11. Ten Dam GB, Yamada S, Kobayashi F, Purushothaman A, van de Westerlo EM, et al. (2009) Dermatan sulfate domains defined by the novel antibody GD3A12, in normal tissues and ovarian adenocarcinomas. HistochemCell Biol 132: 117–127.
12. Wolanska M, Sobolewski K, Bankowski E, Drozdzewicz M (1999) Accumulation of collagen in ovarian benign tumours. Acta Biochim Pol 46: 941–947.
13. Ghosh S, Albitar L, LeBaron R, Welch WR, Samimi G, et al. (2010) Up-regulation of stromal versican expression in advanced stage serous ovarian cancer. GynecolOncol 119: 114–120.
14. Theocharis AD, Tsolakis I, Tzanakakis GN, Karamanos NK (2006) Chondroitin sulfate as a key molecule in the development of atherosclerosis and cancer progression. Adv Pharmacol 53: 281–295.
15. Theocharis AD, Vynios DH, Papageorgakopoulou N, Skandalis SS, Theocharis DA (2003) Altered content composition and structure of glycosaminoglycans and proteoglycans in gastric carcinoma. Int J Biochem Cell Biol 35: 376–390.
16. Kalathas D, Theocharis DA, Bounias D, Kyriakopoulou D, Papageorgakopoulou N, et al. (2009) Alterations of glycosaminoglycan disaccharide content and composition in colorectal cancer: structural and expressional studies. OncolRep 22: 369–375.
17. Lv H, Yu G, Sun L, Zhang Z, Zhao X, et al. (2007) Elevate level of glycosaminoglycans and altered sulfation pattern of chondroitin sulfate are associated with differentiation status and histological type of human primary hepatic carcinoma. Oncology 72: 347–356.
18. Papadas TA, Stylianou M, Mastronikolis NS, Papageorgakopoulou N, Skandalis S, et al. (2002) Alterations in the content and composition of glycosaminoglycans in human laryngeal carcinoma. Acta Otolaryngol 122: 330–337.
19. Vallen MJ, Massuger LF, ten Dam GB, Bulten J, van Kuppevelt TH (2012) Highly sulfated chondroitin sulfates, a novel class of prognostic biomarkers in ovarian cancer tissue. Gynecol Oncol 127: 202–209.
20. Weyers A, Yang B, Park JH, Kim YS, Kim SM, et al. (2013) Microanalysis of stomach cancer glycosaminoglycans. Glycoconj J.
21. Weyers A, Yang B, Yoon DS, Park JH, Zhang F, et al. (2012) A structural analysis of glycosaminoglycans from lethal and nonlethal breast cancer tissues: toward a novel class of theragnostics for personalized medicine in oncology? Omics 16: 79–89. doi: 10.1089/omi.2011.0102
22. Li F, Ten Dam GB, Murugan S, Yamada S, Hashiguchi T, et al. (2008) Involvement of highly sulfated chondroitin sulfate in the metastasis of the Lewis lung carcinoma cells. JBiolChem 283: 34294–34304.
23. Basappa, Murugan S, Sugahara KN, Lee CM, Ten Dam GB, et al. (2009) Involvement of chondroitin sulfate E in the liver tumor focal formation of murine osteosarcoma cells. Glycobiology 19: 735–742.
24. Ohtake S, Ito Y, Fukuta M, Habuchi O (2001) Human N-acetylgalactosamine 4-sulfate 6-O-sulfotransferase cDNA is related to human B cell recombination activating gene-associated gene. J Biol Chem 276: 43894–43900.
25. Ito Y, Watanabe M, Nishizawa T, Omachi T, Kobayashi T, et al. (2007) The utility of formalin-fixed and paraffin-embedded tissue blocks for quantitative analysis of N-acetylgalactosamine 4-sulfate 6-O-sulfotransferase mRNA expressed by colorectal cancer cells. Acta Histochem Cytochem 40: 53–59.
26. Kobayashi T, Yan H, Kurahashi Y, Ito Y, Maeda H, et al. (2013) Role of GalNAc4S-6ST in astrocytic tumor progression. PLoS One 8: e54278.
27. Mizumoto S, Watanabe M, Yamada S, Sugahara K (2013) Expression of N-acetylgalactosamine 4-sulfate 6-O-sulfotransferase involved in chondroitin sulfate synthesis is responsible for pulmonary metastasis. Biomed Res Int 2013: 656319.
28. Heintz AP, Odicino F, Maisonneuve P, Quinn MA, Benedet JL, et al. (2006) Carcinoma of the ovary. FIGO 6th Annual Report on the Results of Treatment in Gynecological Cancer. IntJGynaecolObstet 95 Suppl 1: S161–S192.
29. Seidman JD, Russell P, Kurman RJ (2002) Surface Epithelial Tumor of the Ovary. In: Kurman RJ, editor. Blaustein's Pathology of the Femal Genetal Tract. New York: Springer. pp. 791–904.
30. Smetsers TF, van de Westerlo EM, ten Dam GB, Overes IM, Schalkwijk J, et al. (2004) Human single-chain antibodies reactive with native chondroitin sulfate detect chondroitin sulfate alterations in melanoma and psoriasis. J Invest Dermatol 122: 707–716.
31. Ten Dam GB, van de Westerlo EM, Purushothaman A, Stan RV, Bulten J, et al. (2007) Antibody GD3G7 selected against embryonic glycosaminoglycans defines chondroitin sulfate-E domains highly up-regulated in ovarian cancer and involved in vascular endothelial growth factor binding. Am J Pathol 171: 1324–1333.
32. Rozen S, Skaletsky H (2000) Primer3 on the WWW for general users and for biologist programmers. Methods Mol Biol 132: 365–386.
33. Ambrosius M, Kleesiek K, Gotting C (2009) Quantitative determination and comparison of the glycosaminoglycan Delta-disaccharide composition in 22 different human cell lines. Cell Biol Int 33: 848–852.
34. Korff T, Augustin HG (1998) Integration of endothelial cells in multicellular spheroids prevents apoptosis and induces differentiation. J Cell Biol 143: 1341–1352.
35. Friedl P, Maaser K, Klein CE, Niggemann B, Krohne G, et al. (1997) Migration of highly aggressive MV3 melanoma cells in 3-dimensional collagen lattices results in local matrix reorganization and shedding of alpha2 and beta1 integrins and CD44. Cancer Res 57: 2061–2070.
36. Friedl P, Noble PB, Zanker KS (1993) Lymphocyte locomotion in three-dimensional collagen gels. Comparison of three quantitative methods for analysing cell trajectories. J Immunol Methods 165: 157–165.
37. Wegrowski Y, Maquart FX (2006) Chondroitin sulfate proteoglycans in tumor progression. AdvPharmacol 53: 297–321.
38. Vallen MJ, van der Steen SC, van Tilborg AA, Massuger LF, van Kuppevelt TH (2014) Sulfated sugars in the extracellular matrix orchestrate ovarian cancer development: 'When sweet turns sour'. Gynecol Oncol 23: 01276–01271.
39. Shield K, Ackland ML, Ahmed N, Rice GE (2009) Multicellular spheroids in ovarian cancer metastases: Biology and pathology. Gynecol Oncol 113: 143–148.
40. Sodek KL, Ringuette MJ, Brown TJ (2009) Compact spheroid formation by ovarian cancer cells is associated with contractile behavior and an invasive phenotype. Int J Cancer 124: 2060–2070.
41. Burleson KM, Boente MP, Pambuccian SE, Skubitz AP (2006) Disaggregation and invasion of ovarian carcinoma ascites spheroids. J Transl Med 4: 6.
42. Desoize B, Jardillier J (2000) Multicellular resistance: a paradigm for clinical resistance? Crit Rev Oncol Hematol 36: 193–207.
43. Labiche A, Heutte N, Herlin P, Chasle J, Gauduchon P, et al. (2010) Stromal compartment as a survival prognostic factor in advanced ovarian carcinoma. Int J Gynecol Cancer 20: 28–33.

44. Nederman T, Norling B, Glimelius B, Carlsson J, Brunk U (1984) Demonstration of an extracellular matrix in multicellular tumor spheroids. Cancer Res 44: 3090–3097.
45. Ricciardelli C, Rodgers RJ (2006) Extracellular matrix of ovarian tumors. SeminReprodMed 24: 270–282.
46. Fidler IJ (2003) The pathogenesis of cancer metastasis: the 'seed and soil' hypothesis revisited. Nat Rev Cancer 3: 453–458.
47. Koike T, Izumikawa T, Tamura J, Kitagawa H (2012) Chondroitin sulfate-E fine-tunes osteoblast differentiation via ERK1/2, Smad3 and Smad1/5/8 signaling by binding to N-cadherin and cadherin-11. Biochem Biophys Res Commun 420: 523–529. doi: 510.1016/j.bbrc.2012.1003.1024. Epub 2012 Mar 1013.
48. Deepa SS, Umehara Y, Higashiyama S, Itoh N, Sugahara K (2002) Specific molecular interactions of oversulfated chondroitin sulfate E with various heparin-binding growth factors. Implications as a physiological binding partner in the brain and other tissues. JBiolChem 277: 43707–43716.
49. Casey RC, Oegema TR, Jr., Skubitz KM, Pambuccian SE, Grindle SM, et al. (2003) Cell membrane glycosylation mediates the adhesion, migration, and invasion of ovarian carcinoma cells. ClinExpMetastasis 20: 143–152.
50. Gardner MJ, Catterall JB, Jones LM, Turner GA (1996) Human ovarian tumour cells can bind hyaluronic acid via membrane CD44: a possible step in peritoneal metastasis. Clin Exp Metastasis 14: 325–334.
51. Denholm EM, Lin YQ, Silver PJ (2001) Anti-tumor activities of chondroitinase AC and chondroitinase B: inhibition of angiogenesis, proliferation and invasion. EurJPharmacol 416: 213–221.
52. Prinz RD, Willis CM, Viloria-Petit A, Kluppel M (2011) Elimination of breast tumor-associated chondroitin sulfate promotes metastasis. Genet Mol Res 10: 3901–3913.
53. Takeuchi J (1972) Effect of chondroitinases on the growth of solid Ehrlich ascites tumour. Br J Cancer 26: 115–119.
54. Friedl P, Noble PB, Zanker KS (1993) Lymphocyte locomotion in three-dimensional collagen gels. Comparison of three quantitative methods for analysing cell trajectories. J Immunol Methods 165: 157–165.

Eribulin Mesylate Targets Human Telomerase Reverse Transcriptase in Ovarian Cancer Cells

Satoko Yamaguchi[1], Yoshiko Maida[1], Mami Yasukawa[1], Tomoyasu Kato[2], Masayuki Yoshida[3], Kenkichi Masutomi[1]*

1 Division of Cancer Stem Cell, National Cancer Center Research Institute, Tokyo, Japan, 2 Department of Gynecology, National Cancer Center Hospital, Tokyo, Japan, 3 Department of Pathology and Clinical Laboratories, National Cancer Center Hospital, Tokyo, Japan

Abstract

Treatment of advanced ovarian cancer involves platinum-based chemotherapy. However, chemoresistance is a major obstacle. Cancer stem cells (CSCs) are thought to be one of the causes of chemoresistance, but the underlying mechanism remains elusive. Recently, human telomerase reverse transcriptase (hTERT) has been reported to promote CSC-like traits. In this study, we found that a mitotic inhibitor, eribulin mesylate (eribulin), effectively inhibited growth of platinum-resistant ovarian cancer cell lines. Eribulin-sensitive cells showed a higher efficiency for sphere formation, suggesting that these cells possess an enhanced CSC-like phenotype. Moreover, these cells expressed a higher level of hTERT, and suppression of hTERT expression by siRNA resulted in decreased sensitivity to eribulin, suggesting that hTERT may be a target for eribulin. Indeed, we found that eribulin directly inhibited RNA-dependent RNA polymerase (RdRP) activity, but not telomerase activity of hTERT *in vitro*. We propose that eribulin targets the RdRP activity of hTERT and may be an effective therapeutic option for CSCs. Furthermore, hTERT may be a useful biomarker to predict clinical responses to eribulin.

Editor: Taro Yamashita, Kanazawa University, Japan

Funding: This work was supported by Grant in Aid for Scientific Research (26462544) (to SY) from Japan Society for the Promotion of Science (http://www.jsps.go.jp/english/e-grants/), Funding program for the Next Generation World-Leading Researchers (NEXT program) (to KM) from Japan Society for the Promotion of Science (http://www.jsps.go.jp/english/e-jisedai/), the Mitsubishi Foundation (to KM) (http://www.mitsubishi-zaidan.jp/en/), the Uehara Memorial Foundation (to KM) (http://www.ueharazaidan.or.jp/), and National Cancer Center Research and Development Funds (26-A-5) (to KM) (http://www.ncc.go.jp/jp/about/rinri/kaihatsu/). The funders had no role in study design, data collection and analysis, decision to publish, or preparation of the manuscript.

Competing Interests: The authors have declared that no competing interests exist.

* Email: kmasutom@ncc.go.jp

Introduction

Ovarian cancer is the most lethal of all gynecological malignancies, claiming around 150,000 lives annually worldwide. The majority of ovarian cancers are diagnosed at an advanced stage, and platinum-based chemotherapy is the standard first-line treatment for advanced ovarian cancer patients. However, chemoresistance is a major obstacle in treating ovarian cancer.

Serous adenocarcinoma (SAC), the most common type of ovarian cancer, usually responds well to initial platinum-based chemotherapy, although it will recur and ultimately develop drug resistance. Clear cell carcinoma (CCC), the second most common type in Japan, is often resistant to initial platinum-based chemotherapy [1]. Regardless of whether the resistance is acquired or primary, more promising therapeutic strategies are necessary to overcome chemoresistance and improve the prognosis of ovarian cancer patients.

Recent studies have suggested that cancer stem cells (CSCs) are, at least in part, responsible for chemoresistance in many types of cancers including ovarian cancer [reviewed in [2]]. CSCs are a subpopulation of tumor cells, which are characterized by a self-renewal capacity and ability to differentiate into distinct cell types. The emergence of CSCs occurs at least partly as a result of epithelial-mesenchymal transition (EMT), a process essential for embryonic development, which is induced during cancer progression and crucial for cancer metastasis. CSCs possess the self-renewal feature of normal stem cells, and similar signaling pathways regulate self-renewal of CSCs and normal stem cells [3]. One such pathway involves telomerase reverse transcriptase (TERT), the rate-limiting catalytic subunit of telomerase, which is expressed in the majority of cancers. Recent evidence indicates that TERT regulates stem cell traits in a telomere length-independent manner. For example, TERT activates quiescent epidermal stem cells *in vivo* in a manner independent of the intrinsic RNA component of the telomerase enzyme TERC [4]. In addition, together with the SWItch-Sucrose NonFermentable (SWI-SNF) complex protein brahma-related gene 1 (BRG1), TERT acts as a transcriptional modulator of the Wnt/β-catenin signaling pathway, contributing to self-renewal and proliferation during development [5]. More recently, accumulating evidence indicates that TERT also operates in CSCs and promotes EMT and CSC-like traits. Specifically, overexpression of human TERT (hTERT) results in an enhanced sphere-forming capacity, increased expression of EMT/CSC markers, and increased *in vivo* tumorigenesis caused by hTERT interacting with β-catenin and enhancing its transcriptional activity [6]. Conversely, suppression of hTERT expression results in a decreased sphere-forming capacity and decreased expression of the CSC marker

CD44 [7]. This function of hTERT in promotion of EMT and CSC-like traits appears to be independent of its telomerase activity [6]. Indeed, we have reported that hTERT in a complex with BRG1 and the nucleolar GTP-binding protein nucleostemin (NS) (TBN complex) participates in maintenance of CSCs. Moreover, we found that overexpression of the TBN complex enhances tumorigenicity and expression of EMT/CSC markers in an hTERT-dependent manner but in a telomere length-independent manner [8]. The exact telomerase-independent mechanisms by which the TBN complex regulates CSCs remain elusive. One possible mechanism is via the RNA-dependent RNA polymerase (RdRP) activity of hTERT [9]. RdRP induces RNA interference through production of double-stranded RNAs from single-stranded template RNAs and regulates the assembly of heterochromatin and mitotic progression [10]. Similar to RdRPs in model organisms, we found that the RdRP activities of the TBN complex are high in mitotic cells, and suppression of the TBN complex results in mitotic arrest [11].

To address chemoresistance, therapeutic strategies targeting EMT and CSCs are increasingly attracting attention. Recently, because eribulin mesylate (eribulin) was reported to inhibit metastasis by reversing EMT [12], we speculated that eribulin might target CSCs. Eribulin is a non-taxane inhibitor of microtubule dynamics [13], which induces irreversible mitotic blockade, leading to persistent inactivation of Bcl-2 and subsequent apoptosis [14]. In the United States, eribulin has been approved for treatment of metastatic breast cancer after at least two treatment regimens including an anthracycline and a taxane. Furthermore, eribulin is approved for treatment of inoperable or recurrent breast cancer in Japan.

In this study, we found that eribulin effectively inhibited growth of platinum-resistant ovarian cancer cells. Eribulin-sensitive cells showed enhanced CSC-like characteristics and high hTERT expression. Suppression of hTERT expression resulted in decreased sensitivity to eribulin. Moreover, eribulin inhibited the RdRP activity of hTERT *in vitro*, demonstrating that hTERT is a direct target of eribulin.

Results

Eribulin inhibits growth of cisplatin-resistant ovarian adenocarcinoma cell lines

Fourteen ovarian adenocarcinoma cell lines were investigated for sensitivity to cisplatin [cis-diamminedichloroplatinum(II)], including six SAC cell lines (PEO1, PEO4, PEO14, PEO23, OVKATE, and OVSAHO), six CCC cell lines (RMG-I, ES-2, OVISE, OVMANA, OVTOKO, and TOV21G), and two undifferentiated/unclassified adenocarcinoma cell lines (OVCAR-3 and A2780) (Table S1). As shown in Figure 1A, OVKATE, RMG-I, PEO4, and PEO23 cells were particularly resistant to cisplatin, presumably via different mechanisms. OVKATE cells have been previously reported as resistant to platinum agents with elevated expression of glutathione-S-transferase, a drug-resistance marker [15]. RMG-I cells are also resistant to cisplatin, which involves the extracellular signal-regulated kinase (ERK) pathway [16]. PEO4 and PEO23 cells were derived from the same patients as PEO1 and PEO14 cells, respectively, after development of clinical chemoresistance, and are therefore platinum resistant [17]. BRCA2 mutation has been found to contribute to platinum resistance in PEO4 cells [18].

We screened a series of known anti-cancer compounds for growth inhibition of platinum-resistant ovarian cancer cell lines. We found that eribulin, a mitotic inhibitor that suppresses microtubule dynamics [13], inhibited growth of RMG-I, PEO23, and PEO4 cells (Figure 1B). Strikingly, eribulin was not as effective in some of the cisplatin-sensitive cell lines such as OVTOKO, PEO14, and TOV21G (Figure 1A and 1B). For further characterization, we defined eight cell lines with an IC_{50} of <100 nM for eribulin as "eribulin-sensitive" (Eribulin S) and six cell lines with an IC_{50} of >100 nM for eribulin as "eribulin-resistant" (Eribulin R).

Eribulin-sensitive cell lines show a higher sphere-forming capacity

CSCs are thought to be responsible for chemoresistance, and CSCs have been reported to contribute to cisplatin resistance in several types of cancer [19]. Moreover, it was recently reported that eribulin reverses EMT [12], a phenotype that is highly related to CSCs. Therefore, we investigated whether eribulin-sensitive cells possess an enhanced CSC-like phenotype. Because a sphere-forming capacity is a CSC-like characteristic, we performed sphere formation assays under serum-free conditions, and found that eribulin-sensitive cell lines showed high sphere formation efficiency (Figure 2A and 2B). The sphere formation efficiency of Eribulin S cell lines was significantly higher than that of Eribulin R cell lines (Figure 2C, $p = 0.0013$), suggesting that eribulin-sensitive cell lines possess enhanced CSC-like characteristics.

Since we have recently demonstrated that NS together with hTERT and BRG1 maintains CSCs [8] and we and others have also demonstrated that NS is a useful CSC marker [20–22], we investigated the expression of BRG1 and NS in Eribulin S and Eribulin R cell lines. The protein expression level of BRG1 was significantly higher in Eribulin S cell lines (Figure 2D and 2E, $p = 0.0189$), while only a modest tendency of higher level of NS in Eribulin S cell lines was observed (Figure 2D and 2E, $p = 0.1216$). We did not detect a difference in the expression level of CD133 or CD44 (Figure S1), the cell surface markers implied in some CSCs [23].

Eribulin S cells express higher levels of hTERT protein

Overexpression of hTERT results in an enhanced sphere-forming capacity in gastric cancer cells [6]. Conversely, suppression of hTERT expression results in a decreased sphere-forming capacity in breast cancer cells [7]. Therefore, we determined whether the ovarian cancer cells with a higher sphere-forming capacity express a higher level of hTERT. We observed a tendency in cell lines with high sphere-forming efficiency, such as RMG-I, PEO23, and A2780, to express relatively high levels of hTERT protein, while cell lines with low sphere-forming efficiency, such as TOV21G, OVTOKO, and OVMANA, expressed low levels of hTERT protein, as demonstrated by enzyme-linked immunosorbent assay (ELISA) (Figure 3A). The high level of hTERT expression in RMG-I cells can be accounted for by a gain-of-function mutation (-124 G>A) in the hTERT promoter region (Table S1 and Figure S2). This cancer-specific mutation was recently reported in melanoma and several other types of cancer [24–27], which creates new binding motifs for E-twenty six/ternary complex factors (ETS/TCF) and thus contributes to upregulated hTERT transcription [24,25].

We found that Eribulin S cell lines expressed higher levels of hTERT protein than those in Eribulin R cell lines (Figure 3B, $p = 0.008$).

Suppression of hTERT expression results in decreased sensitivity to eribulin

The correlation between hTERT expression and eribulin sensitivity led us to postulate that eribulin inhibits growth of

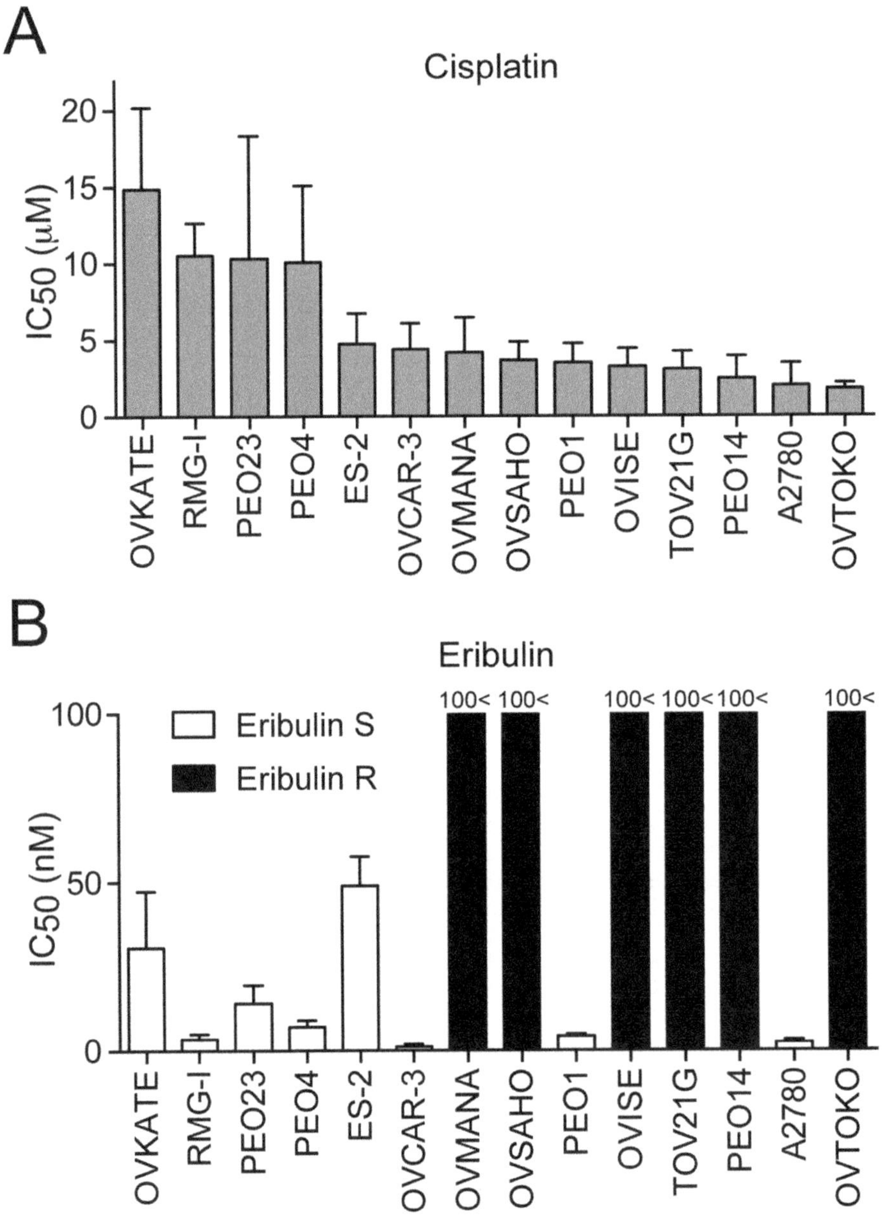

Figure 1. Eribulin inhibits growth of cisplatin-resistant ovarian cancer cells. Cells were treated with cisplatin or eribulin for 72 h, and then cell viability was determined by MTT assays. (A) Mean IC_{50} values for cisplatin (μM). (B) Mean IC_{50} values for eribulin (nM). Eribulin-sensitive (Eribulin S) cell lines are shown as open bars, and eribulin-resistant (Eribulin R) cell lines are shown as closed bars. Error bars represent the SD of at least three independent experiments.

ovarian cancer cells via inhibition of hTERT. To test this hypothesis, we examined whether suppression of hTERT expression in ovarian cancer cells leads to decreased sensitivity to eribulin. Two independent hTERT-specific siRNAs were introduced into A2780 cells, and sensitivity to eribulin was compared with cells expressing control siRNA. As expected, cells expressing hTERT siRNAs showed decreased sensitivity to eribulin (Figure 4A). TERT siRNA1 showed a tendency of stronger suppression of hTERT expression than TERT siRNA2 as demonstrated by ELISA (Figure 4B). This finding may explain why cells expressing TERT siRNA1 tended to be less sensitive to eribulin than those expressing TERT siRNA2 (Figure 4A). Similar results were obtained in ES-2 cells (Figure 4C and 4D). These results suggest that hTERT might be a direct target for eribulin.

Eribulin inhibits RdRP activity of hTERT *in vitro*

It is widely believed that any effect of hTERT suppression is mediated by telomere shortening. However, because we observed decreased sensitivity to eribulin in a relatively short period (Figure 4, 96 h after transfection of siRNA against hTERT), we speculated that this effect is independent of the telomere maintenance function of hTERT. Moreover, the function of hTERT in promotion of EMT and CSC-like traits is independent of its telomerase activity [6]. Together with our recent report showing that hTERT has an RdRP activity independent of telomere maintenance [9], we investigated whether eribulin directly targets hTERT-RdRP activity. We monitored the inhibitory effect of eribulin on hTERT-RdRP activity using an

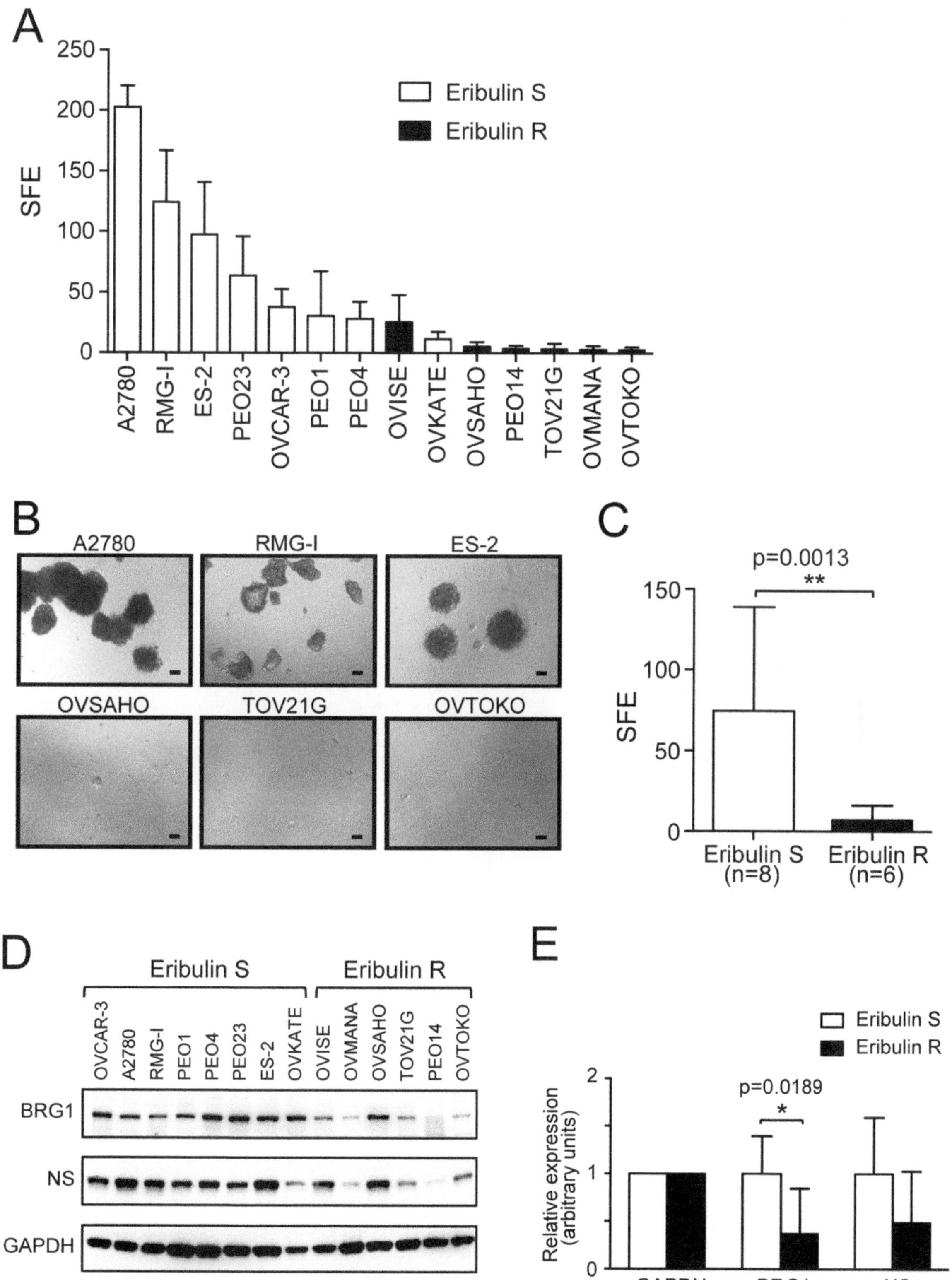

Figure 2. Eribulin-sensitive ovarian cancer cells show high sphere formation efficiency and higher BRG1 expression. (A) Sphere formation efficiency (SFE) of each cell line was indicated per 1,000 cells. Eribulin S cell lines are shown as open bars, and Eribulin R cells are shown as closed bars. Each experiment was performed at least three times, and mean values ± SD are indicated. (B) Morphology of tumorspheres under serum-free conditions. Representative images of spheres formed by A2780, RMG-I, ES-2, OVSAHO, TOV21G, and OVTOKO cells are shown. Scale bar = 50 μm. (C) The mean SFE of Eribulin S cell lines (n = 8) and Eribulin R cell lines (n = 6) shown in (A). Error bars indicate SD. (D) The level of BRG1 and NS protein expression was detected by immunoblotting. GAPDH expression was shown as loading control. (E) Signals in (D) were quantified with ImageJ software and normalized to GAPDH signal. The mean values of relative expression level ± SD are indicated.

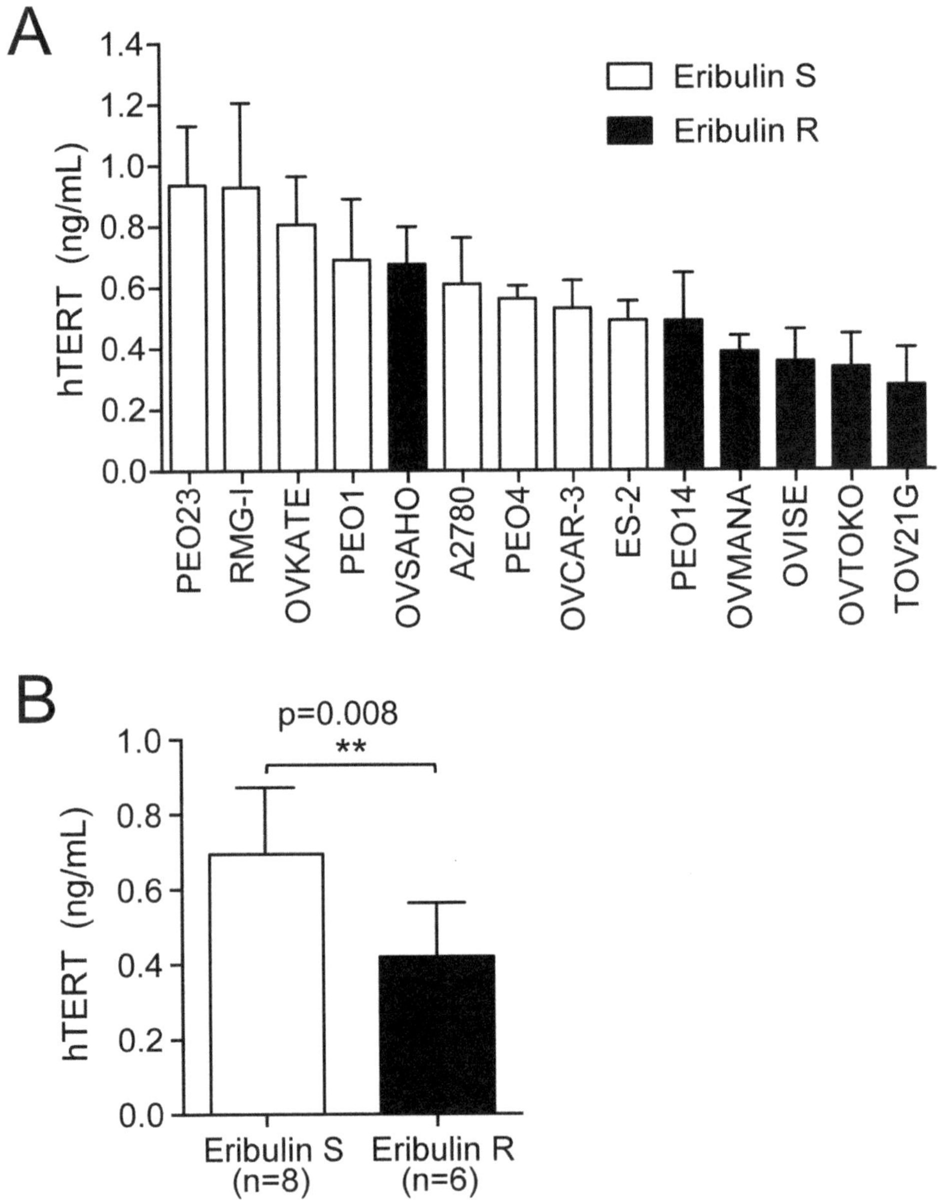

Figure 3. Eribulin-sensitive ovarian cancer cells express higher levels of hTERT protein. (A) The level of hTERT protein expression was determined by ELISA (indicated as ng/ml). Eribulin S cell lines are shown as open bars, and Eribulin R cells are shown as closed bars. Each experiment was performed at least three times, and mean values ± SD are indicated. (B) The mean hTERT level of Eribulin S cell lines (n = 8) and Eribulin R cell lines (n = 6) shown in (A). Error bars indicate SD.

in vitro RdRP assay [11], and found that eribulin inhibited hTERT-RdRP activity *in vitro* at a concentration of 50 μM (Figure 5A). The same concentration of eribulin did not inhibit the telomerase activity of hTERT as shown by telomeric repeat amplification protocol (TRAP) assay (Figure 5B). These results suggest that the effects of eribulin on hTERT are not mediated via telomerase activity, but via RdRP activity. Interestingly, another mitotic inhibitor, paclitaxel, a representative taxane, did not inhibit RdRP activity (Figure 5C), suggesting that eribulin has a specific inhibitory effect on hTERT-RdRP activity.

Discussion

Among gynecological cancers, ovarian cancer is the leading cause of death. In particular, resistance to conventional platinum-based chemotherapy has been a barrier in the improvement of prognoses for ovarian cancer patients, and new therapeutic strategies are urgently required. Here, we found that eribulin was effective to inhibit growth of platinum-resistant ovarian cancer cells. Effects of eribulin were correlated with hTERT expression levels (Figure 3), and suppression of hTERT expression resulted in decreased sensitivity to eribulin (Figure 4), suggesting that hTERT could be a target of eribulin in these cells. Indeed, eribulin inhibited the RdRP activity but not the reverse transcriptase activity of hTERT *in vitro* (Figure 5).

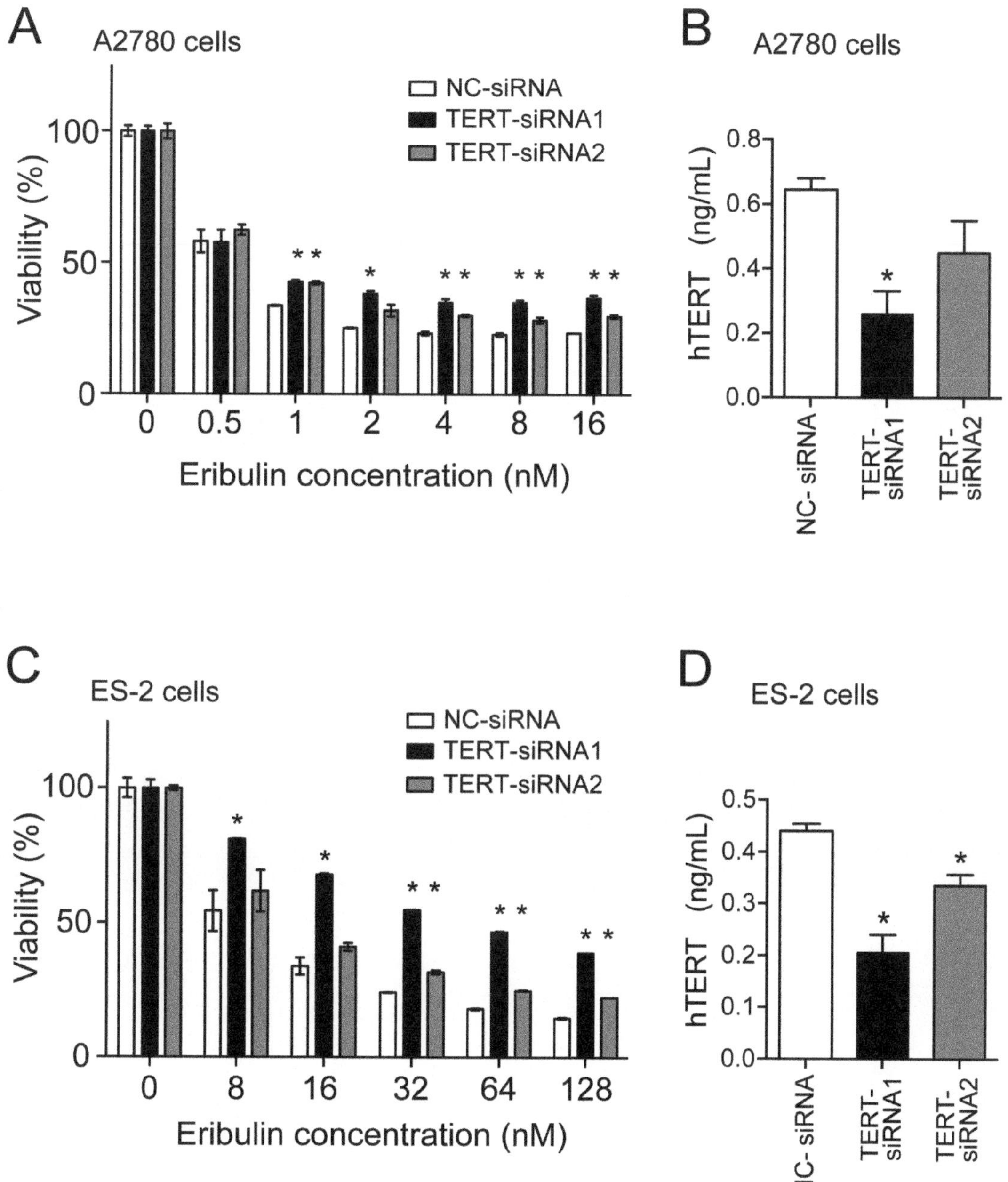

Figure 4. Suppression of hTERT expression by siRNA results in decreased sensitivity to eribulin. (A) A2780 cells expressing control siRNA (open bars), TERT siRNA1 (closed bars), or TERT siRNA2 (shaded bars) were treated with eribulin for 72 h, and then cell viability was determined by MTT assays. *$p<0.05$ vs. cells expressing control siRNA. (B) The level of hTERT protein expression in A2780 cells expressing control siRNA (open bars), TERT siRNA1 (closed bars), or TERT siRNA2 (shaded bars) was determined by ELISA (indicated as ng/ml). (C and D) The experiments described in (A and B) were performed in the same manner using ES-2 cells expressing control siRNA (open bars), TERT siRNA1 (closed bars), or TERT siRNA2 (shaded bars). *$p<0.05$ vs. cells expressing control siRNA.

CSCs and hTERT

CSCs are thought to be involved in chemoresistance, and several pathways have been found to contribute to the promotion or maintenance of CSCs. We and others have shown that hTERT plays an important role in promotion and maintenance of CSCs in telomere maintenance-independent manners [6–8]. Eribulin effectively inhibited growth of platinum-resistant cells (Figure 1). Eribulin-sensitive cells exhibited higher hTERT expression (Figure 3) and a higher sphere-forming capacity (Figure 2), suggesting that these cells have enhanced CSC-like characteristics, possibly due to the high levels of hTERT protein. Consistently, eribulin-sensitive cells exhibited higher BRG1 expression (Figure 2), another component of the TBN complex that maintains CSCs. We did not detect a significant difference in the expression of CD133 or CD44 (Figure S1). Although CD133 and CD44 are thought to be indicative of CSCs in some types of cancer, it remains to be elucidated what markers are appropriate for CSCs in ovarian cancers [23].

Because telomere maintenance by telomerase is indispensable for infinite proliferation of malignant cells, efforts have been made

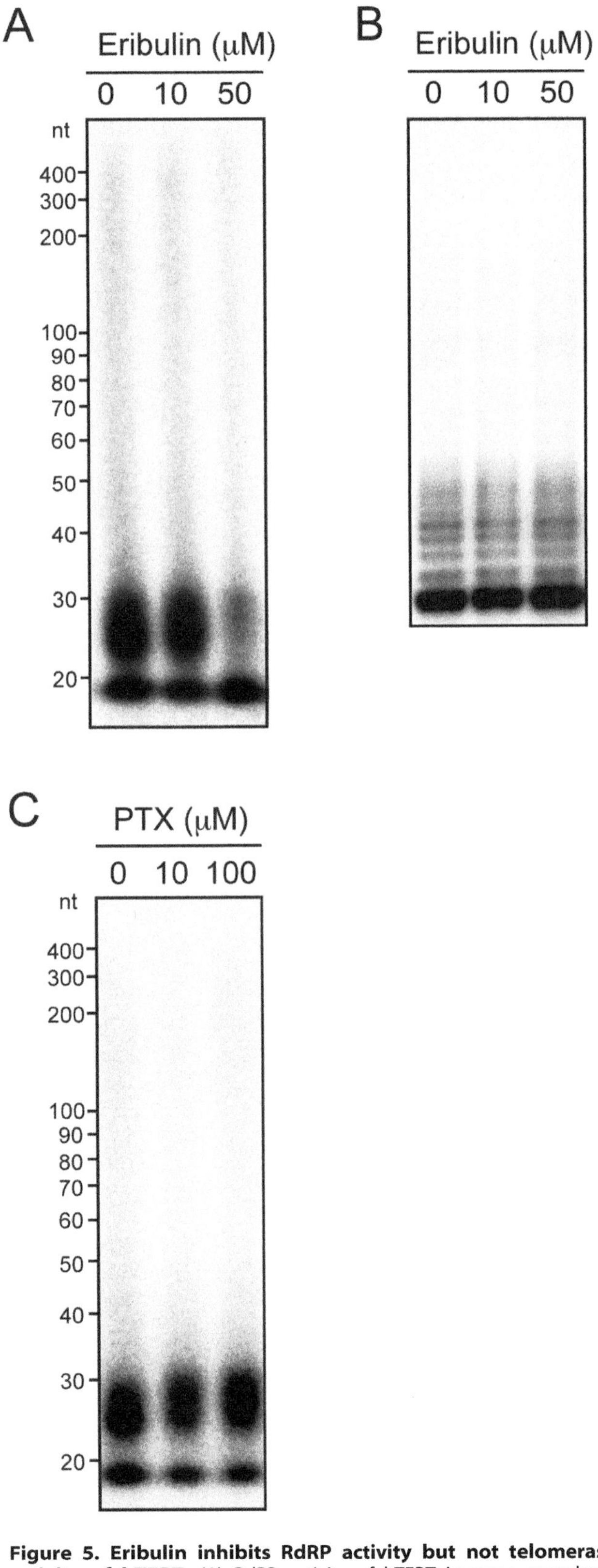

Figure 5. Eribulin inhibits RdRP activity but not telomerase activity of hTERT. (A) RdRP activity of hTERT immune complexes prepared from HeLa cells arrested in the mitotic phase was assayed without or with 10 and 50 μM eribulin. (B) Telomerase activity in HeLa cell extracts was assayed without or with 10 and 50 μM eribulin. (C) RdRP activity of hTERT immune complexes was assayed without or with 10 and 100 μM paclitaxel (PTX).

to develop anticancer therapeutics targeting telomerase. Recent studies indicate that TERT plays functional roles beyond telomere maintenance. Indeed, the function of TERT to activate normal quiescent stem cells or CSC-like traits has been shown to be independent of its telomerase activity [4,6,28]. We have also found that the TBN complex maintains CSCs in a telomere length-independent manner [8]. It is possible that this telomerase-independent mechanism is mediated by the RdRP activity of TERT, because the TBN complex itself is responsible for the RdRP activity and is involved in heterochromatin regulation and mitotic progression [11]. We speculate that the RdRP activity of hTERT is involved in gene expression through heterochromatin regulation in cancer cells, and it could be a novel anticancer therapeutic target. Whether RdRP activity is prerequisite for hTERT function in the promotion of CSCs remains to be determined.

Eribulin and hTERT

Eribulin binds to microtubule plus ends and inhibits the growth phase of microtubule dynamics [29]. Recently, eribulin was shown to reverse EMT by downregulating transforming growth factor-β (TGF-β)-induced Smad phosphorylation [12]. Smad proteins bind to microtubules in the absence of TGF-β and TGF-β triggers dissociation from microtubules and phosphorylation of Smad proteins [30]. Yoshida *et al.* speculated that eribulin inhibits Smad phosphorylation possibly by suppressing Smad dissociation from microtubules [12]. Because we have recently demonstrated that hTERT localizes to mitotic spindles and centromeres during mitosis [11], it is also possible that eribulin inhibits hTERT functions by interfering with the interaction between hTERT and microtubules. Eribulin improves overall survival of patients with metastatic breast cancer, who had prior anthracycline- and taxane-based chemotherapy [31]. A taxane drug, paclitaxel, did not inhibit the RdRP activity of hTERT (Figure 5C), providing one of the potential molecular bases for the different clinical outcomes of taxanes and eribulin. The exact mechanism by which eribulin inhibits hTERT function is yet to be understood.

hTERT as a biomarker

It is important to identify biomarkers to predict responses to anticancer therapies. By determination of hTERT levels in clinical specimens, patients who are likely to respond well to eribulin may be identified before they receive chemotherapy. In particular, an ELISA would be able to measure hTERT levels in clinical practice.

In summary, we found that eribulin inhibits RdRP activity of hTERT, which may contribute to chemoresistance in ovarian cancer by maintaining CSCs. Eribulin inhibited the growth of ovarian cancer cells with high hTERT expression and strong platinum resistance, suggesting it may be a promising therapeutic agent for chemoresistant ovarian cancer. Moreover, hTERT may be a useful biomarker to predict clinical responses to eribulin.

Materials and Methods

Cell lines

RMG-I [32], OVMANA [33], OVTOKO [34], OVISE [34], OVSAHO [33], and OVKATE [33] cells were obtained from the Japanese Collection of Research Bioresources Cell Bank. OV-CAR-3 cells [35] were obtained from the RIKEN BioResource Center. PEO1, PEO4, PEO14, PEO23 [17], and A2780 [36] cells were purchased from the European Collection of Cell Cultures, and TOV21G [37] and ES-2 [38] cells were purchased from the American Type Culture Collection. RMG-I cells were cultured in

Ham's F12 medium supplemented with 10% fetal bovine serum, ES-2 cells in McCoy's 5a medium supplemented with 10% fetal bovine serum, TOV21G cells in MCDB105/Medium 199 (1:1) supplemented with 10% fetal bovine serum, and HeLa cells in Dulbecco's modified Eagle's medium (DMEM) supplemented with 10% fetal bovine serum. All other cell lines (A2780, OVCAR-3, OVMANA, OVTOKO, OVISE, OVSAHO, OVKATE, PEO1, PEO4, PEO14, and PEO23) were cultured in RPMI-1640 medium supplemented with 10% fetal bovine serum and 1 mM sodium pyruvate (Gibco, Grand Island, NY, USA).

Compounds

Cisplatin was purchased from Sigma-Aldrich (St Louis, MO, USA), paclitaxel was purchased from Wako (Osaka, Japan), and eribulin (Halaven) was purchased from Eisai Co., Ltd (Tsukuba, Japan).

MTT assay

Cells (5,000–10,000 per well) were seeded in 96-well plates and then treated with cisplatin or eribulin after 24 h. At 72 h of treatment, an MTT proliferation assay (Cell Proliferation Kit I MTT, Roche Diagnostics, Mannheim, Germany) was performed according to the manufacturer's protocol. Briefly, 10 µl MTT labeling reagent was added to each well, followed by 4 h of incubation. Then, 100 µl solubilization solution was added to each well, followed by overnight incubation. The reaction product was quantified by measuring the absorbance at 570 and 690 nm using a microplate reader (Viento 808, BioTek, Winooski, VT, USA). Cell viability was determined by comparisons to untreated cells.

Sphere formation assay

Single cells were seeded in 96-well ultra low attachment plates (Corning Inc, Corning, NY, USA) at 100–1,000 cells/100 µl medium in each well. Cells were grown in serum-free DMEM/F12 medium (Gibco) supplemented with 20 ng/ml basic fibroblast growth factor (Wako), 20 ng/ml epidermal growth factor (Wako), and B27 supplement (Gibco). Cultures were supplemented with 25 µl of fresh medium every 3–4 days, and the number of spheres was counted on days 7 and 14. Microscopic images were obtained with a CKX41 inverted microscope and DP21 digital camera (Olympus, Tokyo, Japan).

Immunoblotting

Cells were lysed in radioimmunoprecipitation assay (RIPA) buffer containing 1% NP-40, 1 mM EDTA, 50 mM Tris-HCl (pH 7.4) and 150 mM NaCl. After sonication and centrifugation of the lysates, proteins (20 µg) were subjected to SDS-PAGE in 7.5% poly-acrylamide gels, followed by immunoblot analysis. The following antibodies were used: anti-BRG1 (a gift from Dr. Tsutomu Ohta, National Cancer Center, Japan), anti-NS (A300-600A; Bethyl Laboratories, Montgomery, TX, USA), anti-GAPDH (3H12; Medical & Biological Laboratories (MBL), Nagoya, Japan), anti-CD133 (W6B3C1; Miltenyi Biotec, Bergisch Gladbach, Germany) and anti-CD44 (2C5; R&D Systems, Minneapolis, MN, USA). Signals were detected by LAS-3000 (Fujifilm, Tokyo, Japan), quantified with ImageJ software (National Institutes of Health, USA) and normalized using GAPDH loading control.

hTERT ELISA

The hTERT ELISA employed a rabbit anti-hTERT polyclonal antibody as the capture antibody (MBL), and a mouse anti-hTERT monoclonal antibody (mAb) (clone 2E4-5) as the detection antibody (MBL code no. 5340, Ab-Match Assembly Human TERT Kit). The 2E4-5 antibody was generated against recombinant hTERT as an immunogen as described previously [11]. Cells were lysed in RIPA buffer. After sonication and centrifugation of the lysates, 100 µg total protein (100 µl in volume) was added to each well of a 96-well plate (MBL code no. 5310, Ab-Match Universal Kit). The ELISA was performed according to the manufacturer's instructions. Absorbances at 450 and 630 nm were measured by a microplate reader. Each experiment was performed at least three times, and mean values were calculated.

TERT promoter mutation analysis

Genomic DNA was extracted from ovarian cancer cell lines using a Blood and Cell Culture DNA Kit (Qiagen, Hilden, Germany) according to the manufacturer's protocol. The *TERT* promoter region (−146 to −124-bp upstream from the start codon) was amplified by PCR using KOD FX (Toyobo, Osaka, Japan) and the following primers: 5′-GTCCTGCCCCTTCACCTT-3′ and 5′-CAGCGCTGCCTGAAACTC-3′ [25]. PCR was performed under the following conditions: 40 cycles of 98°C for 10 s, 55°C for 30 s, and 68°C for 60 s. Purified PCR products were sequenced by Sanger sequencing.

Transfection of siRNA

Cells were transfected with siRNA by Lipofectamine RNAiMAX (Invitrogen) and then seeded at 5,000–10,000 cells per well in 96-well plates. At 24 h after transfection, the cells were treated with eribulin, and an MTT assay was performed after 72 h of treatment. For the ELISA, 2–5.0×10^6 cells transfected with siRNA were plated in a 10-cm petri dish, and then collected after 48 h of incubation. hTERT siRNA1 and hTERT siRNA2 have been described previously [8]. The negative control siRNA (MISSION siRNA Universal Negative Control; Sigma-Aldrich) was also used.

IP-RdRP assay

In order to detect RdRP activity *in vitro*, the hTERT immune complex was isolated by mAb against hTERT. An IP-RdRP assay has been established in mitotically arrested HeLa cells [11]. Therefore, HeLa cells were used for this assay. To synchronize HeLa cells undergoing mitosis, the cells were cultured in medium containing 2.5 mM thymidine (Nacalai Tesque, Kyoto, Japan) for 24 h. At 6 h after release, the cells were incubated in medium containing 0.1 µg/ml nocodazole (Sigma-Aldrich) for 14 h. After shaking gently, mitotic cells were retrieved. The IP-RdRP assay was performed as described previously [11].

TRAP assay

A TRAP assay was used to detect telomere specific reverse transcriptase activity as described previously [39].

Statistical analysis

Statistical analyses were performed with GraphPad Prism 6 (GraphPad Software, La Jolla, CA, USA). The Student's t-test or Mann Whitney test was used. Two-sided p-values of <0.05 were considered statistically significant.

Supporting Information

Figure S1 CD133 and CD44 expression in Eribulin S and Eribulin R ovarian cancer cells. (A) The level of CD133 and CD44 protein expression was detected by immunoblotting.

Since the data was obtained in the same experiment as Figure 2 panel D, GAPDH gel was identical with Figure 2 panel D. (B) Signals in (A) were quantified with ImageJ software and normalized to GAPDH signal. The mean values of relative expression level ± SD are indicated.

Figure S2 ES-2 and RMG-I cells possess hTERT promoter mutations. The hTERT promoter was sequenced in each cell line. ES-2 cells harbor a -138/-139 GG>AA mutation as described previously [27], and RMG-I cells harbor a -124 G>A mutation. The wild-type sequences of the corresponding regions from OVKATE and OVSAHO cells are shown as controls.

Acknowledgments

We thank Dr. Tsutomu Ohta for the gift of anti-BRG1 antibody, Dr. Koichi Ichimura for technical assistance with promoter mutation analysis, and MBL for their assistance in establishing the ELISA kit for hTERT detection.

Author Contributions

Conceived and designed the experiments: SY KM. Performed the experiments: SY YM M. Yasukawa. Analyzed the data: SY YM. Contributed reagents/materials/analysis tools: TK M. Yoshida. Contributed to the writing of the manuscript: SY YM KM.

References

1. Takano M, Tsuda H, Sugiyama T (2012) Clear cell carcinoma of the ovary: is there a role of histology-specific treatment? J Exp Clin Cancer Res 31: 53.
2. Singh A, Settleman J (2010) EMT, cancer stem cells and drug resistance: an emerging axis of evil in the war on cancer. Oncogene 29: 4741–4751.
3. Pardal R, Clarke MF, Morrison SJ (2003) Applying the principles of stem-cell biology to cancer. Nat Rev Cancer 3: 895–902.
4. Sarin KY, Cheung P, Gilison D, Lee E, Tennen RI, et al. (2005) Conditional telomerase induction causes proliferation of hair follicle stem cells. Nature 436: 1048–1052.
5. Park JI, Venteicher AS, Hong JY, Choi J, Jun S, et al. (2009) Telomerase modulates Wnt signalling by association with target gene chromatin. Nature 460: 66–72.
6. Liu Z, Li Q, Li K, Chen L, Li W, et al. (2013) Telomerase reverse transcriptase promotes epithelial-mesenchymal transition and stem cell-like traits in cancer cells. Oncogene 32: 4203–4213.
7. Chung SS, Aroh C, Vadgama JV (2013) Constitutive Activation of STAT3 Signaling Regulates hTERT and Promotes Stem Cell-Like Traits in Human Breast Cancer Cells. PLoS One 8: e83971.
8. Okamoto N, Yasukawa M, Nguyen C, Kasim V, Maida Y, et al. (2011) Maintenance of tumor initiating cells of defined genetic composition by nucleostemin. Proc Natl Acad Sci U S A 108: 20388–20393.
9. Maida Y, Yasukawa M, Furuuchi M, Lassmann T, Possemato R, et al. (2009) An RNA-dependent RNA polymerase formed by TERT and the RMRP RNA. Nature 461: 230–235.
10. Martienssen RA, Zaratiegui M, Goto DB (2005) RNA interference and heterochromatin in the fission yeast Schizosaccharomyces pombe. Trends Genet 21: 450–456.
11. Maida Y, Yasukawa M, Okamoto N, Ohka S, Kinoshita K, et al. (2014) Involvement of telomerase reverse transcriptase in heterochromatin maintenance. Mol Cell Biol 34: 1576–1593.
12. Yoshida T, Ozawa Y, Kimura T, Sato Y, Kuznetsov G, et al. (2014) Eribulin mesilate suppresses experimental metastasis of breast cancer cells by reversing phenotype from epithelial-mesenchymal transition (EMT) to mesenchymal-epithelial transition (MET) states. Br J Cancer 110: 1497–1505.
13. Towle MJ, Salvato KA, Budrow J, Wels BF, Kuznetsov G, et al. (2001) In vitro and in vivo anticancer activities of synthetic macrocyclic ketone analogues of halichondrin B. Cancer Res 61: 1013–1021.
14. Towle MJ, Salvato KA, Wels BF, Aalfs KK, Zheng W, et al. (2011) Eribulin induces irreversible mitotic blockade: implications of cell-based pharmacodynamics for in vivo efficacy under intermittent dosing conditions. Cancer Res 71: 496–505.
15. Ohta I, Gorai I, Miyamoto Y, Yang J, Zheng JH, et al. (2001) Cyclophosphamide and 5-fluorouracil act synergistically in ovarian clear cell adenocarcinoma cells. Cancer Lett 162: 39–48.
16. Wang J, Zhou JY, Wu GS (2011) Bim protein degradation contributes to cisplatin resistance. J Biol Chem 286: 22384–22392.
17. Langdon SP, Lawrie SS, Hay FG, Hawkes MM, McDonald A, et al. (1988) Characterization and properties of nine human ovarian adenocarcinoma cell lines. Cancer Res 48: 6166–6172.
18. Sakai W, Swisher EM, Jacquemont C, Chandramohan KV, Couch FJ, et al. (2009) Functional restoration of BRCA2 protein by secondary BRCA2 mutations in BRCA2-mutated ovarian carcinoma. Cancer Res 69: 6381–6386.
19. Vidal SJ, Rodriguez-Bravo V, Galsky M, Cordon-Cardo C, Domingo-Domenech J (2014) Targeting cancer stem cells to suppress acquired chemotherapy resistance. Oncogene 33: 4451–4463.
20. Tamase A, Muraguchi T, Naka K, Tanaka S, Kinoshita M, et al. (2009) Identification of tumor-initiating cells in a highly aggressive brain tumor using promoter activity of nucleostemin. Proc Natl Acad Sci U S A 106: 17163–17168.
21. Kobayashi T, Masutomi K, Tamura K, Moriya T, Yamasaki T, et al. (2014) Nucleostemin expression in invasive breast cancer. BMC Cancer 14: 215.
22. Lin T, Meng L, Li Y, Tsai RY (2010) Tumor-initiating function of nucleostemin-enriched mammary tumor cells. Cancer Res 70: 9444–9452.
23. Medema JP (2013) Cancer stem cells: the challenges ahead. Nat Cell Biol 15: 338–344.
24. Huang FW, Hodis E, Xu MJ, Kryukov GV, Chin L, et al. (2013) Highly recurrent TERT promoter mutations in human melanoma. Science 339: 957–959.
25. Horn S, Figl A, Rachakonda PS, Fischer C, Sucker A, et al. (2013) TERT promoter mutations in familial and sporadic melanoma. Science 339: 959–961.
26. Killela PJ, Reitman ZJ, Jiao Y, Bettegowda C, Agrawal N, et al. (2013) TERT promoter mutations occur frequently in gliomas and a subset of tumors derived from cells with low rates of self-renewal. Proc Natl Acad Sci U S A 110: 6021–6026.
27. Wu RC, Ayhan A, Maeda D, Kim KR, Clarke BA, et al. (2013) Frequent somatic mutations of the telomerase reverse transcriptase promoter in ovarian clear cell carcinoma but not in other major types of gynecologic malignancies. J Pathol 232: 473–481.
28. Choi J, Southworth LK, Sarin KY, Venteicher AS, Ma W, et al. (2008) TERT promotes epithelial proliferation through transcriptional control of a Myc- and Wnt-related developmental program. PLoS Genet 4: e10.
29. Smith JA, Wilson L, Azarenko O, Zhu X, Lewis BM, et al. (2010) Eribulin binds at microtubule ends to a single site on tubulin to suppress dynamic instability. Biochemistry 49: 1331–1337.
30. Dong C, Li Z, Alvarez R Jr, Feng XH, Goldschmidt-Clermont PJ (2000) Microtubule binding to Smads may regulate TGF beta activity. Mol Cell 5: 27–34.
31. Cortes J, O'Shaughnessy J, Loesch D, Blum JL, Vahdat LT, et al. (2011) Eribulin monotherapy versus treatment of physician's choice in patients with metastatic breast cancer (EMBRACE): a phase 3 open-label randomised study. Lancet 377: 914–923.
32. Nozawa S, Tsukazaki K, Sakayori M, Jeng CH, Iizuka R (1988) Establishment of a human ovarian clear cell carcinoma cell line (RMG-I) and its single cell cloning–with special reference to the stem cell of the tumor. Hum Cell 1: 426–435.
33. Yanagibashi T, Gorai I, Nakazawa T, Miyagi E, Hirahara F, et al. (1997) Complexity of expression of the intermediate filaments of six new human ovarian carcinoma cell lines: new expression of cytokeratin 20. Br J Cancer 76: 829–835.
34. Gorai I, Nakazawa T, Miyagi E, Hirahara F, Nagashima Y, et al. (1995) Establishment and characterization of two human ovarian clear cell adenocarcinoma lines from metastatic lesions with different properties. Gynecol Oncol 57: 33–46.
35. Hamilton TC, Young RC, McKoy WM, Grotzinger KR, Green JA, et al. (1983) Characterization of a human ovarian carcinoma cell line (NIH:OVCAR-3) with androgen and estrogen receptors. Cancer Res 43: 5379–5389.
36. Hamilton TC, Young RC, Ozols RF (1984) Experimental model systems of ovarian cancer: applications to the design and evaluation of new treatment approaches. Semin Oncol 11: 285–298.
37. Provencher DM, Lounis H, Champoux L, Tetrault M, Manderson EN, et al. (2000) Characterization of four novel epithelial ovarian cancer cell lines. In Vitro Cell Dev Biol Anim 36: 357–361.
38. Lau DH, Lewis AD, Ehsan MN, Sikic BI (1991) Multifactorial mechanisms associated with broad cross-resistance of ovarian carcinoma cells selected by cyanomorpholino doxorubicin. Cancer Res 51: 5181–5187.
39. Kim NW, Piatyszek MA, Prowse KR, Harley CB, West MD, et al. (1994) Specific association of human telomerase activity with immortal cells and cancer. Science 266: 2011–2015.

16

Preclinical Therapeutic Potential of a Nitrosylating Agent in the Treatment of Ovarian Cancer

Shailendra Giri[¤1]*, Ramandeep Rattan[3], Mandar Deshpande[4], Jacie L. Maguire[1], Zachary Johnson[1], Rondell P. Graham[2], Viji Shridhar[1]*

1 Department of Experimental Pathology, Mayo Clinic College of Medicine, Mayo Clinic, Rochester, Minnesota, United States of America, **2** Department of Anatomic/ Clinical Pathology, Mayo Clinic College of Medicine, Mayo Clinic, Rochester, Minnesota, United States of America, **3** Women's Health Services, Henry Ford Health System, Detroit, Michigan, United States of America, **4** Department of Neurology, Henry Ford Health system, Detroit, Michigan, United States of America

Abstract

This study examines the role of s-nitrosylation in the growth of ovarian cancer using cell culture based and *in vivo* approaches. Using the nitrosylating agent, S-nitrosoglutathione (GSNO), a physiological nitric oxide molecule, we show that GSNO treatment inhibited proliferation of chemoresponsive and chemoresistant ovarian cancer cell lines (A2780, C200, SKVO3, ID8, OVCAR3, OVCAR4, OVCAR5, OVCAR7, OVCAR8, OVCAR10, PE01 and PE04) in a dose dependent manner. GSNO treatment abrogated growth factor (HB-EGF) induced signal transduction including phosphorylation of Akt, p42/44 and STAT3, which are known to play critical roles in ovarian cancer growth and progression. To examine the therapeutic potential of GSNO *in vivo*, nude mice bearing intra-peritoneal xenografts of human A2780 ovarian carcinoma cell line (2×10^6) were orally administered GSNO at the dose of 1 mg/kg body weight. Daily oral administration of GSNO significantly attenuated tumor mass ($p<0.001$) in the peritoneal cavity compared to vehicle (phosphate buffered saline) treated group at 4 weeks. GSNO also potentiated cisplatin mediated tumor toxicity in an A2780 ovarian carcinoma nude mouse model. GSNO's nitrosylating ability was reflected in the induced nitrosylation of various known proteins including NFκB p65, Akt and EGFR. As a novel finding, we observed that GSNO also induced nitrosylation with inverse relationship at tyrosine 705 phosphorylation of STAT3, an established player in chemoresistance and cell proliferation in ovarian cancer and in cancer in general. Overall, our study underlines the significance of S-nitrosylation of key cancer promoting proteins in modulating ovarian cancer and proposes the therapeutic potential of nitrosylating agents (like GSNO) for the treatment of ovarian cancer alone or in combination with chemotherapeutic drugs.

Editor: Chih-Pin Chuu, National Health Research Institutes, Taiwan

Funding: This work is supported by Marsha Rivkin Scholar grant and Department of Defense OCRP award W81XWH-12-1-0270 to SG. The funders had no role in study design, data collection and analysis, decision to publish, or preparation of the manuscript.

Competing Interests: The authors have declared that no competing interests exist.

* E-mail: SGiri1@hfhs.org (SG); shridhar.vijayalakshmi@mayo.edu (VS)

¤ Current address: Department of Neurology, Henry Ford Health system, Detroit, Michigan, United States of America

Introduction

Ovarian cancer (OvCa) is the fifth most common cause of death from all cancers among women in the United States and the leading cause of death from gynecological malignancies [1]. The high mortality rates associated with OvCa is due to the majority of patients (75%) presenting with widespread (stage III or greater) disease at the time of diagnosis [2]. The poor 5-year survival (30%) is due to the fact that most OvCa's are inoperable at the time of diagnosis. If detected early, more than 90% of the patients have a better prognosis and respond to therapy compared to patients with an advanced stage of the disease. Consequently, a better understanding of key molecular events playing important roles in OvCa may lead to better diagnosis and treatment.

S-nitrosoglutathione (GSNO) is a nitrosylating agent which mediates the posttranslational process of S-nitrosylation on proteins resulting in modulation of their activity. S-nitrosylation is an important biological reaction of nitric oxide (NO) and refers to the conversion of thiol groups, including cysteine residues in proteins, to form S-nitrosothiols. It is a mechanism for dynamic posttranslational regulation of most or all major classes of protein and is independent of enzyme catalysis, labile modification, on/off switch-like photophosphorylation [3]; however, denitrosylation can be enzymatic or non-enzymatic. An increasing number of proteins have been found to undergo S-nitrosylation *in vivo*, called S-nitrosothiols, and they play an important role in various processes ranging from signal transduction, DNA repair, host defense, and blood pressure control to ion channel regulation and neurotransmission [3]. However, the role of S-nitrosylation in OvCa growth and progression has not been studied.

This study was planned to examine the therapeutic effect of a nitrosylating agent (GSNO) in OvCa using *in vitro* and *in vivo* models and to examine the role of nitrosylation in OvCa.

Methods

Reagents and antibodies

GSNO was purchased from World Precision Instruments (Sarasota, FL) and its purity is <98%. The following antibodies phospho-STAT3 (Y705) (Cat # 9145, used at 1:1000), pAkt

(Ser473) (Cat # 4060, used at 1:1000), p-p42/44 (Thr202/Tyr204) (Cat # 4370, used at 1:1000), STAT3 (Cat # 9139, used at 1:1000), Akt (Cat # 4685, used at 1:1000), p42/44 (Cat # 9107, used at 1:1000) were from Cell Signaling (Danvers, MA). Beta-actin (b-actin) was purchased from Sigma (St. Louis, MO). Fetal bovine serum was purchased from BioAbChem (Ladson, SC). Recombinant STAT3 was purchased from SignalChem (Richmond, Canada).

Cell Culture

Human OvCa cell line SKOV3 and OVCARs were from American Type Culture Collection (Manassas, VA). A2780, C200 and OVCAR4 cell lines were a kind gift from Dr. Tom Hamilton (Fox Chase Cancer Center) [4]. PE01 and PE04 were a kind gift from Dr. Taniguchi (University of Washington, Seattle) [4]. All OvCa cell lines were maintained and cultured in complete Roswell Park Memorial Institute (RPMI) media containing 10% fetal bovine serum and antibiotics.

Animals

Ethics Statement. Six- to eight-week old female nude mice were purchased from the National Cancer Institute-Frederick Cancer Research and Development Center (Frederick, MD). All mice were housed and maintained under specific conditions in facilities at the Mayo Clinic in Rochester, MN. The facilities are approved and inspected by the American Association for Accreditation of Laboratory Animal Care (AAALAC Accreditation # 000717) and in accordance with current regulations and standards of the U.S. Department of Agriculture, U.S. Department of Health and Human Services, and the National Institutes of Health. All studies were approved and supervised by the Mayo Clinic Institutional Animal Care and Use Committee (IACUC) under the protocol number A13909.

Mice were maintained according to Institutional IACUC approved protocol. A2780 cells were washed twice and resuspended in phosphate buffered saline (PBS) at 2×10^6/100 µl and injected into the intraperitoneal cavity of the nude mice (day 0). Treatment with GSNO (1 mg/kg of body weight) was started 3 days after the inoculation of the cells. GSNO was administered by oral gavage in 0.1 mL volume using a 20 gauge feeding needle with ball diameter of 2.25 mm (Braintree Scientific, MA). The control group received PBS as a vehicle. The mice were monitored daily for any discomfort and weighed every third day to check for tumor growth. For combination studies, cisplatin treatment (4 mg/kg of body weight) by intraperitoneal injections was given on days 7, 14 and 21 along with GSNO treatment as described above (day 0 was taken as the day of inoculation of cells). After tumor induction, mice were monitored daily for signs of any distress. Mice were humanly killed with overdose of CO2 at 4 weeks when the tumor burden reached the mandate weight in untreated mice [4,5] and tumors were excised and fixed in formalin for sectioning.

Immunoblot analysis

After the stipulated time of incubation in the presence or absence of indicated amounts of GSNO, immunoblot analysis with specific antibodies was performed as previously described [6–9]. In brief, treated and untreated A2780 or SKOV3 cells were treated with HB-EGF (50 ng/ml) and/or GSNO (2 h pretreatment prior to the addition of HB-EGF on cells) at various time periods (5–20 min) were lysed in lysis buffer [50 mM Tris-HCl (pH 7.5), 250 mM NaCl, 5 mM EDTA, 50 mM NaF, 1 mM DTT, 50 mM Na3VO4 and 0.5% Nonidet P-40] containing a protease inhibitor cocktail (Sigma, St. Louis, MO). Forty µg of proteins were resolved by SDS-PAGE and transferred onto nitrocellulose membrane. The membrane was then blocked for 1 hour in 5% nonfat dry milk TTBS (20 mM Tris, 500 mM NaCl, and 0.1% Tween 20, pH 7.5) and incubated overnight in primary antisera against phosphor-STAT3 (Y705), STAT3, p-p42/44 (Thr202/Y204), p42/44, pAkt (Ser473), Akt or β-actin containing 5% nonfat dry milk or 5% BSA in case of phospho-antibodies. After incubation with HRP-conjugated secondary Ab, blots were developed with an ECL detection system (GE Healthcare, Piscataway, NJ).

Proliferation assays

Cells (2.5–5.0×10^4) were plated in 24-well plate in triplicates and treated with indicated concentrations of GSNO for 48 hours. Inactive oxidized GSNO was used as a control. Inactive oxidized GSNO was prepared by exposing GSNO solution (0.2 mM in DMSO) to light for 7 days. Oxidized GSNO is colorless and does not produce NO when added to cell media alone or with cells unlike unexposed GSNO (**Figure S1A & C**). MTT assay was performed as previously described [8] to ascertain the number of live cells.

Colony Formation Assay

Cells (2×10^3) were plated in triplicates in 6-well plate and after 24 hour, cells were treated with indicated concentrations of GSNO once. The cells were allowed to form colonies for up to 2 weeks and complete media was replaced every fourth day. Colonies were stained with MTT and counted as previously described [8].

Dose-effect analyses

The concentration for 50% inhibition (IC 50) was determined on the basis of dose-response curves from MTT assay and was calculated using CalcuSyn software (Biosoft, Cambridge, UK).

Migration and Invasion Assay

SKOV3 cells were grown in serum-free media overnight. Scratch migration and invasion assays were measured as described before [5]. For wound closure assay, SKOV3 cells were grown to confluence in 24-well plates and kept in low serum conditions (0.2%) overnight. A scratch was created in the middle of the well with a sterile 200 µl tip, and media replaced with the respective treatments. Micrographs were collected at 0 and 24 hour. The pixel distance between the gaps was measured at a pre-determined point at each time point. The distance covered was subtracted from the start time point to estimate the distance covered by the migrating cells [10]. For invasion assay, SKOV3 cells in suspensions (500 µl, 2.5×10^4) were seeded on the top of Matrigel-coated transwell plates (8- µM pore diameter; BD Biosciences). The lower chambers contained serum-free media containing various growth factor including HB-EGF and SDF1 at the concentration of 25 ng/ml. Cells invading the lower surface of the filter coated with a thin layer of Matrigel were stained with 0.5% crystal violet (60% PBS, 40% EtOH) and counted with an inverted microscope. The results from at least two independent experiments in triplicates are presented.

Immunohistochemistry (IHC)

The tumors excised from mice were fixed in 10% paraformaldehyde for 48 hours and paraffin embedded. Four-µm-thick consecutive sections were cut and processed for immunohistochemistry for CD31 (Cat # sc31045, used at 1:100) and Ki-67 (Cat # M7240, used at 1:100). Solutions obtained from Dako Cytomation (Glostrup, Denmark) were used for performing immunostaining. In brief, tissue sections were deparaffinized, unmasked, blocked with avidin-biotin and incubated with primary antibody overnight. Next day the reaction was detected by using chromogen according to the manufacturer's instructions (Dako, Glostrup, Denmark). The positive cells stained brown. The slides were examined under light microscope and representative pictograms were taken from a minimum of 5 or 6 different slides of each group. For CD31 staining, FITC-labeled secondary antibody was used and visualized using fluorescent microscope in 6 sections per group.

Mitotic count and Live Tumor Measurements

The mitotic count was recorded on hematoxylin and eosin stained sections using the Olympus BX-41 light microscope at high power field (HPF; ×400). Cells undergoing mitosis were counted in the tumors, in the most active area ("hot spots") in a minimum of 5 consecutive HPFs. The average number of cells undergoing mitosis per HPF was enumerated. Maximum diameter of viable tumor was calculated by summing the largest unidimensional diameter of each fragment of tumor using the Olympus BX-41 microscope and a micrometer. Similarly, necrotic areas were measured and the composite live tumor size was calculated from each slide as published before [4,5].

Statistical Analysis

Data are expressed as the means + SD and were statistically analyzed using Student's t-test (Prism). $P<0.05$ was considered to be statistically significant.

Results

GSNO inhibits proliferation of OvCa cell lines

To assess the effect of GSNO treatment on OvCa growth, various OvCa cell lines (A2780, C200, PE01, PE04, OV202 and SKOV3) were treated with various concentrations of GSNO (0.1–1 mM). Proliferation was determined by MTT assay after 24 hours. Treatment with GSNO inhibited the proliferation of these OvCa cell lines significantly in a dose-dependent manner (**Fig. 1**) including cisplatin resistant C200 (**Fig. 1B**), taxol resistant PE04 (**Fig. 1D**) and aggressive SKOV3 cell lines (**Fig. 1E**). Addition of GSNO in media released NO in dose dependent manner; however, oxidized GSNO did not produce NO (**Fig. S1B–C**). We also measured IC50 of GSNO on cell proliferation of various OVCA cell lines using CalcuSyn program. IC50 for GSNO were 0.162, 0.385, 0.337, 0.427, 0.196 and 0.235 mmol/L in A2780, C200, PE01, PE04, OV2O2 and SKOV3, respectively (**Table S1**). GSNO treatment also attenuated cell proliferation of other OvCa cell lines including OVCAR-3, -4, 5, -7, -8 and -10 in a dose dependent manner (**Fig. S2**). The IC50 for GSNO in these cell lines were found differentially and listed in table S1. The inactive oxidized form of GSNO had no effect on the proliferation of OvCa cell lines.

To determine if this inhibition was reflected in clonogenic survival, the colony forming ability of A2780, C200, PE01 and PE04 cells were performed. As shown in **Figure 2**, a single treatment of GSNO significantly attenuated clonogenic survival of these OvCa cell lines in a dose dependent manner compared to untreated cells (**Fig. 2**). IC50 for GSNO was found to be 0.122, 0.161, 0.356 and 0.352 mmol/L in in A2780, C200, PE01 and PE04, respectively (**Table S2**). Inactive oxidized form of GSNO had no effect on the colony formation of OvCa cell lines. These results suggest that GSNO treatment can result in a sustained inhibition of proliferation of various OvCa cell lines, including chemoresistant cell lines (C200 and PE04) (**Fig. 2B, C & F**).

GSNO attenuates growth factors induced cell migration and invasion *in vitro*

We next examined the effect of GSNO on growth factor mediated cell migration and invasion. SKOV3 cells grown overnight in low serum (0.2%) containing medium were scratched using a sterile 200 µl pipette tip, once they had reached 90% confluency. Various growth factors including HB-EGF and SDF1 (50 ng and 25 ng/ml, respectively) were added individually to the medium in the presence or absence of GSNO (200 µM). Twenty-four hours later, the rate of wound closure was calculated. As shown in **Figure 3A**, GSNO inhibited all HB-EGF and SDF1 mediated cell migration in SKOV3 cell line. Similar results were obtained for A2780 and C200 cell lines (data not shown). Next we assessed the effect of GSNO in modulating growth factor mediated invasion of SKOV3 cells using Boyden chamber migration assay (BD Bioscience, San Jose, CA) as previously described [11]. **Figure 3B** clearly demonstrates that GSNO treatment significantly inhibited growth factor induced invasion of SKOV3 cells compared to untreated cells. These results indicate that GSNO has the ability to inhibit the migration and invasion of OvCa cells.

GSNO abrogates growth factor induced signaling in OvCa cells

To examine the effect of GSNO on growth factor induced signaling, serum starved A2780 and SKOV3 cells were treated with GSNO followed by HB-EGF treatment for various time periods. Cells were harvested and immunoblotted for various signaling molecules. As shown in **Figure 4**, treatment with GSNO inhibited HB-EGF induced activation of STAT3, Akt and p42/44 as evident from the decreased or lack of phosphorylation detected compared to HB-EGF treated samples. GSNO treatment also reduced the basal levels of phosphorylated form of Akt, STAT3 and p42/44 in A2780 and SKOV3 cells lines (**Fig. 4**). Inactive control (oxidized GSNO) had no effect on the growth factor induced signaling, suggesting the specificity of GSNO in attenuating HB-EGF induced signaling and a possible mechanism by which GSNO mediates attenuation of cell growth, migration and invasion of OvCa cells *in vitro*.

Oral administration of GSNO attenuates tumor growth and enhances the cisplatin induced cytotoxicity *in vivo*

In order to determine if GSNO could attenuate tumor growth *in vivo*, A2780 cells (2×10^6) in PBS were inoculated intraperitoneally in 6-week old female nude mice for establishment of tumors. Mice were assigned to two treatment groups. The first group (untreated) was given 100 µl of PBS as vehicle by gavage. The second group was given GSNO orally in PBS (100 µl) at the dose of 1 mg/kg of body weight every day as described in the material and methods (**Fig. 5A**). At the end of 4 weeks, mice were sacrificed, and the tumor burden was grossly examined, excised and weighed. Daily administration of GSNO significantly reduced the abdominal circumference ($p<0.01$) (**Fig. 5B**), an indication of the tumor burden being carried in the peritoneum. GSNO also reduced tumor growth ($p<0.001$) in the peritoneal cavity of A2780 bearing nude mice compared to the vehicle (PBS) treated group. The mean weights of the excised tumors were approximately 68% less in GSNO (3.35 ± 0.52 gm) treated mice compared to untreated mice (7.91 ± 0.412 gm) (**Fig. 5C**). As previously reported by Shaw et al [12] and us [4], intraperitoneally injected A2780 cells formed mainly solid tumors and presented with ovary-specific metastases (**Fig 5D**, bottom panel). The ovary-associated tumor masses in the GSNO treated mice were much smaller than in the untreated mice (**Fig. 5D**). To further assess the viability of the tumor,

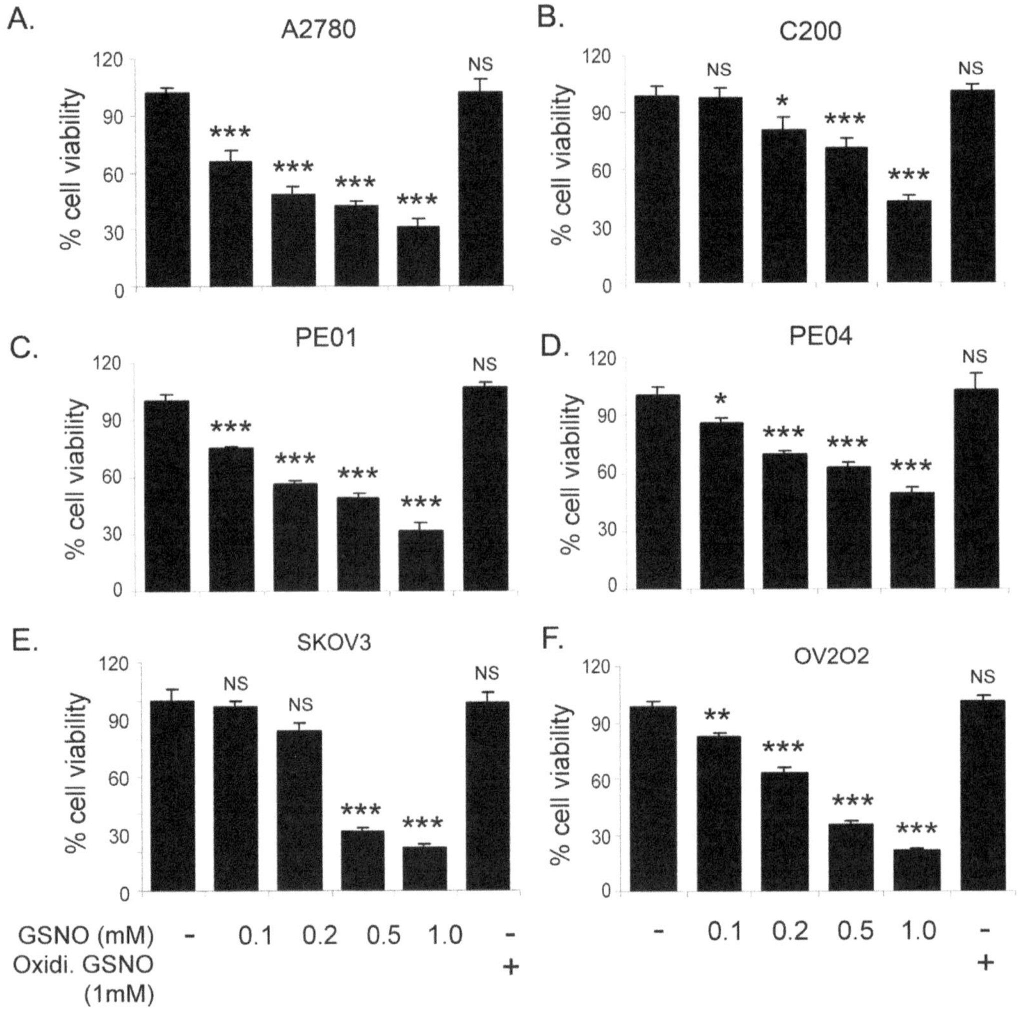

Figure 1. GSNO attenuates cell proliferation in ovarian cancer cell lines. Percentage viability of A2780, C200, PE01, PE04, SKOV3 and OV202 treated with indicated doses of S-nitrosoglutathione (GSNO; 0.1–1 mM) was determined by MTT assay. Inactive GSNO (oxidized, last bar) was used as a control. The data represents 3 individual experiments done in triplicate. ***$p<0.001$; **$p<0.01$; *$p<0.05$ and NS; not significant compared to untreated cells using Student's t-test (Prism).

necrotic and viable tumor size was determined from hematoxylin and eosin stained sections. The ratio of live tumor size to total tumor size was calculated based on the largest unidimensional diameter as described in the methods. As shown in **Figure 5E,** xenografts derived from GSNO treated mice had significantly less viable tumor sizes ($p<0.001$) and increased necrotic regions compared to xenografts derived from untreated mice. Although there was a decreasing trend observed in mitotic and vessel counts of the GSNO treated mice tumors, we could not detect a significant change (**Fig. 5F–G**). Overall, our study strongly suggests the potential of nitrosylating agent in mitigating the growth of OvCa *in vivo* (**Fig. 5**).

We further examined if a combination of GSNO with cisplatin could enhance the cytotoxic effect in tumors. Therefore, following the injection of A2780 cells, 2 sets of mice were treated daily with oral administration of GSNO (1 mg/kg of body weight) and cisplatin (weekly intraperitoneal injection of cisplatin on days 7, 14 and 21) as monotherapy. For combination therapy, one set of mice was treated with GSNO and cisplatin as depicted in **Figure 6A.** Both GSNO and cisplatin were significantly effective in reducing tumor growth and mass as monotherapy in A2780 bearing mice (**Fig. 6B**). However, combination therapy was more effective in inhibiting the tumor growth compared to monotherapy of either drug. Combination of cisplatin (4 mg/kg of body weight) with GSNO (1 mg/kg of body weight) (2.08±0.18 gm) (**Fig. 6B**) significantly reduced tumor growth compared to either GSNO (3.54±0.35 gm) or cisplatin treatment alone (3.15±0.34 gm) or the untreated mice (6.9±0.66 gm). Tumor volume was reduced by ~90% in most of the mice treated with the combination. Collectively, these results suggest that combining GSNO with cisplatin treatment is significantly effective in reducing tumor growth in an OvCa mouse model.

GSNO treatment induced nitrosylation of STAT3

Since, GSNO is a nitrosylating agent and known to mediate the posttranslational process of S-nitrosylation on proteins, which results in modulation of their activity [13]. We examined the effect of GSNO on nitrosylation on various endogenous proteins that are known to be nitrosylated and key players in OvCa including Akt, p65 and EGFR [14–17].

To examine the nitrosylation of various proteins, we employed a sophisticated biotin-switch assay. Basal level of nitrosylated

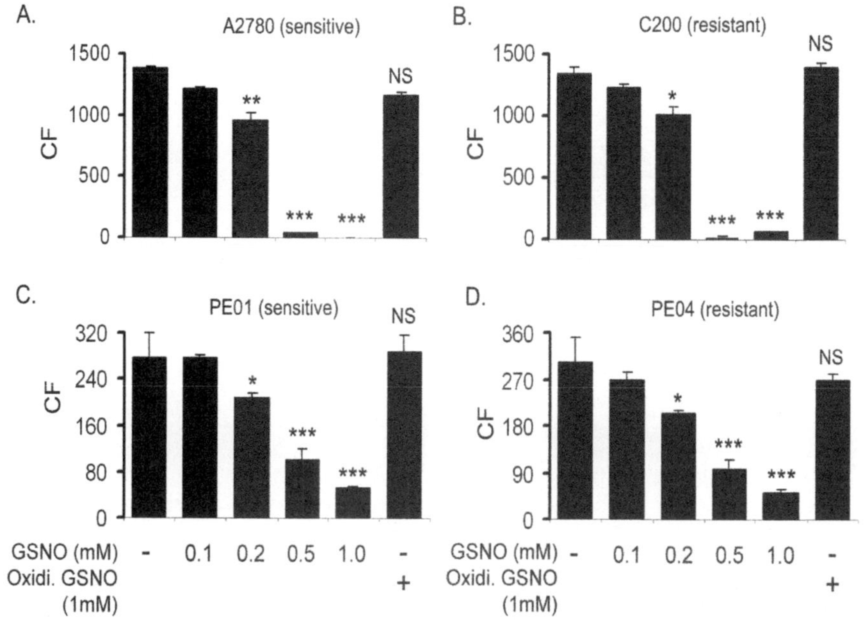

Figure 2. GSNO inhibits colony formation in chemosensitive and chemoresistant ovarian cancer cell line. Cells (2×10^3)/well (A2780, C200, PEO1 and PEO4) were plated in 6-well plates and treated with indicated concentrations of S-nitrosoglutathione (GSNO) once. Oxidized GSNO was used as a negative control (last bar). After 2 weeks, colonies were stained with MTT and counted. Results are shown as mean ± SD of triplicates. *p<0.05, **p<0.01, ***p<0.001 and NS; not significant compared to untreated cells using Student's t-test (Prism).

proteins could be detected ranging from 250 to 35 kd molecular weight in OvCa cells (**Fig. 7A, lane 1**). GSNO treatment potentiated the nitrosylation of endogenous proteins in treated cells with GSNO (0.5 mM) for 2 hours (**Fig. 7A, lane 2**). The specificity of nitrosylation could be achieved by omitting the addition of HPDP-biotin during biotin-switch assay. As shown in **Figure 7A, lane 3**, the omission of the HPDP-biotin step completely blocked the detection of nitrosylation of endogenous proteins, underlining the specificity of nitrosylation method in our laboratory. We further validated the induction of nitrosylation by GSNO by observing for nitrosylation of already reported signaling proteins associated with cancer progression, including ovarian. GSNO treatment induced the nitrosylation of p65, Akt and EGFR as expected (**Fig. 7B**). We further detected the unique observation of STAT3 undergoing nitrosylation upon GSNO treatment (**Fig. 7B, C**). To confirm that STAT3 is nitrosylated, STAT3 was immunoprecipitated after biotin-switch assay using its specific antibody and immunoblotted with anti-biotin-HRP. A similar observation of STAT3 undergoing nitrosylation upon GSNO treatment was seen. These sets of experiments clearly indicate a novel regulation of STAT3 by s-nitrosylation. To further examine if this phenomenon is not just confined to one cell type, we treated various OvCa cell lines including A2780, C200 and SKOV3 with GSNO and oxidized GSNO as a control. After 2 hours of

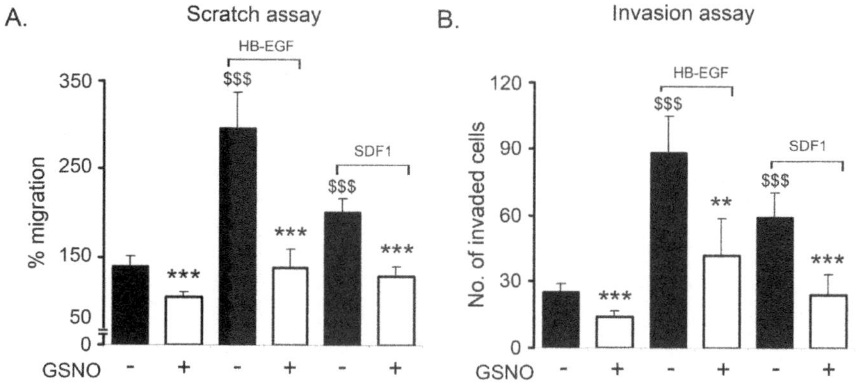

Figure 3. GSNO treatment attenuated cell migration and invasion in ovarian cancer cell line. A. Cells grown with HB-EGF and SDF1 in absence or presence of S-nitrosoglutathione (GSNO) and cell migration were measured by wound closure assay as described in the material and methods. Results are shown as mean ± SD of n = 7. **B.** To examine the effect of GSNO on invasion, 1×10^5 SKOV3 cells were seeded into the upper wells with 0.2 mM GSNO in the upper chamber of transwell in 500 μl culture medium. Various growth factors (HB-EGF and SDF1) (25 ng/ml) was added to the underlying media. Twenty-four hours later, invasion was determined following manufacturer's instructions. Results are shown as mean ± SD of triplicates. $$$ p<0.001 growth factor treated compared to control. *p <0.05; ***p<0.001 GSNO treated compared to growth factor using Student's t-test (Prism).

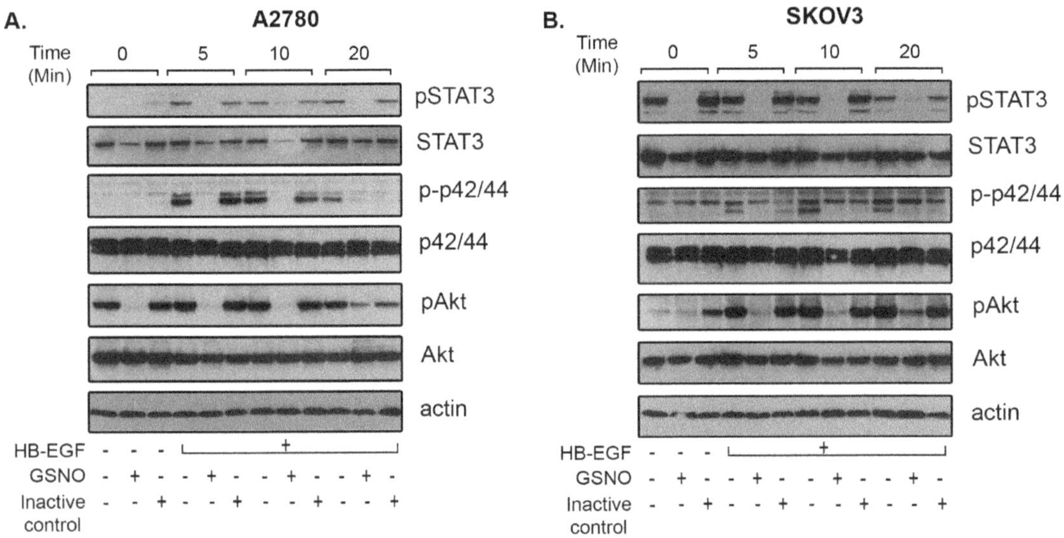

Figure 4. GSNO treatment attenuates STAT3 activation and proliferative signaling in ovarian cancer cell lines. A2780 (**A**) and SKOV3 (**B**) cells were plated, serum starved overnight and treated with S-nitrosoglutathione (GSNO; 0.5 mM) or inactive control (oxidized GSNO; 0.5 mM) in the presence or absence of HB-EGF (50 ng/ml) for various time periods (5–20 min). Cells were harvested at indicated time points and processed for the detection of various signaling molecules including pSTAT3 (Tyr705), pAkt (Ser473) and p-p42/44 (Thr202/Tyr204) using their specific antibodies from Cell Signaling (Danvers, MA). Total STAT3, Akt, p42/44 and β-actin was used for equal loading. Blots are representative of two independently run experiments.

incubation, total cell lysate was processed for the detection of phosphorylation status of STAT3. As shown in **Figure 7D**, GSNO treatment abolished or reduced the tyrosine phosphorylation in all OvCa cell lines without affecting the STAT3 levels. Oxidized GSNO did not affect the pSTAT3 levels in any cell lines. Under similar experimental conditions, we examined the nitrosylation of STAT3 using biotin switch method. GSNO treatment increased the total nitrosylation of multiple proteins with low to high molecular weights compared to untreated and oxidized GSNO treated samples as evident from **Figure 7E**. A similar pattern was observed in nitrosylation of STAT3 suggesting that the GSNO mediated increase in nitrosylation of STAT3 is a general phenomenon in all OvCa cell lines.

GSNO nitrosylates STAT3 and affects its ability to bind DNA

Once we established that STAT3 undergoes nitrosylation in cultured cells, we further examined if STAT3 could be nitrosylated *in vitro* and if it may affect its DNA binding ability. For this, we took two approaches, first we isolated nuclear extract from SKOV3, which exhibits higher basal levels of the phosphorylated form of STAT3 and has the ability to bind STAT3 DNA binding motif without stimulation. We incubated 20 μg of nuclear extract (NE) with GSNO or oxidized GSNO in the presence or absence of DTT for 4 hours. Following incubation, the DNA binding ability of STAT3 was examined by incubating nitrosylated NE with STAT3 gel shift oligonucleotides conjugated with agarose. As shown in **Figure 8A**, the GSNO treated sample showed nitrosylation of STAT3 as evident by biotin switch assay and could not be pulled down by STAT3 gel shift oligonucleotides conjugated with agarose. Inclusion of DTT in samples abolished GSNO mediated nitrosylation of STAT3, resulting in the binding of STAT3 on its DNA binding motif. STAT3 also has been shown to recruit coactivator including p300. We also found that while untreated NE showed recruitment of p300, nitrosylated STAT3 (GSNO treatment) could recruit p300 (**Fig. 8A**), further suggesting the role of nitrosylation in regulating gene transcription in general. As a second approach, we used recombinant STAT3 protein. We nitrosylated recombinant STAT3 for 2 hours with GSNO and pulled down with STAT3 gel shift oligonucleotides conjugated with agarose (**Fig. 8B**). Untreated STAT3 was able to bind to the DNA binding motif and could be observed after pull down; however, GSNO treated STAT3 did not bind, and was not seen bound to the DNA. Treatment with DTT reversed the GSNO mediated inability of recombinant STAT3 to bind DNA motif (**Fig. 8B**), further strengthening the point that STAT3 could be nitrosylated *in vivo* and *in vitro*, which could affect its ability to bind STAT3 DNA motif.

Discussion

The combination of cytoreproductive surgery with cisplatin-centered chemotherapy has significantly enhanced the survival of patients and reduced the mortality of OvCa, but development of chemoresistance and relapsing of OvCa in treated patients is still responsible for the low survival rates. The current major focus is to identify an effective therapeutic treatment which not only reduces tumor mass, but also potentiates the chemotherapy outcome. In the present study we examined the therapeutic potential of a nitrosylating agent, GSNO, using cell culture based and an *in vivo* preclinical mouse model of OvCa studies. We show that GSNO treatment attenuated cell growth of various chemoresistant and chemosensitive OvCa cell lines including A2780, C200, SKVO3, ID8, OVCAR3, OVCAR4, OVCAR5, OVCAR7, OVCAR8, OVCAR10, PE01 and PE04. It also inhibited growth factors induced activation of STAT3, Akt and p42/44 resulting in attenuation of cell invasion and migration of OvCa. Daily oral administration of GSNO at the dose of 1 mg/kg of body weight was not only able to reduce tumor burden, but also enhanced the cisplatin mediated cytotoxic effect in nude mice bearing human ovarian xenografts. Being a nitrosylating agent, GSNO treatment induced the nitrosylation of various known proteins including

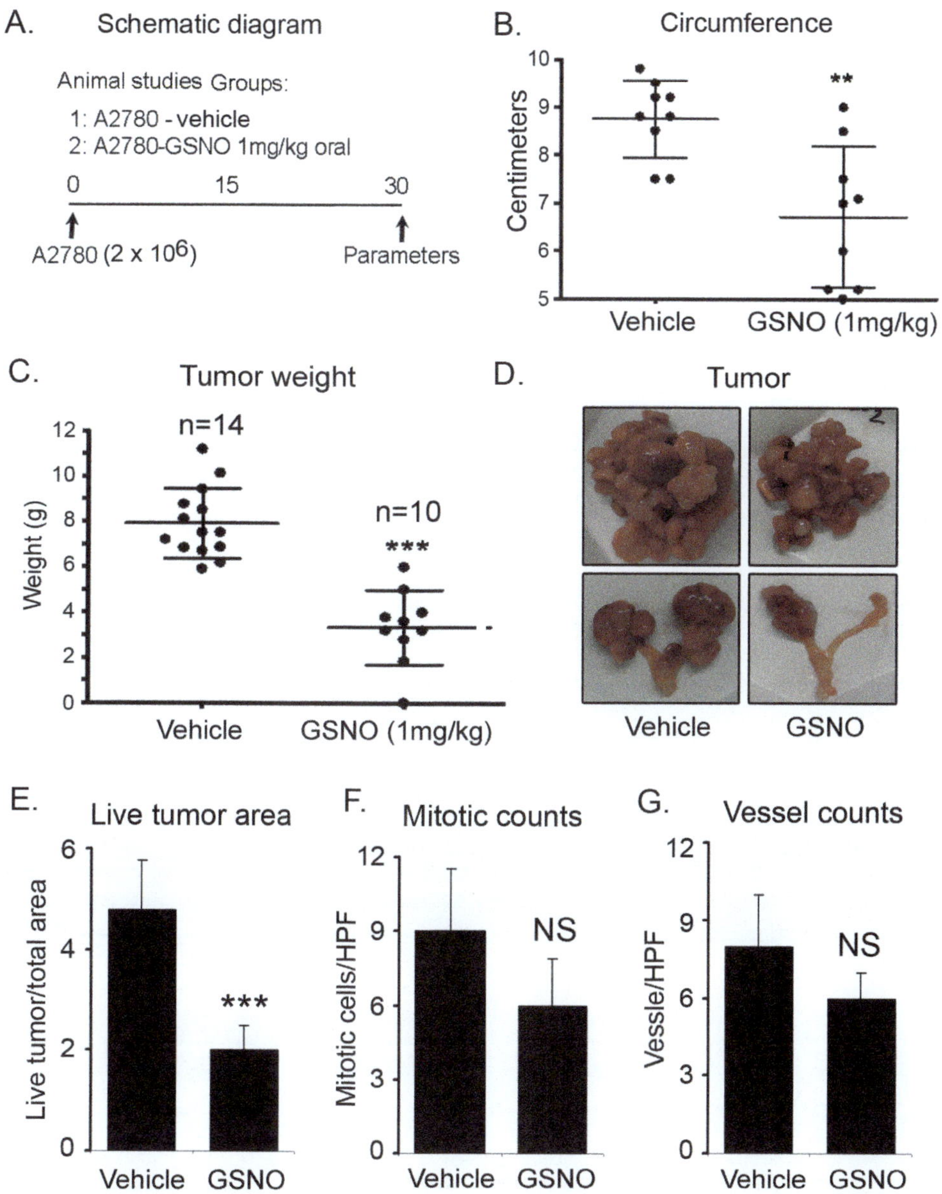

Figure 5. Oral administration of GSNO abrogates tumor growth in A2780 bearing nude mice. A. Schematic diagram of experimental design. In brief, A2780 ovarian cancer cell line was injected interperitoneally in nude mice and S-nitrosoglutathione (GSNO) was given orally daily from day 3 at the dose of 1 mg/kg of body weight till the end of the study. Phosphate buffered saline (PBS) was given as vehicle. **B.** Decreased abdominal circumference of GSNO treated mice compared to vehicle treated groups measured at week 4 (**$p<0.01$ treated compared to vehicle). **C.** Decreased excised tumor weights of GSNO treated mice compared to vehicle treated at week 4 (***$p<0.001$ treated compared to vehicle). Results are shown as mean $\pm$ SD of 10–14 individual animals. **D.** Representative gross morphological picture of tumor mass and tumor associated with ovary of vehicle and GSNO treated mice. **E.** Measurements of viable tumor size of GSNO vs PBS treated mice, as described in methods (***$p<0.001$ treated compared to vehicle). **F.** Count of mitotic cells and **G.** count of CD31 positive vessels per HPF (x400) in GSNO vs PBS treated mice, as described in methods), counts were performed from 5 fields of 3 different tumors from each group. NS; non-significant treated compared to vehicle.

NFκB p65, Akt and EGFR. As a novel finding, we found, GSNO also induced nitrosylation of STAT3, which is a known player in chemoresistance and cell proliferation in OvCa and in cancer in general. Overall, our study presents a novel attribute of a nitrosylating agent, like GSNO, as a tumor suppressor agent, which can be used as a therapeutic in ovarian and other cancers.

NO has been shown to be cytotoxic for tumor cells [18]. NO could be produced in tumors by inducible nitric oxide synthase (iNOS), a pro-inflammatory mediator which is expressed under inflammatory and pathological conditions. Expression of iNOS has been reported in human ovarian tumors [18–20]. Exogenous NO donors, including S-nitroso-N-acetyl-penicillamine (SNAP) and sodium nitroprusside (SNP), have been shown to induce cell death by down regulating the surviving network in OvCa [21]. These NO donors are fast acting and spontaneously release NO in aqueous media irrespective of the presence or absence of cells. In contrast, GSNO being a natural compound releases NO in a slow defined manner. Uncontrolled delivery of NO could not only affect tumor cells, but could also be deleterious to stromal normal cells. Therefore, use of controlled NO releasing molecules seems to

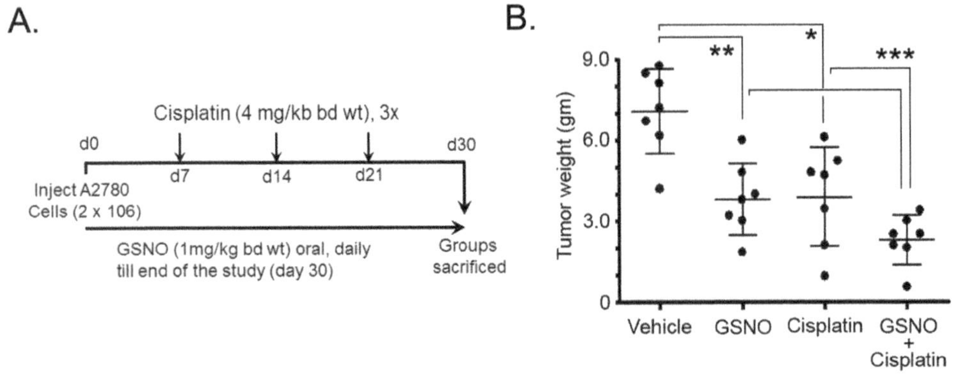

Figure 6. GSNO potentiates cisplatin induced cytotoxicity in A2780 bearing nude mice. A. Schematic diagram of experimental design. **B**. Cumulative excised tumor weight from individual mice at 4 weeks with S-nitrosoglutathione (GSNO; 1 mg/kg of body weight) (panel 2), cisplatin (4 mg/kg of body weight) (panel 3) and GSNO (1 mg/kg of body weight) and cisplatin (4 mg/kg of body weight) combination (panel 4). Cisplatin was given 3 times by intraperitoneal route at day 7, 14 and 21 post-tumor injections. Results are shown as mean ± SD of 7 individual animals. ***$p<0.001$ combination of GSNO + cisplatin treated group compared to untreated or cisplatin alone treated group; **$p<0.01$ GSNO treated group compared to untreated group; *$p<0.05$ cisplatin treated group compared to untreated group; #$p<0.05$ combination of GSNO + cisplatin group compared to GSNO alone group.

be a better approach. Under slow release NO donors, including NO releasing silica nanoparticle and NO-releasing aspirin, have been used in OvCa [22–24]. Our finding shows that slow releasing NO from GSNO attenuated the growth of various OvCa cell lines; however, oxidized GSNO (not able to produce NO) did not show any effect on cell proliferation. Similar to our data, a previous study using NO releasing silica nanoparticles also inhibited anchorage-independent growth of tumor-derived and Ras-transformed OvCa using a cell culture based study [22]. NO releasing aspirin (NCX-4040) has also been shown to attenuate cisplatin-sensitive and cisplatin-resistant OvCa cells *in vivo* and *in vitro* [23,24]. Our results are inconsistent with these findings as GSNO was able to inhibit growth of chemoresistant and chemosensitive OvCa cell lines. GSNO also inhibited activation of EGFR and STAT3 in OvCa, which is consistent with the previous finding using NCX-4040; however, this report did not show the mechanism. Moreover, a higher dose of NCX-4040 (50-100 mg/kg of body weight) was required to show effectiveness in tumor regression in ovarian tumor bearing mice and was given intraperitoneally. However, oral administration of GSNO at the dose of 1 mg/kg of body weight was significantly effective in reducing tumor burden in nude mice bearing human A2780

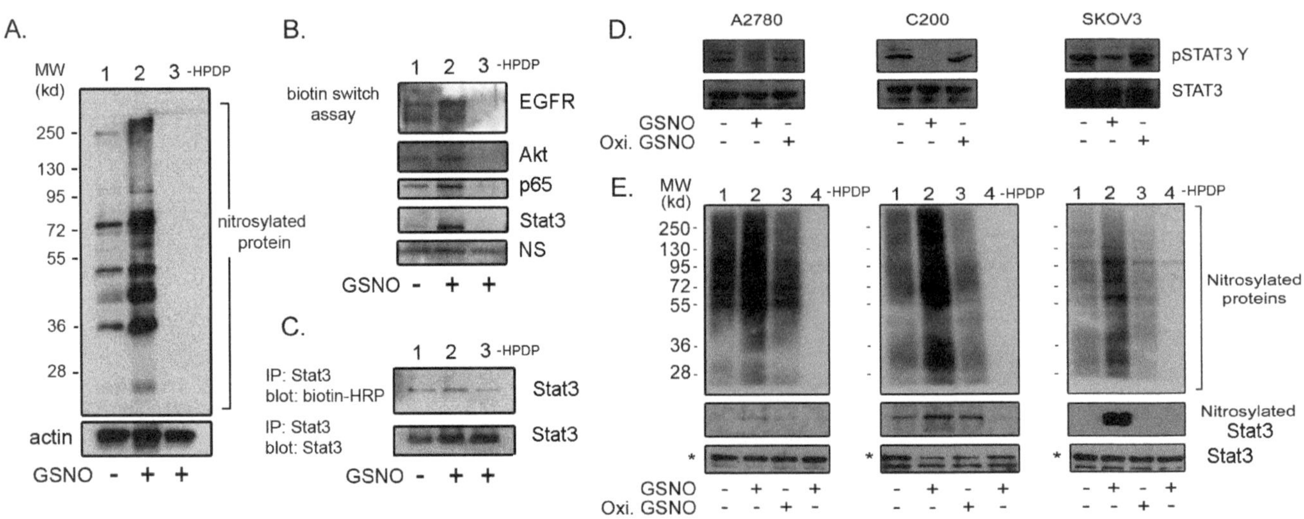

Figure 7. Detection of STAT3 as S-nitrosylating protein by biotin switch method. A. Detection of biotinylated proteins after biotin-switch method in the presence or absence of S-nitrosoglutathione (GSNO; 0.5 mM). Omission of biotin-HPRT indicates the specificity of S-nitrosylation by biotin-switch method. **B**. Detection of nitrosylation of various proteins including EGFR, p65, Akt and STAT3 in ovarian cancer cells upon GSNO treatment. **C**. STAT3 was immunoprecipitated from nitrosylated protein lysate after biotin switch assay and its biotinylation was detected by anti-biotin-HRP using western blot analysis. **D**. A2780, C200 and SKOV3 cell lines were treated with GSNO (0.5 mM) or oxidized GSNO (0.5 mM) as control for 2 hours followed by immunoblot analysis for detection of tyrosine phosphorylation of STAT3 at 705 residue and total STAT3. **E**. Under similar experimental conditions as "D", A2780, C200 and SKOV3 cells were processed for biotin switch method for detection of STAT3. Sample in lane 4 was treated with GSNO as lane 2, except during processing for biotin switch assay; the addition of HPDP was omitted. Upper panel shows the biotinylated proteins after biotin-switch assay. Nitrosylated STAT3 was detected by pulling down biotinylated proteins by streptavidin agarose followed by immunoblot analysis using anti-STAT3 antibody. Lower bands show the total levels of input STAT3 processed for biotin switch assay.

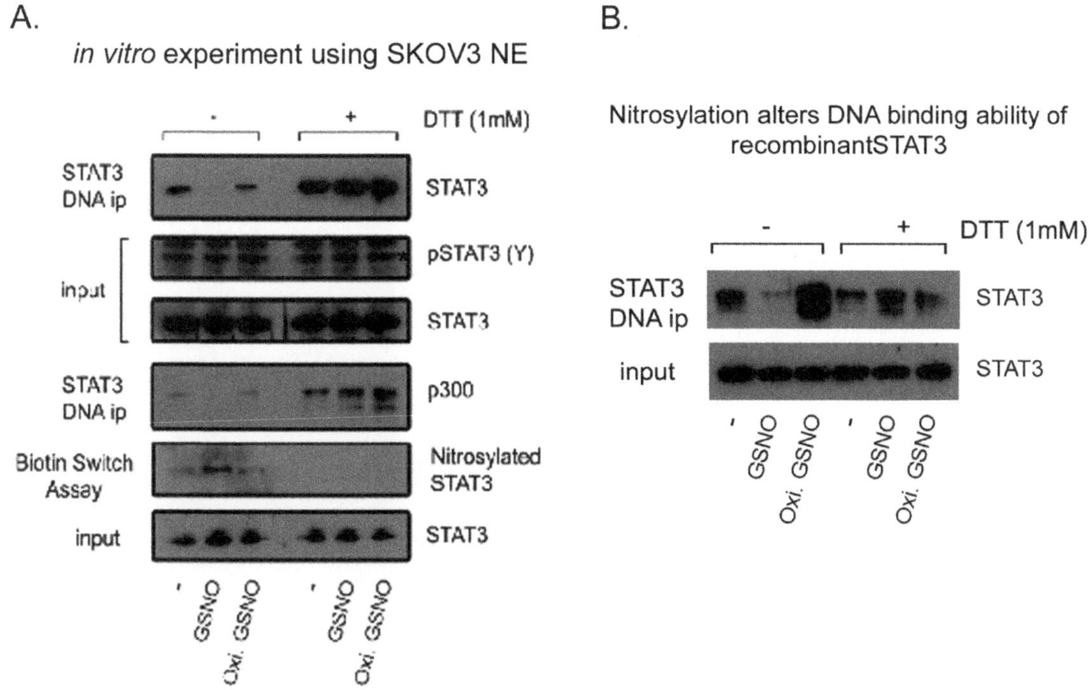

Figure 8. *In vitro* nitrosylation of STAT3 affects its DNA binding ability. A. Nuclear extract (NE) from SKOV3 was isolated and 20 µg was incubated with S-nitrosoglutathione (GSNO) or oxidized GSNO (100 µM) at 4°C in the presence or absence of DTT (1 mM). After 4 hours of incubation, DNA binding ability of nuclear STAT3 was examined by incubating nitrosylated NE with STAT3 gel shift oligonucleotides conjugated with agarose followed by immunoblot analysis with anti-STAT3 antibody. Since STAT3 recruits coactivator, including p300, we also examined the recruitment of p300 under similar experimental conditions. STAT3 and pSTAT3 (Y705) were examined before pulling down STAT3 with gel shift oligonucleotides conjugated with agarose. Nitrosylation of STAT3 was also examined under similar experimental conditions using biotin switch method. Total STAT3 level was examined in the input of NE from SKOV3, which was used to show that an equal protein amount was used in this experiment. **B.** Recombinant STAT3 (1 µg) was incubated with GSNO or oxidized GSNO (0.1 mM) at 4°C in the presence or absence of DTT (1 mM). After 2 hours of incubation, DNA binding ability of recombinant STAT3 is examined by pulling down Stat3 by incubating with gel shift oligonucleotides conjugated with agarose.

carcinoma. GSNO is a naturally-occurring compound in the body that slowly releases NO under physiological conditions, and its main mode of action has been shown to nitrosylate a number of proteins involved in diverse signaling including cell proliferation, migration and chemo resistance.

Protein nitrosylation is a reversible posttranslational modification in which NO moieties are covalently bound to reactive cysteine thiols via the S-nitrosothiol bond. S-nitrosylation has been reported to have a profound effect on several biological molecules involved in normal and pathological signaling in cells, including Akt [14], NFκB [15,16], IKKbeta [25], PTEN [26], phosphatase, EGFR [17] and caspase 3 [27]. GSNO has been shown to provide a cytoprotective effect in ischemia reperfusion injury [28], hemorrhagic shock [29] and in models of autoimmune diseases [16,30]. We report for the first time GSNO mediated nitrosylation of various proteins in OvCa including EGFR, Akt, NFκB p65 and STAT3. NO mediated inactivation of EGFR has been reported previously [31]; however, its nitrosylation and nitrosylation sites (C166 and C305) have only been identified recently [17,32]. Our findings of the loss of phosphorylation of EGFR in response to GSNO treatment and the enhancement of nitrosylation in OvCa are in accordance with these reports. We also observed an increase in the nitrosylation of Akt and p65 in GSNO treated OvCa cells. Akt1 is also nitrosylated at the residue C224 and is inactivated under pathogenesis of iNOS and/or oxidative stress-involved insulin resistance [14]. The p65, an important component of the NFκB pathway, is also reported as being regulated by nitrosylation and impairs its ability to bind NFκB consensus binding site(s) in promoters of NFκB regulated genes [15,16,33,34].

GSNO treatment not only attenuated growth factors mediated activation of signaling molecules involved in cell proliferation including Akt, p42/44 and STAT3 but also inhibited their basal level in A2780 and SKOV3. Abnormal activation of Akt is well documented in human ovarian cancer and play important role in ovarian carcinogenesis [35,36]. Consistent with these reports, the basal activity of Akt was found to be high in A2780 which was completely attenuated by GSNO treatment. In SKOV3 cell line, STAT3 is highly activated at basal level due to over expression of activated EGFR [37]. GSNO treatment also attenuated phosphorylation of STAT3 in SKOV3 in the presence or absence of growth factor. GSNO mediated inhibition of activated Akt and STAT3 in A2780 and SKOV3, respectively, might be responsible for attenuation of cell proliferation in these cell lines as well as other OvCa cell lines used in this study. Attenuation of growth factor induced signaling by GSNO treatment in OvCa cell lines is directly reflecting by the inhibition of cell proliferation in these cell lines. Our data clearly showed that nitrosylation could be one of the important modifications leading the abrogation of phosphorylation of various signaling molecules including EGFR, Akt and STAT3.

Signal transducers and activators of transcription (STATs) are a group of transcription factors that have been increasingly implicated in cancer pathogenesis [38,39]. Of the 7 known STAT proteins, activated STAT3 is reported to be strongly associated with various cancers including OvCa [40–45]. Constitutive activation of STAT3 signaling is observed in a number of neoplasms, including acute leukemia [46], breast cancer [47], squamous cell carcinoma of the head and neck [48], multiple myeloma [49] and OvCa [40–45]. In OvCa, increased STAT3 directed transcription has been implicated in the stimulation of proliferation seen in response to cytokines, including VEGF and IL-6, in invasiveness [44] and as a predictor of poor prognosis [50]. It activates the transcription of a number of genes, including antiapoptotic proteins Bcl-2, Bcl-x_L and Mcl-1 [39,51,52]. Moreover, constitutive activation of the STAT3 pathway has recently been shown to confer resistance to chemotherapy-induced apoptosis in epithelial malignancies [53–56]. Because of the vast data implicating STAT3 activation in cancer pathogenesis, inhibition of the STAT3 signaling pathway has tremendous implications in the treatment as well as reversing the drug resistance seen in OvCa patients [38,39,57–65]. The activity of STAT3 and its interaction with other proteins are modulated by phosphorylation [66,67] and acetylation [68], but other posttranslational modifications, including S nitrosylation, are not reported. Our findings report nitrosylation as a novel modification of STAT3 in GSNO treated OvCa cells. Using biotin switch method, basal level of nitrosylated STAT3 was detected and GSNO treatment enhanced it many folds. This observation was confirmed by detection of biotinylated STAT3 using immunoblot after biotin switch assay followed by immunoprecipitation of STAT3. Currently nitrosylation site(s) in STAT3 is not known. Identification of nitrosylation site(s) in STAT3 and their regulation will lead to a better understanding of the exact underlying biology of STAT3 in the pathogenesis of OvCa.

Overall, our study highlights an important role of nitrosylation as a regulatory process involved in modulation of various proteins in OvCa. Our data also clearly indicates the therapeutic potential of nitrosylating agents like GSNO as a mono-therapy or in combination with chemotherapy for the treatment of OvCa and could modulate a number of oncogenes like EGFR, STAT3, NFκB (p65), Akt and IKK. Therefore, this approach follows the new strategy of "one-drug, multiple-target" therapy in OvCa.

Supporting Information

Figure S1 GSNO mediated release of NO in the medium containing A2780 or SKOV3 cells. A. GSNO solution (0.2 mM in DMSO; pink in color) was exposed to light for 7 days to prepare inactive oxidized GSNO (colorless). **B**. A2780 and SKOV3 cells were plated in 24 well plates at the density of 50×10^3 cells/well. After 24 h incubation, cells were treated with various concentrations of GSNO ranging from 0.01 to 1 mM. After 24 h of treatment, NO was measured in medium with Griess reagent. **C**. NO was measured in medium in oxidized GSNO and GSNO treated A2780 and SKOV3 cells at 24 hour (N = 4).

Figure S2 GSNO treatment attenuated cell proliferation of multiple ovarian cancer cell lines. A-F. Various ovarian cancer cell lines including OVCAR-3, -4, 5, -7, -8 and -10 were treated with various concentration of GSNO (0.1-1 mM). Percent viability of these cell lines were determined by MTT assay after 48 h of treatment. Inactive GSNO (oxidized, last bar) was used as control. The data is represents three individual experiments done in triplicates. ***$p < 0.001$; **$p < 0.01$; *$p < 0.05$ and NS; not significant compared to untreated cells using Student's t-test (Prism).

Table S1 Measurement of IC50 of GSNO mediated effect on cell proliferation of human ovarian cancer (OvCa) cell lines. OvCa cell lines were treated with various concentrations of GSNO and cell viability was measured by MTT. IC 50 was calculated using CalcuSyn software (Biosoft, Cambridge, UK). Values are presented as mean ± SD of three values.

Table S2 Measurement of IC 50 of GSNO mediated effect on clonogenic survival of human ovarian cancer (OvCa) cell lines. OvCa cells (2×10^3) were plated in triplicates in 6-well plate and after 24 hour, cells were treated with indicated concentrations of GSNO once. The cells were allowed to form colonies for up to 2 weeks. Colonies were stained with MTT, counted and IC 50 was calculated using CalcuSyn software (Biosoft, Cambridge, UK). Values are presented as mean ± SD of three values.

Acknowledgments

The authors would like to thank Stephanie Stebens, MLIS, for her assistance with editing and preparing the manuscript.

Author Contributions

Conceived and designed the experiments: SG. Performed the experiments: SG RR JM ZJ MD RG. Analyzed the data: SG RR. Wrote the paper: SG RR. Revised and approved the final version of the paper: SG RR VS.

References

1. Kenny HA, Kaur S, Coussens LM, Lengyel E (2008) The initial steps of ovarian cancer cell metastasis are mediated by MMP-2 cleavage of vitronectin and fibronectin. J Clin Invest 118: 1367–1379.
2. Friedlander ML (1998) Prognostic factors in ovarian cancer. Semin Oncol 25: 305–314.
3. Foster MW, Hess DT, Stamler JS (2009) Protein S-nitrosylation in health and disease: a current perspective. Trends Mol Med 15: 391–404.
4. Rattan R, Graham RP, Maguire JL, Giri S, Shridhar V (2011) Metformin suppresses ovarian cancer growth and metastasis with enhancement of cisplatin cytotoxicity in vivo. Neoplasia 13: 483–491.
5. Giri S, Karakoti A, Graham RP, Maguire JL, Reilly CM, et al. (2013) Nanoceria: a rare-Earth nanoparticle as a novel anti-angiogenic therapeutic agent in ovarian cancer. PLoS One 8: e54578.
6. Prasad R, Giri S, Singh AK, Singh I (2008) 15-deoxy-delta12,14-prostaglandin J2 attenuates endothelial-monocyte interaction: implication for inflammatory diseases. J Inflamm (Lond) 5: 14.
7. Giri S, Khan M, Rattan R, Singh I, Singh AK (2006) Krabbe disease: psychosine-mediated activation of phospholipase A2 in oligodendrocyte cell death. J Lipid Res 47: 1478–1492.
8. Rattan R, Giri S, Hartmann LC, Shridhar V (2011) Metformin attenuates ovarian cancer cell growth in an AMP-kinase dispensable manner. J Cell Mol Med 15: 166–178.
9. Rattan R, Giri S, Singh AK, Singh I (2005) 5-Aminoimidazole-4-carboxamide-1-beta-D-ribofuranoside inhibits cancer cell proliferation in vitro and in vivo via AMP-activated protein kinase. J Biol Chem 280: 39582–39593.
10. Liang CC, Park AY, Guan JL (2007) In vitro scratch assay: a convenient and inexpensive method for analysis of cell migration in vitro. Nat Protoc 2: 329–333.
11. Narita K, Staub J, Chien J, Meyer K, Bauer M, et al. (2006) HSulf-1 inhibits angiogenesis and tumorigenesis in vivo. Cancer Res 66: 6025–6032.
12. Shaw TJ, Senterman MK, Dawson K, Crane CA, Vanderhyden BC (2004) Characterization of intraperitoneal, orthotopic, and metastatic xenograft models of human ovarian cancer. Mol Ther 10: 1032–1042.
13. Hess DT, Stamler JS (2012) Regulation by S-nitrosylation of protein post-translational modification. J Biol Chem 287: 4411–4418.
14. Yasukawa T, Tokunaga E, Ota H, Sugita H, Martyn JA, et al. (2005) S-nitrosylation-dependent inactivation of Akt/protein kinase B in insulin resistance. J Biol Chem 280: 7511–7518.
15. Kelleher ZT, Matsumoto A, Stamler JS, Marshall HE (2007) NOS2 regulation of NF-kappaB by S-nitrosylation of p65. J Biol Chem 282: 30667–30672.

16. Prasad R, Giri S, Nath N, Singh I, Singh AK (2007) GSNO attenuates EAE disease by S-nitrosylation-mediated modulation of endothelial-monocyte interactions. Glia 55: 65–77.
17. Switzer CH, Glynn SA, Cheng RY, Ridnour LA, Green JE, et al. (2012) S-nitrosylation of EGFR and Src activates an oncogenic signaling network in human basal-like breast cancer. Mol Cancer Res 10: 1203–1215.
18. Klimp AH, Hollema H, Kempinga C, van der Zee AG, de Vries EG, et al. (2001) Expression of cyclooxygenase-2 and inducible nitric oxide synthase in human ovarian tumors and tumor-associated macrophages. Cancer Res 61: 7305–7309.
19. Anttila MA, Voutilainen K, Merivalo S, Saarikoski S, Kosma VM (2007) Prognostic significance of iNOS in epithelial ovarian cancer. Gynecol Oncol 105: 97–103.
20. Nomelini RS, de Abreu Ribeiro LC, Tavares-Murta BM, Adad SJ, Murta EF (2008) Production of nitric oxide and expression of inducible nitric oxide synthase in ovarian cystic tumors. Mediators Inflamm 2008: 186584.
21. Engels K, Knauer SK, Loibl S, Fetz V, Harter P, et al. (2008) NO signaling confers cytoprotectivity through the survivin network in ovarian carcinomas. Cancer Res 68: 5159–5166.
22. Stevens EV, Carpenter AW, Shin JH, Liu J, Der CJ, et al. (2010) Nitric oxide-releasing silica nanoparticle inhibition of ovarian cancer cell growth. Mol Pharm 7: 775–785.
23. Bratasz A, Selvendiran K, Wasowicz T, Bobko A, Khramtsov VV, et al. (2008) NCX-4040, a nitric oxide-releasing aspirin, sensitizes drug-resistant human ovarian xenograft tumors to cisplatin by depletion of cellular thiols. J Transl Med 6: 9.
24. Selvendiran K, Bratasz A, Tong L, Ignarro LJ, Kuppusamy P (2008) NCX-4016, a nitro-derivative of aspirin, inhibits EGFR and STAT3 signaling and modulates Bcl-2 proteins in cisplatin-resistant human ovarian cancer cells and xenografts. Cell Cycle 7: 81–88.
25. Reynaert NL, Ckless K, Korn SH, Vos N, Guala AS, et al. (2004) Nitric oxide represses inhibitory kappaB kinase through S-nitrosylation. Proc Natl Acad Sci U S A 101: 8945–8950.
26. Numajiri N, Takasawa K, Nishiya T, Tanaka H, Ohno K, et al. (2011) On-off system for PI3-kinase-Akt signaling through S-nitrosylation of phosphatase with sequence homology to tensin (PTEN). Proc Natl Acad Sci U S A 108: 10349–10354.
27. Matsumoto A, Comatas KE, Liu L, Stamler JS (2003) Screening for nitric oxide-dependent protein-protein interactions. Science 301: 657–661.
28. Khan M, Sekhon B, Giri S, Jatana M, Gilg AG, et al. (2005) S-Nitrosoglutathione reduces inflammation and protects brain against focal cerebral ischemia in a rat model of experimental stroke. J Cereb Blood Flow Metab 25: 177–192.
29. Cabrales P, Tsai AG, Intaglietta M (2009) Exogenous nitric oxide induces protection during hemorrhagic shock. Resuscitation 80: 707–712.
30. Haq E, Rohrer B, Nath N, Crosson CE, Singh I (2007) S-nitrosoglutathione prevents interphotoreceptor retinoid-binding protein (IRBP(161-180))-induced experimental autoimmune uveitis. J Ocul Pharmacol Ther 23: 221–231.
31. Estrada C, Gomez C, Martin-Nieto J, De Frutos T, Jimenez A, et al. (1997) Nitric oxide reversibly inhibits the epidermal growth factor receptor tyrosine kinase. Biochem J 326 (Pt 2): 369–376.
32. Murillo-Carretero M, Torroglosa A, Castro C, Villalobo A, Estrada C (2009) S-Nitrosylation of the epidermal growth factor receptor: a regulatory mechanism of receptor tyrosine kinase activity. Free Radic Biol Med 46: 471–479.
33. Marshall HE, Stamler JS (2001) Inhibition of NF-kappa B by S-nitrosylation. Biochemistry 40: 1688–1693.
34. Chattopadhyay M, Goswami S, Rodes DB, Kodela R, Velazquez CA, et al. (2010) NO-releasing NSAIDs suppress NF-kappaB signaling in vitro and in vivo through S-nitrosylation. Cancer Lett 298: 204–211.
35. Altomare DA, Wang HQ, Skele KL, De Rienzo A, Klein-Szanto AJ, et al. (2004) AKT and mTOR phosphorylation is frequently detected in ovarian cancer and can be targeted to disrupt ovarian tumor cell growth. Oncogene 23: 5853–5857.
36. Gao N, Flynn DC, Zhang Z, Zhong XS, Walker V, et al. (2004) G1 cell cycle progression and the expression of G1 cyclins are regulated by PI3K/AKT/mTOR/p70S6K1 signaling in human ovarian cancer cells. Am J Physiol Cell Physiol 287: C281–291.
37. Zeineldin R, Muller CY, Stack MS, Hudson LG (2010) Targeting the EGF receptor for ovarian cancer therapy. J Oncol 2010: 414676.
38. Germain D, Frank DA (2007) Targeting the cytoplasmic and nuclear functions of signal transducers and activators of transcription 3 for cancer therapy. Clin Cancer Res 13: 5665–5669.
39. Haura EB, Turkson J, Jove R (2005) Mechanisms of disease: Insights into the emerging role of signal transducers and activators of transcription in cancer. Nat Clin Pract Oncol 2: 315–324.
40. Burke WM, Jin X, Lin HJ, Huang M, Liu R, et al. (2001) Inhibition of constitutively active Stat3 suppresses growth of human ovarian and breast cancer cells. Oncogene 20: 7925–7934.
41. Huang F, Tong X, Fu L, Zhang R (2008) Knockdown of STAT3 by shRNA inhibits the growth of CAOV3 ovarian cancer cell line in vitro and in vivo. Acta Biochim Biophys Sin (Shanghai) 40: 519–525.
42. Huang M, Page C, Reynolds RK, Lin J (2000) Constitutive activation of stat 3 oncogene product in human ovarian carcinoma cells. Gynecol Oncol 79: 67–73.
43. Savarese TM, Campbell CL, McQuain C, Mitchell K, Guardiani R, et al. (2002) Coexpression of oncostatin M and its receptors and evidence for STAT3 activation in human ovarian carcinomas. Cytokine 17: 324–334.
44. Silver DL, Naora H, Liu J, Cheng W, Montell DJ (2004) Activated signal transducer and activator of transcription (STAT) 3: localization in focal adhesions and function in ovarian cancer cell motility. Cancer Res 64: 3550–3558.
45. Min H, Wei-hong Z (2009) Constitutive activation of signal transducer and activator of transcription 3 in epithelial ovarian carcinoma. J Obstet Gynaecol Res 35: 918–925.
46. Lin TS, Mahajan S, Frank DA (2000) STAT signaling in the pathogenesis and treatment of leukemias. Oncogene 19: 2496–2504.
47. Garcia R, Bowman TL, Niu G, Yu H, Minton S, et al. (2001) Constitutive activation of Stat3 by the Src and JAK tyrosine kinases participates in growth regulation of human breast carcinoma cells. Oncogene 20: 2499–2513.
48. Song JI, Grandis JR (2000) STAT signaling in head and neck cancer. Oncogene 19: 2489–2495.
49. Catlett-Falcone R, Landowski TH, Oshiro MM, Turkson J, Levitzki A, et al. (1999) Constitutive activation of Stat3 signaling confers resistance to apoptosis in human U266 myeloma cells. Immunity 10: 105–115.
50. Meinhold-Heerlein I, Bauerschlag D, Hilpert F, Dimitrov P, Sapinoso LM, et al. (2005) Molecular and prognostic distinction between serous ovarian carcinomas of varying grade and malignant potential. Oncogene 24: 1053–1065.
51. Bromberg J, Darnell JE Jr (2000) The role of STATs in transcriptional control and their impact on cellular function. Oncogene 19: 2468–2473.
52. Yu H, Jove R (2004) The STATs of cancer—new molecular targets come of age. Nat Rev Cancer 4: 97–105.
53. Ikuta K, Takemura K, Kihara M, Nishimura M, Ueda N, et al. (2005) Overexpression of constitutive signal transducer and activator of transcription 3 mRNA in cisplatin-resistant human non-small cell lung cancer cells. Oncol Rep 13: 217–222.
54. Kato K, Nomoto M, Izumi H, Ise T, Nakano S, et al. (2000) Structure and functional analysis of the human STAT3 gene promoter: alteration of chromatin structure as a possible mechanism for the upregulation in cisplatin-resistant cells. Biochim Biophys Acta 1493: 91–100.
55. Roberts D, Schick J, Conway S, Biade S, Laub PB, et al. (2005) Identification of genes associated with platinum drug sensitivity and resistance in human ovarian cancer cells. Br J Cancer 92: 1149–1158.
56. Song H, Sondak VK, Barber DL, Reid TJ, Lin J (2004) Modulation of Janus kinase 2 by cisplatin in cancer cells. Int J Oncol 24: 1017–1026.
57. Luo C, Laaja P (2004) Inhibitors of JAKs/STATs and the kinases: a possible new cluster of drugs. Drug Discov Today 9: 268–275.
58. Meyer T, Vinkemeier U (2007) STAT nuclear translocation: potential for pharmacological intervention. Expert Opin Ther Targets 11: 1355–1365.
59. Duan Z, Foster R, Bell DA, Mahoney J, Wolak K, et al. (2006) Signal transducers and activators of transcription 3 pathway activation in drug-resistant ovarian cancer. Clin Cancer Res 12: 5055–5063.
60. Jiang Q, Dai L, Cheng L, Chen X, Li Y, et al. (2013) Efficient inhibition of intraperitoneal ovarian cancer growth in nude mice by liposomal delivery of short hairpin RNA against STAT3. J Obstet Gynaecol Res 39: 701–709.
61. Kandala PK, Srivastava SK (2012) Diindolylmethane suppresses ovarian cancer growth and potentiates the effect of cisplatin in tumor mouse model by targeting signal transducer and activator of transcription 3 (STAT3). BMC Med 10: 9.
62. Liu M, Wang F, Wen Z, Shi M, Zhang H (2014) Blockage of STAT3 signaling pathway with a decoy oligodeoxynucleotide inhibits growth of human ovarian cancer cells. Cancer Invest 32: 8–12.
63. Rath KS, Naidu SK, Lata P, Bid HK, Rivera BK, et al. (2014) HO-3867, a Safe STAT3 Inhibitor, Is Selectively Cytotoxic to Ovarian Cancer. Cancer Res.
64. Sun ZL, Tang YJ, Wu WG, Xing J, He YF, et al. (2013) AZD1480 can inhibit the biological behavior of ovarian cancer SKOV3 cells in vitro. Asian Pac J Cancer Prev 14: 4823–4827.
65. Zhao SH, Zhao F, Zheng JY, Gao LF, Zhao XJ, et al. (2011) Knockdown of stat3 expression by RNAi inhibits in vitro growth of human ovarian cancer. Radiol Oncol 45: 196–203.
66. Darnell JE Jr, Kerr IM, Stark GR (1994) Jak-STAT pathways and transcriptional activation in response to IFNs and other extracellular signaling proteins. Science 264: 1415–1421.
67. Zhang X, Blenis J, Li HC, Schindler C, Chen-Kiang S (1995) Requirement of serine phosphorylation for formation of STAT-promoter complexes. Science 267: 1990–1994.
68. Yuan ZL, Guan YJ, Chatterjee D, Chin YE (2005) Stat3 dimerization regulated by reversible acetylation of a single lysine residue. Science 307: 269–273.

Glucocorticoid-Induced Reversal of Interleukin-1β-Stimulated Inflammatory Gene Expression in Human Oviductal Cells

Stéphanie Backman[1]‡, Alexandra Kollara[1,2]‡, Robin Haw[3], Lincoln Stein[3], Theodore J. Brown[1,2]*

1 Department of Obstetrics and Gynecology, University of Toronto, Toronto, Ontario, Canada, **2** Lunenfeld-Tanenbaum Research Institute, Mt. Sinai Hospital, Toronto, Ontario, Canada, **3** Ontario Institute for Cancer Research, Informatics and Bio-Computing, Toronto, Ontario, Canada

Abstract

Studies indicate that high-grade serous ovarian carcinoma (HGSOC), the most common epithelial ovarian carcinoma histotype, originates from the fallopian tube epithelium (FTE). Risk factors for this cancer include reproductive parameters associated with lifetime ovulatory events. Ovulation is an acute inflammatory process during which the FTE is exposed to follicular fluid containing both pro- and anti-inflammatory molecules, such as interleukin-1 (IL1), tumor necrosis factor (TNF), and cortisol. Repeated exposure to inflammatory cytokines may contribute to transforming events in the FTE, with glucocorticoids exerting a protective effect. The global response of FTE cells to inflammatory cytokines or glucocorticoids has not been investigated. To examine the response of FTE cells and the ability of glucocorticoids to oppose this response, an immortalized human FTE cell line, OE-E6/E7, was treated with IL1β, dexamethasone (DEX), IL1β and DEX, or vehicle and genome-wide gene expression profiling was performed. IL1β altered the expression of 47 genes of which 17 were reversed by DEX. DEX treatment alone altered the expression of 590 genes, whereas combined DEX and IL1β treatment altered the expression of 784 genes. Network and pathway enrichment analysis indicated that many genes altered by DEX are involved in cytokine, chemokine, and cell cycle signaling, including NFκ*B* target genes and interacting proteins. Quantitative real time RT-PCR studies validated the gene array data for *IL8, IL23A, PI3* and *TACC2* in OE-E6/E7 cells. Consistent with the array data, Western blot analysis showed increased levels of PTGS2 protein induced by IL1β that was blocked by DEX. A parallel experiment using primary cultured human FTE cells indicated similar effects on *PTGS2, IL8, IL23A, PI3* and *TACC2* transcripts. These findings support the hypothesis that pro-inflammatory signaling is induced in FTE cells by inflammatory mediators and raises the possibility that dysregulation of glucocorticoid signaling could contribute to increased risk for HGSOC.

Editor: Shannon M. Hawkins, Baylor College of Medicine, United States of America

Funding: This work was supported by CIHR (Canadian Institutes of Health Research) MOP106679. The funders had no role in study design, data collection and analysis, decision to publish, or preparation of the manuscript.

Competing Interests: The authors have declared that no competing interests exist.

* E-mail: brown@lunenfeld.ca

‡ These authors contributed equally to this work.

Introduction

High-grade serous ovarian cancer (HGSOC) is the most common of the epithelial ovarian cancer histotypes and almost invariably presents as late stage disease associated with poor prognosis [1]. While traditionally thought to derive from the ovarian surface epithelium, recent studies indicate that HGSOCs likely originate in the fallopian tube epithelium (FTE) [2,3]. Women with germline mutations in breast cancer susceptibility genes 1 or 2 (*BRCA1* or *2*) are at high risk of developing HGSOC and often elect to undergo bilateral salpingoophorectomy to reduce this risk [4]. Histomorphological examination of fallopian tubes from these women has revealed putative HGSOC precursor lesions [3,5]. These include regions of FTE exhibiting strong p53 immunostaining, reflective of *TP53* mutations characteristic of HGSOCs, and tubal intraepithelial carcinomas (TICs), which are occult *in situ* adenocarcinomas [6,7,8]. TICs have been found in more than half of patients presenting with HGSOC [7,9,10,11] and share identical *TP53* mutations with the invasive tumor, supporting the concept that they are clonally related [8].

Risk factors for epithelial ovarian cancer are associated with increased lifetime ovulatory years [12,13,14,15], which have led to the concept that ovulation may contribute to malignant transformation of adnexal epithelia. Ovulation is a localized acute inflammatory event during which fimbrial epithelial cells are exposed to follicular fluid containing a complex combination of inflammatory molecules [16]. Prolonged exposure to pro-inflammatory signaling can result in DNA adduct formation, increasing the incidence of gene mutations that can lead to malignant transformation [17,18,19]. Glucocorticoids have been shown to exert anti-inflammatory effects in several tissues [20]. We have previously shown that *BRCA1* enhances glucocorticoid receptor signaling and found evidence of suppressed glucocorticoid activity in luteal phase FTE from *BRCA1* mutation carriers relative to control patients [21]. However, anti-inflammatory activity of glucocorticoids does not occur in all cell types. For example, a stimulatory rather than inhibitory effect of glucocorticoids on expression of prostaglandin-endoperoxide synthase 2 (PTGS2), the rate-limiting enzyme in prostaglandin production, has been shown

Table 1. List of primers used for RT-qPCR.

Gene ID	Primer sequence	NCBI accession #
PTGS2	F: GTTCCCACCCATGTCAAAAC	NM_000963
	R: ATTCCGGTGTTGAGCAGTT	
IL23A	F: CAAGGACTCAGGGACAACAG	NM_016584
	R: GCTCCCCTGTGAAAATATCC	
IL8	F: CTCTCTTGGCAGCCTTCCT	NM_000584
	R: GGGTGGAAAGGTTTGGAGTA	
PI3	F: ATCGTGGTGGTGTTCCTCAT	NM_002638
	R: ACGGGATCTTGTCCATTGAA	
TACC2	F: TCAGGAGAGCCCTGTCAAGT	NM_206861
	R: GTTTTTCGCAGCAGTGTTCA	
TBP	F: TGCACAGGAGCCAAGAGTGAA	NM_003194
	R: CACATCACAGCTCCCCACCA	
GAPD	F: CGAGCCACATCGCTCAGA	NM_002046
	R: AGTTAAAAGCAGCCCTGGTGA	
B2M	F: CTCCGTGGCCTTAGCTGTG	NM_004048
	R: TTGGAGTACGCTGGATAGCCT	
YWHAZ	F: ACGTCCCTCAAACCTTGCTT	NM_003406
	R: GGCCTTCTGAACCAGCTCAT	

F = forward, R = reverse.

in amnion fibroblasts [22], placental cytotrophoblasts [23], cardiomyocytes [24], and nasal polyps [25].

Human FTE cells have been shown to respond to IL1 with increased IL-8 expression [26], the global response of fallopian epithelial cells to inflammatory cytokines and/or glucocorticoids has not been investigated. In this study, we used an immortalized human oviductal cell line (OE-E6/E7) to assess changes in gene expression induced by Interleukin-1β (IL1β), a pro-inflammatory cytokine, implicated in ovulation [27], and dexamethasone (DEX), a glucocorticoid receptor agonist, to determine whether glucocorticoid signaling alters the response to IL1β in these cells. OE-E6/E7 cells were derived from ampullary tubal epithelial cells of a patient who underwent surgery for uterine fibromyoma and were immortalized using HPV16 E6/E7 [28]. These cells have been extensively characterized and shown to exhibit properties consistent with oviductal secretory epithelial cells [28,29,30]. Thus, these cells serve as a useful model to explore mechanisms that could relate to early carcinogenesis.

Materials and Methods

Cell Culture

OE-E6/E7 cells [28] were obtained from Dr. William S.B. Yeung, University of Hong Kong (Hong Kong, China). BT20 human breast cancer cells were obtained from ATCC (Manassas, VA). Both cell lines were maintained in Dulbecco's Modified Eagle's medium supplemented with 10% fetal bovine serum (FBS), 100 U/ml penicillin and 100 μg/ml streptomycin (all from Invitrogen, Burlington, ON). A human fallopian tube sample was obtained from a patient undergoing prophylactic bilateral salpingoophorectomy for a *BRCA2* mutation at Mount Sinai Hospital (MSH). The tissue collection and use was made with patient informed consent and was approved by the MSH Research Ethics Board. Epithelial cells were derived from the tissue and grown in primary culture on collagen-coated transwell membranes as previously described by Fotheringham at al [31]. All cells were grown in a humidified incubator at 37°C and 5% CO_2. DEX (Sigma, St. Louis, MO) was dissolved in ethanol at 1 mM. Recombinant human IL1β and TNFα (R&D Systems, Minneapolis, MN) were reconstituted in phosphate-buffered saline containing 0.1% bovine serum albumin to 25 μg/ml and 100 μg/ml, respectively. Stock solutions were diluted with culture medium just prior to use to achieve final stated concentrations. Cells were transferred to medium containing 0.5% charcoal-stripped FBS 18 h before initiating hormone or cytokine treatments.

Western Blot Analysis

Cells were collected in RIPA lysis buffer (150 mM NaCl, 50 mM HEPES pH 7.25, 1% Triton X-100, 0.1% SDS, 1% sodium deoxycholate) containing Complete protease inhibitor cocktail (Roche Diagnostics, Laval, QC). Clarified lysates were collected by centrifugation at 20,000 *g* for 15 min at 4°C and total protein was quantified using a BCA protein assay (Pierce, Rockford, IL) following the manufacturer's protocol. Aliquots of lysates containing 15 to 20 μg of total protein were subjected to Western blot analysis as described previously [32] using anti-PTGS2 mouse monoclonal antibody (1:1000; Cayman Chemicals, Ann Arbor, MI) or anti-glucocorticoid receptor rabbit polyclonal (1:500; Abcam, Cambridge, MA) or anti-tubulin mouse monoclonal antibody (1:5000; Sigma). Immunoreactive band intensities were quantified using Molecular Dynamics Image Quant version 5.0 software. Statistical analysis was performed using one-way ANOVA followed by Student-Newman-Keuls post-hoc multiple comparison test (SigmaStat, Systat Software Inc, Chicago, IL). Comparisons were considered statistically significant at $p<0.05$.

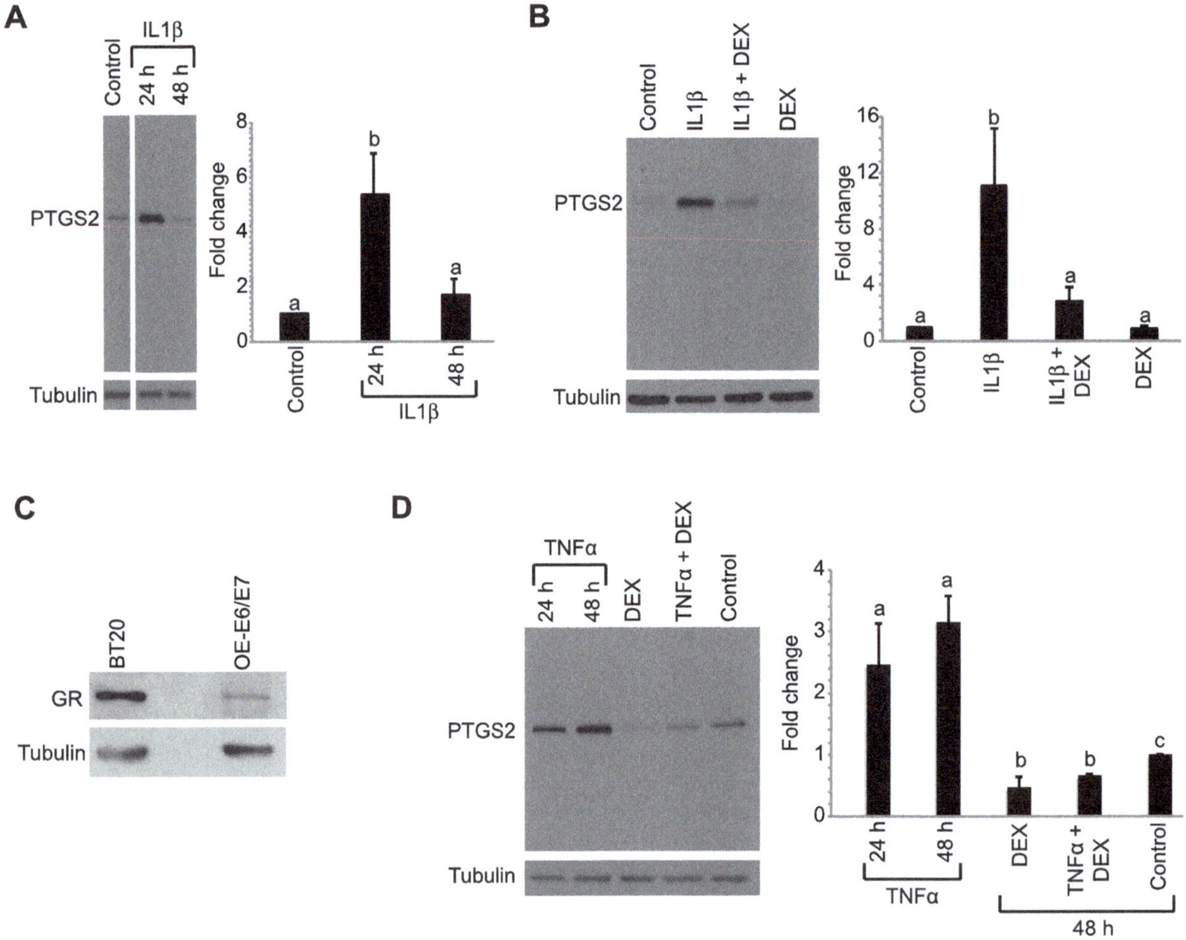

Figure 1. Increased PTGS2 levels in OE-E6/E7 cells by IL1β and TNFα treatment is blocked by DEX. A, Cells were treated with 50 ng/ml IL1β for 24 h or 48 h and Western blot analysis was performed for PTSG2 and tubulin. B, Cells were treated with 10 nM DEX or vehicle 30 h prior to treatment with IL1β or vehicle and harvested 24 h later. Western blot analysis was performed for PTGS2 and tubulin. C, Western blot analysis was performed on OE-E6/E7 cells for glucocorticoid receptor and tubulin levels with BT20 breast cancer cells used as positive control. D, Cells were treated with DEX or vehicle 30 h prior to treatment with TNFα or vehicle. Cells treated with TNFα alone were harvested at 24 and 48 h after treatment and cells treated with DEX+TNFα were harvested at the 48 h time point. Western blot analysis was performed for PTGS2 and tubulin. Histograms summarize quantification of PTGS2 levels normalized to tubulin in 3 to 6 immunoblots. Bars represent the mean ± SEM relative to control. Bars with different letters are statistically different from one another as determined by ANOVA followed by a Student-Newman-Keuls post-hoc multiple comparison test ($p<0.05$).

Gene Expression Analysis

Total RNA extracted using Trizol reagent (Invitrogen) and verified for integrity and purity, was labeled using Illumina TotalPrep RNA amplification kit (Ambion, Austin, TX) as per manufacturer's instructions. The cRNA generated was hybridized to Illumina HT-12 v4.0 BeadChips at 58°C for 18 h. The BeadChips were then washed, stained, and scanned using iScan (Illumina). Data files were quantified in GenomeStudio v2011.1 (Illumina), quantile normalized using the lumi package of Bioconductor [33], and filtered using varFilter to retain the 10% most variable probes. Data for multiple probes targeting the same gene were collapsed to their median value and annotated with gene names using GenePattern [34]. The collapsed data were analyzed using the linear models for microarray analysis (LIMMA) package [35] to identify differentially expressed genes. To understand the relationship among differentially expressed genes further, we performed a network-based analysis using the Reactome Functional Interaction (FI) Network plugin for Cytoscape [36]. The gene expression profiling data can be

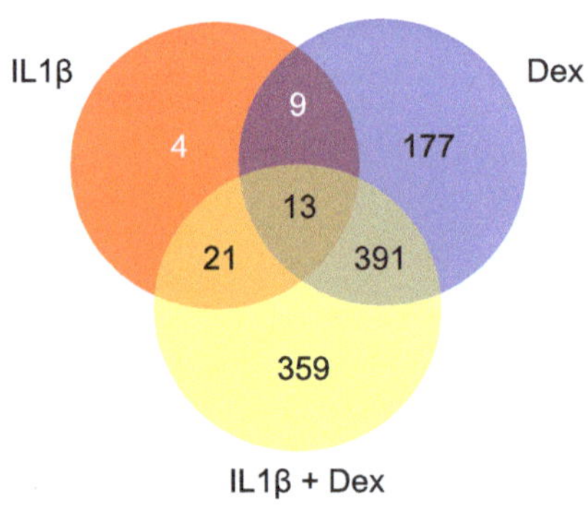

Figure 2. Number and overlap of genes differentially expressed due to IL1β, DEX, and IL1β+DEX treatment. Cells were treated with 10 nM DEX or vehicle 30 h prior to treatment with 50 ng/ml IL1β or vehicle and harvested 18 h later. Total RNA was extracted and gene expression profiling was performed on Illumina HT-12 v4.0 BeadChips. The venn diagram shows the overlap of genes differentially expressed by the different treatments relative to control treated cells.

Table 2. Genes with altered expression due to IL1β treatment.

Gene ID	Gene Name	Log2 Fold-Change*		
		IL1β	DEX	IL1β+DEX
	13 genes altered in all 3 treatment groups			
NGLY1	N-glycanase 1	0.35	0.30	0.43
TRIML2	Tripartite motif family-like 2	0.63	−1.03	−0.67
FOXQ1	Forkhead box Q1	0.97	0.69	1.58
CCL20	Chemokine (C-C motif) ligand 20	0.43	0.49	0.84
C7ORF10	Chromosome 7 open reading frame 10	0.40	1.11	0.98
EBI3	Epstein-Barr virus induced 3	0.46	0.79	1.53
GJB2	Gap junction protein, beta 2	0.75	−0.39	0.36
SYTL2	Synaptotagmin-like 2	−0.85	−1.22	−1.58
PLD5	Phospholipase D family, member 5	−0.73	2.59	2.25
PRSS23	Protease, serine, 23	−0.64	−0.56	−1.53
MAMDC2	MAM domain containing 2	−0.55	−0.59	−1.38
LTB	Lymphotoxin beta	−0.81	−0.88	−1.92
CAMK2N1	Ca^{++}/calmodulin-dependent protein kinase II inhibitor 1	−0.59	0.91	0.38
	21 genes altered by IL1β and by IL1β+Dex			
BATF3	Basic leucine zipper transcription factor, ATF-like 3	0.64	NS	0.91
SAT1	Spermidine/spermine N1-acetyltransferase 1	0.45	NS	0.29
CES1	Carboxylesterase 1	0.81	NS	0.88
E2F2	E2F transcription factor 2	0.71	NS	0.45
ST6GAL1	ST6 beta-galactosamide alpha-2,6-sialyltransferase 1	0.47	NS	0.45
CXCL5	Chemokine (C-X-C motif) ligand 5	0.70	NS	0.71
APPL2	Adaptor protein, phosphotyrosine interaction, PH domain and leucine zipper containing 2	0.37	NS	0.24
CXCL6	Chemokine (C-X-C motif) ligand 6	0.65	NS	0.60
IL17C	Interleukin 17C	1.22	NS	1.45
ARG2	Arginase, type II	0.79	NS	0.68
PI3	Peptidase inhibitor 3	1.18	NS	1.66
RAB38	RAB 38, member RAS oncogene family	0.68	NS	0.68
FLJ10986	FGGY, Carbohydrate kinase domain containing	0.64	NS	0.40
FAM19A3	Chemokine (C-C motif)-like protein TAFA-3	−0.68	NS	−0.84
TMEM166	Transmembrane protein 166	−0.61	NS	−0.40
OXTR	Oxytocin receptor	−0.71	NS	−0.67
SPOCK2	Testican	−0.41	NS	−0.58
CXCL1	Chemokine (C-X3-C motif) ligand 1	−0.99	NS	−0.69
ITGA3	Integrin, alpha 3	−0.50	NS	−0.64
C15ORF52	Chromosome 15 open reading frame 52	−0.34	NS	−0.26
GBP4	Guanylate binding protein 4	−0.62	NS	−0.45
	9 genes altered by IL1β and by DEX			
PTGS2	Prostaglandin-endoperoxide synthase 2	1.10	−1.57	NS
NFKBIZ	I-Kappa-B-zeta	0.46	−0.32	NS
FGFRL1	Fibroblast growth factor receptor-like 1	0.43	−0.31	NS
S100A9	S100 calcium binding protein A9	1.19	−0.96	NS
LOC728454	Similar to Beta-defensin 2 precursor	0.69	−0.83	NS
PTPN20	Protein tyrosine phosphatase, non-receptor type 20	0.51	−0.44	NS
DEFB4	Defensin, beta 4	0.69	−0.76	NS
LI10RB	Interleukin 10 receptor, beta	−0.50	0.42	NS
NFKBIE	I-Kappa-B-epsilon	−0.47	0.45	NS
	4 genes altered by IL1β only			
LXN	Latexin	0.63	NS	NS

Table 2. Cont.

		Log2 Fold-Change*		
Gene ID	**Gene Name**	**IL1β**	**DEX**	**IL1β+DEX**
MAGED1	Melanoma antigen family D, 1	0.40	NS	NS
CCDC24	Coiled-coil domain containing 24	−0.43	NS	NS
IL1R2	Interleukin 1 receptor, type II	−0.52	NS	NS

*Values represent log2 fold change relative to control-treated cells with adjusted p-value <0.05.
NS = non significant (adjusted p-value >0.05).

accessed from the NCBI Gene Expression Omnibus (GEO; http://www.ncbi.nlm.nih.gov/geo. Accessed 2014 May 1), accession number GSE54608.

Quantitative real-time RT-PCR (RT-qPCR)

Total RNA from OE-E6/E7 and primary FTE cells was isolated using Trizol reagent (Invitrogen) following the manufacturer's protocol. Traces of genomic DNA from RNA isolated from OE-E6/E7 cells were removed using a TURBO DNA-free Kit (Applied Biosytems, Foster City, CA) following the manufacturer's protocol. RNA from primary FTE cells was purified using the RNeasy MinElute Clean up kit (Qiagen, Toronto, ON). RNA purity and integrity was determined using a bioanalyzer (Agilent Technologies, Inc, Mississauga, ON) and only samples with a

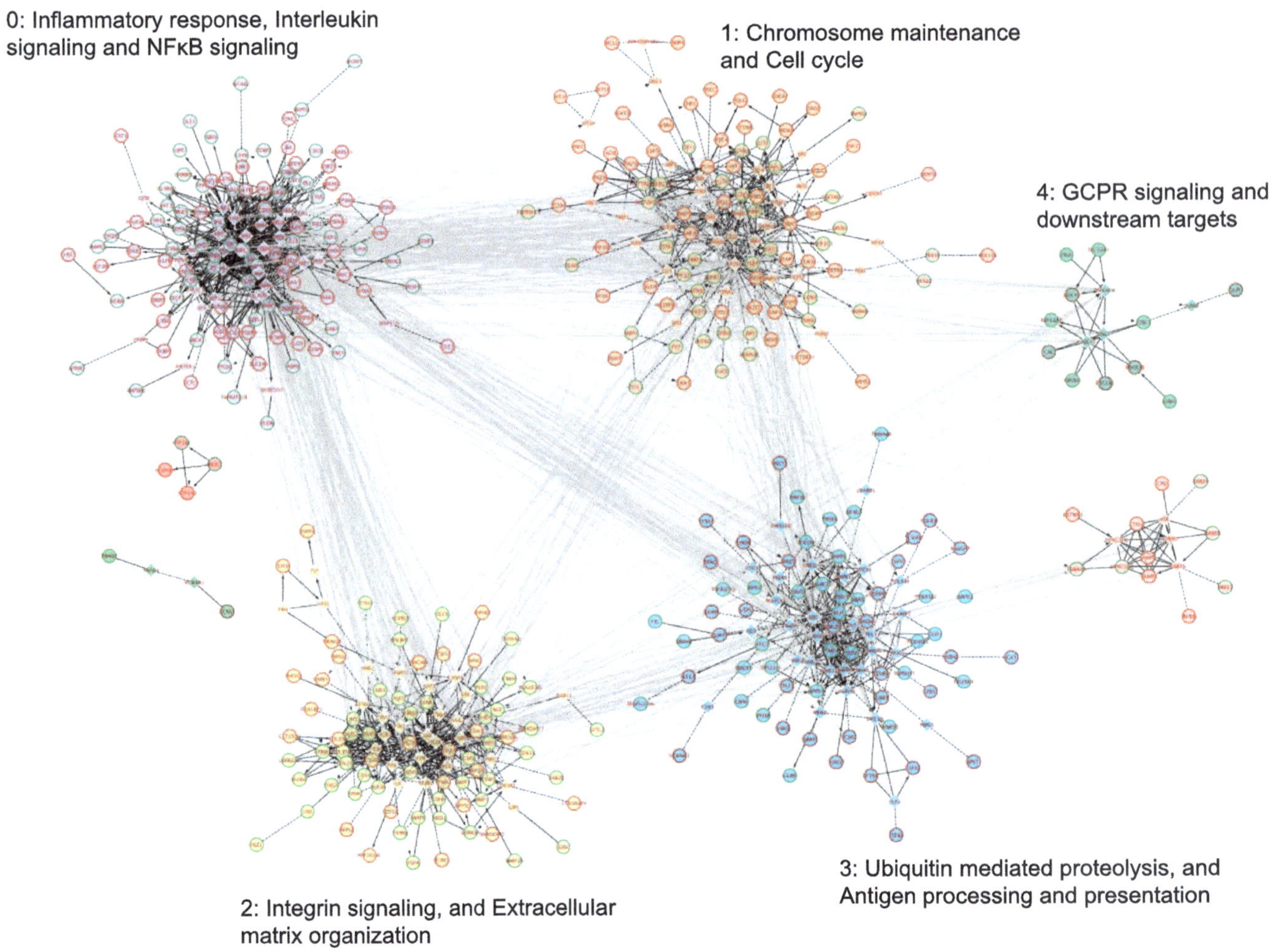

Figure 3. Network analysis of differentially expressed genes in human FTE OE-E6/E7 cells treated with DEX. Module annotations were performed with false discovery rate (FDR)<0.05. Genes up-regulated in human FTE OE-E6/E7 cells treated with DEX are depicted by red outer circles, whereas genes down-regulated in human FTE OE-E6/E7 cells treated with DEX are depicted by green outer circles. Linker genes are depicted as diamond shaped nodes. Direct activating or inhibitory interactions are indicated with the symbols → and -|, respectively. Indirect interactions involving additional proteins are depicted with dashed lines.

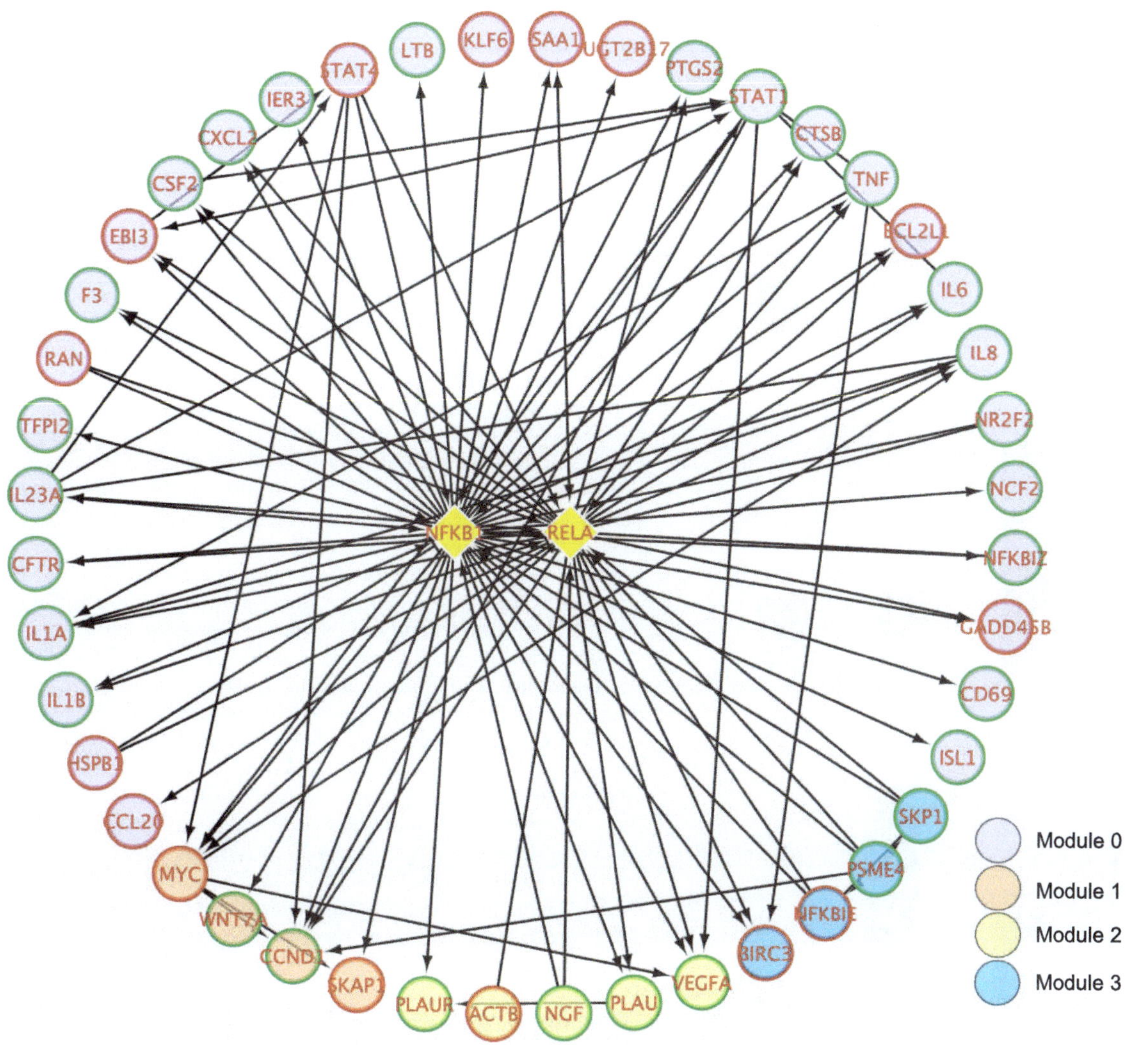

Figure 4. DEX affected NFκB target genes and interacting proteins across four network modules identified by network-based analysis. Genes up-regulated by DEX are depicted by red outer circles, whereas genes down-regulated by DEX are depicted by green outer circles. NFκB subunits are depicted by yellow diamonds. Direct activating or inhibitory interactions are indicated with the symbols → and -|, respectively. Indirect interactions involving additional proteins are depicted with dashed lines.

RNA integrity number greater than 9 were used. The RNA was then reverse transcribed using Superscript III Reverse Transcriptase and random hexamers (Invitrogen) following the manufacturer's protocol. Primers were designed to span an intron/exon boundary using Primer3 (v.0.4.0.) and NCBI Primer-BLAST programs (Table 1) and their specificity was verified by BLAST analysis. Real-time qPCR was performed using a Perkin Elmer-JAMUS automated liquid handling system (Perkin Elmer, Waltham, MA) and a C1000 Thermal cycler (Bio-Rad, Hercules, CA) with LuminoCt SYBER Green (Sigma) detection using a total reaction volume of 5 µl containing 2.5 µl SYBER Green, 300 nM of each primer pair and 75 ng cDNA in 384 well plate. The cycling conditions were 95°C for 30 sec, 95°C for 5 sec, and 60°C for 20 sec. At the end of the PCR cycle, a dissociation curve was performed to confirm amplification of a single product. Each template was run with reference genes (Glyceraldehyde-3-phosphate dehydrogenase, *GAPD*; Beta-2-microglobulin, *B2M*; and Tyrosine 3-monooxygenase/tryptophan 5-monooxygenase activation protein, Zeta polypeptide, *YWHAZ*; and/or TATA-binding protein, *TBP*). RT-qPCR data were analyzed using Bio-Rad CFX manager 2.0 software (Bio-Rad) and the targeted Cq values were normalized to *TBP* (OE-E6/E7 cells) or the geometric mean of *TBP, GAPD, B2M* and *YWHAZ* values using standard curves for each gene to account for any possible differences in primer efficiency. Statistical analysis was performed using two-way ANOVA followed by Student-Newman-Keuls post-hoc multiple comparison test. In cases of inhomogeneity of variance, data were log-transformed or analyzed using Kruskal-Wallis ANOVA on ranks followed by Student-Newman-Keuls post-hoc multiple comparison test. Comparisons were considered statistically significant at $p<0.05$.

Results

We first established that OE-E6/E7 cells respond to IL1β treatment with increased PTGS2 expression. Western blot analysis showed a more than 5-fold increase in levels of PTGS2 at 24 h, but not 48 h after treatment with 50 ng/ml IL1β, relative to

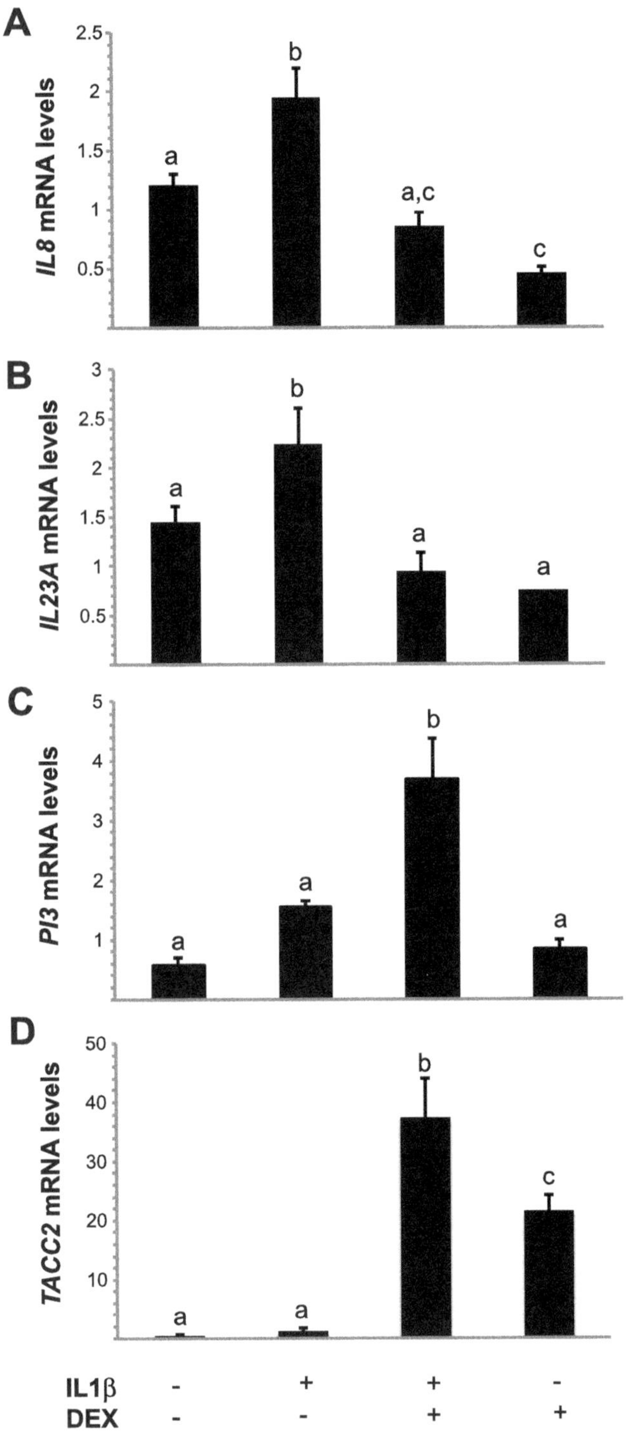

Figure 5. Transcript levels of *IL8, IL23A, PI3* and *TACC2* following IL1β and/or DEX treatment. OE-E6/E7 cells were treated with 10 nM DEX or vehicle 30 h prior to treatment with 50 ng/ml IL1β or vehicle and harvested 18 h later. Total RNA was extracted and RT-qPCR was performed for *IL8* (A), *IL23A* (B), *PI3* (C), *TACC2* (D) and were normalized to *TBP*. Bars represent the mean ± SEM (n = 3 biological replicates performed in triplicate). Bars with different letters are statistically different from one another as determined by ANOVA followed by a Student-Newman-Keuls post-hoc multiple comparison test ($p<0.05$).

control-treated cells (Figure 1A). Pre-treatment of cells with 10 nM DEX reversed the IL1β-induced increase at 24 h but did not affect uninduced PTGS2 levels (Figure 1B). Western blot analysis indicated OE-E6/E7 cells express glucocorticoid receptor but at levels below that of BT20 used as a positive control [37] (Figure 1C). A similar inhibitory effect on PTGS2 was observed with TNFα (Figure 1D). Treatment of cells with 100 ng/ml TNFα increased PTGS2 levels with the highest levels observed at 48 h after treatment. TNFα induction of PTGS2 at 48 h was blocked by pre-treatment with DEX (Figure 1D).

The global impact of IL1β and glucocorticoid treatment on gene expression in OE-E6/E7 cells was determined by whole genome microarray analysis. Cells were treated with DEX or vehicle 30 h prior to treatment with IL1β or vehicle. Cells were harvested 18 h after IL1β treatment and RNA was extracted, labeled, and hybridized to Illumina HT-12 v4.0 BeadChip arrays. Genes differentially expressed between treatment groups and the control group were identified by t-test with correction for multiple testing. Altogether, a statistically significant alteration due to treatment was detected for expression of 974 of the 26,737 genes. Relative to control, IL1β treatment altered the expression of 47 genes, whereas DEX altered the expression of 590 genes (Table S1). Combined IL1β and DEX treatment altered the expression of 784 genes as compared to control-treated cells (Table S1). Of the 47 genes with altered expression due to IL1β treatment, 4 were unique to IL1β and 9 were also altered by DEX alone (Figure 2). IL1β increased the expression of 7 and decreased the expression of 2 of these 9 genes with DEX treatment alone having an opposite effect on their expression relative to control-treated cells (Table 2). None of the 13 genes were altered by combined IL1β and DEX treatment, as compared to control group (Figure 2). Thus, DEX treatment opposed the effect of IL1β on the expression of these 13 genes. Thirteen genes were commonly regulated by all three treatment groups relative to the control group (Figure 2). Pre-treatment with DEX reversed the impact of IL1β on 4 while enhancing the effect on 8 of these 13 genes (Table 2).

Twenty-one genes were common between the IL1β+DEX and IL1β alone versus control comparisons, but not DEX alone versus control (Figure 2 and Table 2). The impact of treatment on the expression of these genes reflects IL1β since DEX neither further enhanced nor inhibited the IL1β effect. This was confirmed by direct comparison of the IL1β alone and IL1β+DEX treatment groups (data not shown).

DEX treatment altered the expression of a greater number of genes than IL1β. We used the Reactome Functional Interaction (FI) Network to explore the relationships among differentially expressed genes in OE-E6/E7 cells treated with DEX [36]. In brief, the FI network covers ~50% of the human proteome representing nearly 210,000 FIs. Of the 590 genes that were differentially expressed in response to DEX, 356 (60%) were projected onto the FI network. The average-shortest path calculation demonstrated that the interactions between the 365 genes were more highly connected with each other than by chance alone ($p<0.001$). A minimum spanning tree algorithm was used to add 128 "linker" genes from the FI network to create a single fully connected subnetwork [38]. A spectral partitioning clustering algorithm was then used to identify clusters of genes that were highly interconnected with each other [39]. The clustering algorithm identified 5 functionally related network modules (0 to 4), which consisted of 11 or more genes (Figure 3 and File S1). All network diagrams were visualized using Cytoscape [40]. Using functional enrichment analysis, the modules were annotated for BioCarta, KEGG, NCI-PID, Panther, and Reactome pathways with a false discovery rate (FDR)<0.05. Of interest were a number

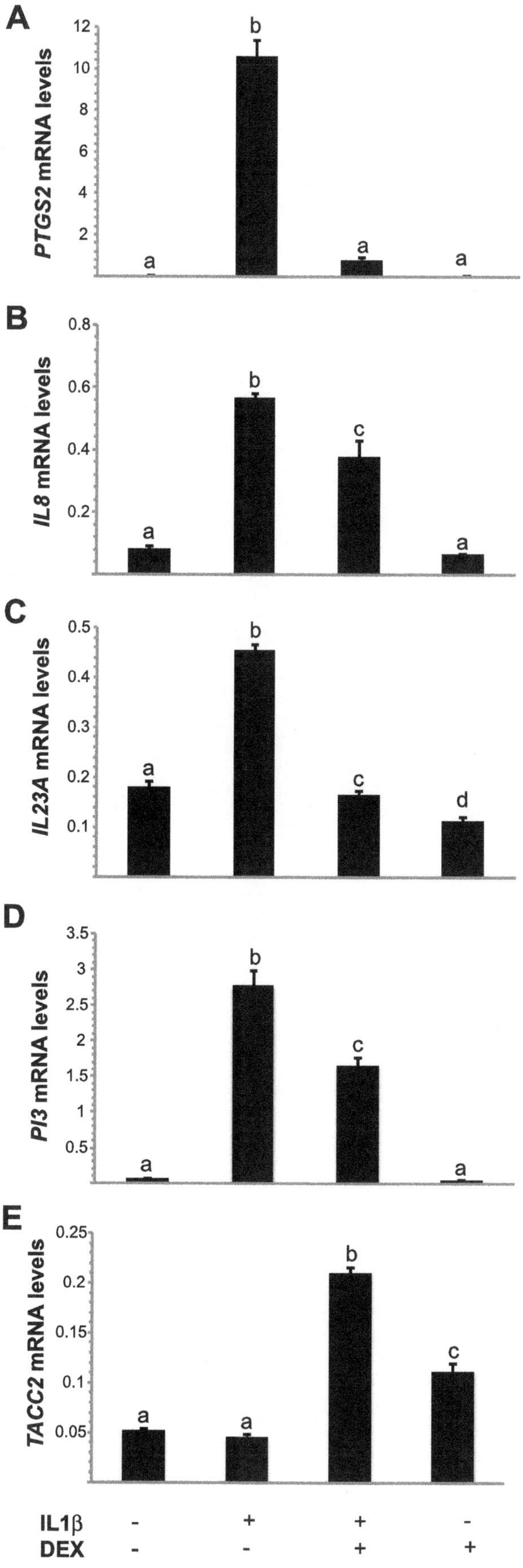

Figure 6. Transcript levels of *PTGS2, IL8, IL23A, PI3* and *TACC2* following IL1β and/or DEX treatment. Primary FTE cells were treated with 10 nM DEX or vehicle 30 h prior to treatment with 50 ng/ml IL1β or vehicle and harvested 18 h later. Total RNA was extracted and RT-qPCR was performed for *PTGS2* (A), *IL8* (B), *IL23A* (C), *PI3* (D), *TACC2* (E) and were normalized to the geometric mean of 4 reference genes. Bars represent the mean ± SEM (n = 3). Bars with different letters are statistically different from one another as determined by ANOVA followed by a Student-Newman-Keuls post-hoc multiple comparison test ($p<0.05$).

of pathways contained within the modules, including inflammatory response, interleukin and NFκB signaling (module 0; Figure S1 in File S1), chromosome maintenance and cell cycle (module 1; Figure S2 in File S1), integrin signaling and extracellular matrix organization (module 2; Figure S3 in File S1), ubiquitin mediated proteolysis and antigen processing/presentation (module 3; Figure S4 in File S1), and G protein coupled receptor signaling and downstream targets (module 4; Figure S5 in File S1). Using *NFKB1* and *RELA1* 'linker' genes of module 0, NFκ*B* target genes and interacting proteins across four network modules were visualized in Cytoscape (Figure 4).

Four genes were selected for validation as differentially expressed genes due to IL1β or DEX treatment based on their potential involvement in carcinogenesis. OE-E6/E7 cells were treated as described for the gene expression profiling study and levels of Interleukin 8 (*IL8*), Interleukin-23 alpha subunit p19 (*IL23A*), Peptidase Inhibitor 3 (*PI3*) and Transforming Acidic Coiled-Coil Containing protein 2 (*TACC2*) transcripts were measured by RT-qPCR. Microarray analysis indicated increased expression of NFκ*B* target gene *IL23A* by IL1β that did not attain statistical significance with a FDR-corrected t-test (P = 0.051, Table S1); however, a statistically significant increase was detected by RT-qPCR (Figure 5B). A similar increase was also observed for the NFκ*B* target gene *IL8* (Figure 5A). Consistent with an anti-inflammatory role, DEX pre-treatment inhibited the IL1β-induced expression of both genes. In agreement with our gene expression profiling data, DEX alone reduced expression of *IL8*. Also consistent with our microarray data, DEX treatment increased *TACC2* expression, which was further increased by IL1β (Figure 5D). *PI3* expression was increased by IL1β in our microarray analysis (Table 1) and the increase detected by RT-qPCR approached statistical significance (P = 0.096; Figure 5C). Consistent with our microarray data, increased *PI3* expression was detected with combined IL1β and DEX treatment.

To determine if similar effects are observed in non-immortalized FTE cells, a primary culture of human FTE cells derived from excess surgical material was treated with IL1β with or without DEX as described for OE-E6/E7 cells and RT-qPCR was performed for *PTGS2, IL8, IL23A, PI3* and *TACC2* transcripts. IL1β treatment increased the expression of *PTGS2, IL8, IL23A, PI3* transcripts and DEX treatment inhibited the IL1β-induced increase (Figure 6). DEX alone had no effect on *PTGS2, IL8*, or *PI3* transcript levels but decreased expression of *IL23A*. Similar to OE-E6/E7 cells, DEX treatment increased *TACC2* transcript levels, which were further elevated by IL1β co-treatment (Figure 6).

Discussion

Inflammation plays an important role in the initiation and progression of several cancers [18,41]. In healthy cycling women, the fallopian tube may be exposed to an inflammatory milieu at the time of ovulation and in the event of retrograde menstruation

[42]. Ovulation is a highly-localized, acute inflammatory event that exposes the distal FTE to follicular fluid containing pro-inflammatory cytokines and mediators, including IL1 and TNF, as well as high concentrations of steroid hormones [43,44]. Likewise, retrograde menstruation can expose the entire length of the fallopian tube to pro-inflammatory agents within the menses. Rapid resolution of inflammatory signaling is thus important to limit cellular damage to the epithelium. Approximately 80% of TICs within the FTE are found in the fimbria or distal portion of the tube [3], consistent with exposure to ovulation-associated inflammation. Molecular profiling of microdissected FTE from *BRCA* mutation carriers and control patients indicated luteal FTE from mutation carriers differed from that of control patients, whereas follicular FTE were highly similar between the two groups [45]. This difference in luteal phase FTE from *BRCA* mutation carriers predominantly reflected a pro-inflammatory gene signature consistent with increased NFκB signaling and diminished glucocorticoid receptor signaling [21,46]. The FTE samples were not obtained immediately following ovulation and the response of tubule epithelial cells to inflammatory cytokine or glucocorticoid exposure has not been characterized.

NFκB, a principal intracellular mediator of pro-inflammatory cytokines, has been proposed as a mechanistic link between inflammation and cancer [47,48] and its pro-inflammatory signaling targets are activated by both IL1 and TNF. Consistent with this, we found well-established direct transcriptional targets of NFκB signaling to be up-regulated by IL1β treatment in OE-E6/E7 cells.

Glucocorticoids exert pleiotropic effects critical to maintaining tissue homeostasis. As such, they play a key role in moderating and resolving inflammatory environments by inhibiting downstream signaling by inflammatory cytokines and by inducing cell-type specific apoptosis of monocytes, macrophages, and T-lymphocytes [49]. In addition to reversing the impact of IL1β on many inflammation-associated genes, our data indicate that glucocorticoid receptor signaling impacts the expression of multiple genes unaffected by IL1β. Activated glucocorticoid receptors heterodimerize with the NFκB subunit RelA, resulting in inhibition of RelA signaling [50,51]. Additionally, the glucocorticoid receptor can affect the expression of anti-inflammatory genes through transactivation. Our pathway analysis indicated genes involved with inflammatory response, cell cycle, extracellular matrix organization, antigen processing, and G-protein coupled receptor signaling are affected by DEX treatment. Many of the genes in these pathways are NFκB target genes or encode NFκB interacting proteins. Several of these were not found to be affected by IL1β treatment, which could reflect differences in NFκ*B* family members involved, the timing of the treatments, or regulation through independent pathways [52,53]. Nonetheless, this finding is consistent with a more generalized anti-inflammatory effect of glucocorticoid receptor activaton that is not restricted to inhibition of IL1β-activated NFκ*B* signaling.

The genes validated in this study – *PTGS2*, *IL8*, *IL23A*, *TACC2* and *PI3* – were selected based upon their differential response to treatment and their implication for cancer initiation. IL1 is a potent stimulator of *PTGS2* expression and prostaglandin production in ovarian tissue. Mice with targeted deletion of *PTGS2* fail to ovulate [54], indicating the importance of prostaglandin production in ovulation. Within the fallopian tube, prostaglandins may play a non-inflammatory role in muscular contraction and the resulting transport of the oocyte/embryo toward the uterus [55]. We found that treatment of OE-E6/E7 cells with peri-ovulatory follicular fluid collected from patients undergoing *in vitro* fertilization increased PTGS2 protein levels (data not shown). PTGS2 is a major inflammatory mediator up-regulated in several cancers, most notably colorectal carcinoma [56,57]. Prostaglandins evoke further cytokine expression to promote the inflammatory response, which could contribute to carcinogenesis. Indeed, a protective effect of PTGS2 inhibition has been shown for certain cancers, such as colorectal cancer [56,57]. Moreover, recent studies suggest aspirin, an inhibitor of both PTGS1 and 2, may exert a protective effect for invasive ovarian cancer [58,59]. In the present study, we found PTGS2 expression was increased by IL1β, an effect that was blocked by glucocorticoid signaling. A stimulatory, rather than inhibitory effect of DEX on PTGS2 expression has been reported in a variety of cell types [22,23,24,25]. While the mechanism underlying this paradoxical response are not fully understood, Wang et al [23] recently showed that DEX treatment of placental cytotrophoblast cells up-regulated expression of *MAP3K14/NIK*, a serine/threonine kinase that mediates activation of non-canonical NFκB signaling by processing NFκB2/p100 to active p52 [52]. In the present study, we did not see evidence of DEX altering the expression of *MAP3K14* or of NFκB subunits in OE-E6/E7 cells.

IL8 accentuates local pro-inflammatory signaling by attracting monocytes, neutrophils and T-cells and its expression is increased in the distal fallopian tube during the peri-ovulatory period [45,60]. IL8 is elevated in the serum of ovarian cancer patients and enhances tumorigenicity of ovarian cancer cell mouse xenographs [61,62]. Since *IL8* is a known downstream target of IL1 [26] and our profiling data indicated an inhibitory effect of DEX, we examined its expression by RT-qPCR. Our results are consistent with IL1β acting upon these cells and primary cultured FTE cells to induce *IL8*, and verified the inhibitory impact of DEX on this expression.

IL23 is a heterodimeric cytokine, consisting of a p19 (IL23A) and p40 (IL12β) subunit, produced by multiple cell types [63]. Although IL23 shares a subunit with IL12, it activates a distinct receptor and exerts effects that differ from those of IL12 [64]. In contrast to IL12, IL23 promotes pro-inflammatory responses and diminishes tumor infiltration of cytotoxic T cells as determined in a DMBA/TPA-induced skin papilloma mouse model [65]. More recently, Teng et al [66] showed IL23 promotes methylcholanthrene-induced fibrosarcoma in mice by antagonizing anti-tumor innate immune responses. This combination of stimulating inflammatory signaling while diminishing immune surveillance would facilitate early events in carcinogenesis. We found that IL1β stimulated expression of *IL23A* in both OE-E6/E7 and primary FTE cells and that this increase was blocked by DEX.

TACC2 is a member of a family of highly conserved proteins that associate with the centrosome-spindle apparatus and are thought to play a role in cell division [67]. In mammals, both TACC2 and 3 function as nuclear receptor coactivators [60,67]. TACC2 associates with retinoic acid receptor RXRβ and with histone acetytransferases and the Switch/sucrose nonfermentable (swi/snf) complex involved with chromatin remodeling and transcription [67,68,69]. While both tumor promoting and suppressive activities of TACC2 have been reported in various cancers [70,71,72], Lauffart et al [73] have shown that TACC2 and 3 interact with the BARD1/BRCA1 complex and may play a role in DNA double-strand break repair. Our data indicate *TACC2* expression is increased by DEX in both OE-E6/E7 cells and primary FTE cells, which is consistent with a previous report showing increased expression of TACC2 by DEX in ovarian cancer cells [74]. The functional impact of this increase remains to be determined.

PI3 encodes a serine protease inhibitor that functions as an anti-inflammatory mediator. Ghosh et al [75] reported that epithelial cells within the female reproductive tract, including the fallopian tube, express PI3 with higher levels observed during the luteal phase. Although PI3 has been shown to reduce neutrophil and macrophage accumulation and increase G-CSF levels, consistent with a role in innate immunity, a role in adaptive immunity has also been suggested [76]. Consistent with our data showing increased PI3 expression by IL1β, other studies have shown increased expression of PI3 in IL1β-treated endocervical cells and in OE-E6/E7 cells exposed to *Chlamydia trachomatis* [77,78], likely through NFκB signaling [79]. Since NFκB signaling is in turn inhibited by PI3 [80] this increase in PI3 may be directed at containing the pro-inflammatory response. Our finding that DEX treatment further increased PI3 expression in the presence of IL1β in OE-E6/E7 cells was surprising, given the inhibitory impact of glucocorticoid activation on NFκB signaling. However, an inhibitory effect of DEX on IL1β-induced *PI3* transcript levels was observed in primary FTE cells.

In summary, we demonstrate that IL1β, a cytokine associated with ovulation, induces a pro-inflammatory gene expression signature in an immortalized human fallopian tube epithelial cell line. Activation of glucocorticoid receptor by a synthetic agonist reversed the expression of several IL1β-induced inflammatory genes and altered the expression of additional inflammation-associated genes. These findings were confirmed for key representative genes in a primary culture of FTE cells. Thus, this study provides support for the hypothesis that pro-inflammatory signaling is induced in FTE cells by inflammatory mediators, such as those present in follicular fluid at the time of ovulation, and that this signaling is opposed by glucocorticoids. Dysregulation of glucocorticoid receptor signaling could therefore contribute to increased risk for HGSOC.

Supporting Information

Table S1 Annotation of Genes in Venn diagram shown in Figure 2.

File S1 Supporting Figures. Figure S1. Network Module 0, representing 'Inflammatory response, Interleukin signaling and NFκB signaling' shown in Figure 3. **Figure S2.** Network Module 1, representing 'Chromosomal maintenance and Cell cycle' shown in Figure 3. **Figure S3.** Network Module 2, representing 'Integrin signaling and Extracellular matrix organization' shown in Figure 3. **Figure S4.** Network Module 3, representing 'Ubiquitin mediated proteolysis and Antigen processing and presentation' shown in Figure 3. **Figure S5.** Network Module 4, representing 'G protein coupled receptor signaling and downstream targets' shown in Figure 3.

Acknowledgments

We thank Dr. Claudio Monetti and Dr. Premalatha Shathasivam for their technical assistance and Carl Virtanen of the OCI Genomics Centre for performing initial quality control assessments on the data and for helpful comments. We also thank Irina Kalatskaya and Paul Krzyzanowski for helpful discussions on network analysis and Thomasina Spybey for helpful comments on the manuscript. We thank Angela Lau for technical assistance with FTE culture.

Author Contributions

Conceived and designed the experiments: SB AK TJB. Performed the experiments: SB AK. Analyzed the data: RH LS SB AK TJB. Contributed reagents/materials/analysis tools: RH LS. Wrote the paper: SB AK RH TJB.

References

1. Soslow RA (2008) Histologic subtypes of ovarian carcinoma: an overview. Int J Gynecol Pathol 27: 161–174.
2. Crum CP, Drapkin R, Miron A, Ince TA, Muto M, et al. (2007) The distal fallopian tube: a new model for pelvic serous carcinogenesis. Curr Opin Obstet Gynecol 19: 3–9.
3. Lee Y, Miron A, Drapkin R, Nucci MR, Medeiros F, et al. (2007) A candidate precursor to serous carcinoma that originates in the distal fallopian tube. J Pathol 211: 26–35.
4. Sogaard M, Kjaer SK, Gayther S (2006) Ovarian cancer and genetic susceptibility in relation to the BRCA1 and BRCA2 genes. Occurrence, clinical importance and intervention. Acta Obstet Gynecol Scand 85: 93–105.
5. Piek JM, van Diest PJ, Zweemer RP, Jansen JW, Poort-Keesom RJ, et al. (2001) Dysplastic changes in prophylactically removed Fallopian tubes of women predisposed to developing ovarian cancer. J Pathol 195: 451–456.
6. Finch A, Shaw P, Rosen B, Murphy J, Narod SA, et al. (2006) Clinical and pathologic findings of prophylactic salpingo-oophorectomies in 159 BRCA1 and BRCA2 carriers. Gynecol Oncol 100: 58–64.
7. Kindelberger DW, Lee Y, Miron A, Hirsch MS, Feltmate C, et al. (2007) Intraepithelial carcinoma of the fimbria and pelvic serous carcinoma: Evidence for a causal relationship. Am J Surg Pathol 31: 161–169.
8. Kuhn E, Kurman RJ, Vang R, Sehdev AS, Han G, et al. (2012) TP53 mutations in serous tubal intraepithelial carcinoma and concurrent pelvic high-grade serous carcinoma—evidence supporting the clonal relationship of the two lesions. J Pathol 226: 421–426.
9. Carlson JW, Miron A, Jarboe EA, Parast MM, Hirsch MS, et al. (2008) Serous tubal intraepithelial carcinoma: its potential role in primary peritoneal serous carcinoma and serous cancer prevention. J Clin Oncol 26: 4160–4165.
10. Seidman JD, Zhao P, Yemelyanova A (2011) "Primary peritoneal" high-grade serous carcinoma is very likely metastatic from serous tubal intraepithelial carcinoma: assessing the new paradigm of ovarian and pelvic serous carcinogenesis and its implications for screening for ovarian cancer. Gynecol Oncol 120: 470–473.
11. Tang S, Onuma K, Deb P, Wang E, Lytwyn A, et al. (2012) Frequency of serous tubal intraepithelial carcinoma in various gynecologic malignancies: a study of 300 consecutive cases. Int J Gynecol Pathol 31: 103–110.
12. Hunn J, Rodriguez GC (2012) Ovarian cancer: etiology, risk factors, and epidemiology. Clin Obstet Gynecol 55: 3–23.
13. McGuire V, Felberg A, Mills M, Ostrow KL, DiCioccio R, et al. (2004) Relation of contraceptive and reproductive history to ovarian cancer risk in carriers and noncarriers of BRCA1 gene mutations. Am J Epidemiol 160: 613–618.
14. McLaughlin JR, Risch HA, Lubinski J, Moller P, Ghadirian P, et al. (2007) Reproductive risk factors for ovarian cancer in carriers of BRCA1 or BRCA2 mutations: a case-control study. Lancet Oncol 8: 26–34.
15. Tung KH, Wilkens LR, Wu AH, McDuffie K, Nomura AM, et al. (2005) Effect of anovulation factors on pre- and postmenopausal ovarian cancer risk: revisiting the incessant ovulation hypothesis. Am J Epidemiol 161: 321–329.
16. Buscher U, Chen FC, Kentenich H, Schmiady H (1999) Cytokines in the follicular fluid of stimulated and non-stimulated human ovaries; is ovulation a suppressed inflammatory reaction? Hum Reprod 14: 162–166.
17. Karihtala P, Soini Y, Vaskivuo L, Bloigu R, Puistola U (2009) DNA adduct 8-hydroxydeoxyguanosine, a novel putative marker of prognostic significance in ovarian carcinoma. Int J Gynecol Cancer 19: 1047–1051.
18. Lu H, Ouyang W, Huang C (2006) Inflammation, a key event in cancer development. Mol Cancer Res 4: 221–233.
19. Valavanidis A, Vlachogianni T, Fiotakis C (2009) 8-hydroxy-2′ -deoxyguanosine (8-OHdG): A critical biomarker of oxidative stress and carcinogenesis. J Environ Sci Health C Environ Carcinog Ecotoxicol Rev 27: 120–139.
20. Singh N, Rieder MJ, Tucker MJ (2004) Mechanisms of glucocorticoid-mediated anti-inflammatory and immunosuppressive action. Paediatric and Perinatal Drug Therapy 6: 107–115.
21. Tone AA, Virtanen C, Shaw P, Brown TJ (2012) Prolonged postovulatory proinflammatory signaling in the fallopian tube epithelium may be mediated through a BRCA1/DAB2 axis. Clin Cancer Res 18: 4334–4344.
22. Zhu XO, Yang Z, Guo CM, Ni XT, Li JN, et al. (2009) Paradoxical stimulation of cyclooxygenase-2 expression by glucocorticoids via a cyclic AMP response element in human amnion fibroblasts. Mol Endocrinol 23: 1839–1849.
23. Wang B, Palomares K, Parobchak N, Cece J, Rosen M, et al. (2012) Glucocorticoid Receptor Signaling Contributes to Constitutive Activation of the Noncanonical NF-kappaB Pathway in Term Human Placenta. Mol Endocrinol 27: 203–211.
24. Sun H, Sheveleva E, Xu B, Inoue H, Bowden TG, et al. (2008) Corticosteroids induce COX-2 expression in cardiomyocytes: role of glucocorticoid receptor and C/EBP-beta. Am J Physiol Cell Physiol 295: C915–922.

25. Pujols L, Benitez P, Alobid I, Martinez-Anton A, Roca-Ferrer J, et al. (2009) Glucocorticoid therapy increases COX-2 gene expression in nasal polyps in vivo. Eur Respir J 33: 502–508.
26. Mulayim N, Palter SF, Selam B, Arici A (2003) Expression and regulation of interleukin-8 in human fallopian tubal cells. American journal of obstetrics and gynecology 188: 651–656.
27. Gerard N, Caillaud M, Martoriati A, Goudet G, Lalmanach AC (2004) The interleukin-1 system and female reproduction. J Endocrinol 180: 203–212.
28. Lee YL, Lee KF, Xu JS, Wang YL, Tsao SW, et al. (2001) Establishment and characterization of an immortalized human oviductal cell line. Mol Reprod Dev 59: 400–409.
29. Monkkonen KS, Aflatoonian R, Lee KF, Yeung WS, Tsao SW, et al. (2007) Hormonal regulation of Galphai2 and mPRalpha in immortalized human oviductal cell line OE-E6/E7. Mol Hum Reprod 13: 845–851.
30. Ling L, Lee YL, Lee KF, Tsao SW, Yeung WS, et al. (2005) Expression of human oviductin in an immortalized human oviductal cell line. Fertil Steril 84 Suppl 2: 1095–1103.
31. Fotheringham S, Levanon K, Drapkin R (2011) Ex vivo culture of primary human fallopian tube epithelial cells. J Vis Exp 51. Available: http://www.jove.com/details.php?id = 2728, doi:10.3791/2728.
32. Kollara A, Brown TJ (2006) Functional interaction of nuclear receptor coactivator 4 with aryl hydrocarbon receptor. Biochem Biophys Res Commun 346: 526–534.
33. Gentleman RC, Carey VJ, Bates DM, Bolstad B, Dettling M, et al. (2004) Bioconductor: open software development for computational biology and bioinformatics. Genome Biol 5: R80.
34. Reich M, Liefeld T, Gould J, Lerner J, Tamayo P, et al. (2006) GenePattern 2.0. Nat Genet 38: 500–501.
35. Wettenhall JM, Smyth GK (2004) limmaGUI: a graphical user interface for linear modeling of microarray data. Bioinformatics 20: 3705–3706.
36. Wu G, Feng X, Stein L (2010) A human functional protein interaction network and its application to cancer data analysis. Genome Biol 11: R53.
37. Mikosz CA, Brickley DR, Sharkey MS, Moran TW, Conzen SD (2001) Glucocorticoid receptor-mediated protection from apoptosis is associated with induction of the serine/threonine survival kinase gene, sgk-1. J Biol Chem 276: 16649–16654.
38. Gross JL, Yellen J (1998) Graph Theory and Its Applications. Boca Raton, FL: CRC Press.
39. Girvan M, Newman ME (2002) Community structure in social and biological networks. Proc Natl Acad Sci USA 99: 7821–7826.
40. Shannon P, Markiel A, Ozier O, Baliga NS, Wang JT, et al. (2003) Cytoscape: a software environment for integrated models of biomolecular interaction networks. Genome Res 13: 2498–2504.
41. Trinchieri G (2012) Cancer and inflammation: an old intuition with rapidly evolving new concepts. Annu Rev Immunol 30: 677–706.
42. Maccio A, Madeddu C (2012) Inflammation and ovarian cancer. Cytokine 58: 133–147.
43. Johnson ML, Murdoch J, Van Kirk EA, Kaltenbach JE, Murdoch WJ (1999) Tumor necrosis factor alpha regulates collagenolytic activity in preovulatory ovine follicles: relationship to cytokine secretion by the oocyte-cumulus cell complex. Biol Reprod 61: 1581–1585.
44. Revelli A, Delle Piane L, Casano S, Molinari E, Massobrio M, et al. (2009) Follicular fluid content and oocyte quality: from single biochemical markers to metabolomics. Reprod Biol Endocrinol 7: 40.
45. Tone AA, Begley H, Sharma M, Murphy J, Rosen B, et al. (2008) Gene expression profiles of luteal phase fallopian tube epithelium from BRCA mutation carriers resemble high-grade serous carcinoma. Clin Cancer Res 14: 4067–4078.
46. Tone AA, Virtanen C, Shaw PA, Brown TJ (2011) Decreased progesterone receptor isoform expression in luteal phase fallopian tube epithelium and high-grade serous carcinoma. Endocr Relat Cancer 18: 221–234.
47. Karin M (2009) NF-kappaB as a critical link between inflammation and cancer. Cold Spring Harb Perspect Biol 1: a000141.
48. Aggarwal BB, Sung B (2011) NF-kappaB in cancer: a matter of life and death. Cancer Discov 1: 469–471.
49. Almawi WY, Beyhum HN, Rahme AA, Rieder MJ (1996) Regulation of cytokine and cytokine receptor expression by glucocorticoids. J Leukoc Biol 60: 563–572.
50. Caldenhoven E, Liden J, Wissink S, Van de Stolpe A, Raaijmakers J, et al. (1995) Negative cross-talk between RelA and the glucocorticoid receptor: a possible mechanism for the antiinflammatory action of glucocorticoids. Mol Endocrinol 9: 401–412.
51. Necela BM, Cidlowski JA (2004) Mechanisms of glucocorticoid receptor action in noninflammatory and inflammatory cells. Proc Am Thorac Soc 1: 239–246.
52. Sen R, Smale ST (2010) Selectivity of the NF-κB response. Cold Spring Harb Perspect Biol 2: a000257.
53. Chaturvedi MM, Sung B, Yadav VR, Kannappan R, Aggarwal BB (2011) NF-kappaB addiction and its role in cancer: 'one size does not fit all'. Oncogene 30: 1615–1630.
54. Lim H, Paria BC, Das SK, Dinchuk JE, Langenbach R, et al. (1997) Multiple female reproductive failures in cyclooxygenase 2-deficient mice. Cell 91: 197–208.
55. Wanggren K, Stavreus-Evers A, Olsson C, Andersson E, Gemzell-Danielsson K (2008) Regulation of muscular contractions in the human Fallopian tube through prostaglandins and progestagens. Hum Reprod 23: 2359–2368.
56. Menter DG, Schilsky RL, DuBois RN (2010) Cyclooxygenase-2 and cancer treatment: understanding the risk should be worth the reward. Clin Cancer Res 16: 1384–1390.
57. Wang D, Dubois RN (2010) The role of COX-2 in intestinal inflammation and colorectal cancer. Oncogene 29: 781–788.
58. Ammundsen HB, Faber MT, Jensen A, Hogdall E, Blaakaer J, et al. (2012) Use of analgesic drugs and risk of ovarian cancer: results from a Danish case-control study. Acta Obstet Gynecol Scand 91: 1094–1102.
59. Baandrup L, Faber MT, Christensen J, Jensen A, Andersen KK, et al. (2013) Nonsteroidal anti-inflammatory drugs and risk of ovarian cancer: systematic review and meta-analysis of observational studies. Acta Obstet Gynecol Scand 92: 245–255.
60. Palter SF, Mulayim N, Senturk L, Arici A (2001) Interleukin-8 in the human fallopian tube. J Clin Endocrinol Metab 86: 2660–2667.
61. Xu L, Fidler IJ (2000) Interleukin 8: an autocrine growth factor for human ovarian cancer. Oncol Res 12: 97–106.
62. Lokshin AE, Winans M, Landsittel D, Marrangoni AM, Velikokhatnaya L, et al. (2006) Circulating IL-8 and anti-IL-8 autoantibody in patients with ovarian cancer. Gynecol Oncol 102: 244–251.
63. Oppmann B, Lesley R, Blom B, Timans JC, Xu Y, et al. (2000) Novel p19 protein engages IL-12p40 to form a cytokine, IL-23, with biological activities similar as well as distinct from IL-12. Immunity 13: 715–725.
64. McKenzie BS, Kastelein RA, Cua DJ (2006) Understanding the IL-23-IL-17 immune pathway. Trends Immunol 27: 17–23.
65. Langowski JL, Zhang X, Wu L, Mattson JD, Chen T, et al. (2006) IL-23 promotes tumour incidence and growth. Nature 442: 461–465.
66. Teng MW, Andrews DM, McLaughlin N, von Scheidt B, Ngiow SF, et al. (2010) IL-23 suppresses innate immune response independently of IL-17A during carcinogenesis and metastasis. Proc Natl Acad Sci USA 107: 8328–8333.
67. Still IH, Vettaikkorumakankauv AK, DiMatteo A, Liang P (2004) Structure-function evolution of the transforming acidic coiled coil genes revealed by analysis of phylogenetically diverse organisms. BMC Evol Biol 4: 16.
68. Gangisetty O, Lauffart B, Sondarva GV, Chelsea DM, Still IH (2004) The transforming acidic coiled coil proteins interact with nuclear histone acetyltransferases. Oncogene 23: 2559–2563.
69. Lauffart B, Gangisetty O, Still IH (2003) Molecular cloning, genomic structure and interactions of the putative breast tumor suppressor TACC2. Genomics 81: 192–201.
70. Takayama K, Horie-Inoue K, Suzuki T, Urano T, Ikeda K, et al. (2012) TACC2 is an androgen-responsive cell cycle regulator promoting androgen-mediated and castration-resistant growth of prostate cancer. Mol Endocrinol 26: 748–761.
71. Cheng S, Douglas-Jones A, Yang X, Mansel RE, Jiang WG (2010) Transforming acidic coiled-coil-containing protein 2 (TACC2) in human breast cancer, expression pattern and clinical/prognostic relevance. Cancer Genomics Proteomics 7: 67–73.
72. Lauffart B, Vaughan MM, Eddy R, Chervinsky D, DiCioccio RA, et al. (2005) Aberrations of TACC1 and TACC3 are associated with ovarian cancer. BMC Womens Health 5: 8.
73. Lauffart B, Gangisetty O, Still IH (2007) Evolutionary conserved interaction of TACC2/TACC3 with BARD1 and BRCA1: potential implications for DNA damage response in breast and ovarian cancer. Cancer Therapy 5: 409–416.
74. Runnebaum IB, Bruning A (2005) Glucocorticoids inhibit cell death in ovarian cancer and up-regulate caspase inhibitor cIAP2. Clin Cancer Res 11: 6325–6332.
75. Ghosh M, Shen Z, Fahey JV, Cu-Uvin S, Mayer K, et al. (2010) Trappin-2/Elafin: a novel innate anti-human immunodeficiency virus-1 molecule of the human female reproductive tract. Immunology 129: 207–219.
76. Roghanian A, Williams SE, Sheldrake TA, Brown TI, Oberheim K, et al. (2006) The antimicrobial/elastase inhibitor elafin regulates lung dendritic cells and adaptive immunity. Am J Respir Cell Mol Biol 34: 634–642.
77. King AE, Wheelhouse N, Cameron S, McDonald SE, Lee KF, et al. (2009) Expression of secretory leukocyte protease inhibitor and elafin in human fallopian tube and in an in-vitro model of Chlamydia trachomatis infection. Hum Reprod 24: 679–686.
78. Stock SJ, Duthie L, Tremaine T, Calder AA, Kelly RW, et al. (2009) Elafin (SKALP/Trappin-2/proteinase inhibitor-3) is produced by the cervix in pregnancy and cervicovaginal levels are diminished in bacterial vaginosis. Reprod Sci 16: 1125–1134.
79. Bingle L, Tetley TD, Bingle CD (2001) Cytokine-mediated induction of the human elafin gene in pulmonary epithelial cells is regulated by nuclear factor-kappaB. Am J Respir Cell Mol Biol 25: 84–91.
80. Henriksen PA, Hitt M, Xing Z, Wang J, Haslett C, et al. (2004) Adenoviral gene delivery of elafin and secretory leukocyte protease inhibitor attenuates NF-kappa B-dependent inflammatory responses of human endothelial cells and macrophages to atherogenic stimuli. J Immunol 172: 4535–4544.

18

The Role of BRCA Status on the Prognosis of Patients with Epithelial Ovarian Cancer

Chaoyang Sun[§], Na Li[§], Dong Ding[§], Danhui Weng, Li Meng, Gang Chen*, Ding Ma*

Department of Obstetrics and Gynaecology, Tongji Hospital, Tongji Medical College, Huazhong University of Science and Technology, Wuhan, Hubei, China

Abstract

Objective: The role of BRCA dysfunction on the prognosis of patients with epithelial ovarian cancer (EOCs) remains controversial. This systematic review tried to assess the role of BRCA dysfunction, including BRCA1/2 germline, somatic mutations, low BRCA1 protein/mRNA expression or BRCA1 promoter methylation, as prognostic factor in EOCs.

Methods: Studies were selected for analysis if they provided an independent assessment of BRCA status and prognosis in EOC. To make it possible to aggregate survival results of the published studies, their methodology was assessed using a modified quality scale.

Results: Of 35 evaluable studies, 23 identified BRCA dysfucntion status as a favourable prognostic factor. No significant differences were detected in the global score of quality assessment. The aggregated hazard ratio (HR) of overall survival (OS) of 34 evaluable studies suggested that BRCA dysfunction status had a favourable impact on OS (HR = 0.69, 95% CI 0.61–0.79), and when these studies were categorised into BRCA1/2 mutation and low protein/mRNA expression of BRCA1 subgroups, all of them demonstrated positive results (HR = 0.67, 95% CI: 0.57–0.78; HR = 0.62, 95% CI: 0.51–0.75; and HR = 0.51, 95% CI: 0.33–0.78, respectively), except for the subgroup of BRCA1 promoter methylation (HR = 1.59, 95% CI: 0.72–3.50). The meta-analysis of progression-free survival (PFS), which included 18 evaluable studies, demonstrated that BRCA dysfunction status was associated with a longer PFS in EOC (HR = 0.69, 95% CI: 0.63–0.76).

Conclusions: Patients with BRCA dysfunction status tend to have a better outcome, but further prospective clinical studies comparing the different BRCA statuses in EOC is urgently needed to specifically define the most effective treatment for the separate patient groups.

Editor: Alexander James Roy Bishop, University of Texas Health Science Center at San Antonio, United States of America

Funding: The authors have no support or funding to report.

Competing Interests: The authors have declared that no competing interests exist.

* E-mail: gumpc@126.com (GC); dma@tjh.tjmu.edu.cn (DM)

§ These authors contributed equally to this work.

Introduction

Epithelial ovarian carcinoma (EOC) is the fifth leading cause of cancer death in women [1], and the five-year relative survival rates for the late stage of EOC were less than 10% between 2004 and 2008 [2]. Despite advances in surgery and the wide use of platinum-based chemotherapy, the long-term outcome remains poor as a result of recurrences and the emergence of drug resistance, necessitating the discovery of biomarkers for predicting which patients will benefit or not benefit from systemic chemotherapy. Moreover, the lack of active therapeutic agents for patients with platinum-resistant cancers impels researchers to discover novel molecular targets helping define subsets of patients who may benefit the most from specific treatment.

In 1996, a detailed case-control analysis reported that BRCA1/2 germline mutations were beneficial prognostic factors for patients with EOC [3]. Since then, many scientists have tried to discover the real association between BRCA1/2 germline mutation status and the prognosis of EOC in subsequent studies, generating conflicting results [3–8]. Although, the mechanism underlying the association between BRCA1/2 germline mutations and survival is not fully understood, *in vitro* experiments have shown that BRCA1/2 deficient cells display a deficiency in repairing double-strand DNA breaks by homologous recombination [9–11]. This biological mechanism may be responsible for increased chemo-sensitivity, which results in a longer progression-free survival (PFS) and overall survival (OS) [12]. More inspiringly, BRCA1/2 mutation carries can obtain an excellent response from targeted therapies, such as the poly (ADP) ribose polymerase (PARP) inhibitor (Olaparib) [13,14]. However, BRCA1/2 germline mutation carriers only account for 10% to 15% of EOCs. Fortunately, recent data suggest that many sporadic EOCs display "BRCAness", or dysfunction of BRCA1/2. Additionally, in sporadic EOCs, low BRCA1 expression detected by immunohistochemistry (IHC) or RT-PCR or BRCA1 promoter methylation had also been reported as a clinically useful tool to provide important information on prognosis [15].

The aim of this study was to assess the role of BRCA dysfunction status, including BRCA1/2 germline/somatic mutations, low BRCA1 protein/mRNA expression or BRCA1 promoter methylation in sporadic EOCs, on prognosis in EOCs by carrying out a systematic review of the literature followed by a meta-analysis, and to estimate to what extent do these BRCA statuses influence patients' prognosis.

Methods

Publication Selection

This study has been registered at the International Prospective Register of Systematic Reviews (PROSPERO, http://www.crd.york.ac.uk/prospero/display_record.asp?ID=CRD42011001747) in 2011. An electronic search of Medline, Embase, and CNKI (China National Knowledge Infrastructure) was used to select articles with the following keywords: 'ovarian neoplasm', 'ovarian tumour', 'ovarian carcinoma', 'ovarian malignance' or 'ovarian cancer' and 'BRCA1', 'BRCA2' or 'BRCA*' and 'prognos*', 'surviv*', 'outcome' or 'marker'. This search strategy was complemented by examining the personal bibliography of the authors. To avoid overlap between patient populations, when authors reported results obtained on the same patient cohorts in several publications, only the most recent report or the most complete one was included in the analysis. The search was updated in September 2013. A study must have been published as a full paper in the English or Chinese language. To be eligible for inclusion, studies had to meet the following criteria: addressed epithelial ovarian cancer and analysed patients' prognosis according to BRCA statuses (assessed BRCA1/2 mutations, assessed BRCA1/2 protein expression through IHC or assessed mRNA level through RT-PCR, and/or assessed BRCA1 promoter methylation in the primary tumour (not in metastatic tissue or in tissue adjacent to the tumour)). The primary outcome was overall survival (OS) and the secondary outcome was progression-free survival (PFS).

Data Extraction and Methodological Assessment

The data retrieved from the reports included authors, years of studies and publications, patients' resources, population size, methods, histology, stage and treatment. To avoid bias in the data abstraction process, three reviewers (Chaoyang Sun, Na Li, Dong Ding) abstracted the data independently and subsequently compared the results. All of the data were checked for internal consistency, and disagreements were resolved by discussion.

To assess methodology, three investigators (Chaoyang Sun, Na Li, Dong Ding) read each publication independently and scored them according to the European Lung Cancer Working Party (ELCWP) scoring scale, with some modification (Method S1 in File S1) [16]. The scores were compared, and a consensus value for each item was reached in meetings attended by at least two investigators. The score evaluates a number of aspects of methodology, which were grouped into four main categories: design, laboratory methods, generalisability of results and the analysis of the study data. Each category had a maximum score of 10 points, giving a theoretical total maximum score of 40 points. The final scores were expressed as percentages ranging from 0 to 100%, with higher values reflecting better methodological quality.

Statistical Methods

A study was considered to be significant if the P-value for the statistical test comparing the survival distributions between the groups of BRCA dysfunction and normal BRCA status was < 0.05. The study was called 'positive' when BRCA dysfunction status was found as a favourable prognostic factor for survival. Other situations were called 'negative', including when a significant survival difference was found, but the group of patients with BRCA dysfunction status fared worse.

Non-parametric tests were used to compare the distribution of the quality scores according to the value of a discrete variable (Mann-Whitney tests).

For the quantitative aggregation of the survival results, we measured the impact of BRCA dysfunction status on prognosis by the hazard ratio (HR) between the survival distributions of the two BRCA status groups. For each study, the HR was extracted or estimated by a method that depended on the results provided in the publication. The most accurate method was to retrieve the HR estimate and its variance from the reported results or to calculate it directly using parameters provided by the authors for univariate analysis: the confidence interval (CI) for the HR, the log-rank statistic, its *P*-value or the O-E statistic (difference between numbers of observed and expected events). If these parameters were not available, we evaluated the total number of events, the number of patients at risk in each group and the log-rank statistic or it's *P*-value, allowing for the calculation of an approximation of the HR estimate. Finally, if the only useful data were in the form of graphical representations of the survival distributions, we extracted survival rates at specified times to reconstruct the HR estimate and its variance, with the assumption that during the study follow-up, the rate of patients censored was constant [17]. If this latter method was used, three independent persons read the curves to reduce imprecision in the reading variations.

If survival was reported separately for particular subgroups, these results were included in the meta-analysis of the corresponding subgroups. The same patients were never considered more than once in each analysis. The individual HR estimates were combined into an overall HR using the method published by Yusuf S and Peto R et al [18]. If the assumption of homogeneity had to be rejected, we used a random-effects model as a second step. By convention, an observed HR <1 implied better survival for the group with BRCA dysfunction status. This impact of BRCA status on survival was considered to be statistically significant if the 95% CI for the overall HR did not include 1.

Horizontal lines indicate the 95% CI, and each box represents the HR point estimate; the box size is proportional to the number of patients included in the study. A funnel plot and Begg's linear regression test were used to investigate any possible publication bias [19].

For all analyses, a two-sided *P* value of <0.05 was considered to be statistically significant. All analyses were performed using SPSS version 13.0 (SPSS, Chicago, IL) and STATA version 10.0 software (Stata Corporation, College Station, TX).

Studies that were eligible for the systematic review were called 'eligible', and those providing data for the meta-analysis were called 'evaluable'.

Results

Study Selection and Characteristics

The primary search yielded a total of 1,231 publications, 1030 of which were excluded by title screening. Abstracts of the remaining 201 papers were reviewed, resulting in 162 being excluded and leaving 39 as candidate articles [3–8,15,20–51]. To reach a final decision on which articles were to be included in the meta-analysis, we examined all 39 papers in detail, which resulted in the further exclusion of 4 papers because survival information was not available for three papers [29,35,46] and one study's [42] subjects overlapped with a subsequent study that the authors published six years later [26] (Figure 1). All eligible articles were reviewed by three independent investigators. The main features of the 39 studies eligible for the systematic review, which were published between 1996 and 2013, are shown in Table S1 in File S1. All of the eligible literatures were case-control studies. A total of 26 studies investigated BRCA1/2 germline and/or somatic mutions, while low BRCA1 protein/mRNA expressions and BRCA1 promoter methylation statuses in sporadic EOCs were studied in nine, two, and two studies, respectively.

As shown in Table 1, 26 studies were performed on BRCA1/2 germline and/or somatic mutions. Twenty-one (21/26, 80.8%) studies investigated the germline BRCA1/2 mutation alone, four (4/26, 15.4%) studies investigated BRCA mutation status including germline and somatic BRCA1/2 mutation together, and the one (1/26, 3.8%) study left investigated BRCA1 dysfunction secondary to germline, somatic BRCA1 mutation or BRCA1 promoter methylation. The detailed information of these 26 studies was listed in Table 1. Eighteen (18/26, 69.2%) papers identified BRCA1/2 mutation as a good prognostic factor for survival, while the remaining eight (8/26, 30.8%) concluded that BRCA1/2 mutation was not a prognostic factor for survival.

Immunohistochemistry (IHC) was used in 9 studies to detect the low expression of BRCA1 protein in sporadic EOCs. The MS110 clone antibody was used in 88.9% (8/9) of the studies. Various experimental procedures were performed with the same cut-off value (<10% positive cells) except for one study [49], and the summary proportion of low expression of BRCA1 (with cut-off value as <10% positive cells) in sporadic ovarian cancer was 55.2% (Table 2).

BRCA1 mRNA expression and BRCA1 promoter methylation in sporadic EOCs were studied in two papers each. Both articles identified the low expression of BRCA1 mRNA as a significantly better predictor of prognosis, while the other two papers on BRCA1 promoter methylation showed negative results (Table 3).

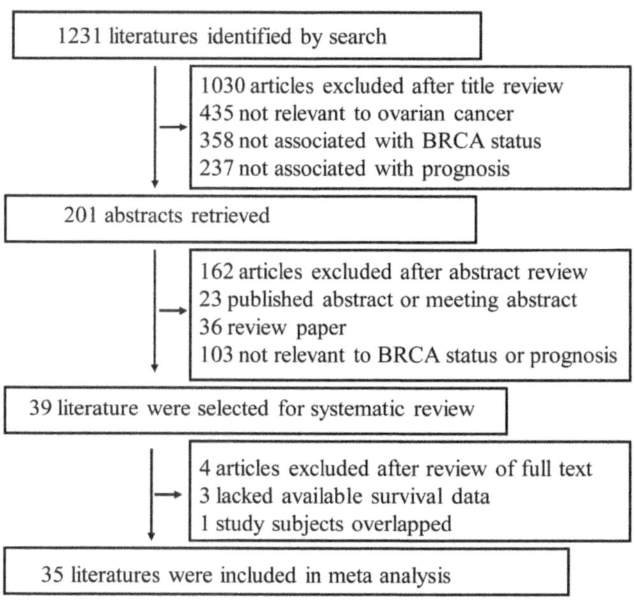

Figure 1. Flow chart of publication selection.

Quality Assessment

Overall, the global quality assessment score, expressed as a percentage, ranged between 36.7% and 89.4%, with a median of 70.6% (Table S2A in File S1, mean ± SD values are shown).

No statistically significant difference of scores were found between the 35 evaluable and 4 non-evaluable studies. There was also no statistically significant difference between the scores of the 26 positive studies and 13 negative studies, except the positive ones had better sub-scores for laboratory methodology ($P = 0.016$). The difference in the global and four subgroup scores between the studies classified according to the types of BRCA dysfunction statuses was not significant.

Table S2B in File S1 shows the scores for the 35 studies classified as evaluable for the meta-analysis. There was no significant difference between significant and not significant studies in the global score, except for the sub-score of generalisability ($P = 0.013$). Moreover, the different types of BRCA dysfunction status did not affect the overall quality assessment or the four subgroup scores.

Meta-analysis of BRCA Status and OS of Ovarian Cancer

The absence of significant qualitative differences between positive and negative trials allowed us to perform a quantitative aggregation of the survival data. Subgroup analysis was performed because the heterogeneity of the trials was obvious: the studies had reported on patients with different BRCA dysfunction statuses (BRCA1/2 germline/somatic mutations, low BRCA1 expression tested by IHC or RT-PCR, and BRCA1 promoter methylation in sporadic EOCs). In this study, we combined studies of germline, somatic BRCA1/2 mutations together as one intervention called the BRCA1/2 mutations in subgroup meta-analysis.

The overall meta-analysis of OS included 34 aggregable studies with 7,986 patients (one studies only provided PFS). The test of overall heterogeneity was significant ($I^2 = 61.7\%$, $P = 0.000$), which primarily came from the BRCA1/2 mutation subgroup ($I^2 = 64.4\%$, $P = 0.000$), while the heterogeneity of the remaining three subgroups (low BRCA1 expression by IHC or RT-PCR and BRCA1 promoter methylation in sporadic EOCs) was not significant. BRCA dysfunction status was associated with a better OS, with HR = 0.69, 95% CI: 0.61–0.79 in random-effects model (HR = 0.72, 95% CI: 0.61–0.79 in fixed-effects model). In the subgroup analyses according to different BRCA statuses, BRCA1/2 mutations (1,686 cases and 4,941 controls) and low BRCA1 expression by IHC (500 cases and 362 controls) or RT-PCR (72 cases and 49 controls) were statistically significantly better prognostic factors for survival (HR = 0.69, 95% CI: 0.59–0.80; HR = 0.62, 95% CI: 0.51–0.75; and HR = 0.51, 95% CI: 0.33–0.78 in the random-effects model, respectively; and HR = 0.72, 95% CI: 0.67–0.78; HR = 0.62, 95% CI: 0.51–0.75; and HR = 0.51, 95% CI: 0.33–0.78 in the fixed-effects model, respectively). However, BRCA1 promoter methylation (62 cases and 196 controls) was not associated with better prognosis (HR = 1.59, 95% CI: 0.72–3.50 in the random-effects model and HR = 1.40, 95% CI: 0.94–2.09 in the fixed-effects model) (Figure 2).

When BRCA mutation was subdivided into BRCA1 or BRCA2 subgroups, the meta-analysis showed that both BRCA1 and BRCA2 mutations predicted better OS (HR = 0.78, 95% CI: 0.69–0.87 and HR = 0.65, 95% CI: 0.50–0.86 in a fixed and random-effects model, respectively) (Figure 3A, 3B).

Meta-analysis of BRCA Status and PFS of Ovarian Cancer

The overall meta-analysis of PFS included 18 evaluable studies with 3,394 patients. The overall heterogeneity and the heteroge-

Table 1. Characteristics of studies of patients with BRCA1/2 mutated ovarian cancer.

First author	Study year, published year	Country	Histology	Stage	No. of cases/ controls	Laboratory methods	BRCA status	Germline/ somatic	Mutation Types	Treatment	Survival result
Aida	1984–1996,1998	Japan	se	I–III	13/29	SCCP,PCR,seq	BRCA1	Germ	Deleterious	2	positive
Alsop	2002–2006,2012	Austrilia	se	I–IV	118/536	PCR,seq, MLPA	BRCA1/2	Germ	Deleterious	2	positive
Artioli	,2010	Italian	all	I–IV	48/40	PCR,seq	BRCA1/2	Germ	Deleterious	1+2	positive
Boyd	1986–1998,2000	U.S.A	all	I–IV	88/100	PCR,seq	BRCA1/2	Germ	Deleterious	2	positive
Brozek	1995–2004,2008	Poland	se+CCC	I–IV	21/130	DHPLC,RFLP,seq	BRCA1/2	Germ	Deleterious+ VUS	2	positive
Buller	1990–2000,2002	U.S.A	all	I–IV	59/59	PTT,SSCP,seq	BRCA1	Mixed	Deleterious+ VUS	2	negative
Cass	1990–2001,2003	U.S.A	all	III–IV	29/25	SSCR,seq	BRCA1/2	Germ	Deleterious	2	positive
Chetrit	1994–1999,2008	Israel	all	I–IV	213/392	PCR,seq	BRCA1/2	Germ	Deleterious	2	positive
David	1994–1999,2002	Israel	all	I–IV	229/549	SCCP,seq	BRCA1/2	Germ+Somatic	Deleterious	2	positive
Dann	1999–2007,2012	U.S.A	all	II–IV	15/38	PCR,seq	BRCA1/2	Germ+Somatic	Deleterious	2	negative
Gallagher	1996–2006,2011	U.S.A	all	III–IV	36/74	PCR,seq	BRCA1/2	Germ	Deleterious	2	positive
Hennessy	1990–2006.2010	U.S.A	all	I–IV	43/192	PCR,seq	BRCA1/2	Germ+Somatic	Deleterious	2	positive
Hyman	2001–2010,2012	U.S.A	se	III–IV	69/298	PCR,seq	BRCA1/2	Germ	Deleterious	2	positive
Johannsson	1958–1995,1998	Swedish	all	I–IV	38/97	PTT,SSCP,seq	BRCA1	Germ	Deleterious	2+3	negative
Lacour	1996–2007,2011	U.S.A	all	III–IV	95/183	PCR,seq	BRCA1/2	Germ	Deleterious	–	positive
Majdak	1997–2002,2005	Poland	se+Mu	I–IV	18/171	F-CSGE,seq	BRCA1	Germ	Deleterious	2	positive
McLaughlin	1995–1995,2002–2004,2012	Canada	all	I–IV	218/1408	PTT, seq,DGGE, DHPLC	BRCA1/2	Germ	Deleterious	2	negative
Pal	2000–2003,2007	West central Florida	all	III–IV	32/177	PCR,seq	BRCA1/2	Germ	Deleterious+ VUS	–	negative
Pharoah	,1999	U.K	all	I–IV	151/119	PTT,SSCP	BRCA1/2	Germ	Deleterious	–	negative
Ramus	1992–1997,2001	Israel	all	I–IV	27/71	SSCP,PCR,seq	BRCA1/2	Germ	Deleterious	–	negative
Rubin	,1996	U.S.A	all	III–IV	43/43	SSCP,PCR,seq	BRCA1	Germ	Deleterious+ VUS	–	positive
Tan	1991–2006,2008	U.K	all	III–IV	22/44	SCCP,seq	BRCA1/2	Germ	Deleterious+ VUS	2	positive
Vencken	1980–2009,2011	Netherlands	all	I–IV	112/222	PCR,seq	BRCA1/2	Germ	unknown	2	positive
Yang	,2011	multi-country	all	III–IV	59/251	exom seq	BRCA1/2	Germ+Somatic	Deleterious+ VUS	2	positive
Zweemer	,1999	Netherlands	–	–	42/84	PTT,PCR	BRCA1/2	Germ	Deleterious	–	positive
Zweemer	,2001	Netherlands	All	I–IV	23/17	PTT,PCR,seq	BRCA1/2	Germ	Deleterious	–	negative

Histology: pathological histology of ovarian cancer, se = serous ovarian cancer, CCC = clear cell cancer of, Mu = mucinous ovarian cancer. all = almost all of the epithelial ovarian cancer types, including serous, mucinous, clear cell cancer, etc.
Laboratory methods: laboratory methods used to detect BRCA1/2 mutation, PTT = Protein truncation test, SSCP = Single-Strand Conformation Polymorphism, seq = sequencing, DGGE = fluorescent multiplex denaturing gradient gel electrophoresis, MLPA = multiplex ligation-dependent probe amplification, DHPLC = Denaturing high performance liquid chromatography, RFLP = Restriction fragment length polymorphisms, F-CSGE = Fluorescence-based Conformation Sensitive Gel Electrophoresis.
Germline/somatic: Germ = germline mutation, Mixed = BRCA1 germline/somatic mutation or BRCA1 promoter methylation.
Mutation types: VUS = variants of unknown significance.
Treatment: chemotherapy used, 1 = only Platinum was used, 2 = Platinum-based chemotherapy, 3 = other agents without Platinum, like Paclitaxel, etc.

Table 2. Characteristics of studies of patients of ovarian cancer with low BRCA1 expression measured by IHC.

First author	Study year, published year	Country	stage	Histology	No. of cases/ controls	Clone	dilution	Retrieval	readers	Double blind	Cut off	Low%	treatment	Survival result
Weberpals	2008,2011	Canada	II–IV	all	75/41	MS110	1:100	–	2	Yes	10%	65%	1	positive
Carser	1998–2004,2011	U.K	I–IV	all	120/172	MS110	–	steam heat	2	Yes	10%	41%	1	positive
Gan	1991–2007,2013	U.K	I–IV	se	112/19	MS110	1:80	microwave	1	Yes	≤70*	84.4%	2	positive
Kaern	1990–1992,2005	Norway	III	all	30/16	MS110	1:200	microwave		No	10%	65.20%	2	negative
Sirisabya	1996–1999,2007	Thailand	I–III	all	87/12	–	–	microwave	1	No	10%	87.80%	1	negative
Thrall	,2006	U.S.A	I–III	all	97/55	MS110	1:50	steam heat	2	Yes	10%	63.8%	1	positive
Swisher	,2009	U.S.A	I–IV	all	39/76	MS110	1:250	steam heat		No	10%	34%	2	positive
Radosa	2000–2005,2011	Germany	III–IV	all	12/15	MS110	1:200	heat	2	Yes	10%	44.40%	1	positive
Yu	1996–1998,2005	China	I–IV	all	35/15	MS110	1:100	–		–	10%	70%	2	negative

Histology: pathological histology of ovarian cancer, all = almost all of the epithelial ovarian cancer types, including serous, mucinous, clear cell cancer, etc, se = serous ovarian cancer.
Treatment: chemotherapy used, 1 = only Platinum was used, 2 = Platinum-based chemotherapy.
*BRCA1 (H-score≤70) defined as the BRCA1-deficient group.

Table 3. Characteristics of studies of patients of ovarian cancer with low BRCA1 mRNA expression or BRCA1 promoter methylation.

	First author	Study year, published year	Country	Histology	stage	No. of cases/controls	Methods of methylation detecting	Treatment	significance
RT-PCR	Quinn	,2007	U.K	all	I–IV	47/23		2	positive
	Weberpals	1997–2005,2009	Canada	all	II–IV	25/26		2	positive
methylation	Wiley	1991–2000,2006	Italy	all	I–IV	44/171	MSP	2	negative
	Chiang	1986–2001,2006	USA	–	I–IV	10/25	MSRE+ Southern blot+ MSP	2	negative

Histology: pathological histology of ovarian cancer, all = almost all of the epithelial ovarian cancer types, including serous, mucinous, clear cell cancer, etc.
Methods of methylation detecting: methods of methylation detecting, MSP = methylation-specific polymerase chain reaction (PCR) analysis, MSRE = methylation-sensitive restriction enzyme digestion.
Treatment: chemotherapy used, 2 = Platinum-based chemotherapy.

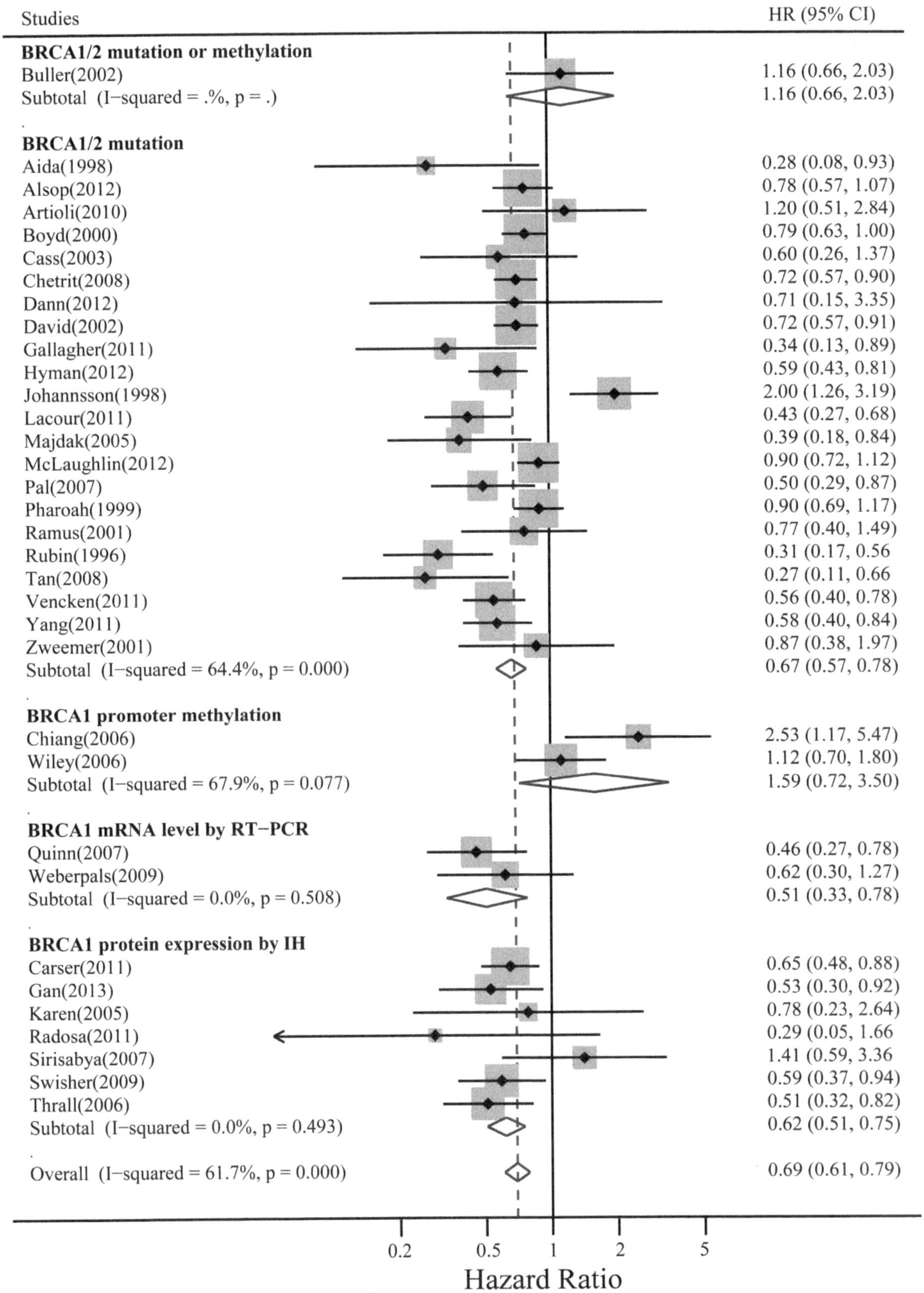

Figure 2. Summary hazard ratios (HRs) and 95% confidence intervals (CIs) of epithelial ovarian cancer OS for BRCA dysfunction status. Horizontal lines represent 95% CIs; diamonds represent summary estimates with corresponding 95% CIs. Test for heterogeneity: $P = .000$, $I^2 = 61.7\%$. A random-effects model was used for analysis.

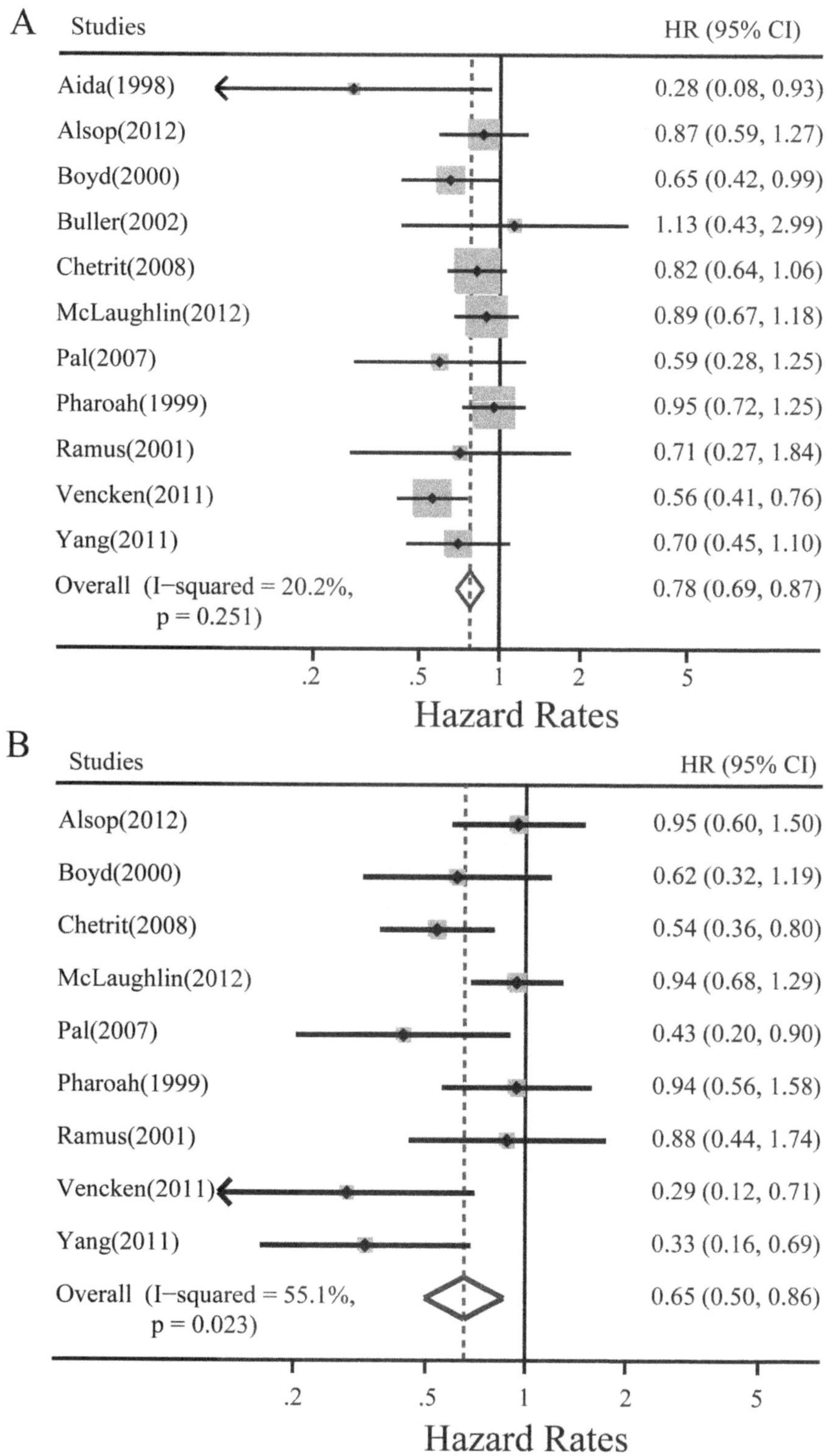

Figure 3. Subgroup meta-analysis of summary hazard ratios (HRs) and 95% confidence intervals (CIs) of ovarian cancer OS for different BRCA mutation statuses. A: BRCA1 mutation. **B:** BRCA2 mutation. Horizontal lines represent 95% CIs; diamonds represent summary estimates with corresponding 95% CIs. Test for heterogeneity: **A:** $P=.251$, $I^2=20.2\%$, a fixed-effects model was used; **B:** $P=.023$, $I^2=55.1\%$, a random-effects model was used.

neity of all subgroups were not significant. BRCA dysfunction status was associated with a better PFS in ovarian cancer, with HR = 0.69 (95% CI: 0.63–0.76, fixed-effect model). In the subgroup analyses according to different BRCA statuses, BRCA1/2 mutation and low BRCA1 expression by IHC were statistically significant predictors for longer PFS (HR = 0.65, 95%

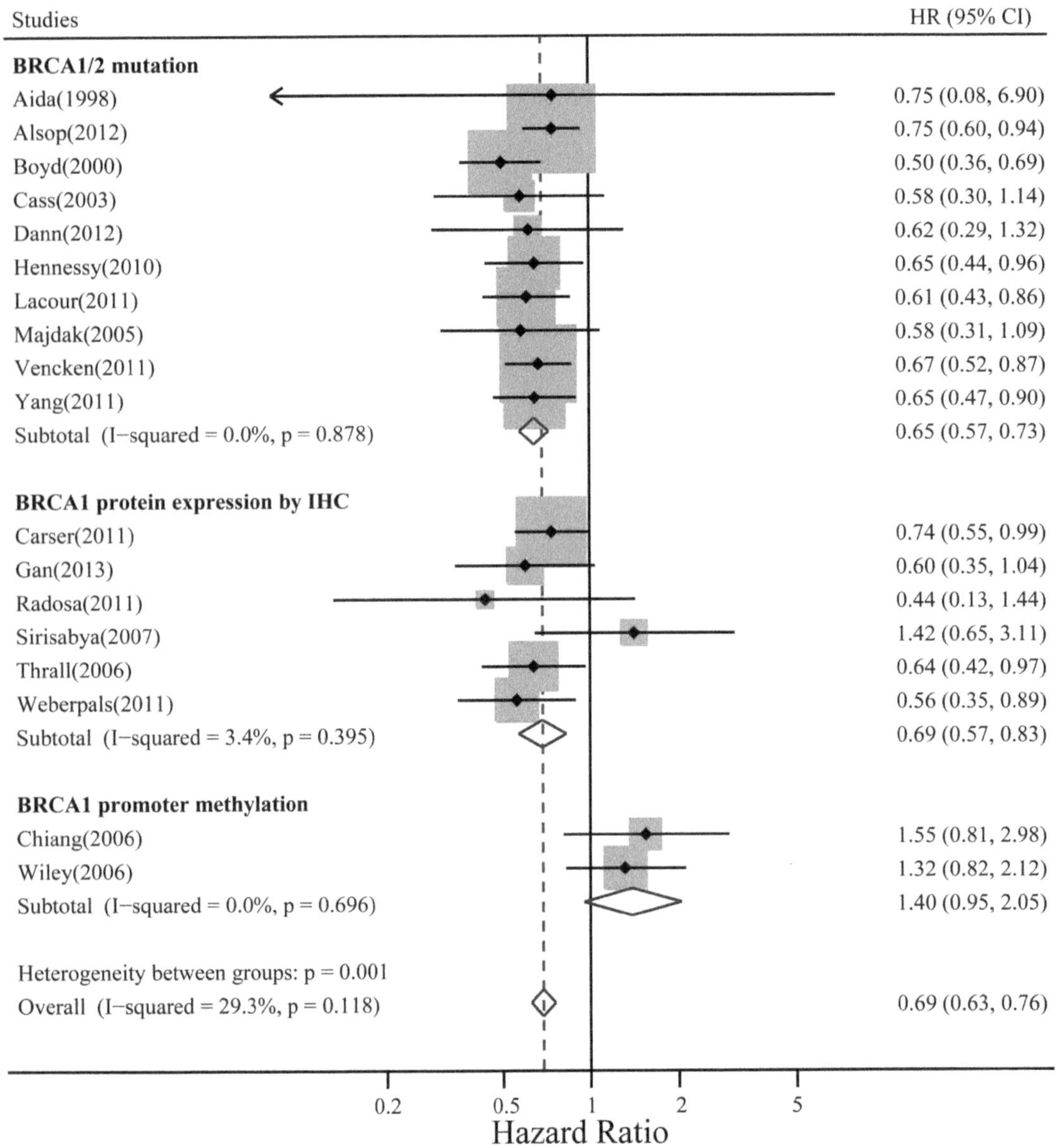

Figure 4. Summary hazard ratios (HRs) and 95% confidence intervals (CIs) of ovarian cancer PFS for BRCA dysfunction status. Horizontal lines represent 95% CIs; diamonds represent summary estimates with corresponding 95% CIs. Test for heterogeneity: $P = .118$, $I^2 = 29.3\%$. A fixed-effects model was used.

CI: 0.57–0.73 and HR = 0.69, 95% CI: 0.57–0.83 in a fixed-effect model, respectively). However, BRCA1 promoter methylation was not associated with better PFS (HR = 1.40, 95% CI: 0.95–2.05) (Figure 4).

Publication Bias

Publication bias statistics were determined using Begg's linear regression test. No publication bias was found for the studies used for the meta-analysis for overall survival (Begg's test, $P = 0.221$) (Figure 5A); moreover, there is no publication bias was found for the studies used for the meta-analysis for PFS (Begg's test, $P = 0.880$) (Figure 5B).

Discussion

Our systematic review of the literature and meta-analysis demonstrate an improved prognosis in patients whose EOC display BRCA1/2 dysfunction, relative to those whose EOC display normal BRCA1/2 function. Although the comparison of prognostic benefit between BRCA1 and BRCA2 mutation was not feasible, the aggregated HRs indicated that patients with a BRCA2 mutation (HR = 0.65) may have a better prognosis than patients with a BRCA1 mutation (HR = 0.78). During the preparation of this manuscript, Bolton et al also reported BRCA1/2 germline mutation was associated with improved survival and BRCA2 carriers had the best prognosis, these findings are consistent with our results [52].

Although BRCA1/2 germline mutation carriers only account for small proportions of EOCs, fortunately, it has been estimated that approximately 50% sporadic EOCs show dysfunction of BRCA1/2 through different mechanisms. Our study is the first meta-analysis, to our knowledge, to assess if low BRCA1/2 expression status of sporadic EOCs could show similar effects on

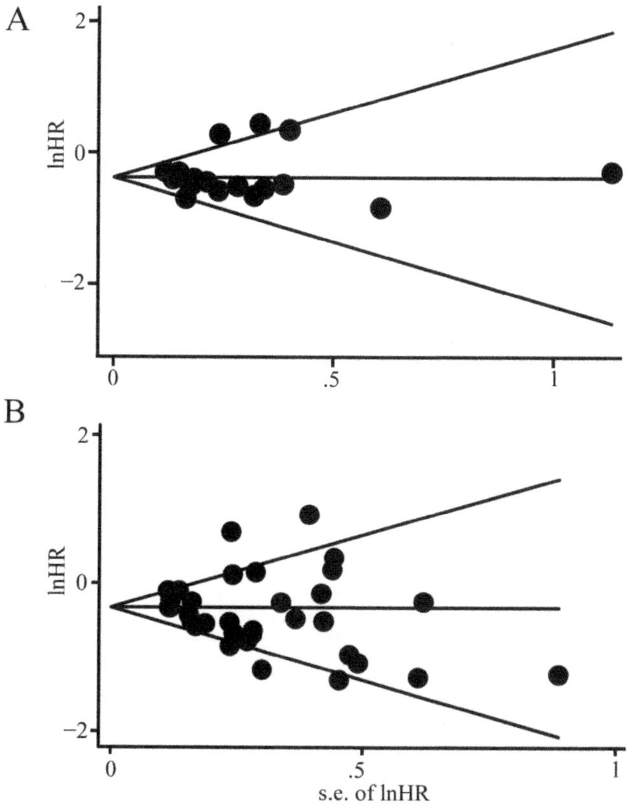

Figure 5. Begg's funnel plots of the natural logarithm of the hazard ratios (HRs) and the SE of the natural logarithm of the HRs for all of the included studies reported with OS and PFS. A: Begg's funnel plots for all of the included studies reported with OS, the dashed line represents 95% confidence intervals (CIs). Circles represent individual studies. Begg's test: $P = 0.221$. B: Begg's funnel plots for all of the included studies reported with PFS, the dashed line represents 95% confidence intervals (CIs). Circles represent individual studies. Begg's test: $P = 0.880$.

prognosis to BRCA1/2 mutation carriers. Our results showed that low BRCA1 expression measured by IHC or RT-PCR but not BRCA1 promoter methylation is a good prognostic factor for both OS and PFS in patients of sporadic EOCs, indicating that low BRCA1 expression status in sporadic EOCs show similar clinical effects on prognosis to germline mutations carriers. However, it is still difficult to draw a definite conclusion because these results were based on small numbers and require confirmation in larger studies, especially for low BRCA1 expression measured by RT-PCR and BRCA1 promoter methylation status. Swisher et al had stated that BRCA1 promoter methylation only occurs in a small proportion of sporadic ovarian cancer with low BRCA1 expression [33], therefore, other mechanisms that could cause low BRCA1 expression need to be further investigated.

In our study, patients whose EOC displays BRCA dysfunction had a favourable prognosis. BRCA1/2 gene products play a pivotal role in DNA repair mechanisms. The better prognosis of patients with BRCA dysfunction may be explained by their inability to repair double-strand DNA breaks caused by platinum-based chemotherapy. As we mentioned above, although the comparison of prognostic benefit between the BRCA1 and BRCA2 mutation was not feasible, the aggregated HR for OS for BRCA2 mutants was lower than that for BRCA1 mutants. It has been established by several research groups that BRCA2-mutated cells are recombination deficient and undergo significantly reduced homologous recombination repair of DNA double-strand breaks [13,53]. Functionally, the primary function of BRCA2 appears to be regulation of the RAD51 protein, which is required for double-strand break repair by homologous recombination [10], indicating that BRCA2 lesions cause more substantial homologous recombination defects than BRCA1 lesions, because BRCA1 is more versatile. However, to date, there are no reports regarding the association between low BRCA2 expression and the prognosis of patients with sporadic EOCs. So, large population-based studies are urgently needed to discover the proportion of low BRCA2 expression patients among sporadic EOCs and the real role of low BRCA2 expression status on survival.

Our results may have important implications for the clinical management of EOCs. Ovarian carcinoma is clinically highly heterogeneous. Our study revealed that both BRCA1/2 mutations and low BRCA1 expression are associated with favourable survival in EOC, so, these BRCA statuses can guide choice of post-operative treatment decisions. Additionally, it has been demonstrated that a deficiency of the BRCA gene confers substantial sensitivity to a new class of agents, namely poly-ADP-ribose polymerase-1 (PARP1) inhibitors [13,14]. A number of phase I and II studies have reported the successful applications of PARP inhibitors in BRCA1/2 mutation carries of ovarian and breast cancer, and phase III studies are underway [13,14,54]. So, routine testing BRCA1/2 germline mutation status of EOCs may now be warranted. A large proportion of sporadic EOCs demonstrate BRCA deficiency, whether these patients could also benefit from PARP1 inhibitor are still unclear. Moreover, a reliable assay to detect these patients is required. Our meta-analysis supports the IHC technique as a promising assay to detect a portion of sporadic ovarian cancer displaying BRCAness. Although RT-PCR may also be a potential assay to discover the BRCAness, the supporting positive literature was limited and without standard experimental protocols and uniform cut-off values. Large prospective clinical trials are expected for further validation.

In conclusion, EOCs patients with BRCA dysfunction status have better outcomes, but more fundamental studies and further prospective clinical studies are urgently needed. Furthermore, EOCs should be stratified by different BRCA statuses to specifically define the most effective treatment for the separate patient groups in further clinical studies.

Supporting Information

File S1 Contains the following files: **Method S1:** The quality score for methodology modified according to the European Lung Cancer Working Party (ELCWP) scoring scale [1]. **Table S1:** Main characteristics and results of eligible studies. **Table S2:** Methodological assessment.

Author Contributions

Conceived and designed the experiments: GC DM. Performed the experiments: NL. Analyzed the data: CYS DHW. Contributed reagents/materials/analysis tools: DD LM. Wrote the paper: CYS.

References

1. Jemal A, Siegel R, Xu J, Ward E (2010) Cancer statistics, 2010. CA Cancer J Clin 60: 277–300.
2. (2011) Ovarian cancer, five-year stage-specific relative survival rates (2004–2008). J Natl Cancer Inst 103: 1287.
3. Rubin SC, Benjamin I, Behbakht K, Takahashi H, Morgan MA, et al. (1996) Clinical and pathological features of ovarian cancer in women with germ- line mutations of BRCA1. New England Journal of Medicine 335: 1413–1416.
4. Gallagher DJ, Konner JA, Bell-McGuinn KM, Bhatia J, Sabbatini P, et al. (2011) Survival in epithelial ovarian cancer: a multivariate analysis incorporating BRCA mutation status and platinum sensitivity. Ann Oncol 22: 1127–1132.
5. Vencken PM, Kriege M, Hoogwerf D, Beugelink S, van der Burg ME, et al. (2011) Chemosensitivity and outcome of BRCA1- and BRCA2-associated ovarian cancer patients after first-line chemotherapy compared with sporadic ovarian cancer patients. Ann Oncol 22: 1346–1352.
6. Johannsson OT, Ranstam J, Borg A, Olsson H (1998) Survival of BRCA1 breast and ovarian cancer patients: a population-based study from southern Sweden. J Clin Oncol 16: 397–404.
7. Tan DS, Rothermundt C, Thomas K, Bancroft E, Eeles R, et al. (2008) "BRCAness" syndrome in ovarian cancer: a case-control study describing the clinical features and outcome of patients with epithelial ovarian cancer associated with BRCA1 and BRCA2 mutations. J Clin Oncol 26: 5530–5536.
8. Yang D, Khan S, Sun Y, Hess K, Shmulevich I, et al. (2011) Association of BRCA1 and BRCA2 mutations with survival, chemotherapy sensitivity, and gene mutator phenotype in patients with ovarian cancer. JAMA 306: 1557–1565.
9. Bhattacharyya A, Ear US, Koller BH, Weichselbaum RR, Bishop DK (2000) The breast cancer susceptibility gene BRCA1 is required for subnuclear assembly of Rad51 and survival following treatment with the DNA cross-linking agent cisplatin. J Biol Chem 275: 23899–23903.
10. Davies AA, Masson JY, McIlwraith MJ, Stasiak AZ, Stasiak A, et al. (2001) Role of BRCA2 in control of the RAD51 recombination and DNA repair protein. Mol Cell 7: 273–282.
11. Kowalczykowski SC (2002) Molecular mimicry connects BRCA2 to Rad51 and recombinational DNA repair. Nat Struct Biol 9: 897–899.
12. Cooke SL, Brenton JD (2011) Evolution of platinum resistance in high-grade serous ovarian cancer. Lancet Oncol 12: 1169–1174.
13. Audeh MW, Carmichael J, Penson RT, Friedlander M, Powell B, et al. (2010) Oral poly(ADP-ribose) polymerase inhibitor olaparib in patients with BRCA1 or BRCA2 mutations and recurrent ovarian cancer: a proof-of-concept trial. Lancet 376: 245–251.
14. Fong PC, Boss DS, Yap TA, Tutt A, Wu P, et al. (2009) Inhibition of poly(ADP-ribose) polymerase in tumors from BRCA mutation carriers. N Engl J Med 361: 123–134.
15. Weberpals JI, Tu D, Squire JA, Amin MS, Islam S, et al. (2011) Breast cancer 1 (BRCA1) protein expression as a prognostic marker in sporadic epithelial ovarian carcinoma: an NCIC CTG OV.16 correlative study. Ann Oncol.
16. Steels E, Paesmans M, Berghmans T, Branle F, Lemaitre F, et al. (2001) Role of p53 as a prognostic factor for survival in lung cancer: a systematic review of the literature with a meta-analysis. Eur Respir J 18: 705–719.
17. Parmar MK, Torri V, Stewart L (1998) Extracting summary statistics to perform meta-analyses of the published literature for survival endpoints. Stat Med 17: 2815–2834.
18. Yusuf S, Peto R, Lewis J, Collins R, Sleight P (1985) Beta blockade during and after myocardial infarction: an overview of the randomized trials. Prog Cardiovasc Dis 27: 335–371.
19. Sterne JA, Egger M (2001) Funnel plots for detecting bias in meta-analysis: guidelines on choice of axis. J Clin Epidemiol 54: 1046–1055.
20. Carser JE, Quinn JE, Michie CO, O'Brien EJ, McCluggage WG, et al. (2011) BRCA1 is both a prognostic and predictive biomarker of response to chemotherapy in sporadic epithelial ovarian cancer. Gynecol Oncol.
21. Kaern J, Aghmesheh M, Nesland JM, Danielsen HE, Sandstad B, et al. (2005) Prognostic factors in ovarian carcinoma stage III patients. Can biomarkers improve the prediction of short- and long-term survivors? International Journal of Gynecological Cancer 15: 1014–1022.
22. Buller RE, Shahin MS, Geisler JP, Zogg M, De Young BR, et al. (2002) Failure of BRCA1 dysfunction to alter ovarian cancer survival. Clinical Cancer Research 8: 1196–1202.
23. Boyd J, Sonoda Y, Federici MG, Bogomolniy F, Rhei E, et al. (2000) Clinicopatholic features of BRCA-linked and sporadic ovarian cancer. Journal of the American Medical Association 283: 2260–2265.
24. Aida H, Takakuwa K, Nagata H, Tsuneki I, Takano M, et al. (1998) Clinical features of ovarian cancer in Japanese women with germ-line mutations of BRCA1. Clinical Cancer Research 4: 235–240.
25. Cass I, Baldwin RL, Varkey T, Moslehi R, Narod SA, et al. (2003) Improved survival in women with BRCA-associated ovarian carcinoma. Cancer 97: 2187–2195.
26. Chetrit A, Hirsh-Yechezkel G, Ben-David Y, Lubin F, Friedman E, et al. (2008) Effect of BRCA1/2 mutations on long-term survival of patients with invasive ovarian cancer: The National Israeli Study of Ovarian Cancer. Journal of Clinical Oncology 26: 20–25.
27. Wiley A, Katsaros D, Chen H, Rigault de la Longrais IA, Beeghly A, et al. (2006) Aberrant promoter methylation of multiple genes in malignant ovarian tumors and in ovarian tumors with low malignant potential. Cancer 107: 299–308.
28. Weberpals J, Garbuio K, O'Brien A, Clark-Knowles K, Doucette S, et al. (2009) The DNA repair proteins BRCA1 and ERCC1 as predictive markers in sporadic ovarian cancer. Int J Cancer 124: 806–815.
29. Zweemer RP, Verheijen RH, Menko FH, Gille JJ, van Diest PJ, et al. (1999) Differences between hereditary and sporadic ovarian cancer. Eur J Obstet Gynecol Reprod Biol 82: 151–153.
30. Chiang JW, Karlan BY, Cass l, Baldwin RL (2006) BRCA1 promoter methylation predicts adverse ovarian cancer prognosis. Gynecologic Oncology 101: 403–410.
31. Quinn JE, James CR, Stewart GE, Mulligan JM, White P, et al. (2007) BRCA1 mRNA expression levels predict for overall survival in ovarian cancer after chemotherapy. Clin Cancer Res 13: 7413–7420.
32. Thrall M, Gallion HH, Kryscio R, Kapali M, Armstrong DK, et al. (2006) BRCA1 expression in a large series of sporadic ovarian carcinomas: a Gynecologic Oncology Group study. Int J Gynecol Cancer 16 Suppl 1: 166–171.
33. Swisher EM, Gonzalez RM, Taniguchi T, Garcia RL, Walsh T, et al. (2009) Methylation and protein expression of DNA repair genes: association with chemotherapy exposure and survival in sporadic ovarian and peritoneal carcinomas. Mol Cancer 8: 48.
34. Pharoah PD, Easton DF, Stockton DL, Gayther S, Ponder BA (1999) Survival in familial, BRCA1-associated, and BRCA2-associated epithelial ovarian cancer. United Kingdom Coordinating Committee for Cancer Research (UKCCCR) Familial Ovarian Cancer Study Group. Cancer Res 59: 868–871.
35. Brozek I, Ochman K, Debniak J, Morzuch L, Ratajska M, et al. (2008) High frequency of BRCA1/2 germline mutations in consecutive ovarian cancer patients in Poland. Gynecologic Oncology 108: 433–437.
36. Zweemer RP, Verheijen RH, Coebergh JW, Jacobs IJ, van Diest PJ, et al. (2001) Survival analysis in familial ovarian cancer, a case control study. European journal of obstetrics, gynecology, and reproductive biology 98: 219–223.
37. Ramus SJ, Fishman A, Pharoah PD, Yarkoni S, Altaras M, et al. (2001) Ovarian cancer survival in Ashkenazi Jewish patients with BRCA1 and BRCA2 mutations. Eur J Surg Oncol 27: 278–281.
38. Radosa MP, Hafner N, Camara O, Diebolder H, Mothes A, et al. (2011) Loss of BRCA1 Protein Expression as Indicator of the BRCAness Phenotype Is Associated With Favorable Overall Survival After Complete Resection of Sporadic Ovarian Cancer. Int J Gynecol Cancer.
39. Artioli G, Borgato L, Cappetta A, Wabersich J, Mocellin S, et al. (2010) Overall survival in BRCA-associated ovarian cancer: Case-control study of an Italian series. European Journal of Gynaecological Oncology 31: 658–661.
40. Lacour RA, Westin SN, Meyer LA, Wingo SN, Schorge JO, et al. (2011) Improved survival in non-Ashkenazi Jewish ovarian cancer patients with BRCA1 and BRCA2 gene mutations. Gynecologic Oncology 121: 358–363.
41. Majdak EJ, Debniak J, Milczek T, Cornelisse CJ, Devilee P, et al. (2005) Prognostic impact of BRCA1 pathogenic and BRCA1/BRCA2 unclassified variant mutations in patients with ovarian carcinoma. Cancer 104: 1004–1012.
42. David YB, Chetrit A, Hirsh-Yechezkel G, Friedman E, Beck BD, et al. (2002) Effect of BRCA mutations on the length of survival in epithelial ovarian tumors. Journal of Clinical Oncology 20: 463–466.
43. Hennessy BTJ, Timms KM, Carey MS, Gutin A, Meyer LA, et al. (2010) Somatic mutations in BRCA1 and BRCA2 could expand the number of patients that benefit from poly (ADP ribose) polymerase inhibitors in ovarian cancer. Journal of Clinical Oncology 28: 3570–3576.
44. Pal T, Permuth-Wey J, Kapoor R, Cantor A, Sutphen R (2007) Improved survival in BRCA2 carriers with ovarian cancer. Familial Cancer 6: 113–119.
45. Sirisabya N, Manchana T, Termrungreunglert W, Triratanachat S, Charuruks N, et al. (2007) Prevalence of BRCA1 expression in epithelial ovarian cancer: Immunohistochemical study. Journal of the Medical Association of Thailand 90: 9–14.
46. Yu M, Hao J, Jiao Z (2005) A study on the expression of BRCA1 & P53 and their correlation in epithelial ovarian cancer. Chinese Journal of Clinical Oncology 32: 18–20.
47. Alsop K, Fereday S, Meldrum C, deFazio A, Emmanuel C, et al. (2012) BRCA mutation frequency and patterns of treatment response in BRCA mutation-positive women with ovarian cancer: a report from the Australian Ovarian Cancer Study Group. J Clin Oncol 30: 2654–2663.
48. Dann RB, DeLoia JA, Timms KM, Zorn KK, Potter J, et al. (2012) BRCA1/2 mutations and expression: response to platinum chemotherapy in patients with advanced stage epithelial ovarian cancer. Gynecol Oncol 125: 677–682.
49. Gan A, Green AR, Nolan CC, Martin S, Deen S (2013) Poly(adenosine diphosphate-ribose) polymerase expression in BRCA-proficient ovarian high-grade serous carcinoma; association with patient survival. Hum Pathol 44: 1638–1647.
50. Hyman DM, Long KC, Tanner EJ, Grisham RN, Arnold AG, et al. (2012) Outcomes of primary surgical cytoreduction in patients with BRCA-associated high-grade serous ovarian carcinoma. Gynecol Oncol 126: 224–228.

51. McLaughlin JR, Rosen B, Moody J, Pal T, Fan I, et al. (2013) Long-term ovarian cancer survival associated with mutation in BRCA1 or BRCA2. J Natl Cancer Inst 105: 141–148.
52. Bolton KL, Chenevix-Trench G, Goh C, Sadetzki S, Ramus SJ, et al. (2012) Association between BRCA1 and BRCA2 mutations and survival in women with invasive epithelial ovarian cancer. JAMA 307: 382–390.
53. Kortmann U, McAlpine JN, Xue H, Guan J, Ha G, et al. (2011) Tumor growth inhibition by olaparib in BRCA2 germline-mutated patient-derived ovarian cancer tissue xenografts. Clin Cancer Res 17: 783–791.
54. Kummar S, Chen A, Ji J, Zhang Y, Reid JM, et al. (2011) Phase I study of PARP inhibitor ABT-888 in combination with topotecan in adults with refractory solid tumors and lymphomas. Cancer Res 71: 5626–5634.

19

Evolution of Pre-Existing versus Acquired Resistance to Platinum Drugs and PARP Inhibitors in BRCA-Associated Cancers

Kimiyo N. Yamamoto[1,2,5], Kouji Hirota[3], Shunichi Takeda[4], Hiroshi Haeno[5]*

1 Department of Information and Computer Sciences, Nara Women's University, Nara, Japan, **2** Japan Society for the Promotion of Science, Tokyo, Japan, **3** Department of Chemistry, Tokyo Metropolitan University, Tokyo, Japan, **4** Department of Radiation Genetics, Graduate School of Medicine, Kyoto University, Kyoto, Japan, **5** Department of Biology, Kyushu University, Fukuoka, Japan

Abstract

Platinum drugs and PARP inhibitors ("PARPis") are considered to be effective in BRCA-associated cancers with impaired DNA repair. These agents cause stalled and collapsed replication forks and create double-strand breaks effectively in the absence of repair mechanisms, resulting in arrest of the cell cycle and induction of cell death. However, recent studies have shown failure of these chemotherapeutic agents due to emerging drug resistance. In this study, we developed a stochastic model of BRCA-associated cancer progression in which there are four cancer populations: those with (i) functional BRCA, (ii) dysfunctional BRCA, (iii) functional BRCA and a growth advantage, and (iv) dysfunctional BRCA and a growth advantage. These four cancer populations expand from one cancer cell with normal repair function until the total cell number reaches a detectable amount. We derived formulas for the probability and expected numbers of each population at the time of detection. Furthermore, we extended the model to consider the tumor dynamics during treatment. Results from the model were validated and showed good agreement with clinical and experimental evidence in BRCA-associated cancers. Based on the model, we investigated conditions in which drug resistance during the treatment course originated from either a pre-existing drug-resistant population or a *de novo* population, due to secondary mutations. Finally, we found that platinum drugs and PARPis were effective if (i) BRCA inactivation is present, (ii) the cancer was diagnosed early, and (iii) tumor growth is rapid. Our results indicate that different types of cancers have a preferential way of acquiring resistance to platinum drugs and PARPis according to their growth and mutational characteristics.

Editor: Peiwen Fei, University of Hawaii Cancer Center, United States of America

Funding: This research was supported by the Aihara Innovative Mathematical Modelling Project, the Japan Society for the Promotion of Science (JSPS) through the "Funding Program for World-Leading Innovative R&D on Science and Technology (FIRST Program)," initiated by the Council for Science and Technology Policy (CSTP) (HH), Grant in Aid for Scientific Research on Innovative Areas "Stem Cell Aging and Disease" from Ministry of Education, Culture, Sports, Science and Technology of Japan (No. 26115006) (HH), JSPS KAKENHI Grant Number 25891019 (HH), 26116518 (KH), and 25281021 (KH), and JSPS Research Fellowship for Young Scientists (PD) (No. 6811) (KNY). The funders had no role in study design, data collection and analysis, decision to publish, or preparation of the manuscript.

Competing Interests: The authors have declared that no competing interests exist.

* Email: haeno@kyushu-u.org

Introduction

The inactivation of BRCA1 or BRCA2 (BRCA1/2) is considered to be an important step in the tumorigenesis of breast and ovarian cancers [1]. BRCA1/2 mutations are also found in a small proportion of prostate, pancreatic, and uterine serous cancers [2–4]. Loss of functional BRCA is strongly associated with the incidence of BRCA-associated cancers, such as basal-like breast cancer [5,6]. Moreover, mutations in BRCA1/2 genes due to several mechanisms, such as germline mutations, somatic mutations, and epigenetic silencing, are present in 33% of ovarian carcinoma samples [7]. However, it has also become evident that biallelic loss of wild-type BRCA is not required for tumorigenesis in some types of BRCA-associated breast cancers [8–10]. Consistently, loss of wild-type BRCA1 is not the initiating step in tumorigenesis in BRCA-associated breast tumors [11]. Additionally, a high level of heterogeneity in loss of heterozygosity (LOH) was observed in breast cancer with BRCA1/2 heterozygotes [12]. These lines of evidence indicate that BRCA-associated cancers undergo two different types of evolutionary trajectories: tumorigenesis with loss of both BRCA alleles and tumorigenesis with BRCA heterozygosity. Other genes, such as TP53 and PIK3CA, are also mutated in BRCA-associated cancers [5]. These mutations confer growth advantages on cancer cells and drive tumorigenesis [13,14].

The BRCA1/2 proteins have essential functions in preserving chromosomal integrity during cell division. DNA replication forks frequently stall even during normal cell proliferation and may generate DNA double-strand breaks (DSBs). These DSBs are repaired by BRCA1/2 via homologous recombination (HR) in an error-free fashion [15]. Without functional BRCA1/2, error-prone repair pathways are selectively stimulated, provoking genetic instability [16,17]. Such genetic instability does not confer growth advantages to cells but accelerates the process of genetic variation that drives carcinogenesis by inducing additional mutational events [18]. Moreover, statistical analyses have shown that there is a correlation between high mutation frequency and DNA repair pathway genes, such as BRCA1/2 [19].

Currently, platinum-based therapy is a major option for BRCA1/2-mutated tumors, such as ovarian cancer [20]. Platinum drugs, such as cisplatin and carboplatin, induce interstrand cross-links (ICLs), inhibiting cellular replication and transcription. BRCA1/2-deficient cells are particularly sensitive to ICL-inducing agents because ICLs are repaired through a Fanconi anemia/ BRCA pathway [21]. Several studies indicate that ovarian cancer patients with BRCA-germline mutations show favorable responses to platinum drugs [7,22,23]. Moreover, poly ADP-ribose polymerase (PARP) inhibitors (PARPis) have gained attention as effective drugs for BRCA-mutated cancers [24]. PARPis leave single-strand breaks (SSBs) unrepaired and induce DSBs. Cancer cells deficient in BRCA1/2 are unable to maintain genomic integrity in the presence of a large number of DSBs, resulting in cell death via a synthetic lethal effect. Cells carrying BRCA mutations are up to 1,000-fold more sensitive to PARPis than wild-type cells [25]. Finally, multiple PARPis are currently in clinical development for cancers deficient in the Fanconi anemia/ BRCA pathway [24].

However, chemotherapy using platinum drugs or PARPis often fails because of the emergence of resistance; indeed, most patients will ultimately have refractory disease [20,24]. Several mechanisms of resistance to platinum drugs have been identified: (i) mutations in cell-membrane transport proteins decrease drug uptake, resulting in reduced intracellular platinum concentrations, (ii) mutations in apoptotic signaling pathways prevent a cell from inducing cell death, and (iii) back mutations to wild-type BRCA1/ 2 result in the restored ability to repair DNA damage generated by platinum drugs [26,27]. Clinical studies have also identified a major mechanism of resistance to PARPis, in which secondary mutations restore BRCA function [28–30].

Resistant mutations can arise either prior to or during chemotherapy. On the one hand, resistant cells may pre-exist in a tumor before treatment and expand under selective pressure after treatment initiation. Indeed, it has been shown that platinum-sensitive and -resistant cells shared a common ancestor during the early stages of tumor development [31]. On the other hand, resistant cells may emerge as a result of novel mutations during treatment and expand under the selective pressure of treatment. The acquisition of secondary mutations has been observed with platinum drug and PARPi treatment [27,28]. Because the emergence of such resistance leads to treatment failure, it is important to investigate conditions in which resistant cells exist before treatment and appear after treatment.

Mathematical investigations have provided insights into how tumor cells drive progression and acquire drug resistance by accumulating mutations. Recently, the emergence of drug-resistant cancer cells from one specific mutation during clonal expansion prior to treatment was considered [32]. Moreover, the evolutionary dynamics of BRCA1-mutated breast cancer initiation were also considered, with the assumption that the number of cells is constant [33]. Breast cancer development caused by inactivation of two tumor suppressor genes has also been investigated [34]. In the case of ovarian cancer progression, a branching process model, accounting for primary, peritoneal, and metastatic cancer populations, was evaluated [35]. Furthermore, the evolution of resistance in cancer cells during continuous and pulsed administration strategies was suggested [36]. The risk of harboring multiple types of resistance at the start of chemotherapy due to various point mutations was studied in chronic myeloid leukemia [37]. In addition, the expected number of mutations conferring drug resistance in colorectal cancer was estimated using a branching process model [38]. Our study is based on a foundation of many previous theoretical studies regarding the accumulation of mutations in cancer cells [39–43].

In this study, we investigated tumor progression mathematically and the evolution of resistance to platinum drugs and PARPis in BRCA1/2-mutated cancers before and during treatment. We focused on the specific effects caused by loss of BRCA1/2 function, which confers (epi)genetic instability in cancer cells. Cancer cells with dysfunctional BRCA1/2 acquire increased mutation rates and become sensitive to platinum drugs and PARPis due to a deficiency in error-free repair mechanisms.

First, we developed a mathematical model of BRCA-associated cancer progression, in which two types of mutations were included: (i) those conferring functional BRCA1/2 inactivation and (ii) those accelerating cell growth by inactivation of cell cycle regulation. Second, we developed analytical formulas for the probability and expected number of cancer cells with (epi)genetic instability and/or a cell growth advantage at the time of diagnosis and validated good agreement between these formulas and exact stochastic computer simulations. Third, we extended the model to consider tumor dynamics during treatment. Fourth, we confirmed that our models strongly represented clinical/experimental findings in BRCA-associated cancers. Finally, we investigated the evolutionary pathways for acquiring drug resistance during tumorigenesis before and during treatment.

We discuss the conditions for effective treatment using platinum drugs and PARPis. This study provides important implications for the evolutionary trajectories of BRCA-associated cancer progression before and during chemotherapy, depending on the growth rate, mutation rate, detection size, and treatment effects.

Models

Clonal expansion of two different types of mutations before diagnosis

We first describe a mathematical model of BRCA-associated cancer progression before diagnosis, considering an exponentially growing population of cancer cells derived from a single tumor-initiating cell (Fig. 1A). In this study, we assume two different types of mutations: one facilitates (epi)genetic mutations due to inactivation of BRCA function, and the other accelerates tumor growth by deregulation of the cell cycle. In BRCA-associated cancer, alterations in genes such as TP53 and PIK3CA are candidates for the latter [5].

Cancer cells with functional BRCA and an intact target for accelerating growth rate are referred to as type-0 cells. During clonal expansion, they give rise to cells harboring either of the two mutations (Fig. 1A). Cells with inactivated BRCA are type-1 cells, which have higher mutation rates than those of type-0 cells due to their error-prone DNA repair mechanisms and (epi)genetic instability. Cells carrying a mutation that accelerates uncontrollable tumor growth are type-2 cells, which grow faster than type-0 or -1 cells. Type-1 and -2 cells may give rise to cells harboring both types of mutations, referred to as type-3 cells. The term 'mutation' here is used collectively to include point mutations, insertions, deletions, inversions, translocations, loss of heterozygosity, and other genetic aberrations that can occur during one cell division.

Each type of population follows a continuous-time branching process. The numbers of type-0, -1, -2, and -3 cells are denoted as w, x, y, and z, respectively. We assume that the growth and death rates of type-0 are the same as those of type-1, r and d, respectively, and those of type-2 are the same as those of type-3, a and b. This assumption is based on experimental observations that

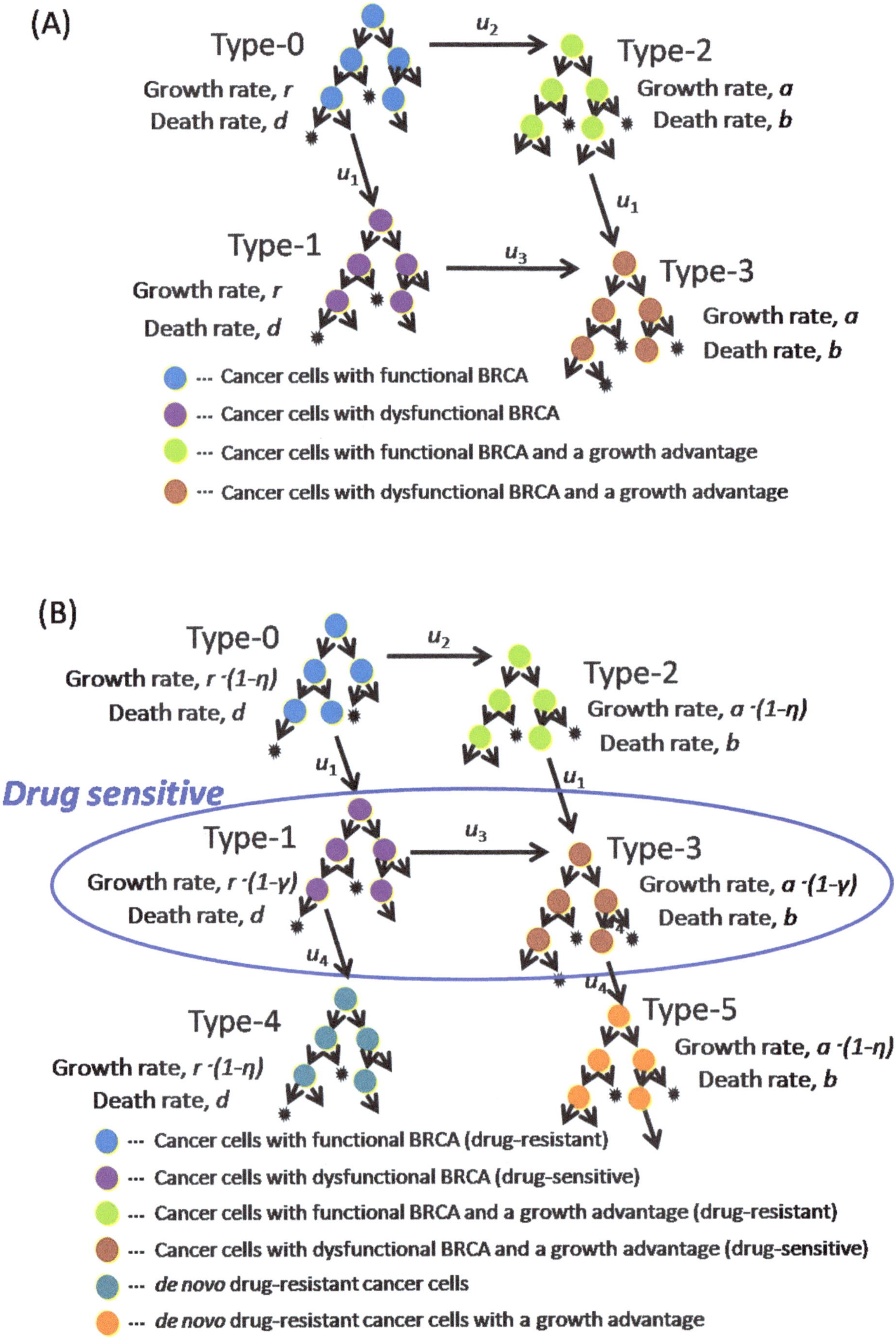
(A)
Type-0
Growth rate, r
Death rate, d
u_2
Type-2
Growth rate, a
Death rate, b
u_1
u_1
Type-1
Growth rate, r
Death rate, d
u_3
Type-3
Growth rate, a
Death rate, b
··· Cancer cells with functional BRCA
··· Cancer cells with dysfunctional BRCA
··· Cancer cells with functional BRCA and a growth advantage
··· Cancer cells with dysfunctional BRCA and a growth advantage
(B)
Type-0
Growth rate, r·(1-η)
Death rate, d
u_2
Type-2
Growth rate, a·(1-η)
Death rate, b
u_1
u_1
Drug sensitive
Type-1
Growth rate, r·(1-γ)
Death rate, d
u_3
Type-3
Growth rate, a·(1-γ)
Death rate, b
u_4
u_4
Type-4
Growth rate, r·(1-η)
Death rate, d
Type-5
Growth rate, a·(1-η)
Death rate, b
··· Cancer cells with functional BRCA (drug-resistant)
··· Cancer cells with dysfunctional BRCA (drug-sensitive)
··· Cancer cells with functional BRCA and a growth advantage (drug-resistant)
··· Cancer cells with dysfunctional BRCA and a growth advantage (drug-sensitive)
··· de novo drug-resistant cancer cells
··· de novo drug-resistant cancer cells with a growth advantage

Figure 1. Mathematical model of BRCA-associated cancer progression (A) until diagnosis and (B) during treatment. (A) We consider an exponentially growing population of cancer cells starting from a single cell that has potential mutation targets within two genomic regions. There are two types of mutations: one facilitates (epi)genetic mutations at rate u_1 and the other accelerates tumor growth at rates u_2 and u_3. Cancer cells with functional BRCA and an intact mutation target site for accelerated growth rates are called type-0. Cells with dysfunctional BRCA and an intact mutation target site for accelerated growth rates are called type-1. Cells carrying a mutation that accelerates uncontrollable tumor growth are called type-2 cells. Type-1 and -2 cells emerge from type-0 cells at mutation rates u_1 and u_2, respectively. Cells harboring both types of mutations are called type-3 cells. Type-3 cells emerge from either type-1 or -2 cells at mutation rates u_3 and u_1, respectively. The growth and death rates of type-0 and -1 cells are r and d, and those of type-2 and -3 cells are a and b, respectively. Once the total cell number reaches a certain size, M, the cancer is diagnosed. (B) To consider the situation during treatment, two populations (type-4 and -5 cells) are added to the model. Type-4 and -5 cells newly arise from type-1 and -3 cells, respectively, at rate u_4 and are resistant to platinum drugs and PARPis after treatment. The growth and death rates of type-4 cells are r and d, and those of type-5 cells are a and b, respectively. The initial numbers within each type of population at diagnosis are calculated by the analytical equations derived in Eq. (S12), Eq. (S13), and Eq. (S22). We assume that neither type-4 nor -5 cells exist at the time of initial treatment. The reduced growth rates of drug-sensitive and -resistant cells caused by drug treatments are given by γ and η, respectively. Once the total cell number reaches a certain size (1.1 M), the cancer is considered to have relapsed.

inactivation of BRCA function does not have much effect on tumor growth [44]. We assume that type-2 and -3 cells have higher net growth rates than type-0 and -1 cells ($a-b>r-d$) since they have an additional mutation that accelerates tumor growth. The rates of mutation (i) from type-0 to -1 cells and from type-2 to -3 cells, (ii) from type-0 to -2 cells, and (iii) from type-1 to -3 cells are denoted by u_1, u_2, and u_3, respectively.

Tumor growth begins from a single type-0 cell, $w=1$, $x=0$, $y=0$, $z=0$. In a short time period, one of the following events occurs: (i) cell division without mutation, (ii) cell division with mutation, (iii) cell death, or (iv) no transition. Tumor cells may become extinct because of stochastic fluctuations or may eventually be detected, once the total population size – the sum number of type-0, -1, -2, and -3 cells – reaches a certain size (see Materials S1 for details of the computer simulations).

Analytical approximations

Let P_1, P_2, and P_3 be the probabilities that type-1, -2, and -3 cells, respectively, exist when the total number of cells reaches M. In a previous study [32], formulas for P_1, and P_2 were given as

$$P_1 = 1 - e^{-Mu_1 \frac{r}{d} \ln \frac{r}{r-d}}. \quad (1)$$

$$P_2 = 1 - e^{-Mu_2 F/(1-d/r)}. \quad (2)$$

Here, $F = \int_0^1 (1-b/a)/(1-(b/a)y^{\alpha})dy$ and $\alpha = (a-b)/(r-d)$.

In our model, there are two paths to the emergence of type-3 cells: through either type-1 or type-2 cells. By considering both cases independently, we derived a formula for P_3 (see Materials S1 for the detailed derivation). Moreover, we consider the expected numbers of type-1, -2, and -3 cells when the total number reaches M to be E_1, E_2, and E_3, respectively (see Materials S1 for the detailed derivations of these quantities).

Emergence of resistance to platinum drugs and PARP inhibitors during treatment

Next, we considered the tumor dynamics during treatment after diagnosis. Type-0 and -2 cells are originally resistant to platinum drugs and PARPis because they can repair ICLs and DNA DSBs created by the drugs through an intact Fanconi anemia/BRCA pathway. In contrast, type-1 and -3 cells are sensitive to the drugs because of the lack of such repair mechanisms. Based on the experimental and clinical observations that secondary mutations in BRCA confer drug resistance to BRCA-deficient cells [26–30], we added two resistant populations, referred to as type-4 and -5 cells (Fig. 1B). Type-4 and -5 populations derive from BRCA-deficient cells (i.e., type-1 and -3 cells, respectively). We did not consider the secondary mutations from type-0 or -2 cells because they have already been defined as resistant cells. We then added two parameters as drug effects: one reduces growth rates in sensitive populations by γ, and the other reduces growth rates in resistant populations by η. In this study, we assumed that the suppression of tumor growth by drugs is achieved by a decrease in the growth rate and not by an increase in the death rate. We also assumed that treatment could decrease the growth rates of resistant cells, but at least one resistant type can increase in number even during treatment.

Based on the model described above, we investigated the cell population composition at relapse and the recurrence time intervals during treatment. We examined various combinations of treatment effects on sensitive and resistant cells, since treatment effects *in situ* have not been identified clearly and are modulated by pharmacokinetics, the tumor micro-environment, and other factors [20]. Once each parameter value is determined, the expected numbers of each population at the start of treatment can be calculated using analytical equations (Eq. (S12), Eq. (S13), and Eq. (S22)). Neither type-4 nor -5 cells exist at the time of the initial treatment. Simulations are stopped when the total number of cells exceeds 110% of the detection size, M, during treatment, which represents recurrence (see Materials S1 for a detailed description of the computer simulations).

Results

Existence probabilities and expected numbers of each cell population at diagnosis

In this section, we investigated the accuracy of the formulas for the existence probabilities as well as the expected numbers of each population at diagnosis and their dependence on each parameter. We evaluated the fit among the predictions using the formulas and the results from the stochastic computer simulations, described in Materials S1.

First, the accuracy of the existence probability formulas and the expected numbers of type-1, -2, and -3 cells at diagnosis (Figs. 2, 3, S1-S4) were evaluated. The Eq. (1), Eq. (2), Eq. (S11), Eq. (S12), Eq. (S13), and Eq. (S22) formulas accurately predicted the results of the stochastic computer simulations. Next, we tested the accuracy of the formulas with large u_1 and u_2 (Figs. S5, S6). The Eq. (1), Eq. (2) and Eq. (S11) formulas accurately predicted the results of the stochastic computer simulations, with the exceptions of P_2 with large u_1 and P_1 with large u_2 (Figs. S5B, S6A). These discrepancies arose because we ignored the effects of u_1 and u_2 in the derivation of P_2 and P_1, respectively. However, when u_1 or u_2 is large, type-2 or -1 cells, respectively, become minor represen-

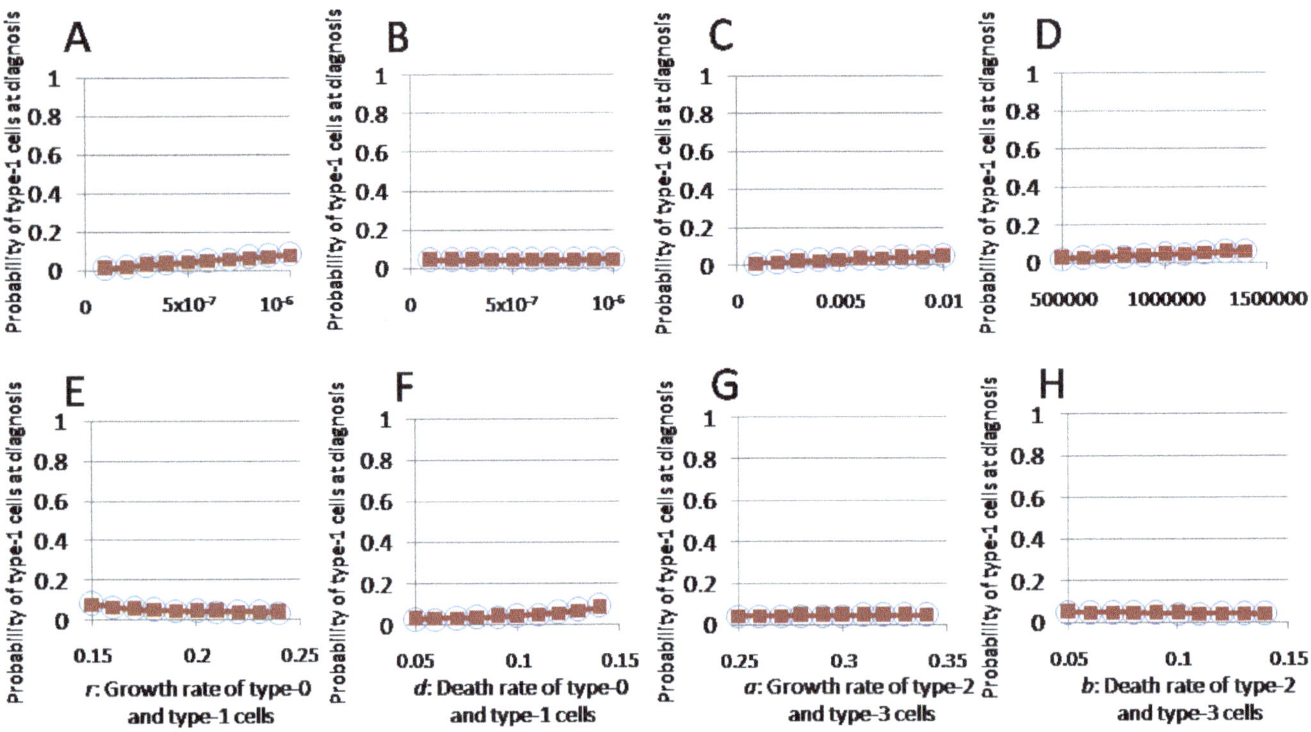

Figure 2. Probability of type-3 cells at diagnosis. The dependence of the probability of type-3 cell existence at diagnosis on various parameters is shown. The curves indicate the predictions of the analytical approximation, Eq. (S11), while the circles indicate the results of the direct computer simulations (system S1). Standard parameter values used in the figure are $u_1 = u_2 = 5.0 \cdot 10^{-7}$, $u_3 = 0.01$, $M = 10^6$, $r = 0.2$, $a = 0.3$, and $d = b = 0.1$.

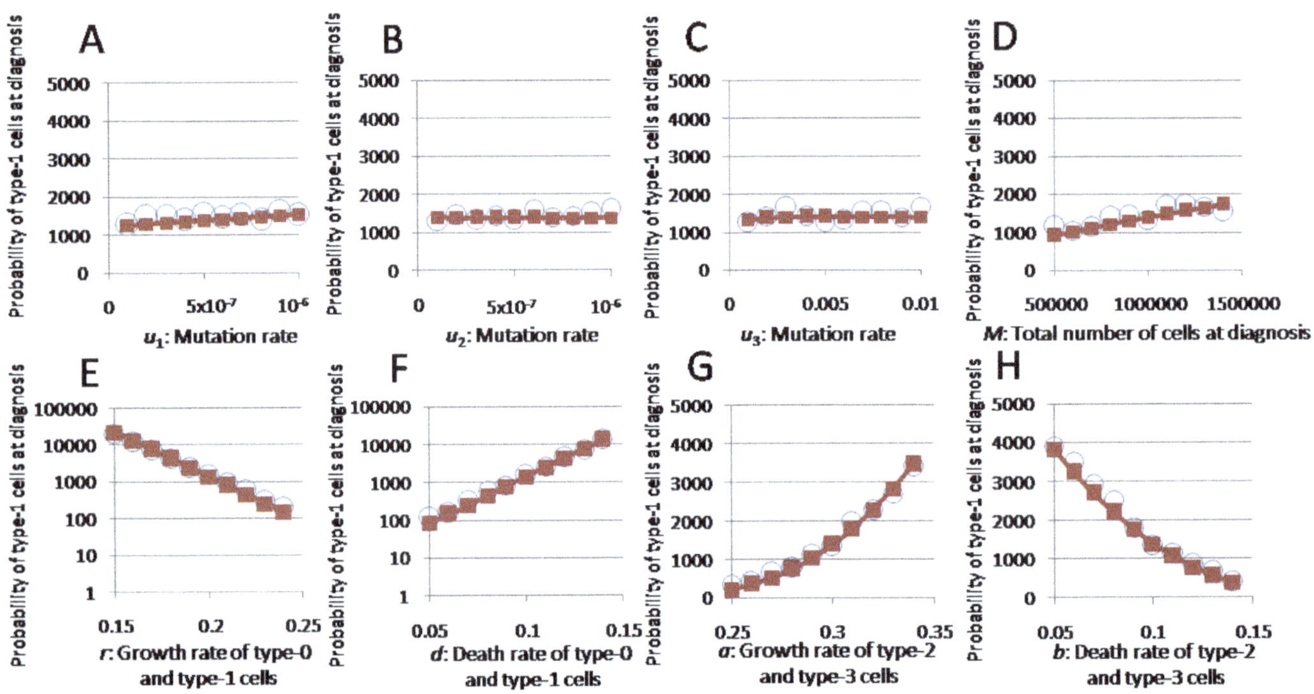

Figure 3. Expected numbers of type-3 cells at diagnosis. The dependence of the expected number of type-3 cells at diagnosis on various parameters is shown. The curves indicate the predictions of the analytical approximation, Eq. (S22), while the circles indicate the results of the direct computer simulations (system S1). Standard parameter values used in the figure are $u_1 = u_2 = 5.0 \cdot 10^{-7}$, $u_3 = 0.01$, $M = 10^6$, $r = 0.2$, $a = 0.3$, and $d = b = 0.1$.

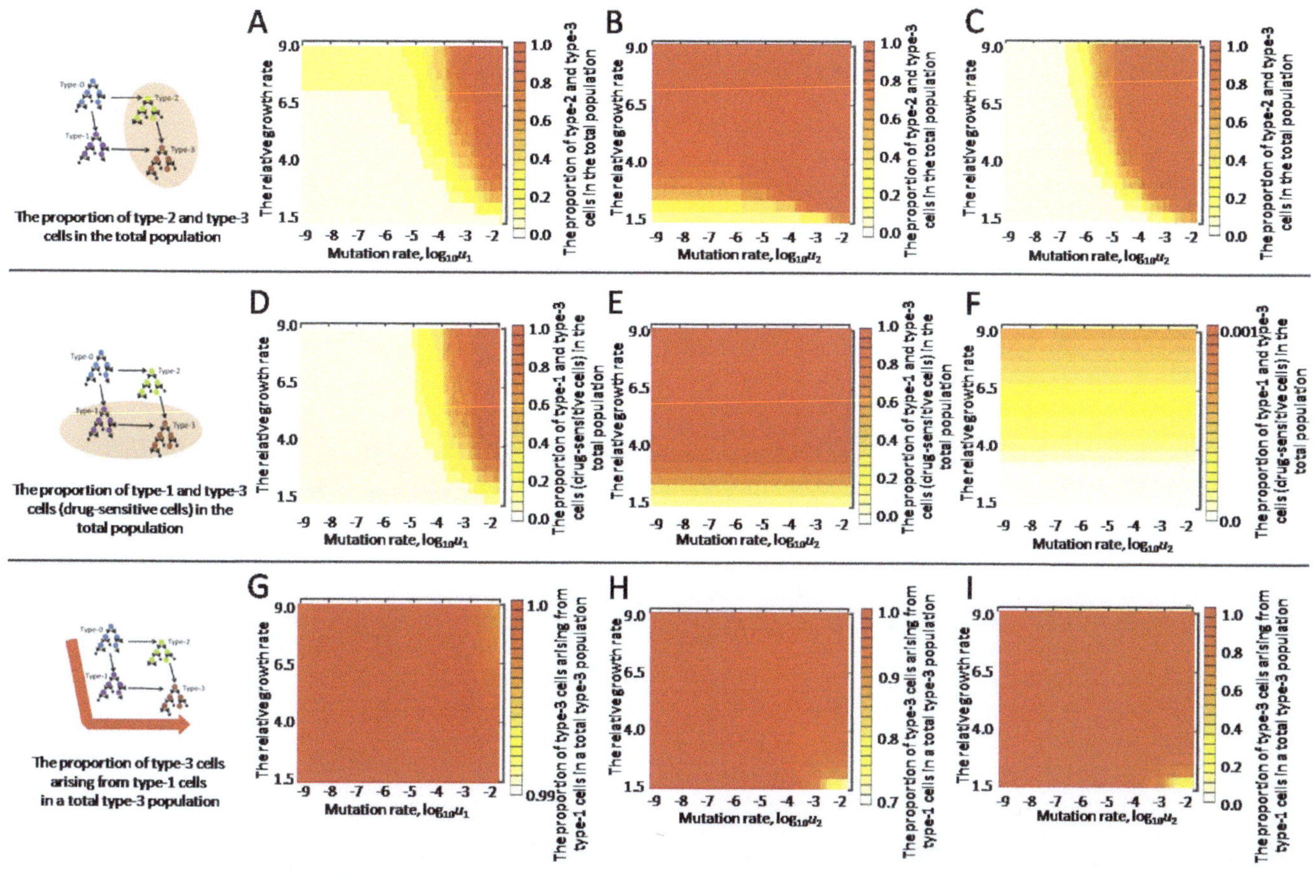

Figure 4. Proportion of clinically significant populations at diagnosis. (A–C) The proportion of type-2 and -3 cells with a growth advantage among the total population at diagnosis is shown over a wide range of u_1, u_2, and the relative growth rate of type-2 and -3 cells to that of type-0 and -1 cells is $(a-b)/(r-d)$. (D–F) The proportion of type-1 and -3 cells (drug-sensitive cells) among the total population is shown. (G–I) The proportion of type-3 cells arising from type-1 cells among the total type-3 population is shown. Each population at diagnosis was calculated by the formulas, Eq. (S12), Eq. (S13), and Eq. (S22). Parameter values used in the figure are $u_2=10^{-7}$, $u_3=0.01$, $M=10^6$, $r=0.2$, $a=0.3$, $d=b=0.1$ (panel A, D, and G), $u_1=10^{-2}$ (panel B, E, and H), and $u_1=10^{-7}$ (panel C, F, and I).

tations of the total population. Thus, this inconsistency has little effect on the expected numbers of each cell type at diagnosis (Figs. S5, S6).

We next investigated the dependence of the formulas on each parameter. The probability that type-1 cells existed at diagnosis increased as u_1, M, and d increased, whereas the probability decreased as r increased. It was not changed by u_2, u_3, a, or b (Fig. S1). The probability that type-2 cells existed at diagnosis increased as u_2, M, d, and a increased, whereas it decreased as r and b increased. It was not changed by u_1 or u_3 (Fig. S2). These results are consistent with those reported previously [32]. The probability that type-3 cells exist at diagnosis increased as u_1, u_3, M, and d increased, whereas it decreased as r increased. It was little changed by u_2, a, or b (Fig. 2). The expected number of type-1 cells under the condition that type-1 cells existed at diagnosis increased as u_1 and M increased, whereas it decreased as u_3 increased. It was not changed greatly by u_2, r, d, a, or b (Fig. S3). The expected number of type-2 cells under the condition that type-2 cells existed at diagnosis increased as u_2, M, d, and a increased, whereas it decreased as r and b increased. It was not changed by u_1 or u_3 (Fig. S4). The expected number of type-3 cells under the condition that type-3 cells existed at diagnosis increased as u_1, u_3, M, d, and a increased, whereas it decreased as r and b increased. It was not changed greatly by u_2 (Fig. 3).

The proportions of the clinically significant populations at diagnosis

In this section, we investigated the following three quantities at diagnosis: (i) the proportion of cell types with high growth rates, (ii) the proportion of drug-sensitive populations, and (iii) the proportion of type-3 cells that arose from type-1 cells. The outcome of anti-tumor therapy is largely affected by the composition of a tumor at the time of therapy. For example, the proportion of cell populations with high growth rates at diagnosis reflects tumor malignancy and thus affects the control of disease by the treatment. Moreover, the proportion of drug-sensitive populations can determine the response to treatment, because platinum drugs and PARPis are effective only in BRCA-deficient cell types. Furthermore, if we specify the evolutionary pathway leading to malignant cells, it would implicate the drug-targeted cells in the prevention of tumor progression.

First, we investigated the proportion of cell populations with high growth rates (i.e., type-2 and -3 cells) among the total population at diagnosis (Figs. 4A–C, S7A–B). This was calculated by dividing the sum of the expected numbers of type-2 and -3 cells by the total number, M. The relative growth rates of type-2 and -3 cells, compared with type-0 and -1 cells, is given by $(a-b)/(r-d)$. The proportions of type-2 and -3 cells increased as the relative growth rate and the mutation rates (u_1 and u_2) increased (Figs. 4A–C, S7A–B). Second, we calculated the proportion of drug-sensitive cell populations (i.e., type-1 and -3 cells; Figs. 4D–F, S7C–D) by dividing the sum of the expected numbers of type-1 and -3 cells by the total number, M. The proportion increased as the relative growth rate and u_1 increased (Figs. 4D, S7C–D) and, interestingly, was greatly affected by the relative growth rate and u_1, but not by u_2 (Figs. 4D–F, S7C–D). Third, we calculated the proportion of type-3 cells that arose from type-1 cells in a total type-3 population (Figs. 4G–I, S7E–F) by dividing the expected numbers of type-3 cells derived from type-1 cells by the expected number of type-3 cells at diagnosis. Type-3 cells emerge from type-1 cells over a wide range of parameter values except in cases where the relative growth rate is low and u_2 is large (Figs. 4G–I, S7E–F). Finally, we investigated those three quantities in cases of small u_3. The proportions of cell populations with high growth rates and drug sensitivity decreased in the region of large u_1, and the proportion of type-3 cells that arose from type-1 cells decreased in the region of large u_2 (Figs. S8, S9). The dependencies of these quantities on the relative growth rate and the mutation rates were similar to the cases of large u_3 (Figs. 4, S7–S9).

Proportion of each cell population at relapse and recurrence time intervals

In this section, we investigated the composition of each cell population in a relapsed tumor and recurrence time intervals. Two scenarios can be considered for the development of resistant populations: (i) a *de novo* resistant population arises from type-1 or -3 cells through secondary mutations during treatment and then expands, or (ii) a resistant population pre-exists in a tumor population before treatment and becomes dominant under selective pressure from the drug. The origin of the resistant population is of great importance because the treatment schedule that will best prolong the time until recurrence would be expected to differ between the two scenarios. Thus, we considered which of the two scenarios occurred preferentially over a wide range of parameter values during treatment.

First, we performed stochastic computer simulations of the model after diagnosis, as described in the MODELS section (Fig. 1B). We determined the composition of each cell population within a tumor at the initial time of treatment with 10 parameter combinations from the formulas Eq. (S12), Eq. (S13), and Eq. (S22) (Table 1). When u_1 is large, type-3 cells become dominant (Table 1A–D). The proportion of type-3 cells becomes large as M increases (Table 1A–D). When u_1 is small, type-0 cells become dominant (Table 1E–I), and when u_2 is large, type-2 cells become dominant (Table 1J). Based on the initial tumor composition, calculated above, hundreds of stochastic simulation runs using the same initial conditions were implemented. For each parameter set listed in Table 1, we examined various drug effects on sensitive and resistant cells, γ and η (Fig. 5). The numbers of each cell type at relapse (the time when the total number reached 1.1 M) and the time until relapse were recorded for each run, and the averaged results are shown in Figure 5. Considering that (epi)genetic instability induced by repair pathway deficiency has a major effect on the ability to induce mutations [19], we assumed that the secondary mutation rate from type-1 and -3 cells to type-4 and -5 cells u_4 was the same as u_3.

We then investigated the proportion of each cell population at the time of recurrence with large u_1 (Fig. 5). The proportion of type-3 cells in a tumor population at relapse is large when η is zero but decreases as η becomes large (Fig. 5A–D). In the former case, resistant cells grow too rapidly for type-3 cells to disappear until tumor relapse; however, in the latter case, slow growth of resistant cells facilitates mutational events from type-3 to -5 cells and also confers a time of elimination by negative selection on type-3 cells. Type-5 cells have more chance of being present at the time of relapse in the latter condition (Fig. 5A–D). The proportion of type-2 cells increases as M, γ, and η increase (Fig. 5A–D). When the tumor size at diagnosis, M, is large, a large proportion of type-2 cells is likely to be present (Table 1), resulting in a large proportion of type-2 cells at relapse. Type-1 and -4 cells are hardly detected at relapse because they are rarely present at the time of initial treatment and grow slower than type-3 and -5 cells.

Furthermore, we investigated the proportion of each cell population at the time of recurrence with small u_1 (Fig. 5). With all treatment effect combinations, type-0 or -2 cells became dominant (Fig. 5E–I), because they were likely to be present in large proportions at diagnosis (Table 1E–J) and are resistant to the drugs. The proportion of type-2 cells at relapse became large when η and u_2 were large (Fig. 5E–J).

Finally, we investigated the length of time between diagnosis and recurrence to find the cases in which platinum drugs and PARPis effectively prolong the time until recurrence. The time until recurrence increased as η increased, whereas it was not changed greatly by γ (Fig. 5). Interestingly, in the case of large u_1 ($=10^{-2}$) and small η ($=0$), the time until recurrence became longer than that with small u_1 ($=10^{-7}$) or small η ($=0$; Fig. 5), because the proportion of drug-sensitive cells becomes dominant at the time of initial treatment when u_1 is large (Table 1A–D). Additionally, we confirmed the robustness of the results over a wide range of u_1 and u_2 (Table S1, Fig. S10).

Agreement between the results and clinical evidence

Next, we investigated whether our models described clinical and experimental observations in BRCA-associated cancers (Table 2). We categorized BRCA-associated cancers into two types in terms of different inactivation rates of BRCA, u_1. BRCA inactivation is induced by LOH in ovarian cancer [7,12] and basal-like breast cancer [5,6], indicating high mutation rates of $u1$. We assume that in this case, u_1 is 10^{-2} at maximum. This value is based on the observation of an inactivated second allele in cells with (epi)genetic instability [45]. In contrast, particularly in breast cancer, biallelic loss of BRCA is not commonly observed at diagnosis, suggesting LOH is not involved in the mutational event [9]. We assume that in this case, u_1 is 10^{-7}. The rate of mutation without LOH has been determined experimentally by investigating DNA replication fidelity [46]. Here, the mutation rate from type-1 to type-3 cells, u_3, is assumed to be as high as the mutation rate induced by LOH, because we took into account the additive (epi)genetic instability effect caused by BRCA inactivation [45]. Additionally, when we considered the agreement between our results and the clinical evidence, we focused on the small treatment effects in resistant populations. This assumption seems reasonable because recurrence during treatment does, in fact, occur in the clinic, and the small effects of platinum drugs and PARPis on resistant cells have been confirmed experimentally [27,29,30,47].

First, we considered the high mutation rate cases, $u_1 = 10^{-2}$, such as ovarian cancer and basal-like breast cancer, in which BRCA inactivation is frequently observed during tumorigenesis (Table 2). In most computer simulation cases, mixed populations coexisted at both diagnosis and relapse, indicating heterogeneity in the tumor (Figs. 4, 5, S7, S8, S9, S10, and Tables 1 and S1). These results are consistent with clinical observations of intra-tumoral genetic heterogeneity in ovarian and breast cancers

Table 1. Parameter sets used for the analysis in Figure 5 and the expected numbers of cells at diagnosis.

(1) $u_1 = 0.01$	Parameter values				Expected Number (Proportion) of Cells at Diagnosis			
	a	u_2	u_3	M	Type-0	Type-1	Type-2	Type-3
A	0.4	10^{-7}	10^{-2}	10^5	52843 (0.53)	3885 (0.03)	31 (0.00)	43249 (0.43)
B				10^6	245500 (0.25)	37102 (0.04)	1446 (0.00)	715950 (0.72)
C				10^7	750925 (0.08)	354324 (0.04)	66724 (0.01)	8828026 (0.88)
D				10^8	0 (0.00)	3383775 (0.03)	3014563 (0.03)	93789333 (0.94)
(2) $u_1 = 10^{-7}$	Parameter values				Expected Number (Proportion) of Cells at Diagnosis			
	a	u_2	u_3	M	Type-0	Type-1	Type-2	Type-3
E	0.4	10^{-7}	10^{-2}	10^5	99967 (1.00)	0 (0.00)	31 (0.00)	2 (0.00)
F				10^6	998468 (1.00)	2 (0.00)	1446 (0.00)	82 (0.00)
G				10^7	9929430 (0.99)	17 (0.00)	66738 (0.01)	3813 (0.00)
H				10^8	96809333 (0.97)	166 (0.00)	3014563 (0.03)	175936 (0.00)
I			10^{-4}	10^6	998549 (1.00)	2 (0.00)	1446 (0.00)	2 (0.00)
J		10^{-2}	10^{-2}	10^6	6149 (0.01)	2 (0.00)	993765 (0.99)	83 (0.00)

The expected numbers of type-1, -2, and -3 cells at diagnosis were calculated using Eq. (S12), Eq. (S13), and Eq. (S22). The remainder of the total number is considered to comprise the number of type-0 cells. The proportion of each type is shown in parentheses. Parameter values used in Figure 5 are $r = 0.2$ and $d = b = 0.1$.

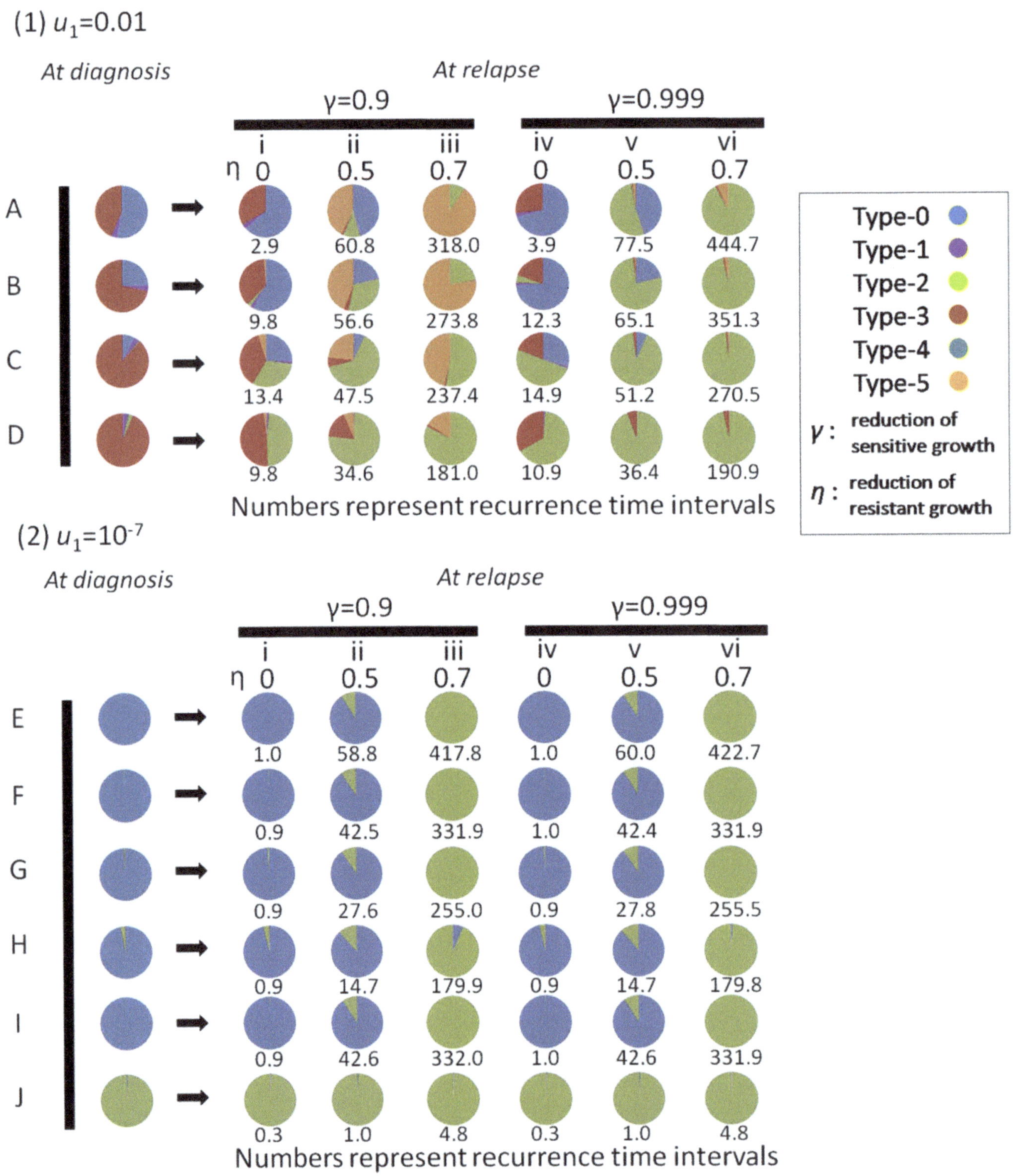

Figure 5. Population composition at relapse and recurrence time intervals. The population compositions at diagnosis (the time of initial treatment) and at the time of recurrence after treatment with 60 parameter sets are shown in the pie charts. The time periods until recurrence after treatment are shown as numbers under the pie charts. The time of recurrence is defined as the time point when the total number has exceeded 10% of the number at diagnosis. Each result is obtained by averaging many trials by stochastic simulations of the model under treatment (system S23). Parameter values used in the simulations, except the treatment effects, γ and η, are listed in Table 1. The letters in Table 1 correspond to those in Figure 5. Treatment effects are shown at the top of the pie charts as the reduction effects on growth rates of sensitive populations (γ) and those on resistant populations (η). We show the results separately by different values of u_1; u_1 is 0.01 in Figure 5(1), and 10^{-7} in Figure 5(2). The parameter values used in the figure, but not shown in Table 1 are $u_4 = 0.01$, and $d = b = 0.1$.

Table 2. Agreements between the results and the clinical and molecular evidence.

Results	Figures and Tables	Clinical and molecular evidence	References
(1)Cases of high mutation rate ($u_1 = 0.01$)			
Coexistence of multiple populations at diagnosis and relapse	Figs. 4, 5, S7, S9, S10, Table 1	Intra-tumor genetic heterogeneity in ovarian and breast cancer	48,49
High frequency of cells with a growth advantage at diagnosis	Figs. 4, S7	Observation of TP53 mutation in more than 90% of ovarian cancers	5,7,50
		Observation of TP53 mutation in more than 80% of basal-like breast cancers	5
High frequency of BRCA-inactivated (drug-sensitive) cells at diagnosis	Figs. 4D, 4E, S7C, S7D	High frequency of (epi)genetic instability in high grade serous ovarian cancer	51,52,53
Ten-fold survival benefit in treatment with platinum drugs and PARPis	Fig. 5A(i)–D(i), E(i)–H(i)	Good prognosis by the platinum-based and PARPis chemotherapy in patients with BRCA mutation.	7,22,23,62
High frequency of drug-sensitive type-3 cells at relapse	Figs. 5A(i)–D(i), A(iv)–D(iv), S10(i), S10(iv)	Some patients can be re-treated with the same drugs which previously showed good sensitivity	54
		Good responses by PARPis to platinum-sensitive relapsed tumors	55
Proportion of type-2 cells increases as tumor detection size increases	Fig. 5A–D, Table 1	Detection in early stage is favorable for overall survival in ovarian cancer	56
(2) Cases of low mutation rate ($u_1 = 10^{-7}$)			
Wide range of aggressiveness at diagnosis	Figs. 4A, 4C, S7A, S7B	Observation of TP53 mutation in 12% to 29% in luminal breast cancers	5
Low frequency of BRCA-inactivated (drug-sensitive) cells at diagnosis	Figs. 4D, 4F, S7C, S7D	Late BRCA1 inactivation in BRCA1-associated breast tumors	11
Early treatment failure due to pre-existing drug-resistant cells	Figs. 5E–J, S10 (i), S10(iv)	Small effects by DNA damaging drugs in BRCA-associated breast cancers	57

[48,49]. When we focused on the aggressiveness of the tumor, the majority of tumor cells at diagnosis had a high proliferation rate under large u_1 conditions (Figs. 4A, 4B, S7A, S7B). The results are consistent with recent reports that TP53 mutations are observed in more than 90% of ovarian cancers [5,7,50] and 80% of basal-like breast cancers [5]. BRCA function is inactivated in a large proportion of tumors at diagnosis with large u_1 (Figs. 4D, 4E, S7C, S7D). Thus, the tumor cells are expected to show (epi)genetic instability and sensitivity to platinum drugs and PARPis while exhibiting a high proliferation rate over a wide range of parameter values (Fig. 4B, 4E). These results fit with the reports of high (epi)genetic instability frequency in high-grade serous ovarian cancer [51,52,53].

Moreover, our results indicate that when there is no treatment effect on resistant cancer cells, platinum drugs and PARPis have a ~10-fold survival benefit for cancers with large u_1 compared with the cases with small u_1 (Fig. 5A(i)–D(i), (i)–H(i)). This observation may explain why clinical cases of ovarian cancer with BRCA mutations show a better prognosis than those with wild-type BRCA during chemotherapy [7,22,23]. Our results support the conventional first-line regimen of platinum-based chemotherapy in BRCA-associated ovarian cancer.

Furthermore, in the case of no treatment effect in resistant cancer cells, drug-sensitive type-3 cells still exist in a large proportion of tumors at relapse (Figs. 5A(i)–D(i), 5A(iv)–D(iv), S10(i), S10(iv)). The results indicate that retreatment with platinum drugs and PARPis after recurrence may still be worthy of consideration. Indeed, this is supported by a recent report in which re-treatment with cisplatin was effective in patients who exhibited good sensitivity to platinum drugs with prior treatment [54], and that PARPis were effective in platinum-sensitive relapsed tumors [55]. Notably, tumors also contain resistant cells in such a situation, and recurrence is inevitable if we simply continue the same strategy as before (Figs. 5A(i)–D(i), A(iv)–D(iv), S10(i), S10(iv)).

Finally, we observed that the proportion of type-2 cells at relapse increased as the total cell number at diagnosis increased (Fig. 5A–D, Table 1). This causes early treatment failure due to the pre-existence of resistant cells. This result is consistent with the clinical evidence that early-stage and smaller residual tumor volumes were favorable characteristics for overall survival in ovarian cancer [56]. Taken together, the model could reproduce the clinical evidence in cases of frequent BRCA inactivation during tumorigenesis, such as in ovarian cancer or basal-like breast cancer.

We also considered the case of a low mutation rate, $u_1 = 10^{-7}$. This represents tumorigenesis in non-basal-like breast cancer with BRCA heterozygotes [10]. Regarding the aggressiveness of the tumor, the results with small u_1 were similar to clinical observations in luminal breast cancer, in which a wide range of aggressiveness occurs (Figs. 4A, 4C, S7A, S7B). Indeed, the prediction may explain the report that TP53 mutations are observed in 12–29% of luminal breast cancers, much lower than that in ovarian or basal-like breast cancers [5]. In marked contrast to the situation with a high mutation rate, $u_1 = 10^{-2}$, the proportion of cells sensitive to platinum drugs and PARPis is very small (<0.002) at diagnosis over the global range of parameter values (Figs. 4D, 4F, S7C, S7D). These results agree well with the finding that TP53 mutations occur first, instead of BRCA1 inactivation, in evolutionary pathways of BRCA1-associated luminal breast tumors [11]. Tumors dominated by resistant populations at diagnosis result in early treatment failure when there is no treatment effect on resistant cells (Figs. 5E–J, S10(i), S10(iv)). These results are consistent with current therapeutic outcomes for BRCA-associated breast cancers, in which DNA-damaging drugs did not show substantial effects with a single agent [57]. These results may also explain why clinical trials on PARPis treatment in patients with triple-negative breast cancer failed, with patients showing no response, in contrast to substantial responses of BRCA-associated ovarian cancers in the same trial [58], because the patient populations with triple-negative breast cancer contained not only basal-like but also non-basal breast cancers [59]. In summary, we have been able to reproduce BRCA-associated cancer types, such as non basal-like breast cancer, in which BRCA inactivation is not frequently observed during tumorigenesis.

Discussion

In this study, we developed mathematical models of BRCA-associated cancer progression before and during treatment with platinum drugs or PARPis. Next, we investigated the frequency of each cell population at diagnosis and the evolution of drug resistance during treatment. We derived analytical approximations for the proportions of drug-sensitive and -resistant cells at diagnosis and explored evolutionary pathways involved in acquiring drug resistance. Recurrence-free intervals were also investigated over a wide parameter range. Moreover, we reproduced clinical/experimental observations successfully. In the parameter settings for ovarian or basal-like breast cancer, in which BRCA inactivation is commonly observed during tumorigenesis, the models succeeded in capturing the following clinical evidence: (i) high tumor heterogeneity and high prevalence of aggressive tumor cells, (ii) high frequency of (epi)genetic instability and sensitivity to platinum drugs and PARPis, (iii) long recurrence-free intervals due to a high frequency of BRCA-mutated cell populations, (iv) possibility of re-treatment with platinum drugs and PARPis, and (v) early treatment failure in the case of large detection size. Moreover, we have reproduced the clinical evidence that a therapy reliant on DNA repair deficiency would not be a promising approach in the case of non-basal-like breast cancer, in which BRCA heterozygosity is sometimes retained during tumorigenesis.

It is clinically important to reveal the trajectory of drug resistance development during the treatment of ovarian carcinoma [60]. In this study, we investigated two possibilities for the evolution of drug resistance in a large u_1 condition: (i) expansion of a pre-existing intrinsic sub-population and (ii) acquisition of drug resistance due to secondary mutations during treatment. When there are 90% growth reducing effects on sensitive cells and no effect on resistant cells, the majority of resistant cells are pre-existing resistant tumor cells, such as type-0 or -2 cells, in a relapsed tumor (Fig. 5A(i)–D(i)). However, when treatment effects on resistant cells are not small, resistant cells may emerge due to secondary mutations in BRCA during treatment (Fig. 5A(iii)–D(iii)). In this case, it takes a long time for *de novo* resistant cells in a relapsed tumor to emerge and become dominant (Fig. 5A(ii), 5A(iii), 5B(ii), 5B(iii), 5C(iii)). Given that large treatment effects on resistant cells in the clinic are less plausible, we suggest that drug resistance acquired by novel mutations during treatment occurs in only a small proportion of patients after long-term exposure to chemotherapy. Indeed, only 6.3% (4/64 patients) of ovarian cancer patients showed *de novo* resistance to treatment [29], and the secondary mutations did not become detectable until more than a decade after chemotherapy for ovarian and breast cancers [29,30]. When there was more than 99% tumor growth reduction on sensitive cells, most of the cells in a relapsed tumor were originally present at the start of therapy (Fig. 5A–D). Collectively, these results indicate that the origin of resistant cells in a relapsed tumor can vary according to the tumor characteristics and treatment effects on both sensitive and resistant cells.

Based on the results from the models, our hypothesis on the evolutionary trajectories of BRCA-associated cancers is illustrated in Figure 6. The frequency of BRCA inactivation is a major determinant in the future sensitivity to platinum drugs and PARPis. If it is high, the drug-sensitive tumor population appears at diagnosis. In this situation, drug-sensitive and -resistant cells may coexist at relapse after treatment, and effective retreatment is conceivable (Fig. 6B). Populations with secondary mutations may emerge after long-term treatment if the drugs effectively suppress the growth of resistant cells as well as sensitive cells (Fig. 6A). If a sufficient growth advantage is not obtained by the mutation to accelerate tumor growth or the tumor is diagnosed at a late phase, the tumor tends to contain drug-resistant cells at the start of therapy (Fig. 6C). If BRCA inactivation does not occur frequently during tumorigenesis, the tumor will be resistant to platinum drugs and PARPis at the start of therapy (Fig. 6D). Taken together, platinum drugs and PARPis should be effective if (i) BRCA inactivation occurs, (ii) treatment is started early, and (iii) tumor growth is rapid. Our results may help determine individualized treatment options for patients with BRCA-associated cancers in the clinic.

This research provides theoretical insights into the therapeutic approaches for different types of cancers that share major mutations in tumorigenesis. Our results suggest that platinum drug and PARPi treatment strategies dependent on the underlying defects in DNA repair mechanisms should be commonly effective in cancers in which BRCA inactivation occurs frequently, such as basal-like breast and ovarian cancers (Fig. 5A–D), as reported [60–62]. In fact, basal-like breast cancer shares molecular features with serous ovarian cancer, but not with other breast cancers [5]. In ovarian cancer, the time interval from completion of platinum-based chemotherapy to disease progression has been conventionally used as an indicator to predict the response to subsequent treatment with platinum-containing regimens [63]. However, our results indicate that the cell population profiles in BRCA-associated cancers at relapse vary largely in accordance with the treatment effects in sensitive and resistant populations (Fig. 5). Thus, assessment of whether the relapsed tumor cells restore HR function, for example, using DNA sequencing and Rad51 foci formation assays, could be key to determining the sequential treatment strategies.

Another important result is the identification of the evolutionary paths leading to tumor cells with malignant characteristics. Interestingly, type-3 cells, which have high mutation and growth rates, emerged exclusively from type-1, and not type-2, cells with high mutation rates regardless of u_1, u_2, or the relative growth rate, $(a–b)/(r–d)$ (Figs. 4G–I, S7E, S7F). These results suggest that even though mutation rates enhanced by dysfunction in DNA repair mechanisms itself do not confer a growth advantage to cells, they subsequently induce additional mutations, some of which may accelerate tumor growth. In this case, the pervasive characteristics of tumor cells regarding dysfunctional BRCA provide a therapeutic opportunity, as seen with platinum drugs and PARPis.

In this study, we considered that tumor cells grow independently during tumorigenesis. In the initial progression of a carcinoma, exponential growth without tumor competition is often assumed. Thus, we adopted the simple growth mode without density effects in the first study regarding the evolution of drug resistance to platinum drugs and PARPis in BRCA-associated cancers. We also considered a simple but feasible dosing strategy of continuous drug

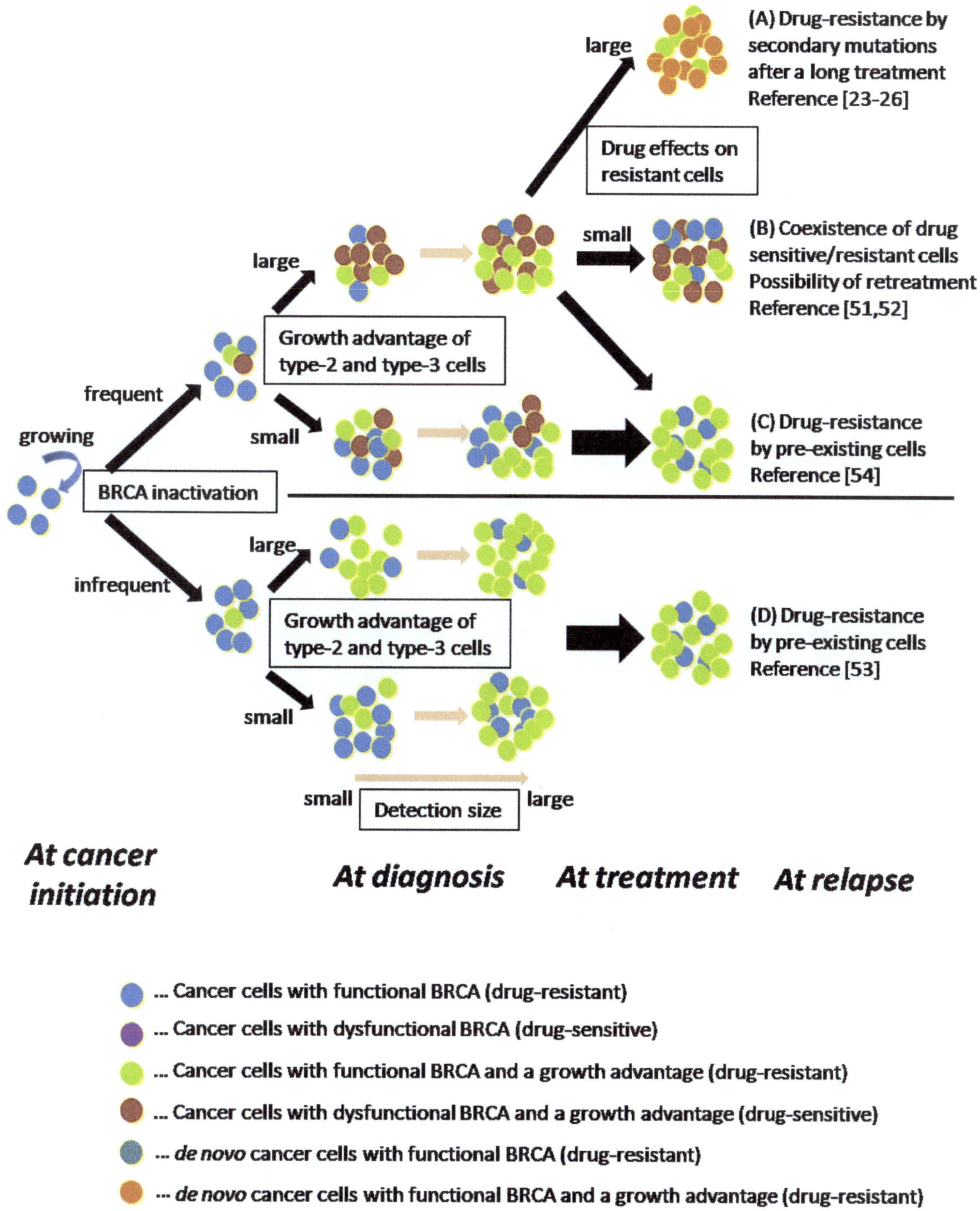

Figure 6. Schematic illustration of evolutionary trajectories of BRCA-associated cancers. The hypothesis on the evolutionary trajectories of BRCA-associated cancers is illustrated. Treatment outcomes are determined by the following four conditions: (i) the frequency of BRCA inactivation, (ii) growth advantage of type-2 and -3 cells, (iii) the detection size, and (iv) drug effects on resistant cells. (A) Drug resistance by secondary mutations emerges after long-term treatment in the case of (i) as high, (ii) as large, (iii) as large, and (iv) as large. (B) Drug-sensitive and -resistant cells coexist at

relapse and retreatment with the same drugs is conceivable in the case of (i) as high, (ii) as large, (iii) as not large, and (iv) as small. (C and D) Drug resistance due to pre-existing resistant cells emerges in the case of (i) as high, (ii) as small, (iii) as large and (iv) as any, or in the case of (i) as small. The reference numbers indicate clinical observations, each of which corresponds to each outcome in the evolutionary trajectories.

administration and assumed the secondary mutation rate u_4 to be the same as u_3. This assumption is based on evidence that (epi)genetic instability induced by deficiency in the repair pathway has a major effect on determining the ability to induce mutations [19]. Moreover, we did not distinguish the treatment effects on several types of resistant cells. Instead, we examined possible situations during treatment over a wide range by considering various parameter combinations of treatment effects on both sensitive and resistant cells. Furthermore, we assumed that secondary mutations before treatment were very rare and that type-4 and -5 populations were introduced only after treatment. This is supported by the evidence that secondary mutations are observed experimentally only when platinum drugs and PARPis are administered to cells [27,28]. Because the effects of inactivation on DNA repair mechanisms vary between BRCA1 and BRCA2, the mutation rate from type-1 to -3 cells, $u3$, can be low [10]. We then investigated the proportions of cell populations at diagnosis with a small $u3$ (Figs. S8, S9). Although parameter dependence shows a similar pattern to that with a large u_3 (Figs. 4, S7, S8, S9), the populations with high growth rates and drug sensitivity (type-3) are less prevalent under these conditions. This result agrees in part with those of clinical cases, in which platinum-resistant cancer recurs in ~25% of ovarian patients within 6 months [7]. These results indicate that, in general, u_3 may not be small [45].

Even though we have focused on BRCA1/2 inactivation in impaired HR function, the frequency of BRCA1/2 mutations does not explain all cases of HR impairment in BRCA-associated cancers. Indeed, 10–20% of ovarian cancers [7] and ~20% of breast cancers show inactivation of BRCA1/2 [5]. However, The Cancer Genome Atlas analysis of serous ovarian cancer documented that ~50% of serous ovarian cases [64] and 20% of triple-negative breast cancers [65] might have disrupted HR repair mechanism(s). Recently, many molecular mutations have been identified that confer BRCA-like characteristics to tumors, such as the Fanconi anemia protein family [66] and PTEN [67]. Thus, there is broad recognition of HR dysfunction in tumorigenesis. Our models can be interpreted as type-1 populations include cells not only with inactivated BRCA1/2 but also with 'BRCAness', that is, HR defects without mutations in BRCA1/2.

Collectively, we considered the evolutionary dynamics of BRCA-associated cancer before and during treatment and identified effective treatment conditions using platinum drugs and PARPis in agreement with clinical and experimental observations. These results may be applied to other BRCA-associated cancers, such as prostate, pancreatic, and uterine serous. The frequency of patients with BRCA mutations is small in these cancers. However, our results indicate that treatment with platinum drugs and PARPis in specific patients with HR impairment due to BRCA mutations might be an effective option essentially as a tailor-made therapy. Furthermore, our method in which we considered different types of cancers (ovarian and breast) in the same model according to the representative mutational status can be applied to other cancers if the major milestones during tumorigenesis are shared among these cancers. This approach will provide novel insights into therapeutic strategies from the viewpoint of pathway-targeted therapy against multiple cancers.

Supporting Information

Figure S1 The probability of type-1 cells at diagnosis. The figure shows the dependence of the probability of the existence of type-1 cells at diagnosis on various parameters. The curves indicate the predictions of the analytical approximation, Eq. (1), while the circles indicate the results of the direct computer simulation (system S1). Standard parameter values used in the figure are $u_1 = u_2 = 5.0 \cdot 10^{-7}$, $u_3 = 0.01$, $M = 10^6$, $r = 0.2$, $a = 0.3$, $d = b = 0.1$.

Figure S2 The probability of type-2 cells at diagnosis. The figure shows the dependence of the probability of the existence of type-2 cells at diagnosis on various parameters. The curves indicate the predictions of the analytical approximation, Eq. (2), while the circles indicate the results of the direct computer simulation (system S1). Standard parameter values used in the figure are $u_1 = u_2 = 5.0 \cdot 10^{-7}$, $u_3 = 0.01$, $M = 10^6$, $r = 0.2$, $a = 0.3$, $d = b = 0.1$.

Figure S3 The expected number of type-1 cells at diagnosis. The figure shows the dependence of the expected number of type-1 cells at diagnosis on various parameters. The curves indicate the predictions of the analytical approximation, Eq. (S12), while the circles indicate the results of the direct computer simulation (system S1). Standard parameter values used in the figure are $u_1 = u_2 = 5.0 \cdot 10^{-7}$, $u_3 = 0.01$, $M = 10^6$, $r = 0.2$, $a = 0.3$, $d = b = 0.1$.

Figure S4 The expected number of type-2 cells at diagnosis. The figure shows the dependence of the expected number of type-2 cells at diagnosis on various parameters. The curves indicate the predictions of the analytical approximation, Eq. (S13), while the circles indicate the results of the direct computer simulation (system S1). Standard parameter values used in the figure are $u_1 = u_2 = 5.0 \cdot 10^{-7}$, $u_3 = 0.01$, $M = 10^6$, $r = 0.2$, $a = 0.3$, $d = b = 0.1$.

Figure S5 The probabilities and the expected numbers of each population at diagnosis with large u_1. The figure shows the probabilities of the existence of type-1, -2, and -3 cells and the expected numbers of type-1, -2, and -3 cells at diagnosis in a region of large u_1. The curves indicate the predictions of the analytical approximations, Eq. (1), Eq. (2), Eq. (S11), Eq. (S12), Eq. (S13), and Eq. (S22), while the circles indicate the results of the direct computer simulations (system S1). Parameter values used in the figure are $u_2 = 5.0 \cdot 10^{-7}$, $u_3 = 0.01$, $M = 10^6$, $r = 0.2$, $a = 0.3$, $d = b = 0.1$.

Figure S6 The probabilities and the expected numbers of each population at diagnosis with large u_2. The figure shows the probabilities of the existence of type-1, -2, and -3 cells and the expected numbers of type-1, -2, and -3 cells at diagnosis in a region of large u_2. The curves indicate the predictions of the analytical approximations, Eq. (1), Eq. (2), Eq. (S11), Eq. (S12), Eq. (S13), and Eq. (S22), while the circles indicate the results of the direct computer simulations (system S1). Parameter values used in

the figure are $u_1 = 5.0 \cdot 10^{-7}$, $u_3 = 0.01$, $M = 10^6$, $r = 0.2$, $a = 0.3$, $d = b = 0.1$.
(TIF)

Figure S7 Proportion of clinically significant populations at diagnosis. (A–B) The proportion of type-2 and -3 cells with a growth advantage in the total population at diagnosis is shown in a wide region of u_1, u_2. (C-D) The proportion of type-1 and -3 cells (drug-sensitive cells) in the total population is shown. (E–F) The proportion of type-3 cells arising from type-1 cells in a total type-3 population is shown. Each population at diagnosis is calculated by the formulas, Eq. (S12), Eq. (S13), and Eq. (S22). Parameter values used in the figure are $u_3 = 10^{-2}$, $M = 10^6$, $r = 0.2$, $a = 0.3$, $d = b = 0.1$ (panel A, C, and E); and $a = 0.6$ (panel B, D, and F).
(TIF)

Figure S8 Proportion of clinically significant populations at diagnosis with a low mutation rate, u_3. (A–C) The proportion of type-2 and -3 cells with a growth advantage in the total population at diagnosis is shown in a wide region of u_1, u_2 and the relative growth rate of type-2 and -3 cells to that of type-0 and -1 cells, $(a–b)/(r–d)$. (D–F) The proportion of type-1 and -3 cells (drug-sensitive cells) in the total population is shown. (G–I) The proportion of type-3 cells arising from type-1 cells in a total type-3 population is shown. Each population at diagnosis is calculated by the formulas, Eq. (S12), Eq. (S13), and Eq. (S22). Parameter values used in the figure are $u_2 = 10^{-7}$, $u_3 = 10^{-4}$, $M = 10^6$, $r = 0.2$, $a = 0.3$, $d = b = 0.1$ (panel A, D, and G); $u_1 = 10^{-2}$ (panel B, E, and H); and $u_1 = 10^{-7}$ (panel C, F, and I).
(TIF)

Figure S9 Proportion of clinically significant populations at diagnosis with a low mutation rate, u_3. (A–B) The proportion of type-2 and -3 cells with a growth advantage in the total population at diagnosis is shown in a wide region of u_1, u_2. (C–D) The proportion of type-1 and -3 cells (drug-sensitive cells) in the total population is shown. (E–F) The proportion of type-3 cells arising from type-1 cells in a total type-3 population is shown. Each population at diagnosis is calculated by the formulas, Eq. (S12), Eq. (S13), and Eq. (S22). Parameter values used in the figure are $u_3 = 10^{-4}$, $M = 10^6$, $r = 0.2$, $a = 0.3$, $d = b = 0.1$ (panel A, C, and E); and $a = 0.6$ (panel B, D, and F).
(TIF)

Figure S10 The population composition at relapse and recurrence time intervals in a wide region of u_1 and u_2. The population compositions at diagnosis (the initial time of treatment) and at the time of recurrence after treatment in a wide region of u_1 and u_2 are shown in pie charts. The time periods until the time of recurrence after treatment are shown as numbers under the pie charts. The time of recurrence is defined as the time point when the total number reaches 10% larger than the number at diagnosis. Each result is obtained by averaging a lot of trials by stochastic simulations of the model under treatment (system S23). The parameter values used in the figure except u_1 and u_2 are $u_3 = u_4 = 0.01$, $M = 10^6$, $a = 0.4$, and $d = b = 0.1$. Treatment effects are shown at the top of pie charts as the reduction effects on growth rates of sensitive populations (γ) and those on resistant populations (η).
(TIF)

Materials S1 Supplementary material.
(DOCX)

Table S1 Parameter sets used for the analysis in Supplementary Figure S10 and expected numbers of cells at diagnosis. The expected numbers of type-1, -2, and -3 cells at diagnosis are calculated by Eq. (S12), Eq. (S13), and Eq. (S22). The number of type-0 cells is considered as the rest of the total number. The proportion of each type is shown in parentheses. The cases where the sum of type-0, type-1, type-2, and type-3 cells exceeded M were excluded. Parameter values used in the figure are $u_3 = 0.01$, $M = 10^6$, $r = 0.2$, $a = 0.4$, $d = b = 0.1$.
(EPS)

Acknowledgments

We thank Akira Nakamura, M.D., Ph.D., for the improvements in computational efficiency. In addition, we would like to thank the anonymous referees for valuable comments and suggestions.

Author Contributions

Conceived and designed the experiments: KNY KH ST HH. Performed the experiments: KNY HH. Analyzed the data: KNY HH. Contributed reagents/materials/analysis tools: KNY HH. Wrote the paper: KNY KH ST HH.

References

1. Fackenthal JD, Olopade OI (2007) Breast cancer risk associated with BRCA1 and BRCA2 in diverse populations. Nat Rev Cancer 7: 937–948.
2. Castro E, Goh C, Olmos D, Saunders E, Leongamornlert D, et al. (2013) Germline BRCA mutations are associated with higher risk of nodal involvement, distant metastasis, and poor survival outcomes in prostate cancer. J Clin Oncol 31: 1748–1757.
3. Skoulidis F, Cassidy LD, Pisupati V, Jonasson JG, Bjarnason H, et al. (2010) Germline Brca2 heterozygosity promotes Kras(G12D) -driven carcinogenesis in a murine model of familial pancreatic cancer. Cancer Cell 18: 499–509.
4. Pennington KP, Walsh T, Lee M, Pennil C, Novetsky AP, et al. (2013) BRCA1, TP53, and CHEK2 germline mutations in uterine serous carcinoma. Cancer 119: 332–338.
5. Cancer Genome Atlas N (2012) Comprehensive molecular portraits of human breast tumours. Nature 490: 61–70.
6. Greenup R, Buchanan A, Lorizio W, Rhoads K, Chan S, et al. (2013) Prevalence of BRCA mutations among women with triple-negative breast cancer (TNBC) in a genetic counseling cohort. Ann Surg Oncol 20: 3254–3258.
7. Cancer Genome Atlas Research N (2011) Integrated genomic analyses of ovarian carcinoma. Nature 474: 609–615.
8. Buchholz TA, Wu X, Hussain A, Tucker SL, Mills GB, et al. (2002) Evidence of haplotype insufficiency in human cells containing a germline mutation in BRCA1 or BRCA2. Int J Cancer 97: 557–561.
9. Rennstam K, Ringberg A, Cunliffe HE, Olsson H, Landberg G, et al. (2010) Genomic alterations in histopathologically normal breast tissue from BRCA1 mutation carriers may be caused by BRCA1 haploinsufficiency. Genes Chromosomes Cancer 49: 78–90.
10. Roy R, Chun J, Powell SN (2012) BRCA1 and BRCA2: different roles in a common pathway of genome protection. Nat Rev Cancer 12: 68–78.
11. Martin RW, Orelli BJ, Yamazoe M, Minn AJ, Takeda S, et al. (2007) RAD51 up-regulation bypasses BRCA1 function and is a common feature of BRCA1-deficient breast tumors. Cancer Res 67: 9658–9665.
12. King TA, Li W, Brogi E, Yee CJ, Gemignani ML, et al. (2007) Heterogenic loss of the wild-type BRCA allele in human breast tumorigenesis. Ann Surg Oncol 14: 2510–2518.
13. Mullany LK, Fan HY, Liu Z, White LD, Marshall A, et al. (2011) Molecular and functional characteristics of ovarian surface epithelial cells transformed by KrasG12D and loss of Pten in a mouse model in vivo. Oncogene 30: 3522–3536.
14. Wu R, Baker SJ, Hu TC, Norman KM, Fearon ER, et al. (2013) Type I to type II ovarian carcinoma progression: mutant Trp53 or Pik3ca confers a more aggressive tumor phenotype in a mouse model of ovarian cancer. Am J Pathol 182: 1391–1399.
15. D'Andrea AD, Grompe M (2003) The Fanconi anaemia/BRCA pathway. Nat Rev Cancer 3: 23–34.
16. Patel KJ, Yu VP, Lee H, Corcoran A, Thistlethwaite FC, et al. (1998) Involvement of Brca2 in DNA repair. Mol Cell 1: 347–357.
17. Shen SX, Weaver Z, Xu X, Li C, Weinstein M, et al. (1998) A targeted disruption of the murine Brca1 gene causes gamma-irradiation hypersensitivity and genetic instability. Oncogene 17: 3115–3124.

18. Alexandrov LB, Nik-Zainal S, Wedge DC, Aparicio SA, Behjati S, et al. (1998) A targeted disruption of the murine Brca1 gene causes gamma-irradiation hypersensitivity and genetic instability. Oncogene 17: 3115–3124.
19. Kandoth C, McLellan MD, Vandin F, Ye K, Niu B, et al. (2013) Mutational landscape and significance across 12 major cancer types. Nature 502: 333–339.
20. Agarwal R, Kaye SB (2003) Ovarian cancer: strategies for overcoming resistance to chemotherapy. Nat Rev Cancer 3: 502–516.
21. Taniguchi T, Tischkowitz M, Ameziane N, Hodgson SV, Mathew CG, et al. (2003) Disruption of the Fanconi anemia-BRCA pathway in cisplatin-sensitive ovarian tumors. Nat Med 9: 568–574.
22. Cass I, Baldwin RL, Varkey T, Moslehi R, Narod SA, et al. (2003) Improved survival in women with BRCA-associated ovarian carcinoma. Cancer 97: 2187–2195.
23. Tan DS, Rothermundt C, Thomas K, Bancroft E, Eeles R, et al. (2008) "BRCAness" syndrome in ovarian cancer: a case-control study describing the clinical features and outcome of patients with epithelial ovarian cancer associated with BRCA1 and BRCA2 mutations. J Clin Oncol 26: 5530–5536.
24. Lee JM, Ledermann JA, Kohn EC (2014) PARP Inhibitors for BRCA1/2 mutation-associated and BRCA-like malignancies. Ann Oncol 25: 32–40.
25. Farmer H, McCabe N, Lord CJ, Tutt AN, Johnson DA, et al. (2005) Targeting the DNA repair defect in BRCA mutant cells as a therapeutic strategy. Nature 434: 917–921.
26. Galluzzi L, Senovilla L, Vitale I, Michels J, Martins I, et al. (2012) Molecular mechanisms of cisplatin resistance. Oncogene 31: 1869–1883.
27. Sakai W, Swisher EM, Karlan BY, Agarwal MK, Higgins J, et al. (2008) Secondary mutations as a mechanism of cisplatin resistance in BRCA2-mutated cancers. Nature 451: 1116–1120.
28. Edwards SL, Brough R, Lord CJ, Natrajan R, Vatcheva R, et al. (2008) Resistance to therapy caused by intragenic deletion in BRCA2. Nature 451: 1111–1115.
29. Norquist B, Wurz KA, Pennil CC, Garcia R, Gross J, et al. (2011) Secondary somatic mutations restoring BRCA1/2 predict chemotherapy resistance in hereditary ovarian carcinomas. J Clin Oncol 29: 3008–3015.
30. Barber LJ, Sandhu S, Chen L, Campbell J, Kozarewa I, et al. (2013) Secondary mutations in BRCA2 associated with clinical resistance to a PARP inhibitor. J Pathol 229: 422–429.
31. Cooke SL, Ng CK, Melnyk N, Garcia MJ, Hardcastle T, et al. (2010) Genomic analysis of genetic heterogeneity and evolution in high-grade serous ovarian carcinoma. Oncogene 29: 4905–4913.
32. Iwasa Y, Nowak MA, Michor F (2006) Evolution of resistance during clonal expansion. Genetics 172: 2557–2566.
33. De Vargas Roditi L, Michor F (2011) Evolutionary dynamics of BRCA1 alterations in breast tumorigenesis. J Theor Biol 273: 207–215.
34. Enderling H, Chaplain MA, Anderson AR, Vaidya JS (2007) A mathematical model of breast cancer development, local treatment and recurrence. J Theor Biol 246: 245–259.
35. Danesh K, Durrett R, Havrilesky LJ, Myers E (2012) A branching process model of ovarian cancer. J Theor Biol 314: 10–15.
36. Foo J, Michor F (2010) Evolution of resistance to anti-cancer therapy during general dosing schedules. J Theor Biol 263: 179–188.
37. Leder K, Foo J, Skaggs B, Gorre M, Sawyers CL, et al. (2011) Fitness conferred by BCR-ABL kinase domain mutations determines the risk of pre-existing resistance in chronic myeloid leukemia. PLoS One 6: e27682.
38. Diaz LA Jr, Williams RT, Wu J, Kinde I, Hecht JR, et al. (2012) The molecular evolution of acquired resistance to targeted EGFR blockade in colorectal cancers. Nature 486: 537–540.
39. van Leeuwen IM, Byrne HM, Jensen OE, King JR (2006) Crypt dynamics and colorectal cancer: advances in mathematical modelling. Cell Prolif 39: 157–181.
40. Johnston MD, Edwards CM, Bodmer WF, Maini PK, Chapman SJ (2007) Mathematical modeling of cell population dynamics in the colonic crypt and in colorectal cancer. Proc Natl Acad Sci U S A 104: 4008–4013.
41. Komarova NL, Wodarz D (2007) Stochastic modeling of cellular colonies with quiescence: an application to drug resistance in cancer. Theor Popul Biol 72: 523–538.
42. Beerenwinkel N, Antal T, Dingli D, Traulsen A, Kinzler KW, et al. (2007) Genetic progression and the waiting time to cancer. PLoS Comput Biol 3: e225.
43. Haeno H, Maruvka YE, Iwasa Y, Michor F (2013) Stochastic Tunneling of Two Mutations in a Population of Cancer Cells. PLoS One 8: e65724.
44. Iijima J, Zeng Z, Takeda S, Taniguchi Y (2010) RAP80 acts independently of BRCA1 in repair of topoisomerase II poison-induced DNA damage. Cancer Res 70: 8467–8474.
45. Lengauer C, Kinzler KW, Vogelstein B (1997) Genetic instability in colorectal cancers. Nature 386: 623–627.
46. Kunkel TA, Bebenek K (2000) DNA replication fidelity. Annu Rev Biochem 69: 497–529.
47. Yamamoto KN, Kobayashi S, Tsuda M, Kurumizaka H, Takata M, et al. (2011) Involvement of SLX4 in interstrand cross-link repair is regulated by the Fanconi anemia pathway. Proc Natl Acad Sci U S A 108: 6492–6496.
48. Khalique L, Ayhan A, Weale ME, Jacobs IJ, Ramus SJ, et al. (2007) Genetic intra-tumour heterogeneity in epithelial ovarian cancer and its implications for molecular diagnosis of tumours. J Pathol 211: 286–295.
49. Torres L, Ribeiro FR, Pandis N, Andersen JA, Heim S, et al. (2007) Intratumor genomic heterogeneity in breast cancer with clonal divergence between primary carcinomas and lymph node metastases. Breast Cancer Res Treat 102: 143–155.
50. Ahmed AA, Etemadmoghadam D, Temple J, Lynch AG, Riad M, et al. (2010) Driver mutations in TP53 are ubiquitous in high grade serous carcinoma of the ovary. J Pathol 221: 49–56.
51. Liu G, Yang D, Sun Y, Shmulevich I, Xue F, et al. (2012) Differing clinical impact of BRCA1 and BRCA2 mutations in serous ovarian cancer. Pharmacogenomics 13: 1523–1535.
52. Noh JM, Han BK, Choi DH, Rhee SJ, Cho EY, et al. (2013) Association between BRCA Mutation Status, Pathological Findings, and Magnetic Resonance Imaging Features in Patients with Breast Cancer at Risk for the Mutation. J Breast Cancer 16: 308–314.
53. Bayani J, Brenton JD, Macgregor PF, Beheshti B, Albert M, et al. (2002) Parallel analysis of sporadic primary ovarian carcinomas by spectral karyotyping, comparative genomic hybridization, and expression microarrays. Cancer Res 62: 3466–3476.
54. Jones R, Ryan M, Friedlander M (2003) Carboplatin hypersensitivity reactions: re-treatment with cisplatin desensitisation. Gynecologic Oncology 89: 112–115.
55. Ledermann J, Harter P, Gourley C, Friedlander M, Vergote I, et al. (2012) Olaparib maintenance therapy in platinum-sensitive relapsed ovarian cancer. N Engl J Med 366: 1382–1392.
56. Omura GA, Brady MF, Homesley HD, Yordan E, Major FJ, et al. (1991) Long-term follow-up and prognostic factor analysis in advanced ovarian carcinoma: the Gynecologic Oncology Group experience. J Clin Oncol. 9: 1138–50.
57. Bayraktar S, Gluck S (2012) Systemic therapy options in BRCA mutation-associated breast cancer. Breast Cancer Res Treat 135: 355–366.
58. Gelmon KA, Tischkowitz M, Mackay H, Swenerton K, Robidoux A, et al. (2011) Olaparib in patients with recurrent high-grade serous or poorly differentiated ovarian carcinoma or triple-negative breast cancer: a phase 2, multicentre, open-label, non-randomised study. The Lancet Oncology 12: 852–861.
59. Shah SP, Roth A, Goya R, Oloumi A, Ha G, et al. (2012) The clonal and mutational evolution spectrum of primary triple-negative breast cancers. Nature 486: 395–399.
60. Lord CJ, Ashworth A (2013) Mechanisms of resistance to therapies targeting BRCA-mutant cancers. Nat Med 19: 1381–1388.
61. Fong PC, Boss DS, Yap TA, Tutt A, Wu P, et al. (2009) Inhibition of poly(ADP-ribose) polymerase in tumors from BRCA mutation carriers. N Engl J Med 361: 123–134.
62. Liu M, Mo QG, Wei CY, Qin QH, Huang Z, et al. (2013) Platinum-based chemotherapy in triple-negative breast cancer: A meta-analysis. Oncol Lett 5: 983–991.
63. Kim A, Ueda Y, Naka T, Enomoto T (2012) Therapeutic strategies in epithelial ovarian cancer. J Exp Clin Cancer Res 31: 14.
64. Dann RB, DeLoia JA, Timms KM, Zorn KK, Potter J, et al. (2012) BRCA1/2 mutations and expression: response to platinum chemotherapy in patients with advanced stage epithelial ovarian cancer. Gynecol Oncol 125: 677–682.
65. Turner NC, Reis-Filho JS, Russell AM, Springall RJ, Ryder K, et al. (2007) BRCA1 dysfunction in sporadic basal-like breast cancer. Oncogene 26: 2126–2132.
66. Wysham WZ, Mhawech-Fauceglia P, Li H, Hays L, Syriac S, et al. (2012) BRCAness profile of sporadic ovarian cancer predicts disease recurrence. PLoS One 7: e30042.
67. Saal LH, Gruvberger-Saal SK, Persson C, Lovgren K, Jumppanen M, et al. (2008) Recurrent gross mutations of the PTEN tumor suppressor gene in breast cancers with deficient DSB repair. Nat Genet 40: 102–107.

Methylseleninic Acid Sensitizes Notch3-Activated OVCA429 Ovarian Cancer Cells to Carboplatin

Tiffany J. Tzeng[1], Lei Cao[2], YangXin Fu[3], Huawei Zeng[4], Wen-Hsing Cheng[1,2]*

1 Department of Nutrition and Food Science, University of Maryland, College Park, Maryland, United States of America, **2** Department of Food Science, Nutrition and Health Promotion, Mississippi State University, Mississippi State, Mississippi, United States of America, **3** Department of Oncology, University of Alberta, Edmonton, Alberta, Canada, **4** USDA, Agriculture Research Service, Grand Forks Human Research Center, Grand Forks, North Dakota, United States of America

Abstract

Ovarian cancer, the deadliest of gynecologic cancers, is usually not diagnosed until advanced stages. Although carboplatin has been popular for treating ovarian cancer for decades, patients eventually develop resistance to this platinum-containing drug. Expression of neurogenic locus notch homolog 3 (Notch3) is associated with chemoresistance and poor overall survival in ovarian cancer patients. Overexpression of NICD3 (the constitutively active form of Notch3) in OVCA429 ovarian cancer cells (OVCA429/NICD3) renders them resistance to carboplatin treatment compared to OVCA429/pCEG cells expressing an empty vector. We have previously shown that methylseleninic acid (MSeA) induces oxidative stress and activates ataxia-telangiectasia mutated and DNA-dependent protein kinase in cancer cells. Here we tested the hypothesis that MSeA and carboplatin exerted a synthetic lethal effect on OVCA429/NICD3 cells. Co-treatment with MSeA synergistically sensitized OVCA429/NICD3 but not OVCA429/pCEG cells to the killing by carboplatin. This synergism was associated with a cell cycle exit at the G2/M phase and the induction of NICD3 target gene *HES1*. Treatment of *N*-acetyl cysteine or inhibitors of the above two kinases did not directly impact on the synergism in OVCA429/NICD3 cells. Taken together, these results suggest that the efficacy of carboplatin in the treatment of high grade ovarian carcinoma can be enhanced by a combinational therapy with MSeA.

Editor: Reiner Albert Veitia, Institut Jacques Monod, France

Funding: This study was partially supported by Maryland Agricultural Experimental Station and Mississippi Agricultural and Forestry Experimental Station (to W.-H. Cheng), and by Women and Children's Health Research Institute with funding donated by the Royal Alexandra Hospital Foundation, Canada (to Y. Fu). The funders had no role in study design, data collection and analysis, decision to publish, or preparation of the manuscript.

Competing Interests: The authors have declared that no competing interests exist.

* Email: wcheng@fsnhp.msstate.edu

Introduction

Results from geographic, animal and clinical studies strongly point to a positive association between selenium and chemoprevention [1–3]. Nonetheless, supranutritional intake of dietary selenium in the form of selenomethionine does not prevent prostate cancer [4]. Among the many selenium compounds, methylseleninic acid (MSeA) has been demonstrated to be exceptionally effective in counteracting prostate, pancreatic and breast cancers in mice [5–8]. The efficacy of selenium chemoprevention also depends on baseline selenium status and genetic background [9]. MSeA is metabolized to methylselenol, eventually resulting in the formation of selenium dioxide, superoxide anion, and hydrogen peroxide [10,11]. Furthermore, MSeA can activate ataxia-telangiectasia mutated (ATM) and the catalytic subunit of DNA-dependent protein kinase (DNA-PK_{cs}), two critical DNA damage response kinases, in cancer cells [12–14].

Mammals express four neurogenic locus notch homolog (Notch) family proteins during tumorigenesis and embryogenesis [15,16]. Unlike many other signaling molecules, activation of the Notch pathway does not require secondary messengers for amplification [17]. Upon ligand binding to the N-terminal EGF-repeat region, the Notch transmembrane receptor undergoes a series of proteolytic cleavages by tumor necrosis factor-α-converting enzyme, metalloprotease, and γ-secretase [18]. γ-Secretase cleavage releases the Notch intraceullular domain (NICD) into cytoplasm, followed by translocation to the nucleus for transactivation of a spectrum of genes involved in tumor development and progression [19–21]. Thus, targeting Notch is considered promising for the improvement of platinum-based chemotherapy [22].

Platinum compounds have been approved by US Food and Drug Administration for cancer treatment since 1979. With reduced side effects, carboplatin [*cis*-diammine (1,1-cyclobutanedicarboxylato) platinum(II)] is the most effective second generation platinum compound for treatment of ovarian and testicular cancer [23,24]. Carboplatin alkylates DNA bases and forms monoadducts, the majority of which eventually are converted into DNA crosslinks [25,26]. Interestingly, cells uptake carboplatin in a manner depending on a copper transporter, CTR1 [27–29].

Most ovarian cancer patients are diagnosed at an advanced stage because of the lack of validated screening tests. Despite of being the most effective drug to treat ovarian cancer, resistance to carboplatin develops in some high grade tumors. Aberrant Notch activation is strongly associated with carboplatin resistance [22,30,31]. In particular, Notch3 is overexpressed in 66% of high grade ovarian carcinoma [32], 22% of which at stages II–IV exhibit altered Notch signaling [33]. Given such findings, the studies reported herein were designed to determine whether MSeA could sensitize Notch3-activated ovarian cancer cells to carboplatin treatment.

Materials and Methods

Cell culture and chemicals

OVCA429 cells were isolated from a patient with late stage, cisplatin-resistant ovarian carcinoma. OVCA429/pCEG cells carrying a green fluorescence protein empty vector and OVCA429/NICD3 cells constitutively expressing green fluorescence protein tagged with NICD3 were sorted by a fluorescence-activated cell sorter and maintained in RPMI 1640 medium (Mediatech Inc, Herndon, VA) supplemented with 10% heat-inactivated fetal bovine serum and 100 U/mL penicillin and streptomycin at 37°C in a 5% CO_2 incubator [34]. *N*-acetyl cysteine (NAC) and MSeA (Sigma-Aldrich, St. Louis, MO) were dissolved in phosphate-buffered saline. NAC is an antioxidant that mainly abolishes hydrogen peroxide. Carboplatin (Enzo Life Sciences, Farmingdale, NY) was dissolved in water. KU 60019 and NU 7026 (Tocris, Ellisville, MO) were dissolved in dimethyl sulfoxide, and were ATP-competitive, selective chemical inhibitors of the kinase activity of ATM and DNA-PK_{cs} [35], respectively.

Cell viability

Sulforhodamine B (SRB) colorimetric assays were performed as described previously [36]. Briefly, cells were seeded (10^5 cells/well) in 96-well plates and allowed for attachment overnight prior to drug treatment. Then, cells were fixed with 10% trichloroacetic acid for 1 h at 4 °C, washed 5 times with water and air dried, and then stained with 0.4% SRB in 1% acetic acid for 20 minutes at room temperature. Unbound dye was removed by gently washing the cells 5 times with 1% acetic acid. After being air dried, cells were incubated with 200 μL of tris(hydroxymethyl)aminomethane buffer (pH 10.5, 10 mmol/L) for 30 minutes at 37 °C. The optical density was measured by a plate reader (BMG LabTech, Cary, NC) at 492 nm. Percent cell viability was calculated using the formula [36]:

% cell viability = $[(\text{meanOD}_{\text{sample}} - \text{meanOD}_{\text{day 0}})/(\text{meanOD}_{\text{neg control}} - \text{meanOD}_{\text{day 0}})] \times 100\%$"

Cell viability was further analyzed by calculating combination index (CI) values with the Calcusyn software (Biosoft) based on the theorem of Chou-Talalay. The synergy CI scale is from 1 to 0 and the antagonism is from 1 to infinity [37].

Immunofluorescence

Immunofluorescent analyses of ATM phosphorylation on Ser-1981 (pATMS1981), DNA-PK_{cs} phosphorylation on Ser-2056 (pDNA-PK_{cs}S2056) and H2AX phosphorylation on Ser-139 (γH2AX) were performed as described previously [14,38,39]. All images were taken under the same parameters of brightness, contrast, and exposure time and processed by deconvolution using AxioVision Release 4.7.2.0 coupled to a Zeiss Axio Observer Z1m fluorescence microscope (Zeiss, Thornwood, NY). Five pictures were randomly taken from each slide (n = 3).

Cell cycle and selenium analyses

Flow cytometric analyses of cell cycle were performed as described previously [12]. Cells were analyzed by a FACScalibur cytometer with CELLQuest program (Becton Dickinson, San Jose, CA). ModFit LT (Version 3.0, Verity Software House, Topsham, ME) was applied for cell cycle analysis on overlaid histograms. Intracellular selenium concentrations were determined as described previously [40,41].

RNA isolation and quantitative RT-PCR (qRT-PCR)

Total RNA was isolated by using chloroform for phase separation, isopropanol for RNA precipitation, 75% ethanol for RNA wash, RNase-free water for RNA resuspension, and DNase-treated before cDNA was synthesized using High-Capacity cDNA Reverse Transcription kit (Life Technologya) in the presence of RNase inhibitor. qRT-PCR was carried out using the SYBR Green method on an Applied Biosystems 7500 Fast Real-time (Applied Biosystems, Foster Ciet, CA). Sequences of the primers for qPCR are listed in Table S1 in File S1.

Statistics

These data were analyzed by using SAS 9.0 (SAS Institute Inc., Cary, NC). Two-tailed student's *t*-test was applied to determine statistical significance ($p < 0.05$) between the treatment and the respective control groups.

Results

Synergistic lethality of MSeA and carboplatin in OVCA429/NICD3 cells

Ovarian carcinomas expressing NICD3 are resistant to platinum therapeutic agents [22,30,31]. We have previously shown that MSeA treatment (LD_{50}, 4 μmol/L) kills HCT116 colorectal, PC-3 prostate and U-2 OS osteosarcoma cells in association with reactive oxygen species (ROS), ATM and DNA-PK_{cs} [12,13]. Because ROS are also implicated in Notch3 signaling pathway [42,43], we tested the hypothesis that MSeA could repress the desensitization of OVCA429/NICD3 ovarian cancer cells to carboplatin. Results from SRB survival assays demonstrated that MSeA (0.25–2 μmol/L, Figure 1A) or carboplatin (1–25 μmol/L, Figure 1B) alone dose-dependently killed more OVCA429/pCEG than OVCA429/NICD3 cells. Results from combinational treatment (Table 1) suggested that MSeA (2 μmol/L) and carboplatin (1-25 μmol/L) synergistically sensitized OVCA429/NICD3 cells (Figure 1D) but not OVCA429/pCEG cells (Figure 1C). Further CI analyses confirmed strong synergism between MSeA (2 μmol/L) and carboplatin (1–25 μmol/L) in OVCA429/NICD3 cells (Table 2). The synergism was linearly enhanced as carboplatin concentrations increased. Interestingly, based on CI values (Table 2), moderate to strong antagonism occurred after co-treatment with MSeA at 2 μmol/L in OVCA429/pCEG cells and ≤ 1 μmol/L in some of the OVCA429/NICD3 cells. In particular, the MSeA (2 μmol/L) and carboplatin (25 μmol/L) co-treatment sensitized the refractory OVCA429/NICD3 cells to an extent reminiscent of that in OVCA429/pCEG cells (36.2 vs. 30.2% survival). Taken together, MSeA can synergistically sensitize Notch3-activated OVCA ovarian cancer cells to the traditional carboplatin treatment at pharmacologically achievable concentrations.

Cell cycle analysis of OVCA429/pCEG and OVCA429/NICD3 cells co-treated with MSeA and carboplatin

In the absence of MSeA and carboplatin, there were greater G2/M and less G1 and S populations ($p < 0.05$) in OVCA429/NICD3 than in OVCA429/pCEG cells (Table 3). Two days after co-treatment of MSeA (2 μmol/L) and carboplatin (5 μmol/L), S and G2/M population was significantly decreased ($p < 0.05$) in OVCA429/pCEG and OVCA429/NICD3 cells, respectively. OVCA429/pCEG and OVCA429/NICD3 cells comparably

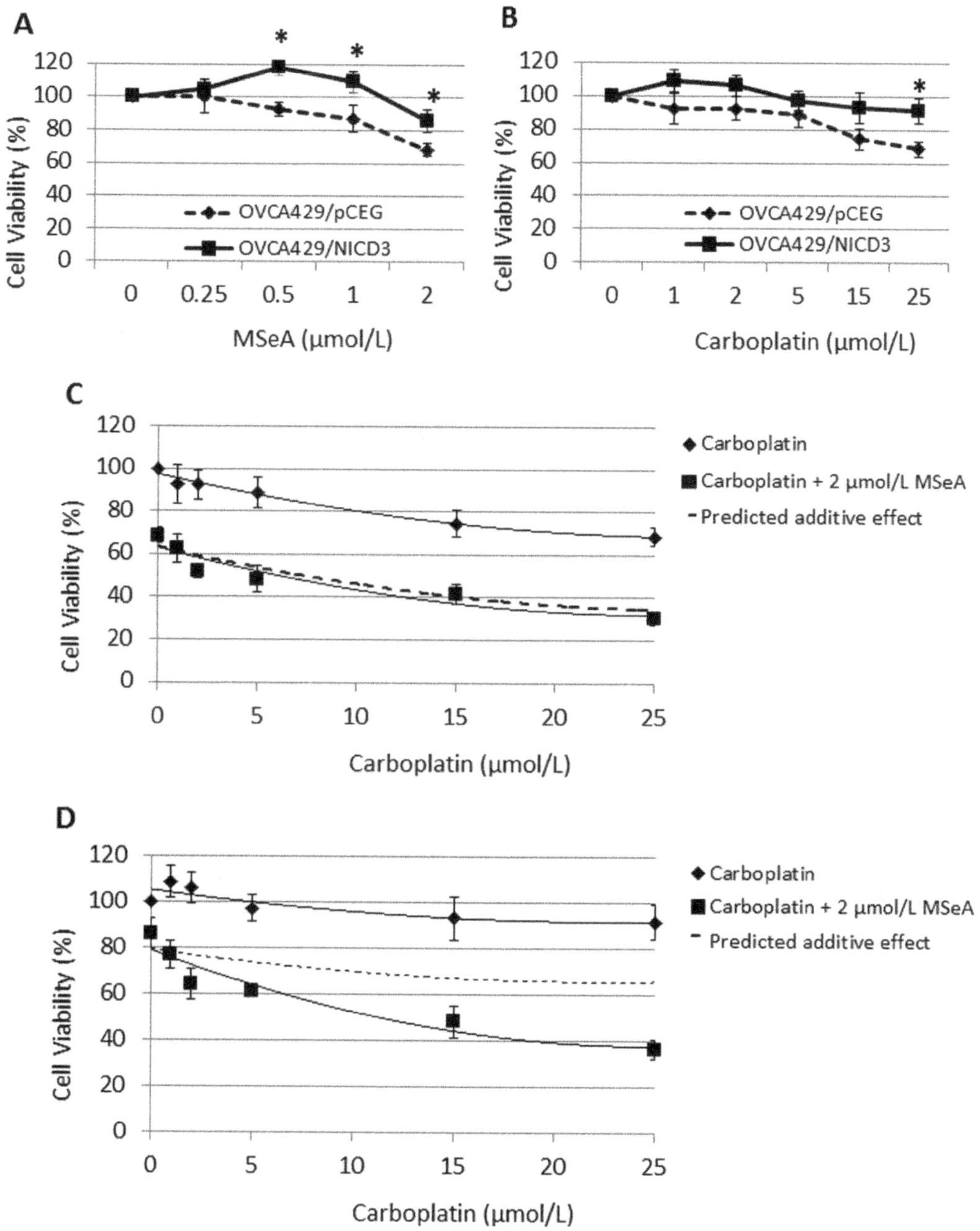

Figure 1. Synergistic effect of MSeA and carboplatin on the killing of OVCA429/NICD3 cells. OVCA429/pCEG and OVCA429/NICD3 cancer cells were treated with a gradient concentration of MSeA (*A*) or carboplatin (*B*) for 2 days. *, $p < 0.05$, compare to OVCA429/pCEG cells. OVCA429/pCEG cells (*C*) and OVCA429/NICD3 cells (*D*) were treated with carboplatin (0–25 μmol/L) in the absence or presence of MSeA (2 μmol/L) for 2 days. Values are mean ± S.E.M. (n = 3). Dashed lines predict the additive effect of MSeA and carboplatin.

displayed a time-dependent induction of DNA fragmentation after the co-treatment as evidenced by sub-G1 populations. These results suggest that the co-treatment differentially target the S phase in OVCA429/pCEG cells and the G2/M phase in OVCA429/NICD3 cells.

Effect of NAC, KU 60019, and NU 7026 on the sensitivity of OVCA429/pCEG and OVCA429/NICD3 cells to the MSeA and carboplatin co-treatment

Next, we determined whether redox status and the kinase activities of ATM and DNA-PK_{cs} were involved in the sensitivity of OVCA429/pCEG and OVCA429/NICD3 cells to the MSeA and carboplatin co-treatment. In the presence of NAC (10 mmol/L), the killing effect of MSeA and carboplatin was greatly alleviated in both cell lines (Figures 2A–2D). In contrast, the presence of KU 60019 (3 μmol/L) or NU 7026 (10 μmol/L) did not alter the sensitivity of OVCA429/pCEG or OVCA429/NICD3 cells to gradient concentrations of MSeA and carboplatin co-treatment (Figure 3). These results suggest that the induction of ROS, but not ATM or DNA-PK_{cs} kinase activities, is involved in the killing effect of MSeA and carboplatin co-treatment.

Table 1. Sensitivity of OVCA429/pCEG and OVCA429/NICD3 ovarian cancer cells to MSeA and carboplatin treatment.

OVCA429/pCEG						
MSeA (μmol/L)	**Carboplatin (μmol/L)**					
	0	**1**	**2**	**5**	**15**	**25**
0	100	92.5±9.4	92.2±7.1	88.8±7.2	74.4±6.1*	68.4±4.3*
0.25	100.2±10.2	90.0±5.4	89.9±7.9	93.5±13.8	75.3±7.2	66.1±11.3
0.5	92.7±4.4	94.1±6.4	89.9±7.5	84.2±8.6	75.2±7.5	63.5±9.6
1	87.1±8.2	82.3±6.5	77.9±6.6	76.5±4.0	61.4±3.6	47.6±0.7$^{\#*}$
2	68.5±3.5$^{\#}$	62.6±6.4	51.7±3.1$^{\#*}$	48.3±6.1$^{\#*}$	41.3±4.6$^{\#*}$	30.3±3.2$^{\#*}$
OVCA429/NICD3						
MSeA (μmol/L)	**Carboplatin (μmol/L)**					
	0	**1**	**2**	**5**	**15**	**25**
0	100	108.5±7.0	106.0±6.4	97.1±5.7	93.2±9.3	91.7±7.5
0.25	104.6±3.5	101.7±5.2	101.8±5.9	105.2±6.8	98.3±5.2	96.5±10.6
0.5	117.8±4.8$^{\#}$	110.3±5.2	118.3±4.6	104.7±4.9	95.8±6.0*	83.6±9.8*
1	109.3±6.5	103.7±4.0	113.3±3.6	98.8±6.6	88.5±5.5	75.4±8.8*
2	86.1±6.8	76.9±6.1$^{\#}$	64.2±6.6$^{\#}$	61.2±1.2$^{\#*}$	48.2±6.9$^{\#*}$	36.2±4.4$^{\#*}$

Cells were cultured in 96-well plates and treated with MSeA and carboplatin at the indicated concentration for 2 days. Cell viability was determined by SRB assay. The condition without MSeA or carboplatin treatment was set as 100%. Values are mean ± S.E.M. (n = 3). #, $p < 0.05$, compared to no MSeA treatment. *, $p < 0.05$, compared to no carboplatin treatment.

Effect of MSeA and carboplatin on the mRNA expression of Notch target genes in OVCA429/pCEG and OVCA429/NICD3 cells

We next determined whether the mRNA expression of Notch target genes can be altered by MSeA and carboplatin treatment. As expected, *HES1 and HEY1*, classical Notch target genes, were up-regulated in OVCA429/NICD3 cells (Figure 4). *HES1* mRNA expression was increased ($p < 0.05$) 6 and 12 h after MSeA treatment in both OVCA429/pCEG and OVCA429/NICD3 cells, the fold-induction of which was greater in the former than the latter. The MSeA-induced *HES1* mRNA expression subsided at 12 h. In contrast, carboplatin treatment resulted in modest and

Table 2. Combination index (CI) values for MSeA and carboplatin treatment in OVCA429/pCEG and OVCA429/NICD3 ovarian cancer cells.

OVCA429/pCEG					
MSeA (μmol/L)	**Carboplatin (μmol/L)**				
	1	**2**	**5**	**15**	**25**
0.25	0.61	0.98	>3.3	1.12	0.90
0.5	1.46	1.20	1.21	1.31	0.96
1	0.93	0.94	1.13	1.04	0.91
2	1.51	1.47	1.47	1.48	1.41
OVCA429/NICD3					
MSeA (μmol/L)	**Carboplatin (μmol/L)**				
	1	**2**	**5**	**15**	**25**
0.25	0.36	0.63	2.64	2.13	2.66
0.5	2.80	>3.3	2.55	1.53	0.59
1	0.96	>3.3	1.13	0.75	0.34
2	0.26	0.16	0.15	0.09	0.05

Based on a refined description made by an inventor of the theorem of Chou-Talalay, the following descriptions of CI values are employed: <0.3, strong synergism; 0.3–0.7, synergism; 0.7–0.9, moderate or slight synergism; 0.9–1.1, nearly additive; 1.1–1.45, slight or moderate antagonism; 1.45–3.3, antagonism; >3.3, strong antagonism [37]. Cell viability and treatment are as described in Table 1.

Table 3. Flow cytometric analyses of the percent G1, S, and G2/M OVCA429/pCEG and OVCA429/NICD3 cells co-treated with MSeA (2 μmol/L) and carboplatin (5 μmol/L) for 1 or 2 days.

	Day		
	0	1	2
Sub G1, %			
OVCA429/pCEG	0.7±0.1*	2.2±0.4#*	8.9±1.0#
OVCA429/NICD3	1.4±0.1	3.4±0.3#	9.1±0.9#
G1, %			
OVCA429/pCEG	32.7±1.0*	34.7±2.7*	34.0±2.7*
OVCA429/NICD3	13.4±0.6	12.7±0.8	15.7±0.3#
S, %			
OVCA429/pCEG	27.1±3.1*	25.1±2.7*	18.2±1.2#*
OVCA429/NICD3	12.3±0.6	13.9±0.7	12.4±0.8
G2/M, %			
OVCA429/pCEG	39.6±2.5*	38.0±0.5*	38.9±2.5*
OVCA429/NICD3	72.9±0.7	70.0±0.8	62.7±1.1#

Values are mean ± S.E.M. (n = 3). *, $p < 0.05$, compared to OVCA429/NICD3 cells. #, $p < 0.05$, compared to Day 0.

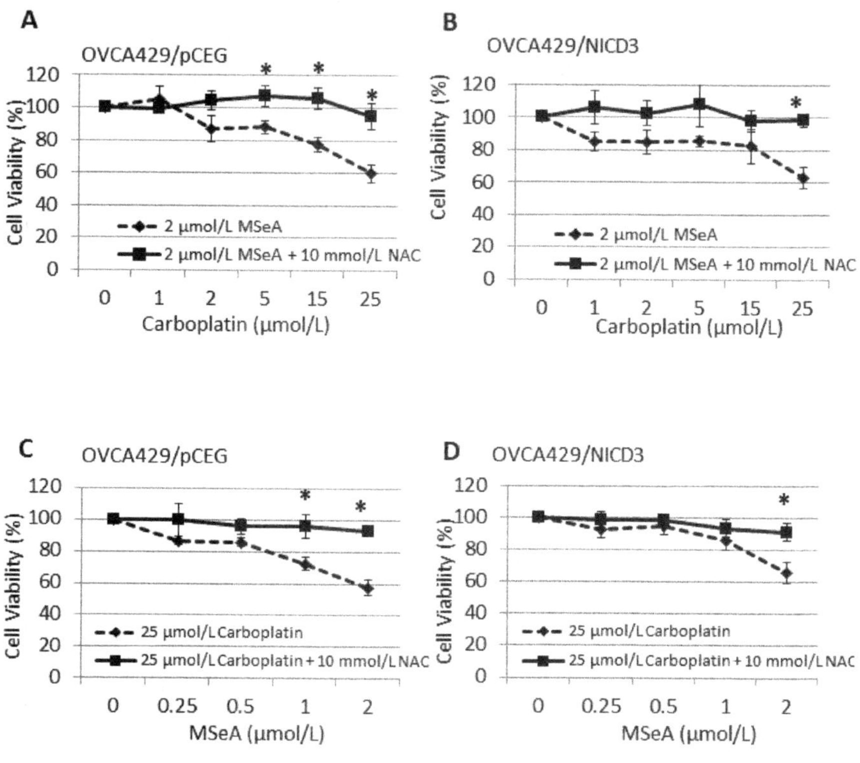

Figure 2. The effect of NAC on the sensitivity of OVCA429/pCEG and OVCA429/NICD3 cells to MSeA and carboplatin co-treatment. OVCA429/pCEG (*A, C*) and OVCA429/NICD3 (*B, D*) cells were treated with MSeA and a gradient concentration of carboplatin (*A, B*) or carboplatin and a gradient concentration of MSeA (*C, D*) in the presence or absence of NAC. Cell viability was determined by SRB assay. Viability of the cells without carboplatin (*A, B*) or MSeA (*C, D*) treatment was set as 100%. Values are mean ± S.E.M. (n = 3). *, $p < 0.05$, compared to MSeA or carboplatin only treatment.

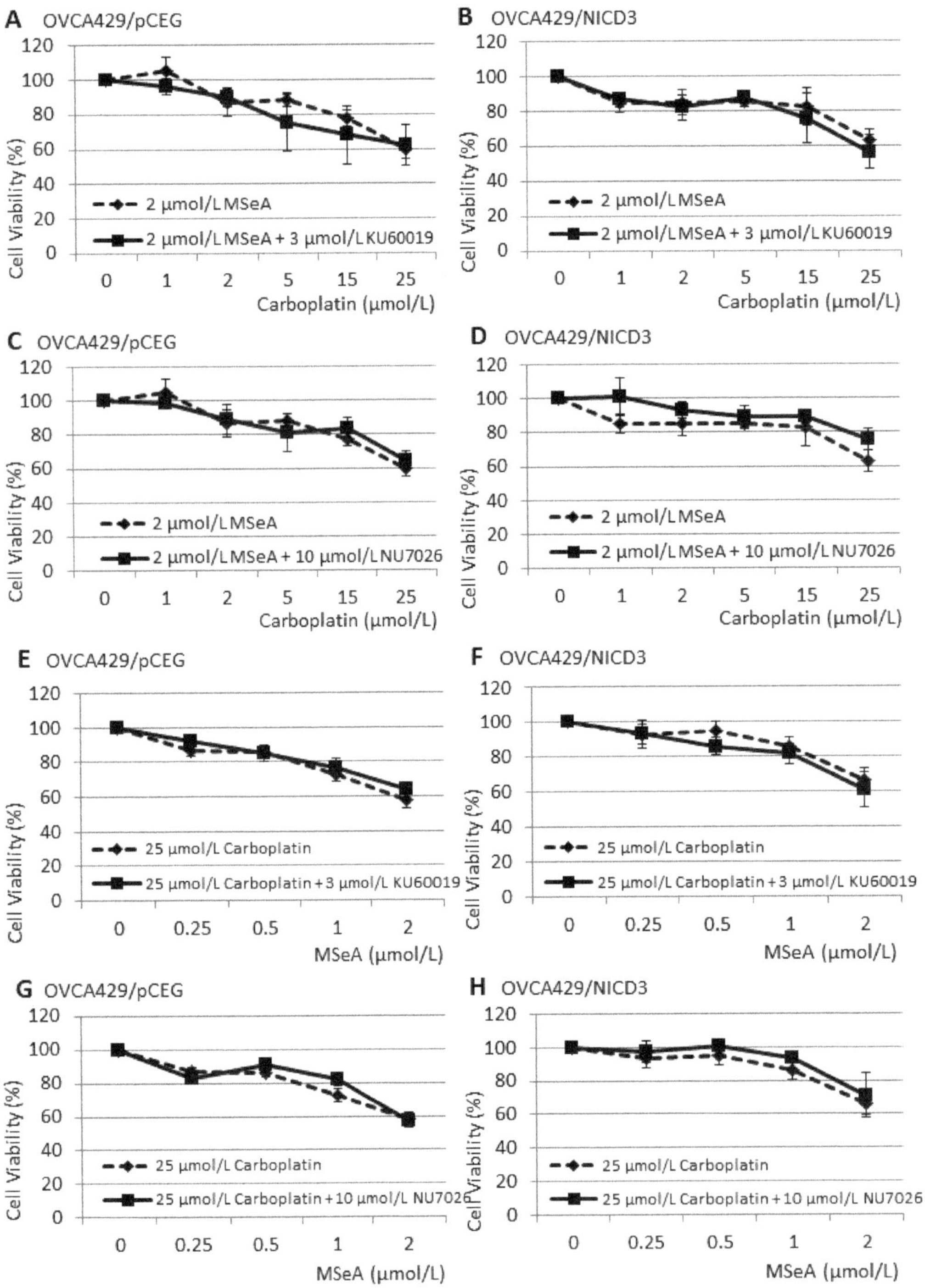

Figure 3. The effect of KU 60019 and NU 7026 on the sensitivity of OVCA429/pCEG and OVCA429/NICD3 cells to MSeA and carboplatin co-treatment. Cells were treated with MSeA and a gradient of carboplatin (*A–D*) or carboplatin and a gradient concentration of MSeA (*E–H*) in the presence or absence of KU 60019 (*A, B, E, F*) and NU 7026 (*C, D, G, H*). Cell viability was determined by SRB assay. Values are mean ± S.E.M. (n = 3).

late induction of *HES1* expression. However, *HEY1* mRNA expression was not affected by MSeA or carboplatin treatment in both OVCA429/pCEG and OVCA429/NICD3 cells. Altogether, MSeA induces the mRNA expression of *HES1* independent of carboplatin or NICD3 expression.

Effect of MSeA and carboplatin co-treatment on the formation of pATMS1981, pDNA-PK$_{cs}$S2056 and γH2AX in OVCA429/pCEG and OVCA429/NICD3 cells

We next assessed cellular DNA damage response to the co-treatment. At 24 h, pDNA-PK$_{cs}$S2056 level rose significantly ($p < 0.05$) and the induction could be completely reversed in the

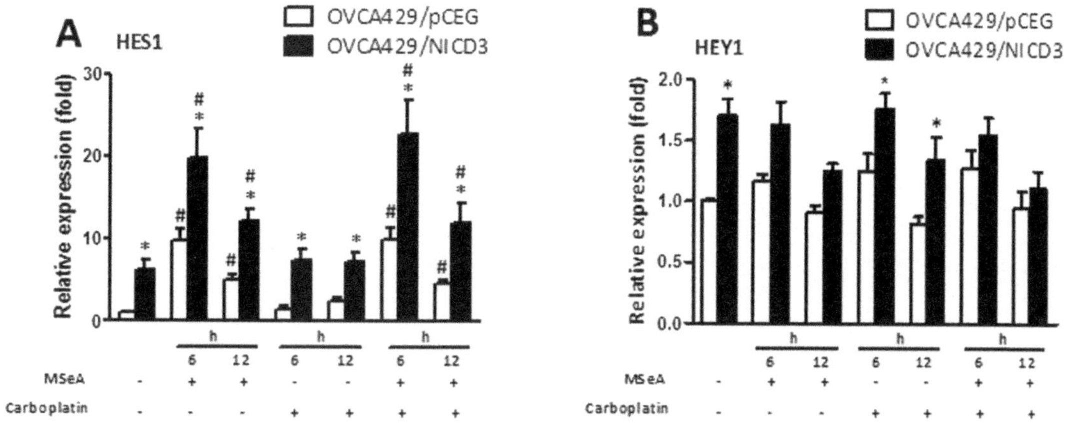

Figure 4. The effect of MSeA and carboplatin on the mRNA expression of *HES1* and *HEY1* in OVCA429/pCEG and OVCA429/NICD3 cells. The mRNA levels were normalized by those of β-actin and presented as fold changes relative to the OVCA429/pCEG cells without MSeA (2 μmol/L) and carboplatin (25 μmol/L) treatment. Values are mean ± S.E.M. (n = 3). *, $p < 0.05$, compared to OVCA429/pCEG cells. #, $p < 0.05$, compared to cells without MSeA and carboplatin treatment.

presence of NU 7026 in both OVCA429/pCEG and OVCA429/NICD3 cells (Figure S1A in File S1). The presence of NAC attenuated pDNA-PK$_{cs}$S2056 expression in OVCA429/pCEG but not in OVCA429/NICD3 cells. On the other hand, pATMS1981 expression was induced ($p < 0.05$) by the co-treatment in OVCA429/pCEG but not in OVCA429/NICD3 cells (Figure S1B in File S1). The induction of pATMS1981 expression was suppressed in the presence of KU 60019 or NAC. The MSeA and carboplatin co-treatment did not induce γH2AX formation (Figure S2 in File S1), which is consistent with previous reports showing that carboplatin treatment, even at a very high dose (100 μmol/L), only slightly induces γH2AX formation in OVCAR-3 ovarian cancer cells [44,45]. Altogether, pDNA-PK$_{cs}$S2056 and pATMS1981 respond differentially to MSeA and carboplatin co-treatment and do not directly correlated with the killing effect in OVCA429/pCEG and OVCA429/NICD3 cells.

Discussion

Results from the present study demonstrate that MSeA can synergistically enhance the efficacy of carboplatin in the killing of OVCA429/NICD3 ovarian cancer cells, suggesting a new strategy to treatment of high grade ovarian carcinoma exhibiting Notch3 activation. Such synergistic effect is likely attributed to the modulation of NICD3 transactivation events regulated by MSeA and carboplatin. Carboplatin treatment or the expression of NICD3 does not affect selenium contents in MSeA-treated cells (OVCA429/pCEG cells, 21.5±2.6 vs. 24.7±1.4 ng/mg protein; OVCA429/NICD3 cells, 26.8±2.9 vs. 25.1±1.4 ng/mg). ROS can contribute to the killing effect of MSeA and carboplatin, but are not required for the synergism in OVCA429/NICD3 cells. Because serum selenium and carboplatin concentrations have been reported to amount 15 and 105 μmol/L, respectively [46,47], the doses of MSeA and carboplatin employed in this study are clinically relevant and pharmacologically achievable. Nonetheless, it is of future interest to confirm the synergism in other Notch3-activated cancer cells and in pre-clinical and clinical settings.

HES1 and *HEY1* are classical NICD3 target genes. HES1 is a transcriptional repressor whose roles in the Notch signaling pathway have begun to be appreciated [30,48]. NICD3 transactivates *HES1* expression by dissociating its co-repressors and allowing co-activators to bind. As a transcriptional repressor, HES1 subsequently can influence cell proliferation. Although HES1 up-regulation is known to promote carcinogenesis [49], there are numerous reports demonstrating down regulation of HES1 in association with prostate cancer progression [50] and in aggressive tumors [51]. Since MSeA induces the mRNA expression of *HES1* but not *HEY1*, MSeA may not directly act on NICD3. Furthermore, MSeA induces a greater *HES1* mRNA expression in OVCA429/pCEG than in OVCA429/NICD3 cells, suggesting that MSeA can stimulate the binding of co-activators independent of NICD3. It is also likely that Notch1 and Notch2 account for the significant HES1 induction in OVCA429/pCEG cells. The differential regulation of MSeA and carboplatin on the mRNA expression of the NICD3 target genes may at least partially explain the synergism in OVCA429/NICD3 cells. However, because treatment with the same doses of MSeA and carboplatin instead result in antagonism in OVCA429/pCEG cells, cautious consideration should be taken pertaining the cell-specific and dose-dependent nature of the synergism. This notion is consistent with the understanding that the range of effective selenium chemoprevention is narrow and cancer-specific [39]. Furthermore, MSeA treatment may promote the expression of some cancer-promoting selenoproteins in OVCA429/pCEG cells [52]. Future studies are needed to elucidate this MSeA-induced transcriptional regulation and to verify the role of HES1 and other Notch target genes in pre-clinical models and clinical samples of ovarian cancer.

Low percent S phase population, as displayed in OVCA429/NICD3 cells, is indicative of rapid DNA replication and poor response to chemotherapy [53,54]. After the MSeA and carboplatin co-treatment, the percent S phase population drops in OVCA429/pCEG cells whereas the percent G2/M population declines in OVCA429/NICD3. The declines amount similarly to the increased sub G1 population, suggesting that the co-treatment may target S phase in OVCA429/pCEG cells and G2/M phase in OVCA429/NICD3 cells for apoptosis. It is possible that the replication stress and DNA breaks induced by carboplatin and MSeA sensitize OVCA429/pCEG cells in the S phase of the cell cycle, but homologous recombination is activated in OVCA429/NICD3 cells. As such, this would require a combinational treatment to induce mitotic stress and target G2/M phase

OVCA429/NICD3 cells to death. Although a combination of gallate and sulforaphane sensitizes advanced stage ovarian cancer cells to cisplatin treatment through G2/M arrest [55], the MSeA and carboplatin co-treatment appears to target S phase OVCA429/pCEG cells and G2/M phase OVCA429/NICD3 cells.

Antioxidant therapy has been proposed to reduce the side effects in association with carboplatin treatment including ototoxicity, nephrotoxicity, and gastrointestinal toxicity [56-59]. However, the impact of oxidative or reductive stress on the treatment of ovarian cancer is not clear. Because NAC treatment desensitizes OVCA429 ovarian cancer cells to carboplatin and MSeA co-treatment independent of NICD3 expression, oxidative stress appears to be a general but not a specific requirement for effective suppression of ovarian cancer cell growth. Consistent with our observation, NAC has been shown to inhibit cisplatin-induced apoptosis in both lung and ovarian cancer cells [56].

It is intriguing that the MSeA and carboplatin co-treatment differentially activates ATM and DNA-PK_{cs} kinases, but inhibition of their kinase activities does not impact on the synergism of MSeA and carboplatin in killing the ovarian cancer cells. After the co-treatment, ROS appear to be required for the activation of ATM but contribute only partially to DNA-PK_{cs} kinase activation in OVCA429/pCEG cells. However, ATM kinase is not activated and DNA-PK_{cs} is activated independent of NAC in OVCA429/NICD3 cells. Although ATM is upstream of DNA-PK_{cs} in the response of MSeA-induced oxidative stress in non-cancerous cells [39], DNA-PK_{cs} activation by the co-treatment in OVCA429/NICD3 cells seems to be independent of ATM activation. Because DNA-PK_{cs} activation can sustain intracellular oxidative stress after MSeA treatment [39], the expression of NICD3 may predispose the cells to oxidative stress. On the other hand, although ATM kinase is activated by oxidative stress in HCT116, PC-3 and U2-OS cancer cells [12-14], it is striking that ATM kinase cannot be activated in OVCA429/NICD3 cells after the co-treatment. Since ovarian cancer stem cells express high levels of ATM [22], the role of ATM in carboplatin-resistant ovarian cancer awaits further verification.

Ovarian cancer is the fifth-leading cause of cancer death among women in the United States. Because most patients are diagnosed at advanced stage due to invalidated screening test and non-specific symptoms presented, they need a combination of debulking surgery and chemotherapy. However, patients typically have recurrent cancer following treatment and even develop chemoresistance. Thus, overcoming the resistance to chemotherapy is one of the promising strategies to treat ovarian cancer. In addition to the combinational effect of MSeA with paclitaxel, curcumin, or ABT-737 in the apoptotic death of prostate and breast cancer cells [60-62], our data provide direct support for a synthetic lethal interaction between MSeA and carboplatin in ovarian cancer cells expressing NICD3 and exhibiting chemoresistance. In conclusion, MSeA and carboplatin synthetic lethality is a promising prospect for late stage ovarian cancer therapy.

Acknowledgments

We thank Changhui Zhao for growing some of the cells, Craig Lacher and William Martin for selenium analysis, and Dr. Nicholas Gaiano for providing the pCEG-NICD3 plasmid.

Approved for publication as Manuscript No. J-12536 of the Mississippi Agricultural and Forestry Experimental Station, Mississippi State University.

Author Contributions

Conceived and designed the experiments: TJT YF WHC. Performed the experiments: TJT LC HZ. Analyzed the data: TJT LC YF HZ WHC. Contributed reagents/materials/analysis tools: YF. Contributed to the writing of the manuscript: TJT WHC.

References

1. Clark LC, Combs GF Jr, Turnbull BW, Slate EH, Chalker DK, et al. (1996) Effects of selenium supplementation for cancer prevention in patients with carcinoma of the skin. A randomized controlled trial. Nutritional Prevention of Cancer Study Group. JAMA 276: 1957–1963.
2. Finley JW, Davis CD, Feng Y (2000) Selenium from high selenium broccoli protects rats from colon cancer. J Nutr 130: 2384–2389.
3. Shamberger RJ, Frost DV (1969) Possible protective effect of selenium against human cancer. Can Med Assoc J 100: 682.
4. Lippman SM, Klein EA, Goodman PJ, Lucia MS, Thompson IM, et al. (2009) Effect of selenium and vitamin E on risk of prostate cancer and other cancers: the Selenium and Vitamin E Cancer Prevention Trial (SELECT). JAMA 301: 39–51.
5. Li GX, Lee HJ, Wang Z, Hu H, Liao JD, et al. (2008) Superior in vivo inhibitory efficacy of methylseleninic acid against human prostate cancer over selenomethionine or selenite. Carcinogenesis 29: 1005–1012.
6. Wang L, Bonorden MJ, Li GX, Lee HJ, Hu H, et al. (2009) Methyl-selenium compounds inhibit prostate carcinogenesis in the transgenic adenocarcinoma of mouse prostate model with survival benefit. Cancer Prev Res (Phila) 2: 484–495.
7. Wang L, Hu H, Wang Z, Xiong H, Cheng Y, et al. (2014) Methylseleninic Acid suppresses pancreatic cancer growth involving multiple pathways. Nutr Cancer 66: 295–307.
8. Wu X, Zhang Y, Pei Z, Chen S, Yang X, et al. (2012) Methylseleninic acid restricts tumor growth in nude mice model of metastatic breast cancer probably via inhibiting angiopoietin-2. BMC Cancer 12: 192.
9. Steinbrenner H, Speckmann B, Sies H (2013) Toward understanding success and failures in the use of selenium for cancer prevention. Antioxid Redox Signal 19: 181–191.
10. Combs GF Jr (2004) Status of selenium in prostate cancer prevention. Br J Cancer 91: 195–199.
11. Zeng H, Combs GF Jr (2008) Selenium as an anticancer nutrient: roles in cell proliferation and tumor cell invasion. J Nutr Biochem 19: 1–7.
12. Cheng WH, Wu RT, Wu M, Rocourt CR, Carrillo JA, et al. (2012) Targeting Werner syndrome protein sensitizes U-2 OS osteosarcoma cells to selenium-induced DNA damage response and necrotic death. Biochem Biophys Res Commun 420: 24–28.
13. Qi Y, Schoene NW, Lartey FM, Cheng WH (2010) Selenium compounds activate ATM-dependent DNA damage response via the mismatch repair protein hMLH1 in colorectal cancer cells. J Biol Chem 285: 33010–33017.
14. Wu M, Kang MM, Schoene NW, Cheng WH (2010) Selenium compounds activate early barriers of tumorigenesis. J Biol Chem 285: 12055–12062.
15. Lobry C, Oh P, Aifantis I (2011) Oncogenic and tumor suppressor functions of Notch in cancer: it's NOTCH what you think. J Exp Med 208: 1931–1935.
16. Maillard I, Pear WS (2003) Notch and cancer: best to avoid the ups and downs. Cancer Cell 3: 203–205.
17. Tien AC, Rajan A, Bellen HJ (2009) A Notch updated. J Cell Biol 184: 621–629.
18. Wang Z, Li Y, Banerjee S, Sarkar FH (2008) Exploitation of the Notch signaling pathway as a novel target for cancer therapy. Anticancer Res 28: 3621–3630.
19. Rizzo P, Osipo C, Foreman K, Golde T, Osborne B, et al. (2008) Rational targeting of Notch signaling in cancer. Oncogene 27: 5124–5131.
20. Wang T, Baron M, Trump D (2008) An overview of Notch3 function in vascular smooth muscle cells. Prog Biophys Mol Biol 96: 499–509.
21. Wang Z, Li Y, Ahmad A, Azmi AS, Banerjee S, et al. (2010) Targeting Notch signaling pathway to overcome drug resistance for cancer therapy. Biochim Biophys Acta 1806: 258–267.
22. McAuliffe SM, Morgan SL, Wyant GA, Tran LT, Muto KW, et al. (2012) Targeting Notch, a key pathway for ovarian cancer stem cells, sensitizes tumors to platinum therapy. Proc Natl Acad Sci U S A 109: E2939–2948.
23. Kelland L (2007) The resurgence of platinum-based cancer chemotherapy. Nat Rev Cancer 7: 573–584.
24. Wheate NJ, Walker S, Craig GE, Oun R (2010) The status of platinum anticancer drugs in the clinic and in clinical trials. Dalton Trans 39: 8113–8127.
25. Cruet-Hennequart S, Villalan S, Kaczmarczyk A, O'Meara E, Sokol AM, et al. (2009) Characterization of the effects of cisplatin and carboplatin on cell cycle

progression and DNA damage response activation in DNA polymerase eta-deficient human cells. Cell Cycle 8: 3039–3050.
26. Deans AJ, West SC (2011) DNA interstrand crosslink repair and cancer. Nat Rev Cancer 11: 467-480.
27. Holzer AK, Manorek GH, Howell SB (2006) Contribution of the major copper influx transporter CTR1 to the cellular accumulation of cisplatin, carboplatin, and oxaliplatin. Mol Pharmacol 70: 1390–1394.
28. Ishida S, Lee J, Thiele DJ, Herskowitz I (2002) Uptake of the anticancer drug cisplatin mediated by the copper transporter Ctr1 in yeast and mammals. Proc Natl Acad Sci U S A 99: 14298–14302.
29. Song IS, Savaraj N, Siddik ZH, Liu P, Wei Y, et al. (2004) Role of human copper transporter Ctr1 in the transport of platinum-based antitumor agents in cisplatin-sensitive and cisplatin-resistant cells. Mol Cancer Ther 3: 1543–1549.
30. Gupta N, Xu Z, El-Sehemy A, Steed H, Fu Y (2013) Notch3 induces epithelial-mesenchymal transition and attenuates carboplatin-induced apoptosis in ovarian cancer cells. Gynecol Oncol 130: 200–206.
31. Park JT, Chen X, Trope CG, Davidson B, Shih Ie M, et al. (2010) Notch3 overexpression is related to the recurrence of ovarian cancer and confers resistance to carboplatin. Am J Pathol 177: 1087–1094.
32. Park JT, Li M, Nakayama K, Mao TL, Davidson B, et al. (2006) Notch3 gene amplification in ovarian cancer. Cancer Res 66: 6312–6318.
33. Cancer Genome Atlas Research N (2011) Integrated genomic analyses of ovarian carcinoma. Nature 474: 609–615.
34. El-Sehemy A, Chang AC, Azad AK, Gupta N, Xu Z, et al. (2013) Notch activation augments nitric oxide/soluble guanylyl cyclase signaling in immortalized ovarian surface epithelial cells and ovarian cancer cells. Cell Signal 25: 2780–2787.
35. Golding SE, Rosenberg E, Valerie N, Hussaini I, Frigerio M, et al. (2009) Improved ATM kinase inhibitor KU-60019 radiosensitizes glioma cells, compromises insulin, AKT and ERK prosurvival signaling, and inhibits migration and invasion. Mol Cancer Ther 8: 2894–2902.
36. Vichai V, Kirtikara K (2006) Sulforhodamine B colorimetric assay for cytotoxicity screening. Nat Protoc 1: 1112–1116.
37. Chou TC (2006) Theoretical basis, experimental design, and computerized simulation of synergism and antagonism in drug combination studies. Pharmacol Rev 58: 621–681.
38. Camphausen K, Brady KJ, Burgan WE, Cerra MA, Russell JS, et al. (2004) Flavopiridol enhances human tumor cell radiosensitivity and prolongs expression of gammaH2AX foci. Mol Cancer Ther 3: 409–416.
39. Rocourt CR, Wu M, Chen BP, Cheng WH (2013) The catalytic subunit of DNA-dependent protein kinase is downstream of ATM and feeds forward oxidative stress in the selenium-induced senescence response. J Nutr Biochem 24: 781–787.
40. Zhang S, Luo Y, Zeng H, Wang Q, Tian F, et al. (2011) Encapsulation of selenium in chitosan nanoparticles improves selenium availability and protects cells from selenium-induced DNA damage response. J Nutr Biochem 22: 1137–1142.
41. Zeng H, Jackson MI, Cheng WH, Combs GF Jr (2011) Chemical form of selenium affects its uptake, transport, and glutathione peroxidase activity in the human intestinal Caco-2 cell model. Biol Trace Elem Res 143: 1209–1218.
42. Chen HH, Chen TW, Lin H (2010) Pravastatin attenuates carboplatin-induced nephrotoxicity in rodents via peroxisome proliferator-activated receptor alpha-regulated heme oxygenase-1. Mol Pharmacol 78: 36–45.
43. Cheng CF, Juan SH, Chen JJ, Chao YC, Chen HH, et al. (2008) Pravastatin attenuates carboplatin-induced cardiotoxicity via inhibition of oxidative stress associated apoptosis. Apoptosis 13: 883–894.
44. Fishel ML, He Y, Smith ML, Kelley MR (2007) Manipulation of base excision repair to sensitize ovarian cancer cells to alkylating agent temozolomide. Clin Cancer Res 13: 260–267.
45. Qian X, LaRochelle WJ, Ara G, Wu F, Petersen KD, et al. (2006) Activity of PXD101, a histone deacetylase inhibitor, in preclinical ovarian cancer studies. Mol Cancer Ther 5: 2086–2095.
46. Fakih MG, Pendyala L, Brady W, Smith PF, Ross ME, et al. (2008) A Phase I and pharmacokinetic study of selenomethionine in combination with a fixed dose of irinotecan in solid tumors. Cancer Chemother Pharmacol 62: 499–508.
47. Oguri S, Sakakibara T, Mase H, Shimizu T, Ishikawa K, et al. (1988) Clinical pharmacokinetics of carboplatin. J Clin Pharmacol 28: 208–215.
48. Kageyama R, Ohtsuka T, Kobayashi T (2007) The Hes gene family: repressors and oscillators that orchestrate embryogenesis. Development 134: 1243–1251.
49. Uchida T, Kitaura J, Nakahara F, Togami K, Inoue D, et al. (2014) Hes1 upregulation contributes to the development of FIP1L1-PDGRA-positive leukemia in blast crisis. Exp Hematol 42: 369–379 e363.
50. Alana L, Sese M, Canovas V, Punyal Y, Fernandez Y, et al. (2014) Prostate tumor OVerexpressed-1 (PTOV1) down-regulates HES1 and HEY1 notch targets genes and promotes prostate cancer progression. Mol Cancer 13: 74.
51. Dailey DD, Anfinsen KP, Pfaff LE, Ehrhart E, Charles JB, et al. (2013) HES1, a target of Notch signaling, is elevated in canine osteosarcoma, but reduced in the most aggressive tumors. BMC Vet Res 9: 130.
52. Hatfield DL, Yoo MH, Carlson BA, Gladyshev VN (2009) Selenoproteins that function in cancer prevention and promotion. Biochim Biophys Acta 1790: 1541–1545.
53. Itamochi H, Kigawa J, Sugiyama T, Kikuchi Y, Suzuki M, et al. (2002) Low proliferation activity may be associated with chemoresistance in clear cell carcinoma of the ovary. Obstet Gynecol 100: 281–287.
54. Kwintkiewicz J, Padilla-Banks E, Jefferson WN, Jacobs IM, Wade PA, et al. (2012) Metastasis-associated protein 3 (MTA3) regulates G2/M progression in proliferating mouse granulosa cells. Biol Reprod 86: 1–8.
55. Chen H, Landen CN, Li Y, Alvarez RD, Tollefsbol TO (2013) Enhancement of Cisplatin-Mediated Apoptosis in Ovarian Cancer Cells through Potentiating G2/M Arrest and p21 Upregulation by Combinatorial Epigallocatechin Gallate and Sulforaphane. J Oncol 2013: 872957.
56. Wu L, Nicholson W, Knobel SM, Steffner RJ, May JM, et al. (2004) Oxidative stress is a mediator of glucose toxicity in insulin-secreting pancreatic islet cell lines. J Biol Chem 279: 12126–12134.
57. Moon IJ, Kim KR, Chu HS, Kim SH, Chung WH, et al. (2011) N-acetylcysteine and N-nitroarginine methyl ester attenuate Carboplatin-induced ototoxicity in dissociated spiral ganglion neuron cultures. Clin Exp Otorhinolaryngol 4: 11–17.
58. Okur E, Kilinc M, Yildirim I, Kilic MA, Tolun FI (2007) Effect of N-acetylcysteine on carboplatin-induced ototoxicity and nitric oxide levels in a rat model. Laryngoscope 117: 2183–2186.
59. Rose SL (2009) Notch signaling pathway in ovarian cancer. Int J Gynecol Cancer 19: 564–566.
60. Guo X, Yin S, Dong Y, Fan L, Ye M, et al. (2013) Enhanced apoptotic effects by the combination of curcumin and methylseleninic acid: potential role of Mcl-1 and FAK. Mol Carcinog 52: 879–889.
61. Qi Y, Fu X, Xiong Z, Zhang H, Hill SM, et al. (2012) Methylseleninic acid enhances paclitaxel efficacy for the treatment of triple-negative breast cancer. PLoS One 7: e31539.
62. Yin S, Dong Y, Li J, Fan L, Wang L, et al. (2012) Methylseleninic acid potentiates multiple types of cancer cells to ABT-737-induced apoptosis by targeting Mcl-1 and Bad. Apoptosis 17: 388–399.

Analysis of FoxP3+ T-Regulatory Cells and CD8+T-Cells in Ovarian Carcinoma: Location and Tumor Infiltration Patterns Are Key Prognostic Markers

Cecilia Hermans[1]*, David Anz[3], Jutta Engel[2], Thomas Kirchner[1], Stefan Endres[3], Doris Mayr[1]

1 Department of Pathology, Ludwig-Maximilians-University, Munich, Germany, 2 Tumorregister Munich, Institute of Medical Informatics, Biometry and Epidemiology, Ludwig-Maximilians-University, Munich, Germany, 3 Center of Integrated Protein Science Munich (CIPS-M) Division of Clinical Pharmacology, Ludwig-Maximilians-University, Munich, Germany

Abstract

Purpose: Tumor infiltrating CD4+CD25+FoxP3+ regulatory immune cells (Treg) have been associated with impaired anti-tumor immune response and unfavorable prognosis for patients affected by ovarian carcinoma, whereas CD8+ T-cells have been found to positively influence survival rates in a large panel of solid tumors. Recently, density, location and tumor infiltration patterns of the respective immune cell subtypes have been identified as key prognostic factors for different types of tumors.

Patients and Methods: We stained 210 human ovarian carcinoma samples immunhistochemically for FoxP3 and CD8 to identify the impact different immune cell patterns have on generally accepted prognostic variables as well as on overall survival.

Results: We found that FoxP3+ cells located within lymphoid aggregates surrounding the tumor were strongly associated with reduced survival time ($P = 0.007$). Central accumulation of CD8+ effector cells within the tumor bed shows a positive effect on survival ($P = 0,001$).

Conclusion: The distribution pattern of immune cells within the tumor environment strongly influences prognosis and overall survival time of patients with ovarian carcinoma.

Editor: Derya Unutmaz, New York University, United States of America

Funding: The authors have no funding or support to report.

Competing Interests: The authors have declared that no competing interests exist.

* Email: Cecilia.Hermans@med.uni-muenchen.de

Introduction

Ovarian cancer has the highest mortality rate of all female genital cancers. Over 200,000 women are diagnosed with primary ovarian cancer every year [1–4]. Most of these cancers are diagnosed at a late stage, over 75% of patients are staged FIGO III or IV at first appearance. Overall five-year survival rates range between devastating 25% and 49% [2,5–8]. Standard therapy, cytoreductive surgery followed by platin and taxan chemotherapy, initially leads to good response rates; however, in over 50% of the cases the disease recurs within the following five years [9,10]. Generally accepted prognostic factors are optimal surgical debulking, histological subtype, tumor grading and staging [2,6]. Nonetheless, these factors fail to predict overall survival rates accurately, since patients with similar clinical and pathological characteristics often differ widely concerning actual outcome and survival.

The correlation between tumor-infiltrating lymphocytes and prognosis of cancer patients has been investigated by numerous papers throughout the past thirty years [11–13]. For ovarian carcinoma Zhang et al. demonstrated as early as 2003 that CD3+ lymphocytes influence the progression-free and overall survival rates of patients [9]. Studies have since aimed at identifying methods to further depict the different cells that are involved in the anti-tumor immune response. As a result, a subpopulation of T-regulatory cells (Treg Cells) has been identified that plays a crucial role in tumor-induced immune suppression [14,15]. The vast majority of Tregs are characterized by expressing CD3, CD4, CD25, the glucocorticoid- induced tumor necrosis factor receptor family related gene (GITR), the cytotoxic T-lymphocyte antigen-4 (CTLA-4) and, most importantly, the transcription factor forkhead box P3 (FoxP3) [16–19].

Treg cells are able to modulate the anti- tumor response of CD8+ effector T-cells and are associated with poor prognosis in ovarian carcinoma [20–24]. Similar results have been reported of numerous other tumors, for example colon carcinoma [25] gastric cancer [26] metastatic melanoma [27]. Curiel at al. showed that human tumor Treg cells suppress tumor-specific T-cell immunity and contribute to tumor growth in vivo. Treg cells were associated

Table 1. Patient and tumor characteristics.

	n
Number of Samples	210
Age (Mean/Range)	60.77(27–87)
Survival Time (Median/Standard Deviation)	48.28 (46,27)
Grading	Result (%)
G1	6 (2.96%)
G2	70 (34.48%)
G3+ G4	127 (62.56%)
Histological subtype	
Serous	162 (77.1%)
Mucinous	3 (1.4%)
Endometroid	17 (8.1%)
Adenocarcinoma (NOS)	11 (5.3%)
Undifferentiated	7 (3.3%)
Unknown	10 (4.8%)
Optimal Surgical Debulking	
Radical operation	49 (23.3%)
Remaining tumor < = 2 cm	68 (32.4%)
Remaining tumor >2 cm	43 (20.5%)
Unknown	47 (22.4%)
Sample laparotomy	2 (1%)

with a high mortality risk and reduced survival for patients with ovarian carcinoma [15]. Other authors have focused on the influence other subsets of T- lymphocytes have on the tumor environment. High numbers of and intratumoral penetration by CD8+ effector T-cells were found to slow down tumor growth and have been identified as independent prognostic factors for serous ovarian carcinoma [22]. On a similar note, a high CD8+ effector T-cell-to-Treg cell ratio, rather than the absolute number of each, has been suggested as an independent predictor of survival for patients affected by ovarian carcinoma [14] as well as breast cancer [28].

Apart from the determination of the mere presence of a distinct cell type within the tumor environment, increasing evidence suggests that the exact location and tumor infiltration pattern need to be considered [23,27,29]. Other authors have claimed the lymphoid clusters surrounding the carcinomata to be the actual site of Treg cell activation. The accumulation of FoxP3+ cells within lymphoid cell clusters was associated with a significantly worse prognosis than samples with high numbers of Treg cells [30–32].

This study is based upon the assumption that FoxP3 is a valid Treg cell marker. However, there have been publications that have questioned this assumption in the past [33,34]. There also have been several reports of FoxP3 expression through tumor cells themselves, which has been interpreted as a specific tumor escape mechanism [35–37]. Some evidence also suggests that FoxP3+ Treg cell subpopulations may also be involved in tumor suppressive functions [38,39]. The interaction of FoxP3 and the transcription factor NFAT are subject to further investigation to ultimately understand FoxP3 function [40]. Moreover, other immune cells are known to be able to exert immunsuppresive mechanisms, but do not express FoxP3 [41,42,43]. However, the single legitimate Treg cell marker still remains to be discovered

Table 2. Antibodys used in this study.

Antibody	Type	Dilution	Incubation Time	Source
Anti- Human FoxP3 (Catalog Number ab20034)	Monoclonal; Mouse (Klon 236A/E7)	1:180	60 min	Biocare medical systems, Abcam, Cambridge, UK
Anti-Human CD8 (Catalog Number MS 457)	Monoclonal; Mouse (Klon C8\144 B)	1:50	24 min	LAB Vision, Fremont, USA
Anti-Human CD20 (Catalog Number M0755)	Monoclonal; Mouse (Klon L26)	1:400		DAKO North America Inc., Carpinteria, USA
Anti-Human CD4 (Catalog Number NCL-CD4-368)	Monoclonal; Mouse (Klon 4B12)	1:10		Leica Biosystems, Nussloch, Germany

Table 3. Scoring System.

	Group1	Group2	Group3	Group4
CD8	0–4	5–14	15–24	>25
FoxP3	0–4	5–14	15–24	>25

and for now FoxP3 remains to be the most established and understood Treg cell marker we know [17,27,44–47].

Material and Methods

Patient characteristics

210 tumor tissue samples were selected from the archives of the Institute of Pathology of the Ludwig-Maximilians University, Munich, Germany. All patients had undergone debulking surgery at the Department of Obstetrics and Gynecology, Maistrasse, University Clinic Munich, between 1989 and 2002. The patients were between 27 and 87 years of age at diagnosis, with a median age of 60.1. Tumors were graded according to the Silverberg grading system. Most tumors were graded class 3+4 (62.2%) and only very few class 1 (2.96%). Only samples classified as stage III cancers, according to the International Federation of Gynecology and Obstetrics (FIGO), were included. All histological types of epithelial ovarian carcinoma were selected, but the serous (77.1%), endometroid (8.1%) and adenocarcinoma NOS (5.3%) were by far the most commonly represented types (Table 1).

Histology and immunohistochemistry

The formalin-fixed, paraffin- bedded blocks were cut into approximately <2 μm thick slices and mounted on SuperFrost Plus microscope slides (Menzel Gläser, Braunschweig, Germany). After deparaffinization and rehydration, sections were immersed into Dako Target Retrieval solution (Dako North America Inc., Carpinteria, USA), pH 6, 1:10, incubated at 97°C–99°C at 750 Watt for 2x 15 minutes, and allowed to cool to room temperature for 20 minutes. Endogenous peroxidase activity was blocked by 10-minute incubation in 7.5% hydrogen-peroxide solution (Hydroxen Peroxide Solution, Sigma Aldrich Co., Munich, Germany). Immunohistochemical staining for FoxP3 was performed according to standard procedure using MACH-3 mouse alkalic phosphatase polymer detection kit from Biocare Medical Systems (Concord, USA). The slides were incubated with monoclonal mouse antibody. Chromogen Red (Dako North Amerika Inc., Carpinteria, USA) was used as chromogen for FoxP3 staining, and lastly hematoxylin counterstaining was done (Vector Laboratories, Burlingam, USA). An independent set of slides was selected to perform immunhistochemical staining for CD8+ T-cells. These specimens were automatically stained using Ventana Benchmark XT according to standard operating procedure with monoclonal mouse antibody (Anti- Human CD8- AB-1 Antigen, Vision, Fremont, USA). Additional single serial staining was performed for CD4 and CD20 automatically using Ventana Benchmark XT with monoclonal mouse antibody according to the XT ultraView DAB procedure (Table 2).

Cells were first quantified by counting absolute numbers of 100 power fields per specimen (two independent investigators). After adequate group boundaries were defined, all remaining 110 specimens, as well as the initial 100 samples, were reevaluated semi-quantitatively. At least 35–40 high power fields were counted at 20- or 40-fold magnification (Axiovert Inverse Microscope, Carl Zeiss, Jena, Germany). The amount of cells was categorized according to a specific scoring system (Table 3).

Preferred cell location (central vs peripheral) and finally, the infiltration of immune cells into the tumor tissue were checked (no infiltration vs. infiltration). Per definition, only cells surrounded by at least three tumor cells were counted as infiltrating the tumor.

Statistical analysis

Statistical analysis was done by Superior Performance Software Systems Statistics Software (SPSS). Correlations between clinico-biological data and the FoxP3+ and CD8+ cell content were determined using a χ^2 test. Survival curves were plotted using the Kaplan-Meier method and compared using the log-rank test. Multivariate analyses of prognostic factors for survival were performed using a Cox Proportional Hazard Model.

Ethics Statement

Following the requirement of an ethics statement for publication of our manuscript in your journal, we would like to declare that the presented data were the result of a retrospective analysis on anonymized biopsy material. The material was sampled for diagnostic purposes. At all times we acted in accordance with the legal requirements concerning confidential medical communication as well as the data protection act. Consequently, we were sure before starting our investigation in 2009 that consulting the Institutional Review Board of out University was not required.

Results

a) Amount, Location, Infiltration of CD8+ and FoxP3+

CD8+ and FoxP3+ cells were detected in nearly all specimens, with CD8+ and FoxP3+ staining exclusively found on lymphocytes (Table 4). The amount of CD8+ cells mostly varied between 5 and 25 cells per field. In 53.8% of the examined specimens, CD8+ cells mainly accumulated in the peripheral stroma surrounding the

Table 4. Amount of cells.

	Group1	Group2	Group3	Group4	Missing
CD8	54 (25.7%)	78 (37.1%)	68 (32.4%)	8 (3.8%)	2 (1%)
FoxP3	65 (31.0%)	50 (23.8%)	59 (28.1%)	27 (12.9%)	9 (4.3%)

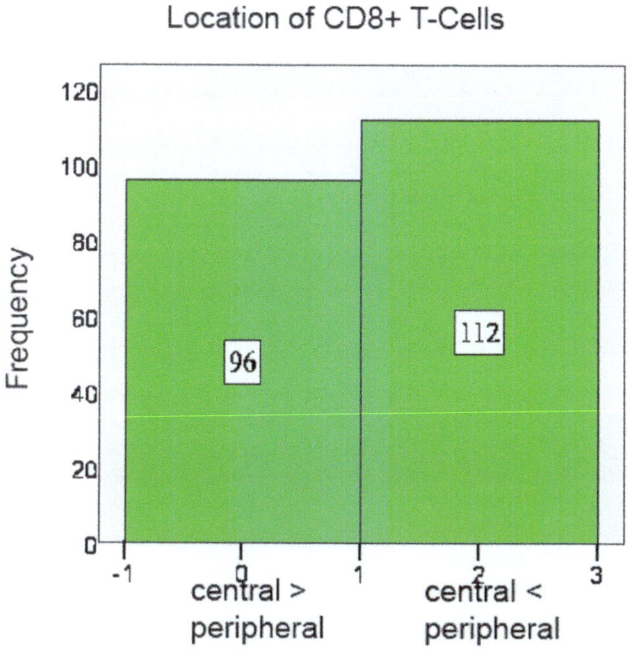

Figure 1. CD8+ T-cells: Location.

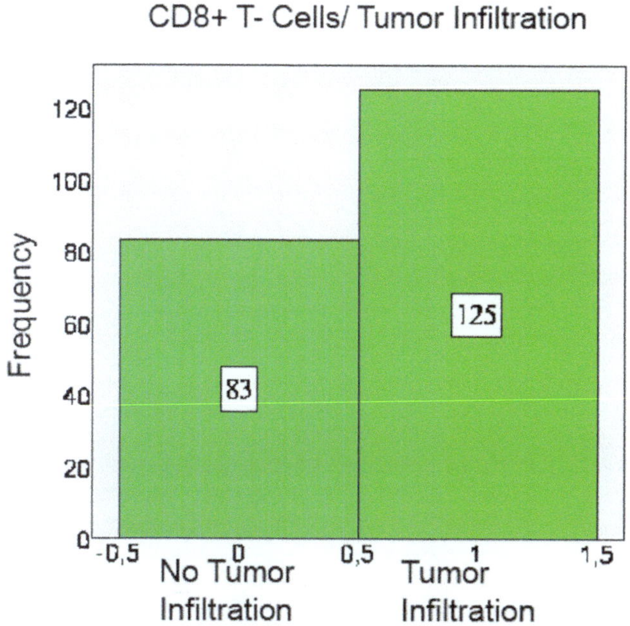

Figure 3. CD8+ T-cells: Tumor infiltration pattern.

tumor tissue and in 46.2% they spread equally throughout the tissue (Figure 1). A mere 60.1% of cases showed tumor-infiltrating CD8+ cells (Figures 2 and 3).

FoxP3+ cell count mainly ranged between 5 and 25 cells per field as well, but overall more FoxP3+ than CD8+ cells were counted in the specimens. Moreover, FoxP3+ cells accumulated relatively more often within the centre of the specimen than in the peripheral stroma (63.3%) (Figures 4 and 5). FoxP3+ cells usually infiltrated the tumor tissue (94.4% positive tumor infiltration) (Figure 6) (Tables 5 and 6).

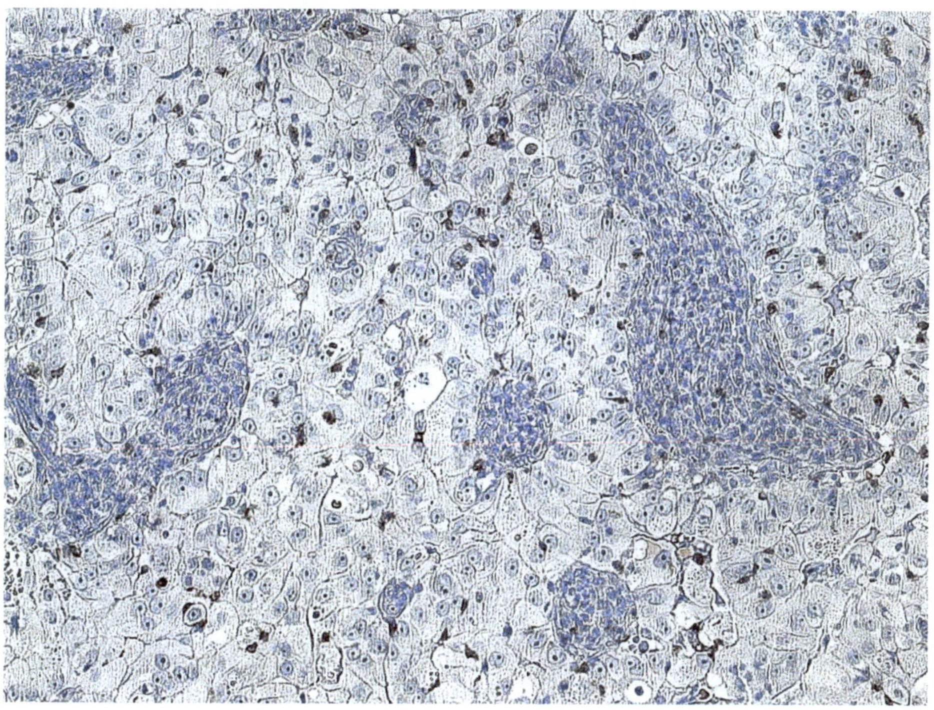

Figure 2. CD8+ T-cells infiltrating tumor tissue. Microscope: Carl Zeiss, Jena, Germany, 20-fold magnification, room temperature, Adobe Photoshop.

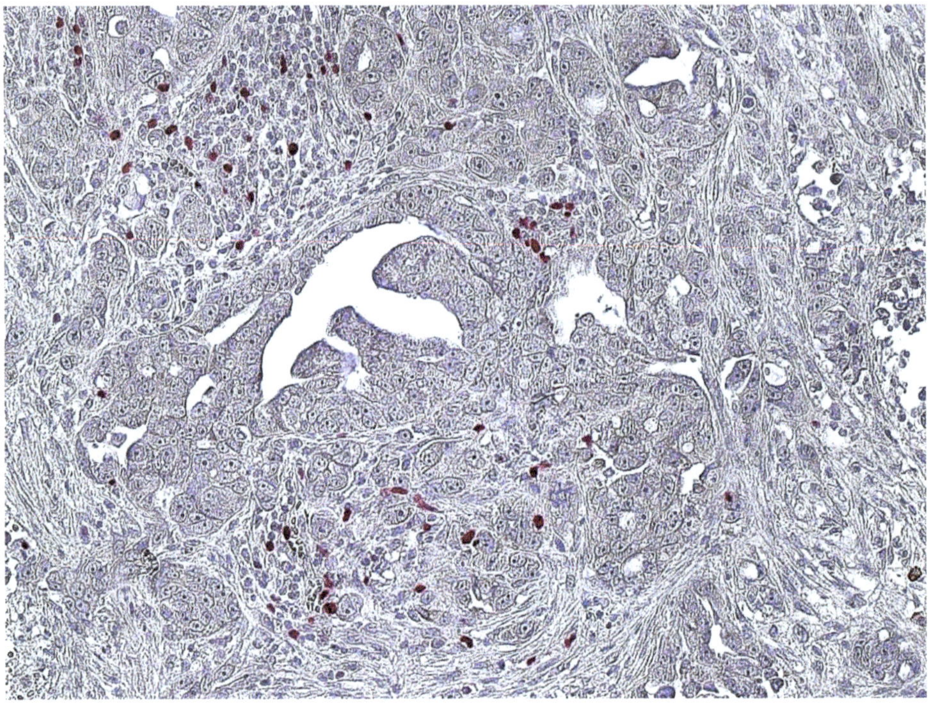

Figure 4. FoxP3+ cells mainly accumulate centrally. Carl Zeiss, Jena, Germany, 20-fold magnification, room temperature, Adobe Photoshop.

b) Correlation analysis

The amount of CD8+ cells within the specimen strongly correlates with the amount of FoxP3+ cells ($p = 0.0001$). Also, high numbers of CD8+ T-cells are positively linked to tumor infiltration of CD8+ cells ($p = 0.001$).

Increased numbers of FoxP3+ cells are associated with tumor infiltration of FoxP3+ cells, thus implying a benchmark number of Treg cells necessary for invasion into the tumor tissue ($p = 0.001$). Moreover, the ratio of CD8+T-cells to FoxP3+ cells strongly correlates with FoxP3+ cell location: a high CD8-to-FoxP3 ratio is associated with peripheral location of FoxP3+ cells. They mainly accumulate in lymphoid clusters surrounding the tumor. A low CD8+ to-FoxP3+ ratio, however, is associated with tumor infiltration of FoxP3+ cells. As soon as FoxP3+ cells outweigh CD8+ cells, they will infiltrate into the tumor and spread throughout the specimen.

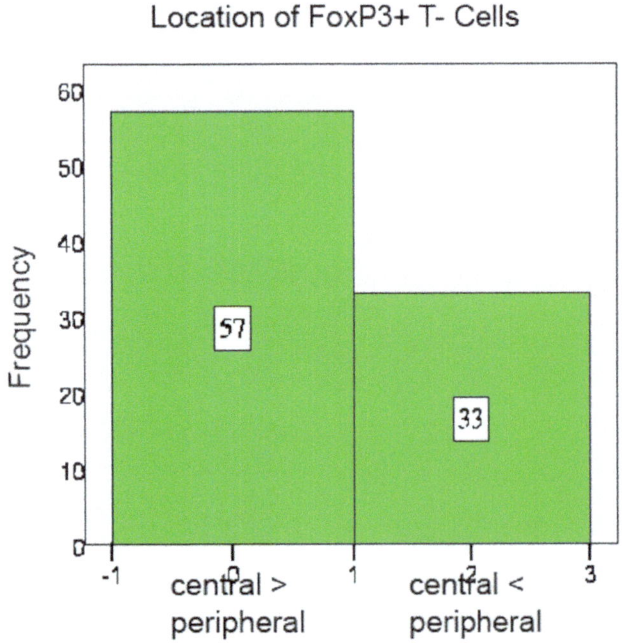

Figure 5. FoxP3+ cells: Location.

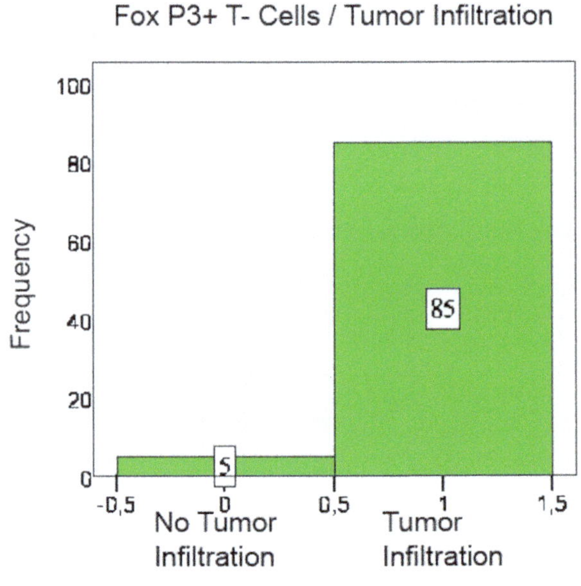

Figure 6. FoxP3+ cells: Tumor infiltration pattern.

Table 5. Localisation of cells.

	Central>=Peripheral	Central<Peripheral	Missing
CD8	96 (45.7%)	112 (53.3%)	2 (1%)
FoxP3	57 (27.1%)	33 (15.7%)	120 (57.1%)

The correlation tables reveal a significant relationship between "grading" level and FoxP3+ cell density, implying that high levels of FoxP3+ Treg cells are associated with significantly worse grading according to the Silverberg grading classification scheme ($p = 0.004$). This relationship is further emphasized by the negative correlation found between the CD8-to-FoxP3+ cell ratio and grading. Relatively low levels of CD8+ effector cells in comparison to FoxP3+ Treg cells are significantly associated with lower histological tumor grading ($p = 0.001$). Surprisingly, the parameter of "location of FoxP3+ cells" individually influences survival time ($p = 0.007$). Peripheral accumulation of Treg cells in lymphoid clusters surrounding the tumor bed is consequently associated with significantly less overall survival time than central accumulation within the tumor bed.

In order to quantify the influence generally accepted prognostic factors have on the prognostic model, statistical analysis was also done for common prognostic variables. "Age" ($p = 0.001$), "grading" ($p = 0.001$) and "optimal surgical debulking" ($p = 0.007$) showed significant effects on survival time, while neither the "employed neo-adjuvant therapy" nor "histological subtype" did. The lack of influence the parameter "histological subtype" shows is probably due to the lack of homogeneity of histological subtypes within the population.

c) Cox Proportional Hazard Model

Using the Cox Proportional Hazard Model eliminated the statistical effects of the prognostic factors age, grading and surgical debulking. Three major individual prognostic factors for patients with ovarian carcinoma were then revealed. Firstly, the location of CD8+ T-cells within the specimen is an individual prognostic factor for patients with ovarian carcinoma ($p = 0.001$). Centralized accumulation of CD8+ effector cells in the tumor bed leads to prolonged survival time. Secondly, peripheral accumulation of FoxP3+ Treg cells in lymphoid clusters is a strongly significant negative prognostic factor for patients suffering from ovarian carcinoma (Table 7).

d) Kaplan-Meier Curves and Log-Rank Test

The significant influence the location of CD8+ T effector cells as well as the location of FoxP3+ Treg cells within the specimen have on the overall survival time of a patient was reinforced by using the Kaplan-Meier Model ($p = 0.049$ and $p = 0.056$) (Figures 7 and 8).

Discussion

This study examined the tissue of 210 patients with ovarian carcinoma for the infiltration of CD8+ effector T-cells and FoxP3+ T regulatory cells (Treg). In addition to the calculation of the respective frequencies, special attention was paid to the exact locations of the immune cells and to their capacity to infiltrate into the tumor bed. In order to adjust for known prognostic factors, multivariate analysis was done using the Cox Proportional Hazards Model introducing classical histophathological parameters such as grading, age at diagnosis, and surgical debulking success.

The current paradigm in tumor immunity suggests that tumor-associated antigens are captured by professional dendritic cells, which in turn prime naive T-cells to become antigen-specific anti tumor effector T-cells [48]. Ultimately, a large number of activated CD8+ effector T-cells should thus be able to attack the tumor tissue and eradicate the tumor. Unfortunately, as tumors actively fight to suppress effector cell function by producing immunosuppressive factors such as IL-10, TGFß, and VEGF, effective tumor eradication is rarely successful [49–52]. Moreover, the immunosuppressive function Treg cells exert on CD4+ and CD8+ T-cells have been identified as a crucial variable limiting an effective anti- tumor immune response. Yet, the mechanisms of suppression Treg cells make use of still remain to be fully understood.

The results of our study signify that the invasion of great numbers of CD8+ T effector cells is in fact one of the major prognostic factors for patients with ovarian carcinoma. This has previously been suggested for ovarian carcinoma as well as breast cancer by numerous authors [10,14,28,53], but the focus of attention has so far not been placed on the location of the cells within the examined material, but on the mere amount of CD8+ T-cells and the ratio of CD8+ to other immune cells, respectively. The location, however, seems to be of greatest importance for an effective tumor attack. High numbers of CD8+ effector cells are also strongly associated with lower levels of histopathological grading, which strengthens the case that sufficient numbers of CD8+ T-cells within the tumor bed are actually able to keep tumor growth in check.

FoxP3+ Treg cells were mainly present within the tumor area, but less frequently they gathered in groups surrounding the tumor. In order to determine what cell types comprise these aggregates of immune cells we performed additional single serial staining for CD4 and CD20. We thereby could identify these peripheral

Table 6. Tumor infiltration of cells.

	Tumor not Infiltrated	Tumor infiltrated	Missing
CD8	83 (39.9%)	125 (59.5%)	2 (1%)
FoxP3	5 (2.4%)	85 (40.5%)	120 (57.1%)

Table 7. Biomarkers and their influence on overall survival.

Biomarkers	No. Positive (%)	Overall survival (P)	Morphological pattern
CD8+ cells			
central	46.2	0.049	Central Location of CD8+ cells increases survival
peripheral	53.8	NS	
FoxP3+ cells			
central	63.3	NS	Peripheral Location of FoxP3+ cells reduces survival
peripheral	36.7	0.056	

NS: Not significant.

immune cell aggregates as lymphoid structures. FoxP3+ expression in these lymphoid aggregates surrounding the tumor bed was found to be an independent prognostic factor for patients with ovarian carcinoma. Therefore, the presence of Treg cells within these lymphoid infiltrates is associated with a significantly higher risk of relapse and death. This finding has previously been reported for patients with breast carcinoma [31] as well as for follicular lymphoma [30]. Supposedly, this clinical observation results from the selective activation of Treg cells within these aggregates surrounding the tumor bed. Here, mature dendritic cells present tumor-specific antigens to peripheral naive FoxP3+ Treg cells, which then proliferate in situ and are thereafter capable of suppressing the anti tumor immune response of CD8+ effector T-cells through heterogeneous mechanisms including IL-10 and TGF-ß [32,48,51,54]. This thesis was further strengthened by Gobert's finding that only Treg cells located in these lymphoid aggregates actually expressed activation markers such as HCA-DR, GITR and ICOS, while FoxP3+Treg cells located within the tumor tissue itself did not [31]. Previously, other authors have reported the expression of B7-H1 by dendritic cells within these aggregates, a receptor by which dendritic cells are able to prime the conversion of peripheral T-cells to functional Treg cells [48]. The accumulation of FoxP3+Treg cells within lymphocyte clusters surrounding the tumor, as well as abundant B7-H1 expression within this region, have lately also been reported for patients with prostate cancer [29]. Thus, it seems to be crucial not only to determine the density of FoxP3+ cells, but their exact location in the examined tissue. In order to influence the tumor microenvironment, the B7-H1 receptor seems to be one key mechanism which controls Treg cell activation.

On a different note but in accordance with the findings of this study, Jaffee et al. revealed that CD8+FoxP3+ cells are present in tumors only if there is an existing pool of tumor-rejecting effector CD8+ T-cells. Therefore, the accumulation and likely the tumor infiltration of FoxP3+ T-cells mark the presence of tumor-rejecting antigen-specific CD8+ T cells, which in turn serves as a marker for an effective T-cell response [55]. Similar results were presented by Nishikawa et al. as well as Rahir et al. [56,57]. Overall, recent

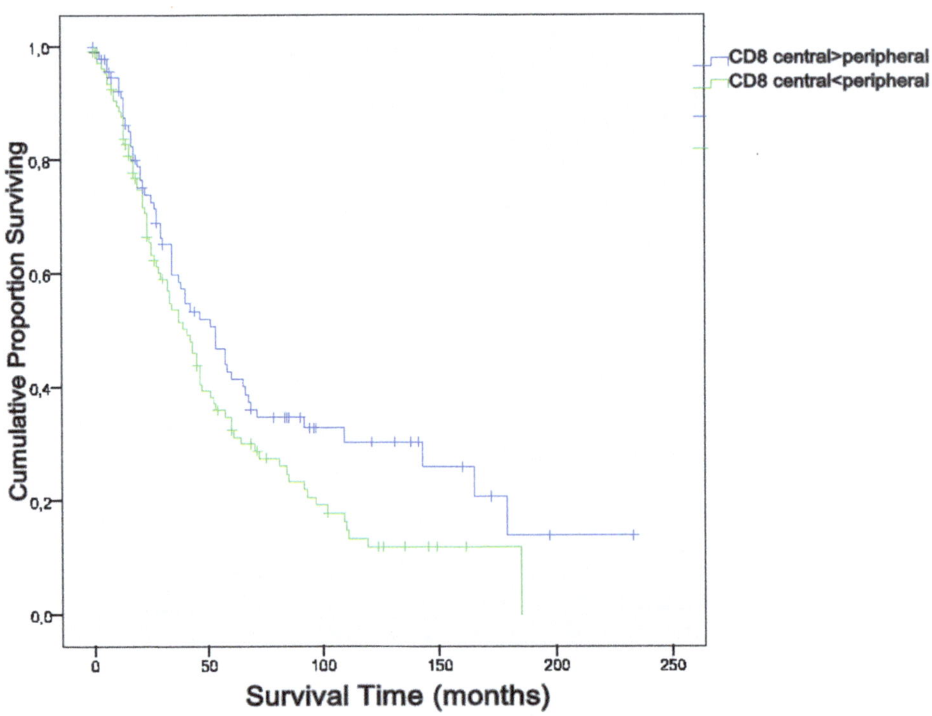

Figure 7. Log-Rank-Test CD8+. Central accumulation of CD8+ T cells is significally associated with survival (p = 0.049).

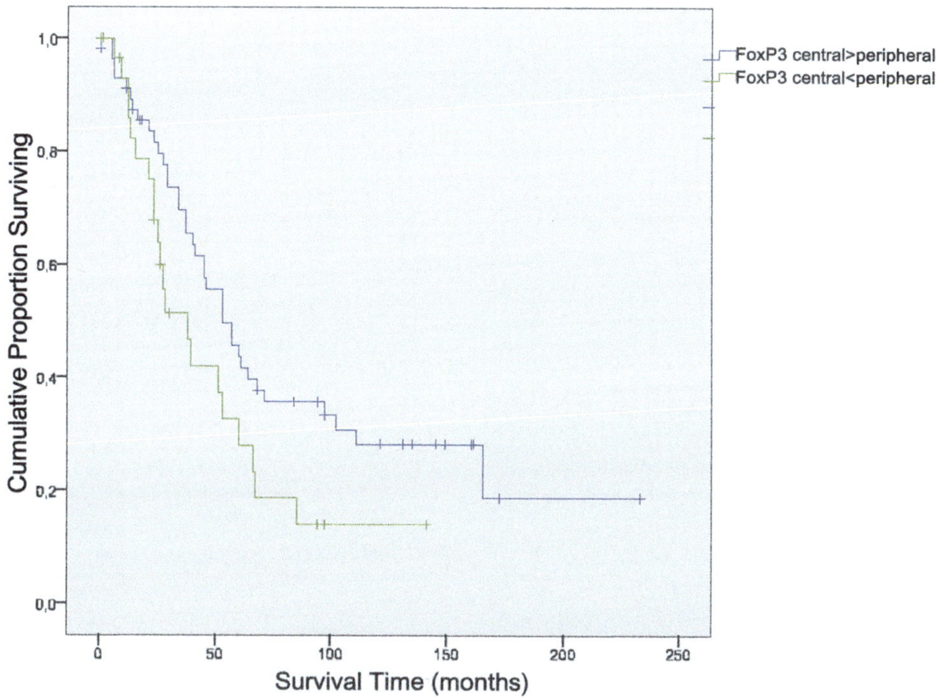

Figure 8. Log-Rank-Test FoxP3+. Peripheral accumulation of FoxP3+ Cells leads to reduced survival (p = 0.056).

data is suggesting that a unique effector subset of FoxP3+ cells may exist which influences the tumor microenvironment in a favorable way and contributes to overall antitumor response. Given the multifaceted influence Tregs play in cancer progression, further research is urgently needed to develop targeted therapies.

Acknowledgments

We thank Andrea Sendelhofert and Anja Heier for expert technical assistance.

Author Contributions

Conceived and designed the experiments: CJLH DM DA SE. Performed the experiments: CJLH DM. Analyzed the data: CJLH DM JE. Contributed reagents/materials/analysis tools: DM TK DA SE. Contributed to the writing of the manuscript: CJLH DM DA.

References

1. WHO WHO (2009) World Health Observatory. Geneva: World Health Organization.
2. Fachgesellschaften AdWM (2007) Diagnostik und Therapie maligner Ovarialtumoren. AWMF.
3. Tavassoli FA, Devilee P, editors (2004) Pathology& Genetics: Tumours of the Breast and Female Genital Organs: World Health Organization Classification of Tumours.
4. Koch-Institut R (2010) Verbreitung von Krebserkrankungen in Deutschland. Entwicklung der Prävalenzen zwischen 1990 und 2010. Beiträge zur Gesundheitsberichterstattung des Bundes. Berlin: Robert Koch Institut.
5. Woodward ER, Sleightholme HV, Considine AM, Williamson S, McHugo JM, et al. (2007) Annual surveillance by CA125 and transvaginal ultrasound for ovarian cancer in both high-risk and population risk women is ineffective. Bjogan International Journal of Obstetrics and Gynaecology 114: 1500–1509.
6. DeutscheKrebsgesellschaft (2006) Interdisziplinäre S2k- Leitlinie für die Diagnostik und Therapie maligner Ovarialtumore. München: W. Zuckschwerdt Verlag. pp. 76.
7. Schmalfeldt B, editor (2007) Manual maligne Ovarialtumore. München: Tumorzentrum München und W. Zuckschwerdt Verlag München. 124 p.
8. Jacobs I, Davies AP, Bridges J, Stabile I, Fay T, et al. (1993) Prevalence Screening for Ovarian-Cancer in Postmenopausal Women by Ca 125 Measurement and Ultrasonography. British Medical Journal 306: 1030–1034.
9. Zhang L, Conejo-Garcia JR, Katsaros D, Gimotty PA, Massobrio M, et al. (2003) Intratumoral T cells, recurrence, and survival in epithelial ovarian cancer. New England Journal of Medicine 348: 203–213.
10. Milne K, Kobel M, Kalloger SE, Barnes RO, Gao D, et al. (2009) Systematic analysis of immune infiltrates in high-grade serous ovarian cancer reveals CD20, FoxP3 and TIA-1 as positive prognostic factors. PLoS One 4: e6412.
11. North RJ, Bursuker I (1984) Generation and decay of the immune response to a progressive fibrosarcoma. I. Ly-1+2- suppressor T cells down-regulate the generation of Ly-1-2+ effector T cells. J Exp Med 159: 1295–1311.
12. Awwad M, North RJ (1988) Immunologically mediated regression of a murine lymphoma after treatment with anti-L3T4 antibody. A consequence of removing L3T4+ suppressor T cells from a host generating predominantly Lyt-2+ T cell-mediated immunity. J Exp Med 168: 2193–2206.
13. Ropponen KM, Eskelinen MJ, Lipponen PK, Alhava E, Kosma VM (1997) Prognostic value of tumour-infiltrating lymphocytes (TILs) in colorectal cancer. J Pathol 182: 318–324.
14. Sato E, Olson SH, Ahn J, Bundy B, Nishikawa H, et al. (2005) Intraepithelial CD8(+) tumor-infiltrating lymphocytes and a high CD8(+)/regulatory T cell ratio are associated with favorable prognosis in ovarian cancer. Proceedings of the National Academy of Sciences of the United States of America 102: 18538–18543.
15. Curiel TJ, Coukos G, Zou LH, Alvarez X, Cheng P, et al. (2004) Specific recruitment of regulatory T cells in ovarian carcinoma fosters immune privilege and predicts reduced survival. Nature Medicine 10: 942–949.
16. Sakaguchi S, Sakaguchi N, Asano M, Itoh M, Toda M (1995) immunological self-tolerance maintained by activated t-cells expressing il-2 receptor alpha-chains (cd25) - breakdown of a single mechanism of self-tolerance causes various autoimmune-diseases. Journal of Immunology 155: 1151–1164.
17. Fontenot JD, Gavin MA, Rudensky AY (2003) Foxp3 programs the development and function of CD4(+)CD25(+) regulatory T cells. Nature Immunology 4: 330–336.
18. Hori S, Nomura T, Sakaguchi S (2003) Control of regulatory T cell development by the transcription factor Foxp3. Science 299: 1057–1061.
19. Shimizu Y, Kamoi S, Amada S, Hasumi K, Akiyama F, et al. (1998) Toward the development of a universal grading system for ovarian epithelial carcinoma - I.

Prognostic significance of histopathologic features - Problems involved in the architectural grading system. Gynecologic Oncology 70: 2–12.
20. Wang L, Ma Q, Chen X, Guo K, Li J, et al. (2010) Clinical significance of b7-h1 and b7-1 expressions in pancreatic carcinoma. World J Surg 34: 1059–1065.
21. Oleinika K, Nibbs RJ, Graham GJ, Fraser AR (2013) Suppression, subversion and escape: the role of regulatory T cells in cancer progression. Clinical and Experimental Immunology 171: 36–45.
22. Clarke SL, Betts GJ, Plant A, Wright KL, El-Shanawany TM, et al. (2006) CD4+CD25+FOXP3+ regulatory T cells suppress anti-tumor immune responses in patients with colorectal cancer. PLoS One 1: e129.
23. Galon J, Costes A, Sanchez-Cabo F, Kirilovsky A, Mlecnik B, et al. (2006) Type, density, and location of immune cells within human colorectal tumors predict clinical outcome. Science 313: 1960–1964.
24. Facciabene A, Motz GT, Coukos G (2012) T-Regulatory Cells: Key Players in Tumor Immune Escape and Angiogenesis. Cancer Research 72: 2162–2171.
25. Chaput N, Louafi S, Bardier A, Charlotte F, Vaillant JC, et al. (2009) Identification of CD8(+)CD25(+)Foxp3(+) suppressive T cells in colorectal cancer tissue. Gut 58: 520–529.
26. Mizukami Y, Kono K, Kawaguchi Y, Akaike H, Kamimura K, et al. (2008) CCL17 and CCL22 chemokines within tumor microenvironment are related to accumulation of Foxp3(+) regulatory T cells in gastric cancer. International Journal of Cancer 122: 2286–2293.
27. Ahmadzadeh M, Felipe-Silva A, Heemskerk B, Powell DJ, Wunderlich JR, et al. (2008) FOXP3 expression accurately defines the population of intratumoral regulatory T cells that selectively accumulate in metastatic melanoma lesions. Blood 112: 4953–4960.
28. Anz D, Koelzer VH, Moder S, Thaler R, Schwerd T, et al. (2010) Immunostimulatory RNA Blocks Suppression by Regulatory T Cells. Journal of Immunology 184: 939–946.
29. Ebelt K, Babaryka G, Frankenberger B, Stief CG, Eisenmenger W, et al. (2009) Prostate cancer lesions are surrounded by FOXP3(+), PD-1(+) and B7-H1(+) lymphocyte clusters. European Journal of Cancer 45: 1664–1672.
30. Farinha P, Al-Tourah A, Gill K, Klasa R, Connors JM, et al. (2010) The architectural pattern of FOXP3-positive T cells in follicular lymphoma is an independent predictor of survival and histologic transformation. Blood 115: 289–295.
31. Gobert M, Treilleux I, Bendriss-Vermare N, Bachelot T, Goddard-Leon S, et al. (2009) Regulatory T Cells Recruited through CCL22/CCR4 Are Selectively Activated in Lymphoid Infiltrates Surrounding Primary Breast Tumors and Lead to an Adverse Clinical Outcome. Cancer Research 69: 2000–2009.
32. Menetrier-Caux C, Gobert M, Caux C (2009) Differences in Tumor Regulatory T-Cell Localization and Activation Status Impact Patient Outcome. Cancer Research 69: 7895–7898.
33. Beyer M, Schultze JL (2006) Regulatory T cells in cancer. Blood 108: 804–811.
34. Wing K, Sakaguchi S (2010) Regulatory T cells exert checks and balances on self tolerance and autoimmunity. Nature Immunology 11: 7–13.
35. Hinz S, Pagerols-Raluy L, Oberg H-H, Ammerpohl O, Grussel S, et al. (2007) Foxp3 expression in pancreatic carcinoma cells as a novel mechanism of immune evasion in cancer. Cancer Res 67: 8344–8350.
36. Ebert LM, Tan BS, Browning J, Svobodova S, Russell SE, et al. (2008) The regulatory T cell-associated transcription factor FoxP3 is expressed by tumor cells. Cancer Res 68: 3001–3009.
37. Karanikas V, Speletas M, Zamanakou M, Kalala F, Loules G, et al. (2008) Foxp3 expression in human cancer cells. J Transl Med 6: 19.
38. Zhang H-Y, Sun H (2010) Up-regulation of Foxp3 inhibits cell proliferation, migration and invasion in epithelial ovarian cancer. Cancer Letters 287: 91–97.
39. Zuo T, Wang L, Morrison C, Chang X, Zhang H, et al. (2007) FOXP3 is an X-linked breast cancer suppressor gene and an important repressor of the HER-2/ErbB2 oncogene. Cell 129: 1275–1286.
40. Wu YQ, Borde M, Heissmeyer V, Feuerer M, Lapan AD, et al. (2006) FOXP3 controls regulatory T cell function through cooperation with NFAT. Cell 126: 375–387.
41. Shevach EM (2006) From vanilla to 28 flavors: Multiple varieties of T regulatory cells. Immunity 25: 195–201.
42. Sakaguchi S (2008) Regulatory T cells in the past and for the future. European Journal of Immunology 38: 901–903.
43. Kryczek I, Zou L, Rodriguez P, Zhu G, Wei S, et al. (2006) B7-H4 expression identifies a novel suppressive macrophage population in human ovarian carcinoma. Journal of Experimental Medicine 203: 871–881.
44. Clarke B, Tinker AV, Lee C-H, Subramanian S, van de Rijn M, et al. (2009) Intraepithelial T cells and prognosis in ovarian carcinoma: novel associations with stage, tumor type, and BRCA1 loss. Modern Pathology 22: 393–402.
45. Feyler S, von Lilienfeld-Toal M, Jarmin S, Marles L, Rawstron A, et al. (2009) CD4(+)CD25(+)FoxP3(+) regulatory T cells are increased whilst CD3(+)CD4(−)CD8(−)alpha beta TCR+ Double Negative T cells are decreased in the peripheral blood of patients with multiple myeloma which correlates with disease burden. British Journal of Haematology 144: 686–695.
46. Chen WJ, Jin WW, Hardegen N, Lei KJ, Li L, et al. (2003) Conversion of peripheral CD4(+)CD25(−) naive T cells to CD4(+)CD25(+) regulatory T cells by TGF-beta induction of transcription factor Foxp3. Journal of Experimental Medicine 198: 1875–1886.
47. Kmieciak M, Gowda M, Graham L, Godder K, Bear HD, et al. (2009) Human T cells express CD25 and Foxp3 upon activation and exhibit effector/memory phenotypes without any regulatory/suppressor function. Journal of Translational Medicine 7.
48. Curiel TJ (2007) Tregs and rethinking cancer immunotherapy. Journal of Clinical Investigation 117: 1167–1174.
49. Dunn GP, Bruce AT, Ikeda H, Old LJ, Schreiber RD (2002) Cancer immunoediting: from immunosurveillance to tumor escape. Nat Immunol 3: 991–998.
50. Dunn GP, Ikeda H, Bruce AT, Koebel C, Uppaluri R, et al. (2005) Interferon-gamma and cancer immunoediting. Immunol Res 32: 231–245.
51. Larmonier N, Marron M, Zeng Y, Cantrell J, Romanoski A, et al. (2007) Tumor-derived CD4(+)CD25(+) regulatory T cell suppression of dendritic cell function involves TGF-beta and IL-10. Cancer Immunol Immunother 56: 48–59.
52. Liu VC, Wong LY, Jang T, Shah AH, Park I, et al. (2007) Tumor evasion of the immune system by converting CD4(+) CD25(−) T cells into CD4(+) CD25(+) T regulatory cells: Role of tumor-derived TGF-beta. Journal of Immunology 178: 2883–2892.
53. Clarke B, Tinker AV, Lee CH, Subramanian S, van de Rijn M, et al. (2009) Intraepithelial T cells and prognosis in ovarian carcinoma: novel associations with stage, tumor type, and BRCA1 loss. Modern Pathology 22: 393–402.
54. Zou WP (2005) Immunosuppressive networks in the tumour environment and their therapeutic relevance. Nature Reviews Cancer 5: 263–274.
55. Le DT, Ladle BH, Lee T, Weiss V, Yao XS, et al. (2011) CD8(+)Foxp3(+) tumor infiltrating lymphocytes accumulate in the context of an effective anti-tumor response. International Journal of Cancer 129: 636–647.
56. Nishikawa H, Sakaguchi S (2010) Regulatory T cells in tumor immunity. International Journal of Cancer 127: 759–767.
57. Rahir G, Moser M (2012) Tumor microenvironment and lymphocyte infiltration. Cancer Immunology Immunotherapy 61: 751–759.

Differential Antigen Expression Profile Predicts Immunoreactive Subset of Advanced Ovarian Cancers

Kevin H. Eng[1]*, Takemasa Tsuji[2]

1 Department of Biostatistics and Bioinformatics, Roswell Park Cancer Institute, Buffalo, NY, United States of America, 2 Center for Immunotherapy, Roswell Park Cancer Institute, Buffalo, NY, United States of America

Abstract

The presence and composition of lymphocytes characterizing an immune response has been connected to prognosis in advanced ovarian cancer. Our aim is to establish novel associations between prognosis and the expression of immune-related genes through a focused screen utilizing publicly available high-throughput assays. We consider transcriptome profiles from $n = 1137$ advanced ovarian cancer patients observed in four separate studies divided into discovery/validation sets ($n = 503/n = 634$). We focus on a subset of lymphocyte markers, antigen presentation and processing genes, T cell receptor associated co-stimulatory/repressor genes and cancer testis (CT) antigens. We modeled differential expression and co-expression using these subsets and tested for association with overall survival. Fifteen of 64 immune-related genes are associated with survival of which 5 are reproduced in the validation set. The expression of these genes defines an immunoreactive (IR) subgroup of patients with a favorable prognosis. Phenotypic characterization of the immune compartment signal includes upregulation of markers of $CD8^+$ T-cell activation in these patients. Using multivariate model building, we find that the expression of 6 CT antigens can predict IR status in the discovery and validation sets. These analyses confirm that a genomic approach can reproducibly detect lymphocyte signals in tumor tissue suggesting a novel way to study the tumor microenvironment. Our search has identified new candidate prognostic markers associated with immune components and uncovered preliminary evidence of prognostic subgroups associated with different immune mechanisms.

Editor: Rolf Müller, Philipps University, Germany

Funding: CA016056 www.cancer.gov National Cancer Institute core grant to Roswell Park Cancer Institute. Roswell Park Alliance Foundation www.roswellpark.org/giving award to KHE. The funders had no role in study design, data collection and analysis, decision to publish, or preparation of the manuscript.

Competing Interests: The authors have declared that no competing interests exist.

* Email: kevin.eng@roswellpark.org

Introduction

Recent, high-throughput gene expression profiling studies in ovarian cancer have identified a theme of differentially regulated immune signaling molecules related to prognosis [1,2]. The finding is consistent with mounting evidence that ovarian cancers are strongly immunogenic: spontaneous humoral and cellular immune reactions develop in response to disease [3], form characteristic epitopes [4], and are subject to complex up- and down-regulation by immune processes [5,6]. The degree of tumor infiltration by host immune cells has been associated with good prognosis [7] as well as the balance of lymphocyte subtypes.

Subtypes of lymphocytes have diverse functions related to antigen recognition and immune suppression [8] and are thought to indicate a dynamic and evolving response to cancer [9]. For example, an increase in $CD8^+$ T cells was found to be associated with good prognosis, but a rise in regulatory T cells was found to counteract this benefit [10]. Thus, studying components of the ovarian tumor microenvironment [11] is a critical angle for identifying prognostic associations [12].

However, few array-based expression studies have sampled both the host's reaction as well as the tumor. Most large observational studies [1,2,13,14] considered only tumor tissue because their goal was prognostic modeling; immune associations were made *post hoc* based only on enrichment inferred from a small number of significant immune genes. Other array-based studies that focused on immune characterization were small and observational (n = 38) [15] or case control (n = 25, n = 25) [16]. These studies showed positive associations between lymphocyte-specific markers and prognosis implying that the sampled tissue contained some microenvironment signal.

Recent work in expression arrays is able to computationally separate tumor, stromal and immune components of these complex tissues. For example, the ESTIMATE algorithm [17] uses 141 genes to estimate the fraction of expression signal attributable to the immune compartment. While this approach is useful for eliminating the noise due to impure samples, this study noted that the immune signals did seem to carry mild association with clinical outcomes. Based on the presence and potential prognostic value of immune markers, we conjecture that the apparent associations can be traced to residual lymphocyte RNA and that further analysis of these markers can be attributed to signal from the microenvironment. As such, we might simply model markers that we suspect are highly likely to be immune-specific *a priori*.

We rely on two large cohorts of public data organized into a discovery set and a validation set: 503 biobanked high-grade serous ovarian cancer samples from the Cancer Genome Atlas (TCGA) [2] form a focused training and exploration set and a more clinically-representative mix of 634 samples from 3 Gene Expression Omnibus (GEO) studies [1,13,14] form the validation set. The clinical features of the data are described in their original papers, but briefly, all of the patients in these studies have advanced, primary ovarian cancer (a small number of primary peritoneal and fallopian tube in the validation set) and received adjuvant platinum and taxane treatments following surgery.

We study first the specificity of immune-related genes to lymphocyte tissues and then explore univariate prognostic associations. Using clustering algorithms, we identify a subset of cancer cases with high adaptive immunity signals and we show that this subset can be predicted by the tumor expression of cancer-testis antigens. Taken together, these results imply that significant prognostic value remains untapped in the tumor microenvironment.

Methods

Clinical and Gene Expression Data

TCGA is a biorepository study of $n=503$ high-grade serous ovarian cancers from multiple centers in the United States and is described extensively in the original article [2]. Relevant to our analysis, this study strictly included ovarian primaries and papillary serous histologies. Samples were originally assessed as Stage III-IV and Grade 2,3 (later re-staged by a TCGA pathologist) and the patient received adjuvant platinum and taxane based chemotherapy. We adopt the view that these cases reflect a biased but homogenous clinical presentation more likely to yield a consistent biological mechanism.

Three clinical datasets were downloaded from the NCBI GEO database and are described below. Table 1 is a summary of clinically relevant differences between the studies.

GEO:GSE9891 is an Australian observational study [14] of $n=285$ mostly serous (227) ovarian cancer including some peritoneal (34) and fallopian (5) primaries. Conditioning on patients receiving platinum/taxol and removing the LMP samples, we analyze $n=240$ samples. For reproducibility purposes, we work with normalized data from GEO.

GEO:GSE32062 is a Japanese observational study [1] of $n=270$ samples including 10 control samples, 193 recurrences, 121 deaths yielding $n=260$ samples to analyze. An adjuvant platinum/taxol regimen was recorded for all patients.

GEO:GSE3149 is an observational study [13] of $n=134$ arrays after combining redundant ones. Significant work has been have been published on the difficulties in the original analysis of this data [18]; we have implemented the recommended similarity checks and averaged arrays when they appear to come from the same patient. This analysis begins with the GEO banked data and should be immune to data conversion problems.

A biological dataset, NCI-60 cell line data were taken from GEO:GSE5846 [19] where all of the cell lines were measured under untreated conditions. As positive controls, ovary cell lines, IGROV-1, OVCAR-3, OVCAR-4, OVCAR-5, OVCAR-8, SK-OV-3 and NCI/ADR-RES; should express no immune markers. For negative controls, we also study leukemia lines CCRF-CEM, HL-60(TB), MOLT-4, RPMI-8226, SR, and K-562.

Candidate Immune-related and Cancer-Testis Antigen Genes

Candidate genes were selected from KEGG:Antigen processing and presentation (hsa04612) focusing on surface receptors and genes involved in plasma membrane transport. Surface markers and co-regulatory molecules of the T-cell receptor signaling pathway (hsa04660) were added, excluding the internal signaling mechanisms (for example: phospholipases, secondary messengers, and the kinase cascades) as these are non-specific and related to other signaling pathways. Cancer-testis antigen genes were defined based on overlap with the CT Database [20]. The full gene list is provided in Tables S1 and S4.

All genes were aligned using official gene names mapped using the provided GEO platform annotation (i.e., an associated GPL file) and R package hthgu133a.db-2.8.0 [21]. Expression values were scaled and centered for comparability across genes. Note that the highly variable parts of the T-cell receptor (TCA, TCB) cannot be measured on the hybridization-based oligonucleotide arrays.

Table 1. Descriptive statistics for data sets used in this study.

	Discovery	Validation		
Study	**TCGA [2]**	**Australian [14]**	**Japanese [1]**	**US [13]**
n	503	240	260	134
GEO Array Type	GPL570*	GPL570	GPL6480	GPL96
GEO identifier	NA	GSE9891	GSE32062	GSE3149
Age (Range)	59.7 (30–89)	60.2 (23–80)	NA	NA
Stage (% III, IV)	92%	5%	100%	NA
Grade (% 3,4)	87%	61%	50%	NA
Residual Disease (% None)	23%	27%	40%	NA
Neoadjuvant (% Yes)	0%	7%	0%	NA
Median Months OS	44 (40–48)	44 (38–57)	60 (50–80)	74 (35–98)
Median Months PFS	18 (15–19)	15 (14–18)	19 (18–23)	NA

* TCGA uses 3 array types. Only the Affymetrix array was used for completeness.

Computational Methods

Univariate associations were performed with proportional hazards regression. No time truncation, to reduce the effect of long survivors, was performed. Significance was cut at $p<0.05$ and was adjusted for multiple testing unless otherwise noted. The reported FDR calculation is based on the expected number of false positives assuming all tests are null.

Clustering analysis in the TCGA data is based on complete hierarchical clustering under Euclidean distance. Subgroups were picked by splitting the tree at 4 leaves based on visual inspection and a within/between group sum of squares criterion. Cluster centers were used to seed a k-means clustering algorithm in the validation data and the p-value is reported for a study-stratified 4-group log-rank test.

The volcano plot uses literature-based surface markers and co-regulators based on a simple t-test. Highlighted genes were significant above the Bonferroni $p<0.001$ mark and had biologically extreme fold change values.

Partial correlations were computed using the class averages for genes assigned to CD4, CD8, CD3, MHCI and MHCII-based sets. The GeneNet algorithm [22] using FDR <0.05 and hard thresholding at absolute correlation 0.15 was used to infer Gaussian graphical models.

To infer the missing nodes in the GGM, a hidden node must satisfy three properties. Using MHCII - X - CD8 as an example: MHCII and CD8 must be conditionally independent given Gene X ($p>0.05$); MHCII and Gene X must be conditionally dependent given all other genes (Bonferroni $p<0.05$); CD8 and Gene X must be conditionally dependent given other genes (Bonferroni $p<0.05$). Each of these can be reduced to a p-value statement using standard linear model theory and added variable analysis.

Predictions from a multivariate logistic regression model were categorized into immunoreactive class calls based on thresholding the predicted value from the model. This threshold was chosen using the sensitivity/specificity intersection point across all validation datasets.

All statistical analysis was performed in the R statistical programming language.

Results

Expression of genes specific to lymphocytes is measurable in tumor samples

We observed that selected lymphocyte specific markers are present in measurable quantities in sampled tumor tissue from our discovery set. The distribution of average expression (Figure 1A) shows the typical multimodal pattern in expression arrays: the lower peak reflects the background noise for genes that are not expressed in the sample and the higher peak represents signal. The lymphocyte marker CD45 is in the signal peak and is relatively highly expressed (Table S2). We conjecture that a measurable portion of the cells in each sample contain lymphocyte RNA which would represent the tumor microenvironment.

Comparison with the GeneAtlas tissues [23] confirms that the nominal action of these expression array probes is lymphocyte-specific. We considered probe expression in ovarian NCI-60 cell lines [19] to exclude the possibility that genes are normally expressed in tumor tissue (Table S2). Considering the mean quantile of expression versus other probes, surface markers CD64, CD1D, CD14, CD33, CD8A, CD16b, CD45 maintain a low level in cell lines versus microdissected tumor (all lower than the 35th quantile, $p<0.05$). The near absence of IL6, IL12, IFNB1, and IFNG (between the 2nd and 25th quantile) suggests that the ability to measure cytokine signaling is lost in this in vitro system; notably, the IL12 receptor is measurable, so surface markers do appear. The exception to this pattern is that CD4 is over-expressed (51st and 61st quantiles in tumor and cell line samples respectively).

This establishes that a reproducible immune signal can be measured in sampled tumor tissue and we proceed assuming that these markers form a representative cross-section of tumor and immune system interaction.

Reproducible associations between candidate genes and overall survival

Of the 64 candidate genes, 15 have univariate associations (score test p-value<0.05) with overall survival (OS) following surgery and primary chemotherapy in the TCGA study (Table S1). A further 5 of these can be validated in the withheld independent studies ($FDR=0.032$).

The validated set can be organized by function: major histocompatibility complex (MHC) I genes, HLA-F, and HLA-G; an MHCII gene, HLA-DOB; the MHCI associated transporter, TAP1; and the co-receptor complex subunit, CD3D (TCR-δ). Increasing expression of each of these transcripts is associated with better survival (Table 2). T-cell related genes are highly correlated, which likely accounts for an indirect but positive association between the suppressor HLA-DOB and survival (Univariate HR = 0.74, 95% CI: 0.65–0.85, $p<0.0001$). We will examine the multivariate expression of these genes next.

Using a hierarchical clustering algorithm, the discovery set patients can be divided into four groups (Figure 1B) associated with OS (p = 1.2e-05). Represented in the heatmap in Figure 1C, the simultaneous expression of all five genes (colored purple) confers the most benefit. The simultaneous expression of all five genes is consistent with T cell activation, so we deem the high expressing subgroup an immunoreactive (IR) subset.

The degree of expression is not associated with variation in poor prognosis: the low expression of all genes (orange) does no worse than a heterogenous pattern of high and medium expression (yellow) or uniformly medium expression (green subgroup). This suggests that the deficient expression of any one gene is sufficient to lead to poor prognosis.

We assign validation patients to their most similar discovery set subgroup by k-means clustering. In the second heatmap (Figure 1D), the patients (columns) are ordered by hierarchical clustering within the validation data set. So, the clustered subgroups are strengthened by the observation that the class labels are preserved in the validation set.

In the discovery data, the survival benefit for the high expressers (n = 55, 10%) is a median of 70.9 months (95% CI: 58.1–98.0) versus 41.4 (36.9–45, p = 3.5e-05) OS; the median progression free survival (PFS) benefit is significant (p = 3.1e-04) at 30.4 (18.2–91.3) months versus 16.4 (14.7–18). This subgroup accounts for 5% of the deaths observed in the dataset and 7% of the recurrent cases. This benefit is weakly reproduced in the validation data: (p = 0.0335) with a difference of 64.0 months versus 51 months median OS. The PFS difference was not significant in the validation set.

Association with immunoreactive subgroup and immune markers

The TCGA analysis confirmed a set of genetic subsets [2] identified in a previous study [14]. Our high expression subgroup (purple, n = 55) is associated with their IR subgroup (38/55, 69%) ($p<0.0001$) (Table 3). The orange subgroup (n = 39) is mostly proliferative (31/37, 84%). Both of these associations hold in the

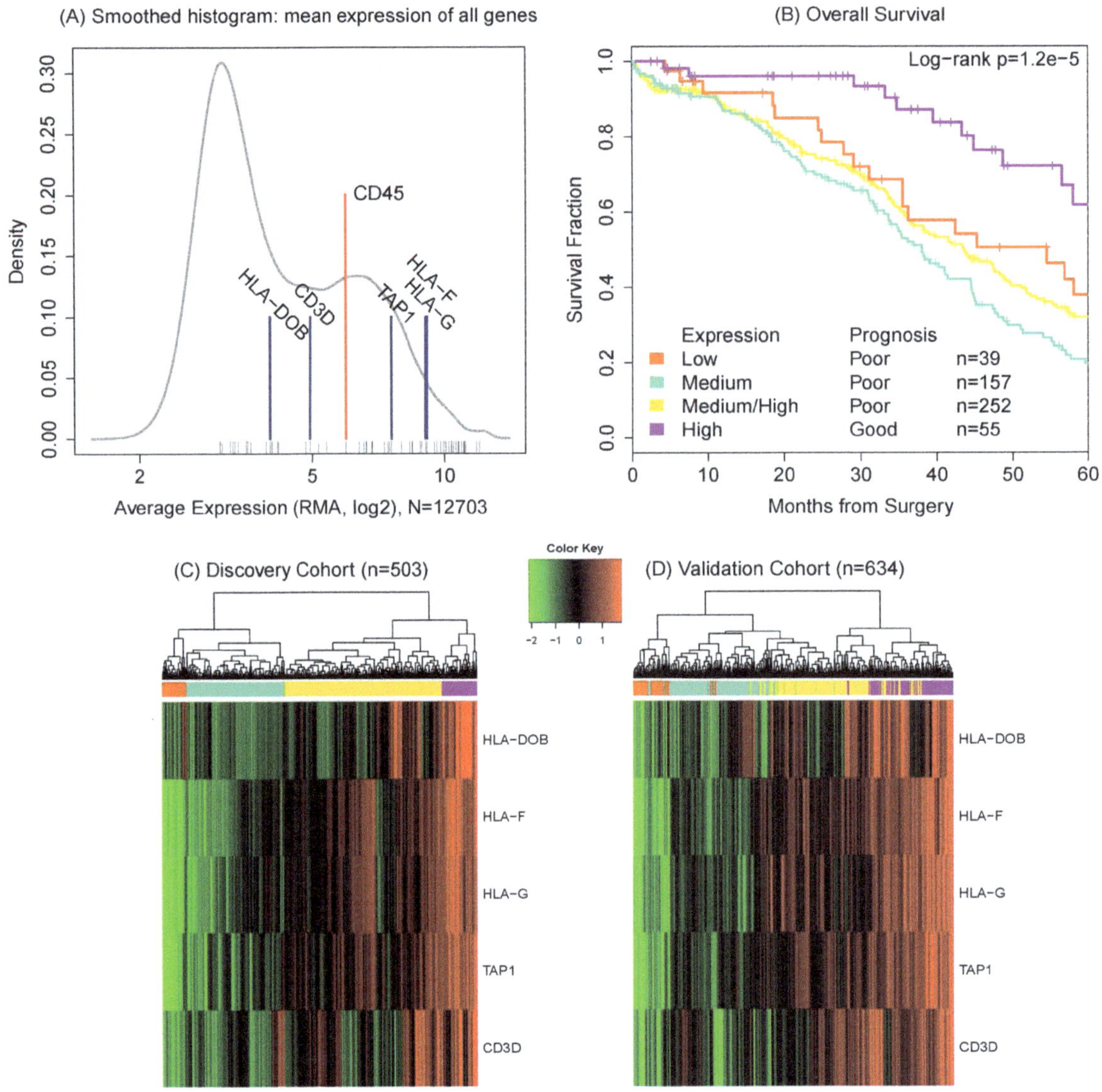

Figure 1. Mean relative expression of the selected genes confirms that they are all expressed in the samples (A). Black ticks indicate the mean expression of immune-related genes. CD45 is highlighted as a lymphocyte specific marker indicating the presence of lymphocytes. Subgroup-based survival estimates (B) are shown for the TCGA data based on hierarchical clustering of relative expression of selected T-cell genes (C and D). The four color bar on the left identifies the subgroups. The purple subset (n = 55, 11%) represents a significant survival benefit associated with the expression of all five genes.

Table 2. Validated immune genes related to overall survival and their correlation structure.

			Correlation			
Gene Name	**HR (95% CI)**	**p-value**	**HLA-G**	**HLA-DOB**	**TAP1**	**CD3D**
HLA-F	0.89 (0.79–1.00)	0.0429	0.95	0.51	0.84	0.60
HLA-G	0.88 (0.79–0.99)	0.0282		0.48	0.81	0.54
HLA-DOB	0.74 (0.65–0.85)	<0.0001			0.57	0.41
TAP1	0.88 (0.79–0.98)	0.0238				0.58
CD3D	0.85 (0.75–0.96)	0.0087				

Table 3. Association between derived subgroups and previously identified TCGA subgroups in discovery and validation sets.

Class	Purple	Yellow	Aqua	Orange
n	55	252	157	39
Overall Survival				p = 1.2e-05
median months	71	43	38	55
Progression-Free Survival				p = 6.7e-04
median months	30	18	15	17
Age				p = 6.2e-03
Mean Years	58	57	61	63
Stage				p = 2.8e-05
I/II	7	13	3	1
III/IV	48	239	154	38
Debulking Status				p = 3.2e-03
Optimal	17	51	21	13
Suboptimal	29	170	124	25
Platinum Status				p = n/s
Resistant	7	42	34	7
Sensitive	20	103	59	14
TCGA Class				p < 2.2e-16
Immunoreactive	38	59	7	0
Other	12	184	141	37
TCGA Class (Validation set)				p = 6.4e-11
Immunoreactive	35	27	8	0
Other	15	52	58	29

The colors are consistent with Figure 1. Note that only one study in the validation set had predicted TCGA classes and totals may not sum to 503 due to missing data.

validation data with TCGA subtypes. Altogether, this suggests that the hierarchical clustering derived subgroup is meaningful and that it nuances the TCGA subtypes as the latter were found to have no significant survival associations. Note that our study focuses on the IR subset and we make no attempt to model the other TCGA subtypes.

We examined the differential expression of standard immunology markers in the good prognosis subgroup. Figure 2 plots the change in expression across prognosis subgroups versus the

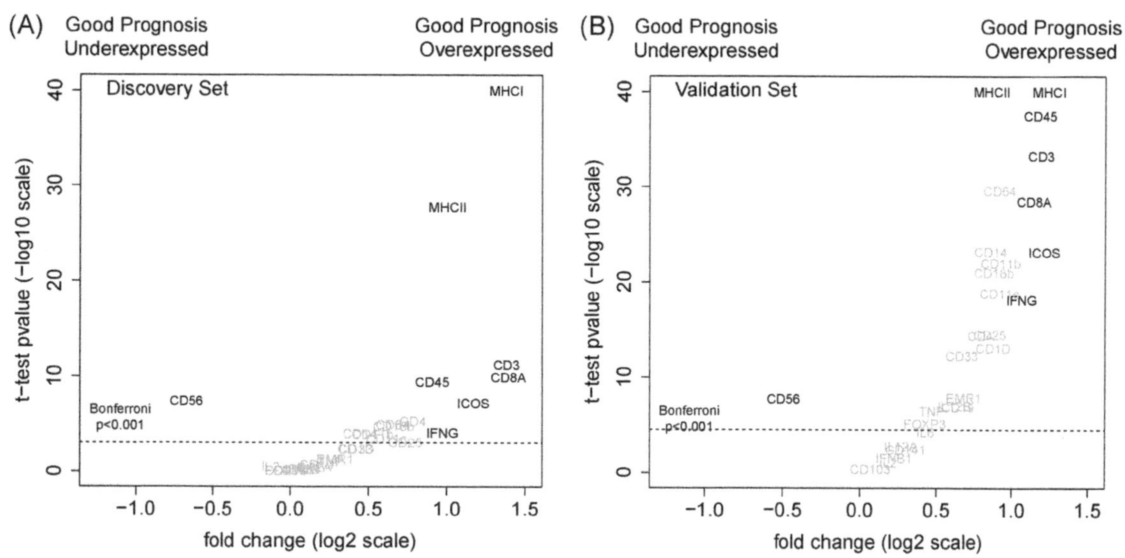

Figure 2. Differential expression of immunological markers in discovery (n = 503) and validation (n = 634) sets. Markers with strong biological and statistical significance (t-test Bonferroni p < 0.001) are chosen in the discovery set and highlighted in both plots.

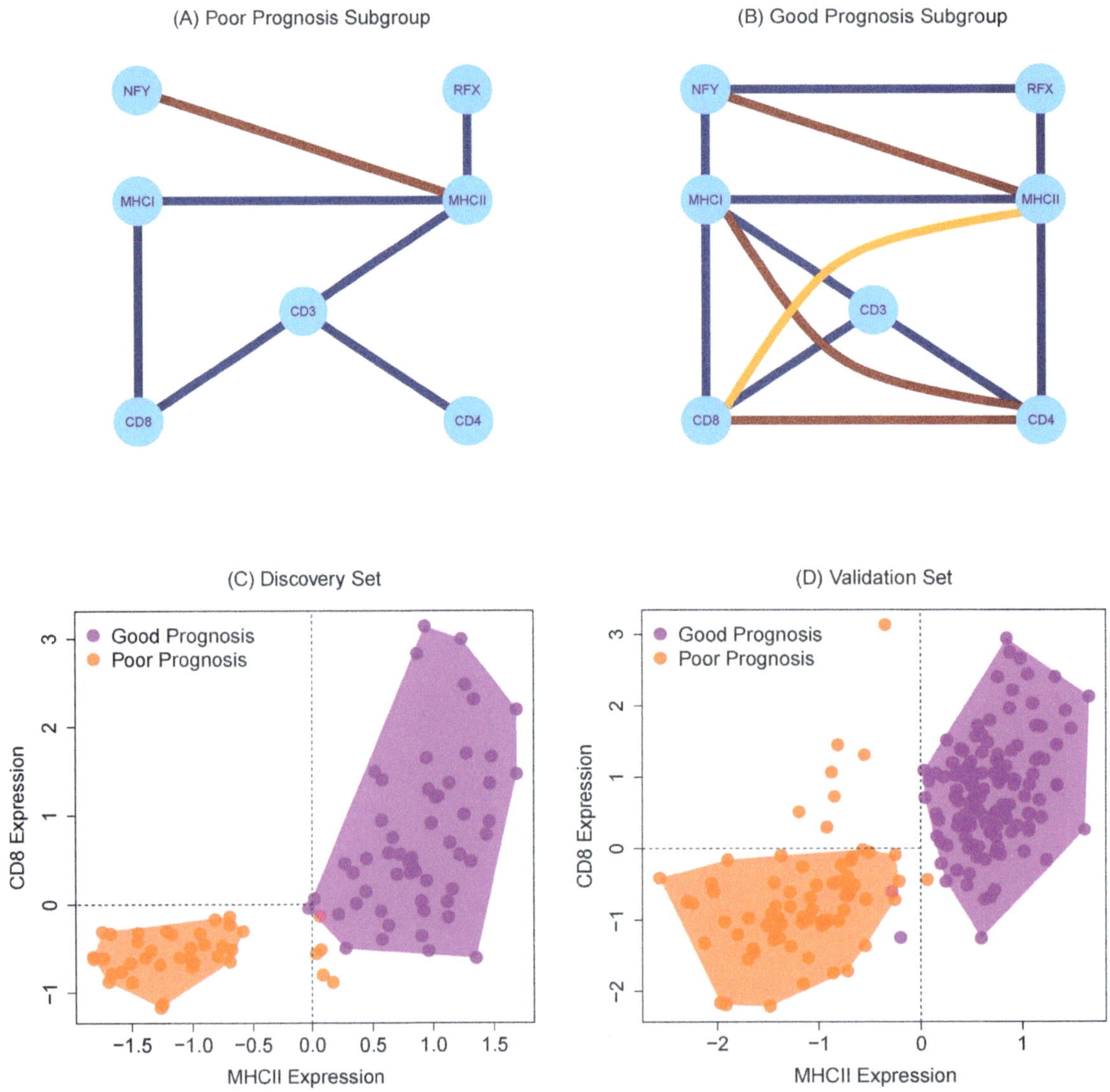

Figure 3. Partial correlation graphs indicating conditional relationships between genes in poor prognosis (n = 39)(A) and good prognosis (n = 55)(B) subgroups. Blue edges are positive associations and red are inhibitory associations. The highlighted orange edge can be removed by considering an independent set of genes. CD8 and MHCII array expression separate good and poor prognosis subgroups in discovery (C) and validation (D) data sets. MHCII expression is positively prognostic but appears in CD8 expressing samples. Shading is added for emphasis.

statistical evidence in both datasets. These markers imply an inflammatory response mediated by the recruitment of $CD45^+$ cells: $CD8^+$ cells and antigen-presenting cells (APC). No change in CD4 expression suggests that there is likely to be an latent background presence of $CD4^+$ T-cells and that the different action is attributable to activation (represented by differential *ICOS* expression). Absent are the NK cells ($CD56^+$) reinforcing the idea that the process is part of adaptive immunity.

We conjecture that these observations are consistent with an immunoediting concept. The good prognosis group represents equilibrium where a prevalence of APCs and activated $CD4^+$ cells recruit $CD8^+$ T-cells to maintain adaptive immunity.

Prognostic co-expression suggests T-cell activation

To infer functional interactions between immune-related genes, we performed a co-expression analysis which summarizes correlation in the IR subgroup and the poor prognosis subgroups graphically. Edges in these Gaussian graphical models (GGMs) represent statistical dependence between immune components (Figure 3A, 3B); positive dependence implies that both components are present and are likely to be interacting while negative edges imply mutually exclusive function or repression.

As in the differential expression analysis, CD4 and MHCII are correlated in the IR subgroup and not in the poor prognosis subgroups. Consistent with its reported function, RFX family (*RFX5*, *RFXANK*, *RFXAP*) of transcription factors' expression increases concordantly with the rise in MHCII expression [24]. In the IR subgroup, two edges imply anti-correlation between CD4 and MHCI which implies mutually exclusive function; and correlation between CD8 and MHCII (Figure 3C, 3D) which appears contrary to the specificity of MHC classes.

To explain this effect, we searched for missing genes whose inclusion in the graph would remove these edges. A missing link between CD8 and MHCII is *GZMA* a protease reflecting the activity of cytolytic T-cells. Between CD4 and MHCI we infer that CCR5, a cytokine receptor related to the activation of the T-cells,

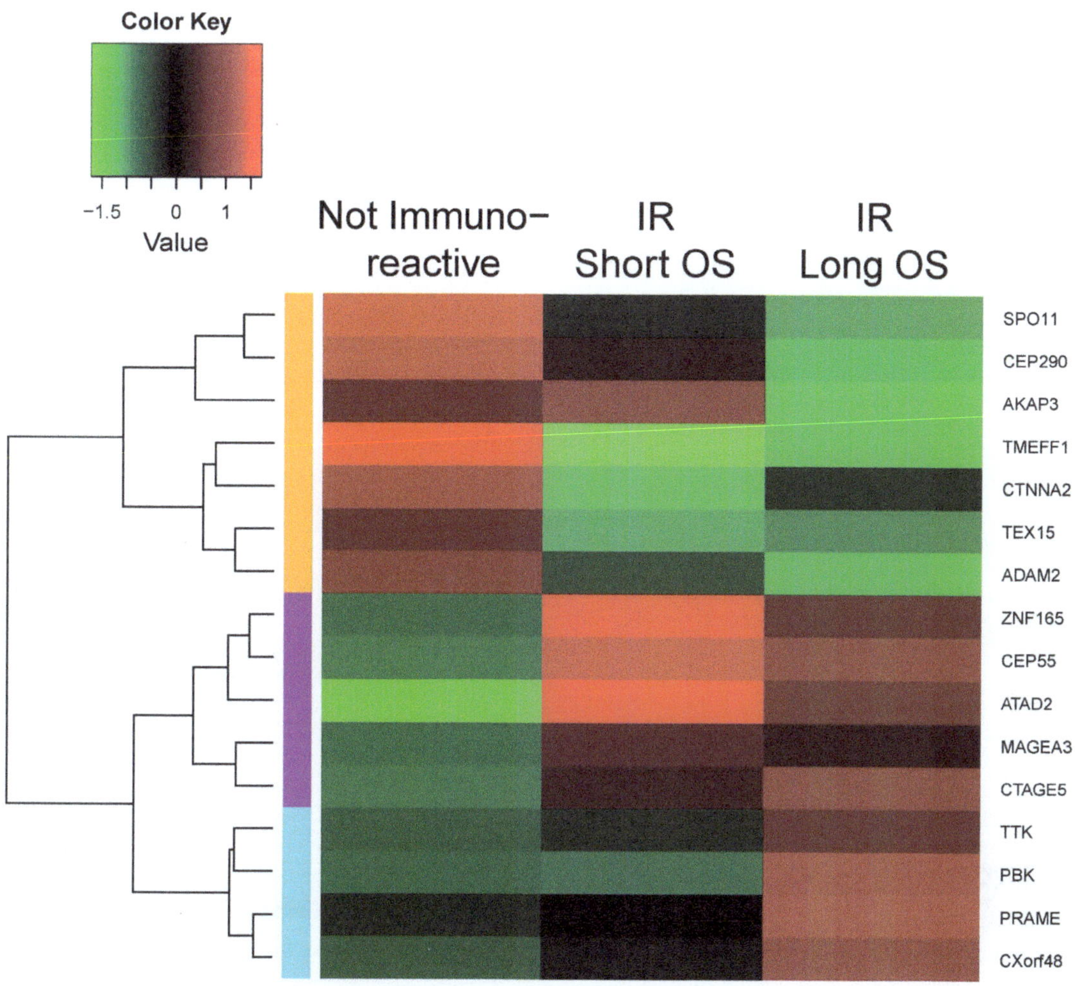

Figure 4. Cancer testis antigens associated with prognosis or immunoreactive (IR) subgroup can be divided into three classes: non-IR (orange), IR (purple) and immune stimulatory (cyan).

is missing. The common observation is that transcript associations likely need to be considered alongside measures of T-cell activation. The relevance of these genes is supported by the statistical significance of the transcriptome-wide search (adjusted $p<.05$) and the specificity of the selected genes' expression in lymphocyte tissues.

Focusing on CD8 and MHCII expression, we note that the good prognosis group can be defined by high MHCII expression where CD8 expression varies; CD8 expression is restricted when MHCII expression is low. Therefore, we hypothesize that MHC class II-mediated activation of $CD4^+$ T-cells are required for infiltration by $CD8^+$ T-cells that provide protection.

Immunoreactivity predicted by cancer-testis antigen profiles

We investigated the association of the IR subgroup with the cancer testis (CT) family of antigens [20]. These genes are frequently over-expressed in cancer cells and induce spontaneous immune responses, which make them a primary target for immunotherapy [25]. In particular, CT antigen expression is believed to influence the IR subset by regulating T-cell responses in the ovarian tumor microenvironment. The discovery set arrays measured 98 CT antigens (Table S4) of which 3 were associated with the IR subset (Bonferroni $p<0.05$): *CEP290*, *CTNNA2*, *TMEFF1*.

Because membership in the IR class is binary, we used logistic regression to model the multivariate set of antigens associated with IR status. Table S3 is the regression table for a model fit using BIC-based stepwise selection. Here, *CEP290*, *CTNNA2*, *TMEFF1*, and *TEX15* expression decreases the likelihood that a patient is in the IR class. Antigens *ZNF164* and *MAGEA3* increase the chance. Other than *CTNNA2*, which is twice as important as *MAGEA3*, the other genes have about the same effect. In the independent data, predictions from this model are strongly associated with the k-means derived associations (HR = 3.96, 95% CI: 2.59–6.14, p = 1.47e-11) tuned for equal sensitivity and specificity (0.66) given a moderate prevalence (140/634, 20.5%).

We further stratified patients in IR subgroup into good and poor prognosis based on OS to 33.5 months (overall study population median OS). A set of 16 antigens includes the union of the 3 IR subset genes and antigens associated with the difference in survival. Figure 4 is a heatmap comprising the mean expression of the 16 genes organized into three classes. The first class (orange) is expressed in non-IR cases and may reflect the activity of immunosuppressive elements. The second set (purple) is expressed in IR cancers but is unrelated to prognosis. The third (cyan) is expressed strongly in IR cases with good prognosis and may indicated immune stimulatory effects. A viable hypothesis might be to see if T cells responding to the second set of antigens (*ZNF165*, *CEP55*, *ATAD2*, *MAGEZ3*, *CTAGE5*) have regulatory phenotypes.

Discussion

We have analyzed the expression of 64 T-cell co-receptor and antigen presentation/processing genes in advanced serous ovarian cancer using a standard univariate screen and an analysis of their co-expression. These analyses define a subset of ovarian cancer cases with prognostically meaningful expression associated with T-cell activation and a previously defined immunoreactive subgroup [2]. In contrast to previous work [17,26], the subgroup can be identified reproducibly with just 5 genes versus over a hundred. This efficiency comes from our initial immunologic perspective. We reduce significantly the extraneous genes, but trade the ability to make a pan-ovarian cancer genetic characterization. As a result, we make no claim about or attempt to model non-immunologic signals.

We now have a small set of markers and antigens that may make translational and biomarker work more feasible for immunotherapy. With respect to the use of CT antigens, we have found a set which predicts non-immunogenic cancers (putatively, ones with low T-cell activation) and a set that might be targeted for blockade type immunotherapy. Both biological studies to verify regulatory activity of T cells in these cases and retrospective clinical studies may be the next investigative step. We speculate that the set of IR specific CT antigens stimulate immune responses (e.g., recruiting activated T cells), but are insufficiently immunogenic to induce tumor eradicating immune reaction. Alternatively, this group may prompt mixed effects: inducing immune responses while promoting tumor progression.

Inferentially, we have adopted a discovery/validation framework that allows us to make preliminary confirmations and to avoid over-interpreting high-dimensional artifacts. The data are limited by the nature of expression data from tumor samples; we rely on the conjecture that even after microdissection, assayed samples retain a portion of lymphocyte genetic material. Because this effect appears independently in multiple studies, these observations may be applicable to assays using this platform and are less likely to be subject to batch effect bias. Additionally, this work motivates the investigation of a structured way to analyze residual stromal signal from the tumor samples and therefore infer genetic interaction in the tumor microenvironment.

Supporting Information

Table S1 Univariate associations between genes and overall survival measured by score test p-value.

Table S2 Tissue specific quantiles of expression of lymphocyte specific markers. Low quantiles imply relatively low or no expression.

Acknowledgments

The results published here are in whole or part based upon data generated by The Cancer Genome Atlas pilot project established by the NCI and NHGRI. Information about TCGA and the investigators and institutions who constitute the TCGA research network can be found at http://cancergenome.nih.gov/.

Author Contributions

Conceived and designed the experiments: KHE TT. Performed the experiments: KHE. Analyzed the data: KHE TT. Contributed reagents/materials/analysis tools: KHE. Wrote the paper: KHE TT.

References

1. Yoshihara K, Tsunoda T, Shigemizu D, Fujiwara H, Hatae M, et al. (2012) High-risk ovarian cancer based on 126-gene expression signature is uniquely characterized by downregulation of antigen presentation pathway. Clinical Cancer Research 18: 1374–1385.
2. The Cancer Genome Atlas Research Network (2011) Integrated genomic analyses of ovarian carcinoma. Nature 474: 609–615.
3. Gnjatic S, Ritter E, Büchler MW, Giese NA, Brors B, et al. (2010) Seromic profiling of ovarian and pancreatic cancer. Proceedings of the National Academy of Sciences 107: 5088–5093.
4. Matsuzaki J, Gnjatic S, Mhawech-Fauceglia P, Beck A, Miller A, et al. (2010) Tumor-infiltrating NY-ESO-1-specific CD8+ t cells are negatively regulated by LAG-3 and PD-1 in human ovarian cancer. Proceedings of the National Academy of Sciences 107: 7875–7880.
5. Curiel TJ, Coukos G, Zou L, Alvarez X, Cheng P, et al. (2004) Specific recruitment of regulatory T cells in ovarian carcinoma fosters immune privilege and predicts reduced survival. Nature Medicine 10: 942–949.
6. Qian F, Gnjatic S, Jager E, Santiago D, Jungbluth A, et al. (2004) Th1/Th2 CD4+ T cell responses against NY-ESO-1 in HLA-DPB1*0401/0402 patients with epithelial ovarian cancer. Cancer Immunology 4: 12.
7. Zhang L, Conejo-Garcia JR, Katsaros D, Gimotty PA, Massobrio M, et al. (2003) Intratumoral T cells, recurrence, and survival in epithelial ovarian cancer. New England Journal of Medicine 348: 203–213.
8. Preston CC, Goode EL, Hartmann LC, Kalli KR, Knutson KL (2011) Immunity and immune suppression in human ovarian cancer. Immunotherapy 3: 539–556.
9. Dunn GP, Old LJ, Schreiber RD (2004) The immunobiology of cancer immunosurveillance and immunoediting. Immunity 21: 137–148.
10. Sato E, Olson SH, Ahn J, Bundy B, Nishikawa H, et al. (2005) Intraepithelial CD8+ tumor-infiltrating lymphocytes and a high cd8+/regulatory t cell ratio are associated with favorable prognosis in ovarian cancer. Proceedings of the National Academy of Sciences 102: 18538–18543.
11. Matsuzaki J, Qian F, Luescher I, Lele S, Ritter G, et al. (2008) Recognition of naturally processed and ovarian cancer reactive CD8+ t cell epitopes within a promiscuous HLA class II T-helper region of NY-ESO-1. Cancer Immunology Immunotherapy 57: 1185–1195.
12. Vaughan S, Coward JI, Bast RC, Berchuck A, Berek JS, et al. (2011) Rethinking ovarian cancer: recommendations for improving outcomes. Nature Reviews Cancer 11: 719–725.
13. Dressman HK, Berchuck A, Chan G, Zhai J, Bild A, et al. (2007) An integrated genomic-based approach to individualized treatment of patients with advanced-stage ovarian cancer. Journal of Clinical Oncology 25: 517–525.
14. Tothill RW, Tinker AV, George J, Brown R, Fox SB, et al. (2008) Novel molecular subtypes of serous and endometrioid ovarian cancer linked to clinical outcome. Clinical Cancer Research 14: 5198–5208.
15. Callahan MJ, Nagymanyoki Z, Bonome T, Johnson ME, Litkouhi B, et al. (2008) Increased hla-dmb expression in the tumor epithelium is associated with increased ctl infiltration and improved prognosis in advanced-stage serous ovarian cancer. Clinical Cancer Research 14: 7667–7673.
16. Leffers N, Fehrmann R, Gooden M, Schulze U, Ten Hoor K, et al. (2010) Identification of genes and pathways associated with cytotoxic T lymphocyte infiltration of serous ovarian cancer. British Journal of Cancer 103: 685–692.
17. Yoshihara K, Shahmoradgoli M, Martínez E, Vegesna R, Kim H, et al. (2013) Inferring tumour purity and stromal and immune cell admixture from expression data. Nature communications 4.
18. Baggerly KA, Coombes KR, Neeley ES (2008) Run batch effects potentially compromise the usefulness of genomic signatures for ovarian cancer. Journal of Clinical Oncology 26: 1186–1187.
19. Lee JK, Havaleshko DM, Cho H, Weinstein JN, Kaldjian EP, et al. (2007) A strategy for predicting the chemosensitivity of human cancers and its application to drug discovery. Proceedings of the National Academy of Sciences 104: 13086–13091.

20. Almeida LG, Sakabe NJ, Silva MCC, Mundstein AS, Cohen T, et al. (2009) CTdatabase: a knowledge-base of high-throughput and curated data on cancer-testis antigens. Nucleic Acids Research 37: D816–D819.
21. Carlson M (2014) hthgu133a.db: Affymetrix HT Human Genome U133 Array Plate Set annotation data (chip hthgu133a). R package version 2.8.0.
22. Schaefer J, Opgen-Rhein R, Strimmer K (2013) GeneNet: Modeling and Inferring Gene Networks. URL http://CRAN.R-project.org/package=GeneNet. R package version 1.2.8.
23. Su AI, Wiltshire T, Batalov S, Lapp H, Ching KA, et al. (2004) A gene atlas of the mouse and human protein-encoding transcriptomes. Proceedings of the National Academy of Sciences 101: 6062–6067.
24. Emery P, Durand B, Mach B, Reith W (1996) RFX proteins, a novel family of DNA binding proteins conserved in the eukaryotic kingdom. Nucleic Acids Research 24: 803–807.
25. Simpson AJ, Caballero OL, Jungbluth A, Chen YT, Old LJ (2005) Cancer/testis antigens, gametogenesis and cancer. Nature Reviews Cancer 5: 615–625.
26. Verhaak RG, Tamayo P, Yang JY, Hubbard D, Zhang H, et al. (2013) Prognostically relevant gene signatures of high-grade serous ovarian carcinoma. The Journal of clinical investigation 123: 517–525.

Permissions

All chapters in this book were first published in PLOS ONE, by The Public Library of Science; hereby published with permission under the Creative Commons Attribution License or equivalent. Every chapter published in this book has been scrutinized by our experts. Their significance has been extensively debated. The topics covered herein carry significant findings which will fuel the growth of the discipline. They may even be implemented as practical applications or may be referred to as a beginning point for another development.

The contributors of this book come from diverse backgrounds, making this book a truly international effort. This book will bring forth new frontiers with its revolutionizing research information and detailed analysis of the nascent developments around the world.

We would like to thank all the contributing authors for lending their expertise to make the book truly unique. They have played a crucial role in the development of this book. Without their invaluable contributions this book wouldn't have been possible. They have made vital efforts to compile up to date information on the varied aspects of this subject to make this book a valuable addition to the collection of many professionals and students.

This book was conceptualized with the vision of imparting up-to-date information and advanced data in this field. To ensure the same, a matchless editorial board was set up. Every individual on the board went through rigorous rounds of assessment to prove their worth. After which they invested a large part of their time researching and compiling the most relevant data for our readers.

The editorial board has been involved in producing this book since its inception. They have spent rigorous hours researching and exploring the diverse topics which have resulted in the successful publishing of this book. They have passed on their knowledge of decades through this book. To expedite this challenging task, the publisher supported the team at every step. A small team of assistant editors was also appointed to further simplify the editing procedure and attain best results for the readers.

Apart from the editorial board, the designing team has also invested a significant amount of their time in understanding the subject and creating the most relevant covers. They scrutinized every image to scout for the most suitable representation of the subject and create an appropriate cover for the book.

The publishing team has been an ardent support to the editorial, designing and production team. Their endless efforts to recruit the best for this project, has resulted in the accomplishment of this book. They are a veteran in the field of academics and their pool of knowledge is as vast as their experience in printing. Their expertise and guidance has proved useful at every step. Their uncompromising quality standards have made this book an exceptional effort. Their encouragement from time to time has been an inspiration for everyone.

The publisher and the editorial board hope that this book will prove to be a valuable piece of knowledge for researchers, students, practitioners and scholars across the globe.

List of Contributors

Fatma Valiyeva
Comprehensive Cancer Center, University of Puerto Rico, San Juan, Puerto Rico

Ileabett M. Echevarría-Vargas and Pablo E. Vivas-Mejía
Comprehensive Cancer Center, University of Puerto Rico, San Juan, Puerto Rico
Department of Biochemistry, University of Puerto Rico, San Juan, Puerto Rico

Charles J. d'Adhemar, Cathy D. Spillane, Michael F. Gallagher, Mark Bates, Paul C Smyth, Aoife A. Cooke, Brendan Ffrench, Cara M. Martin, Britta Stordal, Stephen Finn, Brian Flood and Orla Sheils
Department of Histopathology, Trinity College Dublin, Dublin, Ireland

Sharon O'Toole
Department of Histopathology, Trinity College Dublin, Dublin, Ireland
Department of Obstetrics and Gynaecology, Trinity College Dublin, Dublin, Ireland

John J. O'Leary
Department of Histopathology, Trinity College Dublin, Dublin, Ireland
Department of Pathology, Coombe Women's & Infants University Hospital, Dublin, Ireland

Katie M. Costello, Jacqui Barry-O'Crowley, Niamh Kernan and Ciara Murphy
Department of Pathology, Coombe Women's & Infants University Hospital, Dublin, Ireland

Kathryn Haley, Noreen Gleeson and Tom D'Arcy
Department of Obstetrics and Gynaecology, Trinity College Dublin, Dublin, Ireland

Ken O'Byrne
Translational Research Institute, Princess Alexandra Hospital, Brisbane, Australia

Stephen Pennington and Amanda McCann
College of Health Sciences, University College Dublin, Belfield, Dublin, Ireland

Dearbhaile O'Donnell
Department of Medical Oncology, St. James's Hospital, Dublin, Ireland

Bryan Hennessy
Department of Medical Oncology, Royal College of Surgeons, Dublin, Ireland

Luke A. J. O'Neill
Department of Biochemistry, Trinity College Dublin, Ireland

Xingchen Zhou, Yuan Hu, Lan Dai, Yunfei Wang, Jinhua Zhou, WenWen Wang, Wen Di and Lihua Qiu
Department of Gynecology and Obstetrics, Renji Hospital, School of Medicine, Shanghai Jiao Tong University, Shanghai, China
Shanghai Key Laboratory of Gynecologic Oncology, Shanghai, China

Shu Ly Lim and Frank Grützner
Robinson Research Institute, School of Molecular and Biomedical Sciences, University of Adelaide, Adelaide, SA, Australia

Carmela Ricciardelli, Martin K. Oehler, Izza M. D. De Arao Tan and Darryl Russell
Discipline of Obstetrics and Gynaecology, Robinson Research Institute, University of Adelaide, Adelaide, SA, Australia

Wouter Wegdam, Gemma G. Kenter, Marrije R. Buist and Danielle Meijer
Department of Gynecology, Academic Medical Center, University of Amsterdam, Amsterdam, the Netherlands

Carmen A. Argmann
Department of Genetics and Genomic Sciences, Icahn Institute for Genomics and Multiscale Biology, Icahn School of Medicine at Mount Sinai, New York, New York, United States of America

Gertjan Kramer and Johannes M. F. G. Aerts
Clinical Proteomics Group, Department of Medical Biochemistry, Academic Medical Center, University of Amsterdam, Amsterdam, the Netherlands

Johannes P. Vissers
Waters Corporation MS Technologies Center, Manchester, United Kingdom

Perry D. Moerland
Bioinformatics Laboratory, Department of Clinical Epidemiology, Biostatistics and Bioinformatics, Academic Medical Center, University of Amsterdam, Amsterdam, the Netherlands

Zoltán Dezső, Judith Oestreicher, Amy Weaver, Stephanie Santiago, Sergei Agoulnik, Jesse Chow, Yoshiya Oda and Yasuhiro Funahashi
Biomarkers and Personalized Medicine Core Function Unit, Eisai Product Creation Systems, Eisai Inc., Andover, Massachusetts, United States of America

Zixuan Chen
Department of Pathology and Laboratory Medicine, University of Tennessee Health Science Center, Memphis, Tennessee, United States of America
Center for Cancer Research, University of Tennessee Health Science Center, Memphis, Tennessee, United States of America
Southern Medical University, Guangzhou, P. R. China

Yinan Wang and Wen Liu
Department of Pathology and Laboratory Medicine, University of Tennessee Health Science Center, Memphis, Tennessee, United States of America
Center for Cancer Research, University of Tennessee Health Science Center, Memphis, Tennessee, United States of America
Department of Physiology, University of Tennessee Health Science Center, Memphis, Tennessee, United States of America

Guannan Zhao
Department of Pathology and Laboratory Medicine, University of Tennessee Health Science Center, Memphis, Tennessee, United States of America
Center for Cancer Research, University of Tennessee Health Science Center, Memphis, Tennessee, United States of America
The Third Affiliated Hospital, Zhengzhou University, Zhengzhou, P. R. China

Junming Yue
Department of Pathology and Laboratory Medicine, University of Tennessee Health Science Center, Memphis, Tennessee, United States of America
Center for Cancer Research, University of Tennessee Health Science Center, Memphis, Tennessee, United States of America

Chengyao Li
Southern Medical University, Guangzhou, P. R. China

Suechin Lee, Andrea Balogh, Weiwang Gu and Gabor Tigyi
Department of Physiology, University of Tennessee Health Science Center, Memphis, Tennessee, United States of America

Yuqi Guo and Zhan Zhang
The Third Affiliated Hospital, Zhengzhou University, Zhengzhou, P. R. China

Yanan Zou
The Second Affiliated Hospital of Harbin Medical University, Harbin, P. R. China

Bayarbaatar Amgalan and Hyunju Lee
School of Information and Communications, Gwangju Institute of Science and Technology, Gwangju, South Korea

Loes Olde Loohuis
Center for Neurobehavioral Genetics, University of California Los Angeles, Los Angeles, United States of America

Giulio Caravagna, Alex Graudenzi, Daniele Ramazzotti, Giancarlo Mauri, and Marco Antoniotti
Dipartimento di Informatica Sistemistica e Comunicazione, Universita` degli Studi, Milano-Bicocca, Milano, Italy

Bud Mishra
Courant Institute of Mathematical Sciences, New York University, New York, United States of America

Sham S. Kakar and Sanjay K. Singh
Department of Physiology and Biophysics, University of Louisville, Louisville, Kentucky, United States of America
James Graham Brown Cancer Center, University of Louisville, Louisville, Kentucky, United States of America

Mariusz Z. Ratajczak and Donald M. Miller
James Graham Brown Cancer Center, University of Louisville, Louisville, Kentucky, United States of America

Department of Medicine, University of Louisville, Louisville, Kentucky, United States of America

Karen S. Powell
Research Resources Center, University of Louisville, Louisville, Kentucky, United States of America

Mana Moghadamfalahi
Department of Pathology, University of Louisville, Louisville, Kentucky, United
States of America

Surinder K. Batra
Department of Biochemistry and Molecular Biology, Eppley Institute for Research in Cancer and Allied Diseases, University of Nebraska Medical Center, Omaha, Nebraska, United States of America

Jing Cai, Tao Li, Hui Ding, Weihong Dong, Man Xiao, Ling Liu and Zehua Wang
Department of Obstetrics and Gynecology, Union Hospital, Tongji Medical College, Huazhong University of Science and Technology, Wuhan, China

Bangxing Huang
Department of Obstetrics and Gynecology, Union Hospital, Tongji Medical College, Huazhong University of Science and Technology, Wuhan, China
Department of Pathology, Union Hospital, Tongji Medical College, Huazhong University of Science and Technology, Wuhan, China

Henghui Cheng
Department of Pathology, Tongji Hospital, Tongji Medical College, Huazhong University of Science and Technology, Wuhan, China

Wensheng Zhang, Andrea Edwards and Kun Zhang
Department of Computer Science, Xavier University of Louisiana, New Orleans, Louisiana, United States of America

Erik Flemington
Tulane Cancer Center, Tulane School of Medicine, New Orleans, Louisiana, United States of America

Ruth Holm
Departments of Pathology, The Norwegian Radium Hospital, Oslo University Hospital, Oslo, Norway

Ruixia Huang, Zhenhe Suo, Xiaoran Li and Jahn M. Nesland
Departments of Pathology, The Norwegian Radium Hospital, Oslo University Hospital, Oslo, Norway
Department of Pathology, Institute of Clinical Medicine, Faculty of Medicine, University of Oslo, Oslo, Norway

Dan Wu
Department of Gynecology, International Peace Maternity and Child Health Hospital, Medical College of Shanghai, Jiaotong University, Shanghai, China

Yuan Yuan
Department of Pathology, Capital Medical University, Beijing, China

Claes G. Trope
Department of Gynecology, Institute of Clinical Medicine, Faculty of Medicine, University of Oslo, Oslo, Norway, Department of Gynecology, The Norwegian Radium Hospital, Oslo University Hospital, Oslo, Norway

Arie Oosterhof and Toin H. van Kuppevelt
Department of Biochemistry, Radboud Institute for Molecular Life Sciences, Radboud University Medical Center, Nijmegen, The Netherlands

Myrtille J. E. Vallen
Department of Biochemistry, Radboud Institute for Molecular Life Sciences, Radboud University Medical Center, Nijmegen, The Netherlands
Department of Obstetrics and Gynaecology, Radboud University Medical Center, Nijmegen, The Netherlands

Leon F. A. G. Massuger
Department of Obstetrics and Gynaecology, Radboud University Medical Center, Nijmegen, The Netherlands

Samuel Schmidt
Department of Cell Biology, Nijmegen Center for Molecular Life Sciences, Radboud
University Medical Center, Nijmegen, The Netherlands

Johan Bulten
Department of Pathology, Radboud University Medical Center, Nijmegen, The Netherlands

Satoko Yamaguchi, Yoshiko Maida, Mami Yasukawa and Kenkichi Masutomi
Division of Cancer Stem Cell, National Cancer Center Research Institute, Tokyo, Japan

Tomoyasu Kato
Department of Gynecology, National Cancer Center Hospital, Tokyo, Japan

Masayuki Yoshida
Department of Pathology and Clinical Laboratories, National Cancer Center Hospital, Tokyo, Japan

Shailendra Giri, Jacie L. Maguire, Zachary Johnson and Viji Shridhar
Department of Experimental Pathology, Mayo Clinic College of Medicine, Mayo Clinic, Rochester, Minnesota, United States of America

Ramandeep Rattan
Women's Health Services, Henry Ford Health System, Detroit, Michigan, United States of America

Mandar Deshpande
Department of Neurology, Henry Ford Health system, Detroit, Michigan, United States of America

Rondell P. Graham
Department of Anatomic/Clinical Pathology, Mayo Clinic College of Medicine, Mayo Clinic, Rochester, Minnesota, United States of America

Stéphanie Backman
Department of Obstetrics and Gynecology, University of Toronto, Toronto, Ontario, Canada

Alexandra Kollara and Theodore J. Brown
Lunenfeld-Tanenbaum Research Institute, Mt. Sinai Hospital, Toronto, Ontario, Canada

Robin Haw and Lincoln Stein
Ontario Institute for Cancer Research, Informatics and Bio-Computing, Toronto, Ontario, Canada

Chaoyang Sun, Na Li, Dong Ding, Danhui Weng, Li Meng, Gang Chen and Ding Ma
Department of Obstetrics and Gynaecology, Tongji Hospital, Tongji Medical College, Huazhong University of Science and Technology, Wuhan, Hubei, China

Kimiyo N. Yamamoto
Department of Information and Computer Sciences, Nara Women's University, Nara, Japan
Japan Society for the Promotion of Science, Tokyo, Japan
Department of Biology, Kyushu University, Fukuoka, Japan

Kouji Hirota
Department of Chemistry, Tokyo Metropolitan University, Tokyo, Japan

Shunichi Takeda
Department of Radiation Genetics, Graduate School of Medicine, Kyoto University, Kyoto, Japan

Hiroshi Haeno
Department of Biology, Kyushu University, Fukuoka, Japan

Tiffany J. Tzeng
Department of Nutrition and Food Science, University of Maryland, College Park, Maryland, United States of America

Wen-Hsing Cheng
Department of Nutrition and Food Science, University of Maryland, College Park, Maryland, United States of America
Department of Food Science, Nutrition and Health Promotion, Mississippi State University, Mississippi State, Mississippi, United States of America

Lei Cao
Department of Food Science, Nutrition and Health Promotion, Mississippi State University, Mississippi State, Mississippi, United States of America

YangXin Fu
Department of Oncology, University of Alberta, Edmonton, Alberta, Canada

Huawei Zeng
USDA, Agriculture Research Service, Grand Forks Human Research Center, Grand Forks, North Dakota, United States of America

Cecilia Hermans, Doris Mayr and Thomas Kirchner
Department of Pathology, Ludwig-Maximilians-University, Munich, Germany

Jutta Engel
Tumorregister Munich, Institute of Medical Informatics, Biometry and Epidemiology, Ludwig-Maximilians-University, Munich, Germany

David Anz and Stefan Endres
Center of Integrated Protein Science Munich (CIPS-M) Division of Clinical Pharmacology, Ludwig-Maximilians- University, Munich, Germany

Kevin H. Eng
Department of Biostatistics and Bioinformatics, Roswell Park Cancer Institute, Buffalo, NY, United States of America

Takemasa Tsuji
Center for Immunotherapy, Roswell Park Cancer Institute, Buffalo, NY, United States of America

Index